History of the Specialty of Allergy and Immunology at the University of South Florida Morsani College of Medicine

History of the Specialty of Allergy and Immunology at the University of South Florida Morsani College of Medicine

Firsthand Accounts of the Founding of the Division, Department of Internal Medicine, and Its Evolution

Richard F. Lockey, M.D.
Peggy Lee Hales

KNIGHTSBRIDGE
Genealogy Services

2022

First Printing: 2022

Library of Congress Control Number: 2022903163

ISBN: 978-0-9862134-5-8 (Hardback with color illustrations)

Authors:
Richard F. Lockey, M.D.
Peggy Lee Hales

Publisher:
Knightsbridge Genealogy Services
Tampa, Florida 33613
www.MyGenealogyConsultant.com
info@MyGenealogyConsultant.com

Ordering Information:
Discounts are available on quantity purchases. Contact publisher or order direct from the printer, Lulu, at https://www.lulu.com

Cover Photo:
Live Oak, one of eleven species of oak trees in Central Florida. Oak trees are wind pollinated and cause an epidemic of allergic problems (rhinitis, conjunctivitis, asthma and other diseases) from January through April each year.

In memory of

Samuel C. Bukantz, M.D.

and

Robert A. Good, M.D., Ph.D., D.Sc.

Contents

Dedication

Foreword by Charles (Charly) J. Lockwood, MD

Foreword by John T. Sinnott MD, FACP

Foreword by Allan L. Goldman, MD

Preface by Richard F. Lockey, MD, MS

Chapter 1:	The Division	1
Chapter 2:	Historical Overview as of 2006	53
Chapter 3:	Faculty Throughout the Years	59
Chapter 4:	Department of Internal Medicine, Allergy and Immunology Fellows	77
Chapter 5:	Additional Pictures of Internal Medicine Allergy and Immunology Fellows	85
Chapter 6:	Department of Pediatrics, Allergy and Immunology Fellows	111
Chapter 7:	All Children's Hospital Allergy and Immunology Pediatric and Internal Medicine Fellows	121
Chapter 8:	Division Group Pictures	125
Chapter 9:	The Clinical Research Unit (CRU): A Collection of Memories Including Pictures and Brochures	137
Chapter 10:	International Visitors	151
Chapter 11:	USF Research Personnel	159
Chapter 12:	VA and USF Research Personnel	171
Chapter 13:	Allergy and Immunology Postgraduate Programs Sponsored by the Division	177
Chapter 14:	Select Commemorative Publications	207
Chapter 15:	American Academy of Allergy Asthma & Immunology Meetings	231
Chapter 16:	Christmas and New Year's Celebrations	251
Chapter 17:	Division Celebrations	265

Dedication

With gratitude, this book is dedicated to all colleagues and trainees who made the Division successful; especially to Roger W. Fox, MD and Dennis K. Ledford, MD; brothers in medicine, who played an instrumental role in sculpting the Division into a premier program in the specialty of allergy and immunology.

Richard F. Lockey, MD, MS

Left to right: Roger W. Fox, MD; Richard F. Lockey, MD; Dennis K. Ledford, MD; circa 2000.

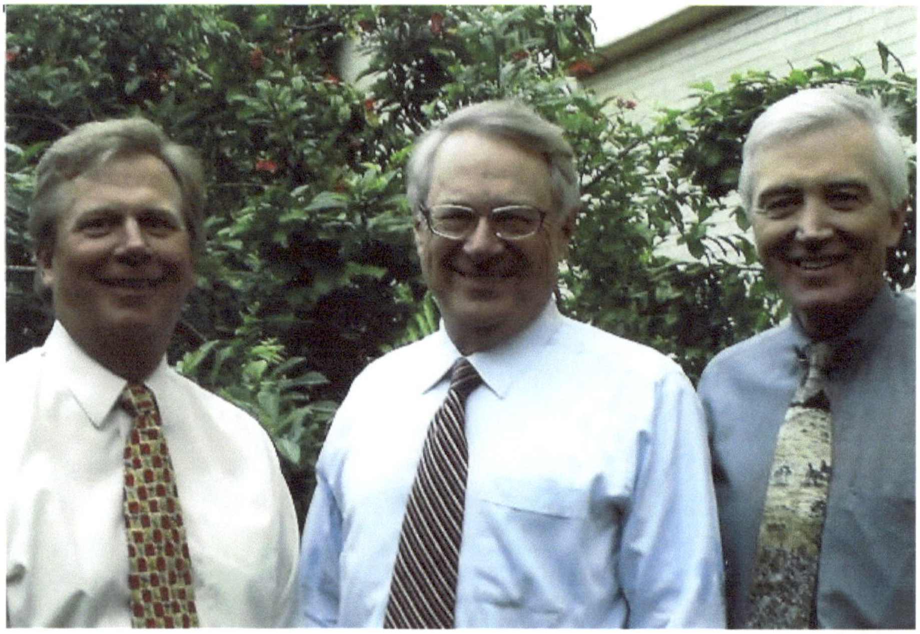

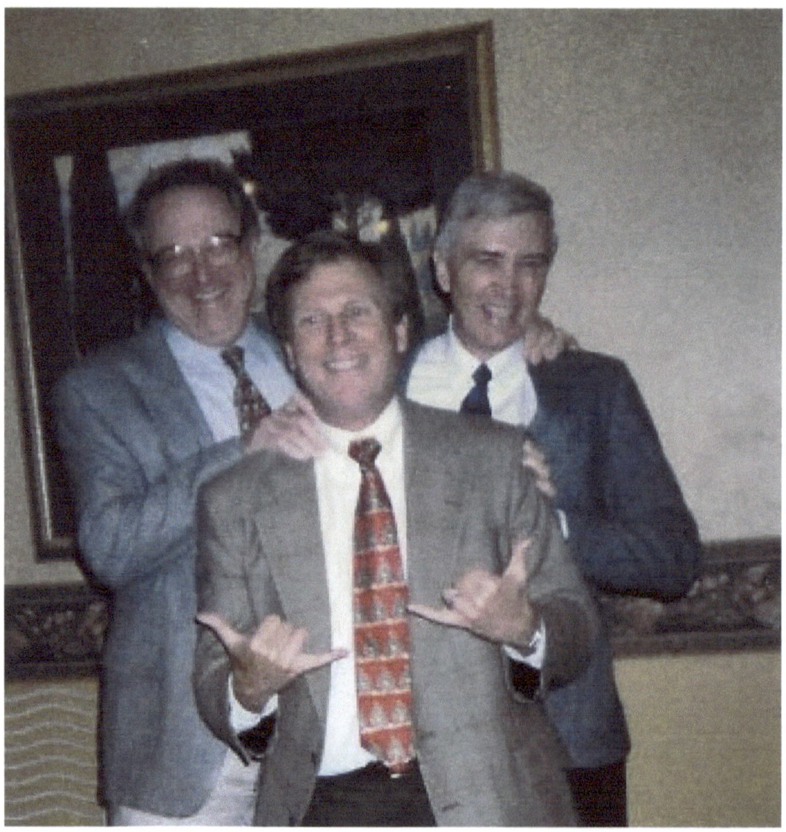

Left to right: Richard F. Lockey, MD; Roger W. Fox, MD; Dennis K. Ledford, MD; circa 2005.

Foreword

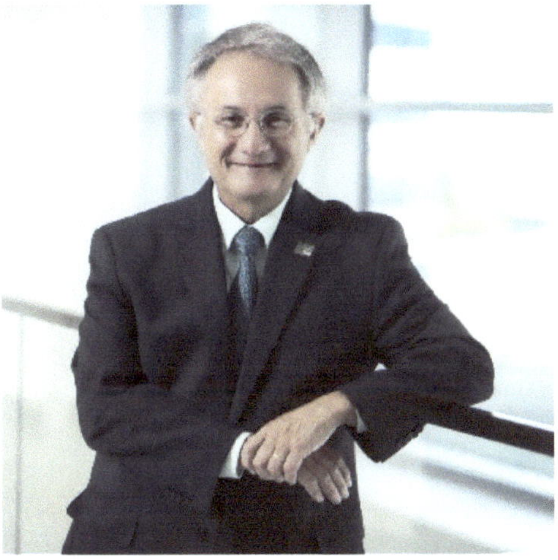

By Charles (Charly) J. Lockwood, MD
Senior Vice President, USF Health
Dean, USF Health Morsani College of Medicine

Too often, those of us at successful institutions take for granted the hard-earned achievements of our predecessors. That is why this volume from Dr. Richard Lockey, a founding faculty member of the University of South Florida College of Medicine and Chief of our Department of Internal Medicine's Division of Allergy and Immunology, and Peggy Hales, the Division's longtime Chief Administrative Assistant, is so important. It catalogues the painstaking work and visionary leadership of the faculty, staff, and fellows who built the Division of Allergy and Immunology from the ground up. It also brings to life the many vibrant personalities and watershed moments that characterized its history.

In just fifty years, the USF Health Morsani College of Medicine has been transformed from a fledging community-based medical school to a robust, nationally ranked, research-intensive medical school delivering world-class research, education, and patient care to the region. This book is the story of the school's humble beginnings and the pioneers who made it possible, told through an in-depth look at one of the College's most decorated divisions. Established in 1972, the Division has produced over 130 physicians and scholars while growing to include the Joy McCann Culverhouse Clinical Airway Disease Research Center, a physician training program, and earning designation as one of only eight World Allergy Organization (WAO) Centers of Excellence. The large ensemble of faculty, staff, residents, fellows, and students who have called the Division home have added incredible value to our patients' lives, the medical school's reputation, and our region's well-being, and I am glad to see so many of their accomplishments recognized and profiled on these pages. Their story is one of dedication, discipline, and daily acts of heroism. Their achievements, and the vigorous academic health of the Division today, are a testament to its original brilliant and dedicated faculty who came together with a shared vision and labored tirelessly to make it a reality.

This history has lessons for us today. Health care is at cross-roads, and vast changes to the system—including rapidly accelerating scientific knowledge, the growing reliance on artificial intelligence and digital technologies, the prohibitively expensive cost of novel pharmaceutical agents, and intractable social disparities in health outcomes—are redefining the practice of medicine and challenging many of our long-held assumptions. And all this was true before the global COVID-19 pandemic disrupted life as we knew it and transformed the health landscape almost beyond recognition.

These challenges resist easy answers. But for us to properly adapt and understand where we are going, we must understand where we have been. Thus, this volume not only preserves our venerated history but should serve as a source of inspiration and guidance for us today. In those early days of the USF College of Medicine and the Division of Allergy and Immunology, it took individuals of steadfast conviction, boldness, and supreme optimism to establish an entirely new institution committed to scientific excellence and compassionate, patient-centered care. It will fall to the present generation to carry that torch forward, building upon the giants who came before, and solidifying the College's place as one the nation's health care leaders. I hope that looking back on our history, and the wisdom offered by our forebearers, will furnish us with the vision we need to rise to the formidable challenges of our own time.

Foreword

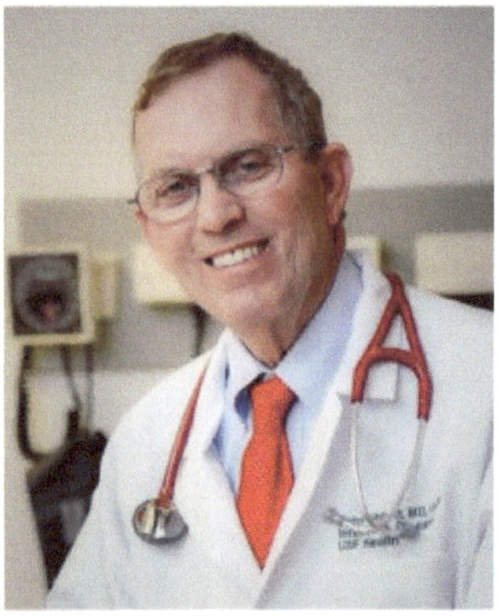

By John T. Sinnott MD, FACP
Professor and Chairman
Department of Internal Medicine
Morsani College of Medicine

This book paints a history of success of the Division of Allergy and Immunology, Department of Internal Medicine, at the Morsani College of Medicine. Its style ranges from broad brush strokes to fine detail and we benefit from each. Secondly, it provides a road map for those seeking to build or enhance any division of allergy and immunology, no matter where.

While allergies were first described 150 years ago by Dr. Charles Blackley, my own experience dates to the summer of 1973, when I first met Dr. Samuel Bukantz in the James A. Haley VA Research Building. This was the same time that Dr. Lockey joined as an assistant professor fresh out of the US Air Force at Caswell AFB Hospital in Ft. Worth, Texas. At that time, Dr. Bukantz was a world acknowledged expert, and I was being introduced to research. He was not just an allergist/immunologist, but a Renaissance man. He was widely read, enjoyed classical music and the arts, and eagerly shared his vast knowledge.

In the 1970's, progress in allergy and immunology was exploding. Fortuitously, we had Dr. Bukantz as the cornerstone of a new division in a new medical school – how incredibly fortunate. Dr. Bukantz recruited Dr. Richard Lockey, a rising star in allergy/immunology, who would go on to a brilliant future. This nexus of quality and energy led to rapid growth. Each year, faculty recruitment, research, and patient care progressively coalesced into one of the top 10 programs in the country.

Dr. Lockey assumed directorship in 1982 and carried Dr. Bukantz's dream into a new millennium. He recruited Drs. Roger Fox, Dennis Ledford, and many more faculty members. More recently, researchers such as Drs. Seong Cho, Narasaiah Kolliputi, Michael Teng, and the nationally respected clinical researcher, Thomas Casale, have joined the faculty. In the 1st century AD, Lucretius noted that food to one man is poison to another. Dr. Casale has pursued food allergies and carved a new path on the national level. Dr. Cho does basic and clinical research in chronic rhinosinusitis; Dr. Teng, respiratory syncytial virus; Dr. Kolliputi, interstitial lung disease; and one of our newest recruits, Dr. Juan Cardet, diseases of the airways.

Advances in allergy/immunology have either taken place in Dr. Lockey's Division or have been readily embraced. We could not be more excited about the future. Monoclonal antibodies to treat asthma, chronic rhinosinusitis and nasal polyposis, atopic eczema, and eosinophilic-driven diseases; medications like AR101 (Palforzia®, Aimmune Therapeutics, Brisbane, CA), an oral peanut-protein for immunotherapy to treat peanut allergic patients; and, finally, the role of appropriate immunotherapy to different allergens to decrease the allergic response, i.e., to create immune tolerance have come to the fore.

This book is an inspiring story of the founding of the Divisions of Allergy and Immunology, first, in the Department of Internal Medicine, and later, in the Department of Pediatrics. It is a tribute to the faculty and trainees and their expert patient care and commitment to research. It exemplifies the art of science of medicine.

Foreword

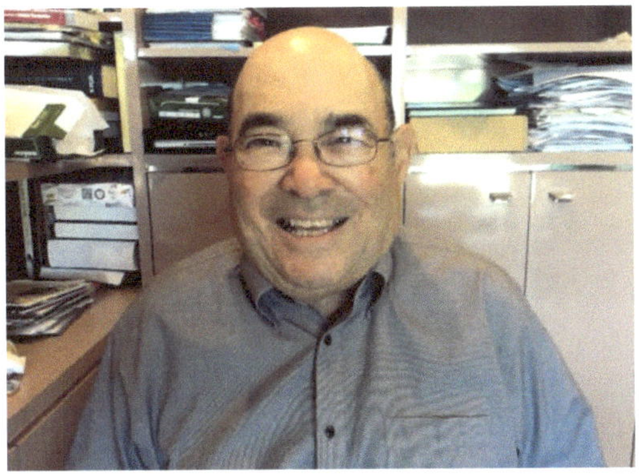

By Allan L. Goldman, MD
Professor and Chairman Emeritus
Department of Internal Medicine
University of South Florida
Morsani College of Medicine

It was 1973. There was a new medical school in Tampa at the University of South Florida. I was asked to come interview to become the founding director of the pulmonary division. Being a new medical school, faculty and divisions were limited, but there was one division that stood out … the Division of Allergy and Immunology. The Division consisted of two faculty members, one well-known physician in the specialty, Samuel C. Bukantz, MD, and one young dynamic physician, Richard F. Lockey, MD. Dr. Lockey set up a highbred Division where the clinical faculty received a very small University or VA stipend. And, at the same time, Dr. Lockey established a thriving part-time clinical practice independent of the University. The clinical practice helped to support salaries as well as other division and educational expenses. It was the only Division organized in this fashion which allowed it to grow and prosper without significant University support. Dr. Lockey soon added two clinical faculty members, Roger W. Fox, MD and Dennis K. Ledford, MD.

I served as the Division Director of the Division of Pulmonary Medicine from 1974 to 1996 and was Chairman of the Department of Internal Medicine from 1994 to 2012. The Division of Allergy and Immunology had grown and developed into a national powerhouse for research, education, and clinical training and practice. Under Dr. Lockey's leadership, it greatly expanded its research activities due to revenue from clinical activities and two Division endowments, the Joy McCann Culverhouse and the Mabel and Ellsworth Simmons Endowments. Research continued to prosper with little to no University support.

This hybrid model was under constant scrutiny by university administrators who questioned its modus operandi. In my role as Department Chair, I fully supported Dr. Lockey and, today, the Division continues to thrive under his devoted leadership.

Today, the Division of Allergy and Immunology is a research powerhouse with numerous research faculty and various federal, private, and pharmaceutical research grants. It is one of the strongest divisions in the Department of Internal Medicine. It is an exemplar for other divisions of allergy and immunology throughout the nation due in large part to the foresight, hard work, capabilities, and dedication of Dr. Lockey and other members of the Division. It has been a pleasure to work with Dr. Lockey and his faculty, and I have no doubt that the Division will prosper for years to come.

Preface

To Friends and Colleagues:

Information contained in this history is from a variety of different sources and recollections of individuals who have worked in Allergy and Immunology, University of South Florida, Morsani College of Medicine from 1972-1973 to the present. There may be names and information which unintentionally is inaccurate or inadvertently omitted.

The purpose of this historical narrative is to provide a description of the past- and present-day structure of allergy and immunology, faculty, fellows, researchers, and staff who have contributed their skills to provide vigor and to advance the academic, research, teaching, and clinical excellence of the specialty. The preeminent reputation of the University of South Florida Morsani College of Medicine Allergy and Immunology is a combined effort of all individuals who have previously or continue to work there.

The Division of Allergy and Immunology, Department of Internal Medicine faculty and researchers have trained hundreds of physicians, graduates, post-graduates, and exchange visitors. They have also published thousands of scientific articles including abstracts, review and scientific articles, book chapters, and books as listed at "https://health.usf.edu/medicine/internalmedicine/allergy". The Division's Annual Reports can also be reviewed at this site. Publications prior to listed Annual Reports can be obtained on PubMed at "https://pubmed.ncbi.nlm.nih.gov".

I am extremely grateful to Ms. Peggy Lee Hales, who joined the Division in 1983 and was chief administrative assistant until she retired in 2019, for taking the initiative to help write and edit this historical document. I am also grateful and thank all those who have contributed to the excellence of the specialty since the Division was founded in 1972-1973.

To quote Cicero: "Nescire autem quid antea quani natus sis acciderit, id est semper esse puerum."

Translated: "Not to know the events which happened before one was born, that is to remain always a boy."

Kind regards,

Richard F. Lockey, MD, MS

Richard F. Lockey, MD, MS

Distinguished University Health Professor
Professor of Medicine, Pediatrics and Public Health
Director, Division of Allergy and Immunology
Department of Internal Medicine
Joy McCann Culverhouse Chair in Allergy and Immunology
1973 – present

Chapter 1: The Division

Samuel C. Bukantz, MD, affectionately known as "Dr. B.", was the founding Director of the Division of Allergy and Immunology. The distinguished career of Dr. Bukantz in academic medicine spanned more than 60 years and helped build USF's Division of Allergy and Immunology, Department of Internal Medicine, into one of the largest, most well-respected in the world.

Prior to coming to Tampa, Dr. B. was Medical and Research Director at Jewish National Home for Asthmatic Children and Children's Asthma Research Institute and Hospital in Denver, 1958 – 1963. Thereafter, he was Associate Clinical Professor of Medicine at NYU College of Medicine from 1964 to 1972. Upon the advice of a former colleague of Dr. Bukantz, Dr. Judith Szentivanyi, who had recently moved to Tampa with her husband, Andor Szentivanyi, MD, DSc, the founding chairman of the USF Department of Pharmacology, Dr. B. met with Mr. George Hiskey, Director of the VA Hospital, which was just opening. Dr. Szentivanyi and Roy Behnke, MD, Founding Chairman of USF Department of Internal Medicine, appointed Dr. B. as Chief of the Division of Allergy and Immunology. He also was appointed Section Chief of Allergy and Immunology at the VA Hospital.

In late 1972, the opening of the James A. Haley Veterans' Administration preceded the admission of house staff or medical students to the medical school. Soon thereafter, the first class was admitted to the medical school and the hospital admitted its first patients. Dr. Bukantz humbly served as house staff at that time and took night call until 1973, sleeping at the hospital to care for patients on the medical service. Dr. Bukantz organized the VA Allergy and Immunology Clinic and recruited Richard F. Lockey, MD, MS as his associate in the Division of Allergy and Immunology and James A. Haley Veterans' Hospital beginning February 1, 1973. Dr. Lockey's appointment was half-time at the VA for which he was paid $14,000.

Actual acceptance of the position by Dr. Lockey took place on October 10, 1972, by letter on the Air Force stationery. He was completing his two years of service as Major in the U.S. Air Force at Carswell Air Force Base Hospital, Fort Worth, Texas. The formal offer of the position originated from Roy H. Behnke, MD, Founding Chair of the USF Department of Medicine. After joining the Division of Allergy and Immunology as a half-time but full tenure-earning faculty member in 1973, Dr. Lockey considered two possible locations, one in north and one south Tampa, and established a single-physician clinic at 3000 Medical Park Drive (1,200 square feet) in Tampa, opposite University Community Hospital (now Advent Hospital). A new patient visit was $45 and a return visit $15. He practiced in that office until 1979. Thereafter, the practice moved to its current location at 13801 Bruce B. Downs Blvd., Suite 502, Tampa, Florida.

Dr. Roger Fox joined the practice in 1980 and Dr. Dennis Ledford in 1986. It continued as the Lockey, Fox, and Ledford, MD, PA, University of South Florida Affiliated Clinic until 2019. All trainees have trained in this Clinic from the beginning of their fellowship. This Clinic is now a 9,000 square-foot facility which is an up-to-date state-of-the-art clinic to diagnose and treat patients with allergic and immunologic diseases. The clinic also has an affiliated clinic located on Platt Street in Tampa, Florida. Mark C. Glaum, MD, PhD, joined the practice in 2004, Seong Cho, MD in 2015, and Amber N. Pepper, MD in 2018. Dona Shearer, RN, joined the practice in 1979, first as a nurse, and then became the office manager. Ms. Shearer is the essential link in the practice enabling Drs. Lockey, Fox (retired from this clinic, 2019), Ledford (retired from this clinic, 2020), Glaum, Cho, and Pepper to participate in academic medicine and practice state-of-the-art allergy and immunology in this USF- affiliated clinic. Without her managerial skills, excellence in patient care and collaboration with the University's affiliated hospitals and the USF Division of Allergy and Immunology Clinical Research Unit, would not have occurred.

Through an early affiliation with the American Academy of Allergy Asthma & Immunology (AAAAI), Dr. Lockey heard about Samuel C. Bukantz, MD and a new university just opening in Tampa. After contacting him, they met for lunch at the then Holiday Inn on Fowler Avenue. Dr. Lockey vividly remembers this autumn day in 1972 as they lunched at a table next to a window facing Fowler Avenue where the sun was brightly shining. With vigorous encouragement, Drs. Bukantz and Behnke (Chief of Internal Medicine) were able to recruit him to USF.

Before he decided to come to Tampa, Dr. Lockey spent several days partaking in many frank and honest conversations with them. Influencing this decision was: 1) Dr. Behnke agreed that he should have a part-time clinical practice as well as a full-time tenure earning appointment at the College of Medicine. New part-time, full-time, faculty members were common at that time because of limited funding; 2) the University was a new and growing entity and Dr. Lockey felt optimistic about its future; 3) he also liked the Tampa Bay area and; 4) wanted to contribute to academic medicine. He drove his green Ford Pinto, packed to the ceiling, from Fort Worth, Texas. At that time, there was an “oil shortage”, the world was “running out of oil”, accounting for the drive in this very small and potentially dangerous but economic compact car. He and his wife had put a down-payment on a house in Carrollwood, located about 15 to 20 minutes from the University, VA, and clinical practice. At that time, there was minimal traffic in north Tampa and Bruce B. Downs Blvd. was a two-lane road that stopped approximately one-half mile north of Fletcher Ave.

Reminiscing about USF, Dr. Lockey recalls that "It was easy to cross Bruce B. Downs, for it was a two-lane street, on which the just new Veterans' Hospital and USF Medical School were located. We walked to and from the two institutions throughout the year, before the bridge was built. Most faculty were originally at the VA, the primary teaching hospital at the start. Half-time and full-time salaries were available from the VA and University. The Division started an allergy and immunology clinic at TGH; Dr. Samuel Bukantz and his wife, Jewell, staffed it. He and I also staffed the VA Allergy/Immunology Clinics and rounded on the VA wards regularly as the attending physicians. Most of the money initially generated for the USF College of Medicine was through inpatient care, not outpatient, and the Colleges of Nursing and Pharmacy and a teaching program in physical therapy did not exist. I was the fifth or sixth faculty member in the Department of Internal Medicine, and as new faculty arrived, regardless of their specialty, all became acquainted. Most everyone staffed both the VA and Tampa General Hospitals. Many in the Department were half-time, because of the limitation of funds. They established their own practices, which helped promote the presence of a new college of medicine. I practiced in a 1,200 square foot clinic, one block north of the University, which is no longer there, and ran the clinic as a single practitioner. So, too, did many others.

My wife and family had dinner at Dr. Behnke's home (Dr. Roy Behnke was the first chief of internal medicine) on multiple occasions. Entertainment at the homes of faculty was the rule, regardless of specialty. If a family's home could accommodate large numbers of guests, so be it. These activities enabled faculty and their families to become acquainted with the spouses and families of colleagues as they joined the faculty. There were always multiple parties to attend during the Christmas and New Year Holiday Season.

An example of faculty hospitality shown to my family and me was in the early 1970s by Dr. James Ingram, an early chief of obstetrics and gynecology, and his wife, and Dr. Irv Essrig, a general surgeon, and his wife. We were weekend guests in Boca Grande, an undiscovered fishing and holiday paradise, two hours south of Tampa. I thought, gee whiz, any place else in the world, this island would look like Miami. It was a small island, just beginning to be transformed from a fishing village to a vacation resort. I thought to myself, not only can I help make the USF College of Medicine grow, I love the outdoors and love to fish, this is a great place to live. This helped introduce a northern and ex-major in the US Air Force to Tampa, USF, and the College of Medicine.

I was told that the land on which USF is located cost $250.00 an acre and was destined to become an outstanding university and college of medicine because of its location, general public interest, and a growing state. The entire area north of University land was ranch land, devoid of people, and the University was located in the ‘north’.

Change, tremendous change, in no time flat took place. USF and its Morsani College of Medicine has always been one of the fastest growing universities in the USA, built and started by the founding faculty members, all fascinated with the idea of helping to build a new and outstanding medical school.”

DEPARTMENT OF THE AIR FORCE

UNITED STATES AIR FORCE REGIONAL HOSPITAL, CARSWELL (SAC)
CARSWELL AIR FORCE BASE, TEXAS 76127

10 October 1972

Samuel Bukantz, M.D.
Chief of Allergy
Veterans Administration Hospital
University of Southern Florida Campus
Tampa, Florida 33620

Dear Dr. Bukantz:

I have accepted the appointment offered to me by Dr. Behnke at the University of Southern Florida.

I look forward to seeing you on several occasions prior to my coming there at the beginning of January 1973. Ann and I want to thank both you and your wife for the exceptional kindness you showed us during our recent visit in Tampa. I will be in contact with you in the near future regarding my next trip to Tampa to begin to solidify a location for a practice. I am also beginning a "crash program" to learn what literature is available on the various allergens which are important in Florida. I know you have looked into this problem already and I will be interested in going over your data on my next visit to Tampa.

My best wishes.

Sincerely yours,

Dick

Dick Lockey

Above: Richard F. Lockey, MD's October 10, 1972 letter of acceptance (on Department of the Air Force stationary) to Samuel C. Bukantz, MD (note the word "Southern" rather than "South", a common error at that time).

October 19, 1972 673/111

Richard Lockey, M. D.
Department of the Air Force
U. S. Air Force Regional Hospital, Carswell (SAC)
Carswell Air Force Base, Texas 76127

Dear Dick:

Many thanks for your letter of October 10th and my congradulations on your acceptance of the appointment to the University of South Florida.

I too, am looking forward to your next visit and hope you will let me know when you will next come. I will definitely want to take some space with you after the first of the year, if the price is right.

Please give my best regards to Ann.

Cordially yours,

SAMUEL C. BUKANTZ, M.D.
Chief of Allergy
Medical Service

Above: Dr. Bukantz's reply of October 19, 1972.

Drs. Bukantz and Lockey staffed the VA Allergy and Immunology Clinics and saw all patients. They also spent much of their time as attending physicians on the VA wards with medical interns and residents. Dr. Lockey usually made rounds at 6:00 AM, when that was permitted, so he could attend the allergy and immunology clinics with Dr. Bukantz at 8:00 AM. The first years were spent in clinics rotating on the internal medicine wards and educating internal medicine residents and trying to meet criteria to start a residency training program in allergy and immunology. First papers published by these two faculty members include the following: 1) Bukantz SC, Lockey RF: Reversible small airway obstruction and asthma. *Adv Asthma Allergy* 1974; 1:7-11;2) Lockey RF, Bukantz SC: Allergic emergencies. *Medical Clinics of North America* 1974; 58(1):147-156; 3) Bukantz SC, Lockey RF: Controversial techniques, protocols for evaluation. *Hospital Practice* 1981; 16(7):11-12; 4) Lockey RF, Bukantz SC: Allergy and immunology. *JAMA* 1986; 256: 2076-2077. Dr. Bukantz remained an active faculty member and VA staff member until he retired in 1983. Thereafter, he was a volunteer faculty member and participated in teaching and research.

Ultimately, an allergy and immunology training program was established in 1976 and the first two allergy and immunology fellows recruited. From the initial organization of the training program, Dr. Lockey has assumed the commitment of strategically managing it. As their association continued, Dr. Bukantz remained Chief of the Division at the College of Medicine and the VA while Dr. Lockey enthusiastically assumed the position of Associate Chief at both facilities. About five or six years later,

Dr. Bukantz remained Director of the USF Division while appointing Dr. Lockey as Chief of the VA Section. Retiring in 1983, Dr. Bukantz relinquished his responsibilities as Director of the USF Division to Dr. Lockey who has since admirably served the Division with great reverence and leadership. He retired from his position at the VA Hospital in 2016 and now volunteers at the same facility. Dr. Dennis Ledford assumed the position of Chief, VA Section of Allergy and Immunology, following Dr. Lockey's retirement as Chief.

In Loving Memory of Samuel C. Bukantz, MD and His Wife, Jewell

By Richard F. Lockey, MD, MS

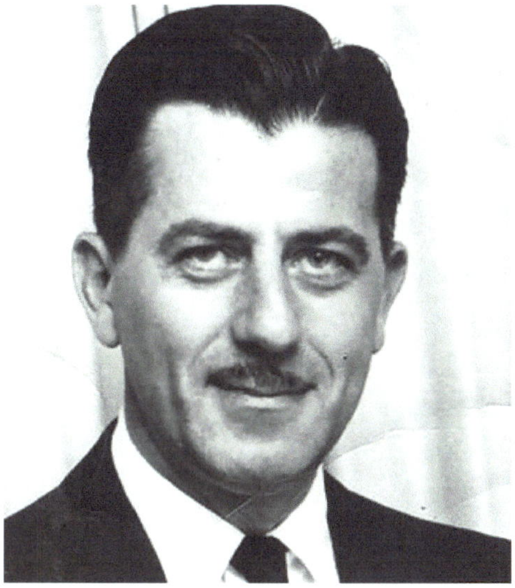

Samuel C. Bukantz, MD

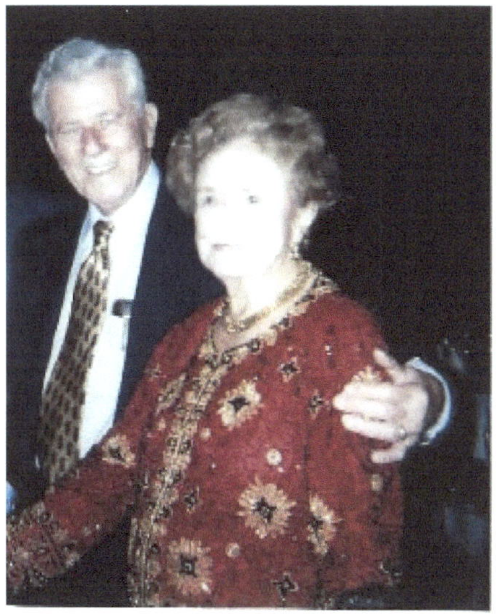

Samuel C. Bukantz, MD and wife, Jewell

Samuel Charles Bukantz, MD was Professor Emeritus and Founding Director of the University of South Florida Division of Allergy and Immunology, Department of Internal Medicine. His distinguished career in academic medicine spanned more than 60 years and helped build USF's fledgling Division of Allergy and Immunology, Department of Internal Medicine, into one of the largest, most well-respected in the world.

He was born Sept. 12, 1911 and died on October 19, 2008, age 97. Dr. Bukantz attended NYC public elementary and high schools from 1917-1926 and Washington Square College, NYU, graduating in 1930. Admitted to NYU College of Medicine in 1930, he won a gold medal for excellence in pathology. He was also elected president of his class and of Alpha Omega Alpha in his junior year and of the student organization in his senior year. At graduation, in 1934, he was awarded the Alpha Omega Alpha (AOA) prize for highest academic standing in his class.

From 1934 to 1938 he was an intern and resident at the Mount Sinai Hospital in NYC in pathology, microbiology and internal medicine. He was president of the house staff and chairman of the Economics Committee of the Intern Council of America. The Committee met with Mayor Fiorello LaGuardia and succeeded in creating the first salary for interns in the United States, $15 a month. More importantly, he met and wooed his late wife, Jewell Williams (Bukantz), a student nurse at Mt. Sinai School of Nursing, and they were married in 1941.

In 1938, Dr. Bukantz entered private practice and was awarded a part-time fellowship in pneumonia research at Harlem Hospital by Dr. Jesse G.M. Bullowa's Pneumonia Research Unit. From 1938 to 1940, he published several papers on the biology of pneumococcus and treatment of pneumococcal pneumonia. He was awarded a Parmalee Fellowship at Emergency Hospital, Washington, D.C., in 1940, where he completed an in vitro study of sulfonamide sensitivity.

In October 1941, he enlisted in the U.S. Army Medical Corps and was assigned to the Medical Department Professional Service School at the Army Medical Center in Washington, D.C. The bombing of Pearl Harbor occurred December 7 that same year and everyone his age either volunteered or was drafted into the US Armed Services. There he developed studies on the immunology of typhus fever and malaria and developed a method to preserve sheep blood for use in complement fixation. He was discharged from the military service in October 1945.

He was awarded a fellowship in allergy in 1946 under Dr. Harry Alexander at Washington University Medical School in St. Louis, became certified in allergy and immunology, and was appointed to the faculty. He spent part of his time as Chief of Internal Medicine at the Jefferson Barracks V.A. Hospital staffed by Washington and St. Louis Universities where he published papers on ragweed sensitivity. He also worked with Drs. Frank Dixon, David Talmage, and Gustav Dammin on the use of radioisotopes in the study of antigen distribution in animals and studied the immunologic characteristics of sputum of severely asthmatic subjects. Detection of large quantities of blood group substance in their sputum led to later investigations of the role of these substances in synthesis of antibodies to the blood groups.

Dr. Bukantz (from 1958 to 1963) was Medical and Research Director of the Children's Asthma Research Institute and Hospital in Denver, CO. In 1963, he was appointed Director of Clinical Research of the Schering Corporation of New Jersey and in 1965, Chief of Clinical Research at Hoffman-LaRoche. In 1967 he became Associate Professor of Medicine at NYU and began private practice in allergy/immunology at the faculty practice offices.

He then joined the USF College of Medicine in 1972 as the first director of the Division of Allergy and Immunology, Department of Internal Medicine, and Chief of the Section of Allergy and Immunology at James A. Haley Veterans' Hospital. His wife Jewell, a nurse, worked with him at the USF Clinics and helped trained some of the earliest USF fellows in the specialty.

Again, when Dr. Bukantz stepped down as Division Director in 1983, he was succeeded by his protégé, Richard F. Lockey, MD, MS. He remained active in teaching for the next twenty years.

"He has been an excellent mentor, great physician and my best friend," said Dr. Lockey, Distinguished University Health Professor, Joy McCann Culverhouse Chair in Allergy and Immunology, and Director of the USF Division of Allergy and Immunology. "Dr. Bukantz is one of the brightest people I've had the pleasure to know and the best at teaching me how to write concisely for scientific publications. He always offered invaluable feedback. The Division of Allergy and Immunology will not be the same without him. He will be sincerely missed and remembered with respect, affection, and gratitude."

Dr. Bukantz had said that one of his proudest accomplishments was helping build USF's fledgling Allergy and Immunology Division into one of the largest and well-respected in the world. "Our fellowship program has trained many physicians in the specialty of allergy and immunology who practice in Florida and are leaders in the field," he said. The Division's faculty members have trained scientists who are involved in allergy and immunology research throughout the world.

Dr. Bukantz earned a lifetime of awards for his outstanding contributions to research in allergy and immunology, medical education, and community service. In 1992, he was named Laureate of the Florida Chapter of the American College of Physicians — the state chapter's highest honor. Other awards include the Distinguished Clinician Award from the American Academy of Allergy & Immunology in 1991, the USF Distinguished Professor of Medicine Award, and the Henry Hyde Salter Award from the American College of Allergy and Clinical Immunology in 1979. Dr. Bukantz served on the editorial board of the *Journal of Allergy and Immunology* and as the editor of *Hospital Practice*. He has edited numerous books with Dr. Lockey, including *Fundamentals of Immunology and Allergy*, W.B. Saunders Co., Philadelphia, Pennsylvania, 1987; *Principles of Immunology and Allergy,* W.B. Saunders Co., Philadelphia, Pennsylvania, 1987; and the first, second, and third editions of *Allergens and*

Allergen Immunotherapy, Marcel Dekker, New York, New York, 1991, 1999, and 2004, respectively, a text used extensively by allergy/immunology training programs worldwide and now in its sixth edition, the latter edited by Drs. Lockey and Dennis K. Ledford.

In June 2004, Dr. Bukantz formally retired following a distinguished career in academic medicine spanning more than 60 years. He remained socially active in the Division until the year before his death.

Samuel C. Bukantz, MD Allergy/Immunology Outstanding Research/Leadership Achievement Award

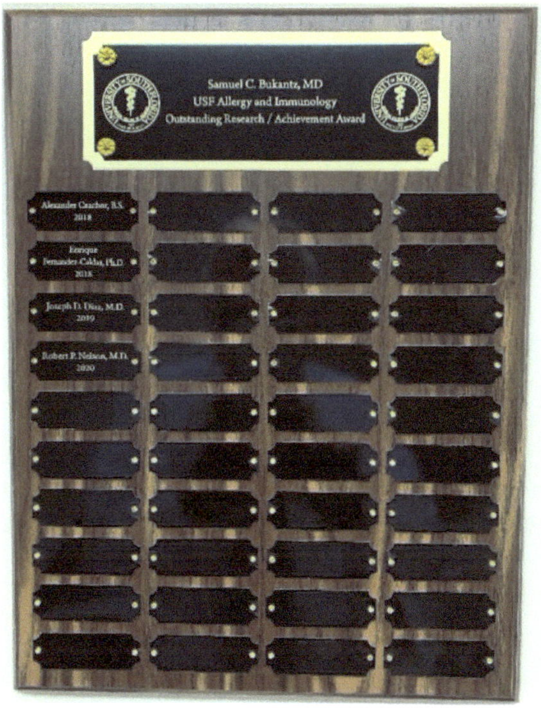

Celebrated Recipients

2018 Alexander Czachor, BS

2018 Enrique Fernandez-Caldas, PhD

2019 Joseph D. Diaz, MD

2020 Robert P. Nelson, MD

2021 Rosa Codina, PhD

The "Samuel C. Bukantz Allergy/Immunology Outstanding Research/Leadership Achievement Award" was inaugurated in 2018 in honor of Founding Division Director, Samuel C. Bukantz, MD.

The award is presented whenever there is a noteworthy candidate, but not more than once a year. Award time-line consideration will be from March to April of each year and nominations will be submitted to the Division Award Committee by May 1st.

A nominee can be anyone who is part of the USF Allergy and Immunology Division, Departments of Internal Medicine or Pediatrics, or who has graduated from or been affiliated with the Division. The award is presented for excellence in clinical medicine, research, and/or service, to be nominated and approved by the faculty of the Division of Allergy and Immunology, Department of Internal Medicine, USF Morsani College of Medicine.

Nominations will be reviewed by the Division's Award Committee. The Committee's recommendations will be provided to the Division Director to be presented to and voted on by the faculty. The award ceremony will take place during the annual USF Department of Internal Medicine graduation program in June or at a more appropriate venue, depending on the locale and convenience of the recipient. The recipient will receive an award recognition plaque and their name will be engraved on the Division's award plaque which is displayed in the Division Director's office.

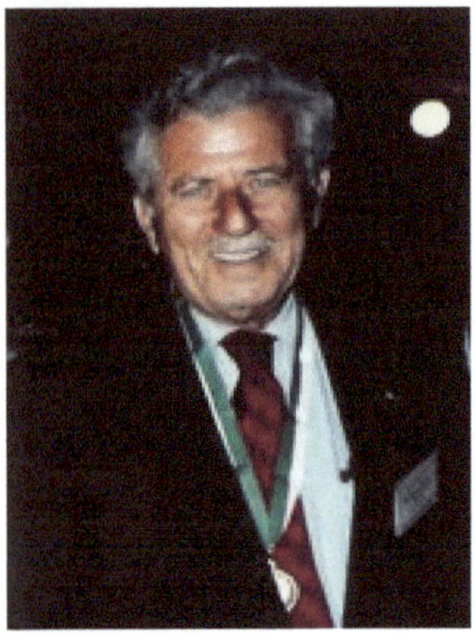

Recollections of Samuel C. Bukantz, M.D. and the Division

by Gerald A. Bucholtz, M.D.

Fellow, USF Division of Allergy and Immunology, 1980-1982. Assistant Professor of Medicine, USF College of Medicine, Division of Allergy and Immunology, Department of Internal Medicine, 1982 -1991.

I had the pleasure and honor of having Samuel C. Bukantz, MD as my attending twice during my USF Internal Medicine Residency. Dr. Bukantz had a tradition of taking his house staff out to dinner at least once per rotation. While on his service, I had ordered a biopsy that required a specific stain of a fresh frozen specimen for diagnosis and the only place that could do the stain was in California, requiring it to be sent priority airmail. Sometime after that, Dr. Bukantz began receiving the first of many shipping bills which he kept handing to me "to take care of". It was many months before that was straightened out and I got called on the carpet for it. After my residency, I worked ERs for four years, 24-hour shifts on and 48-hours off. I decided to get a better job and applied for the newly created USF Allergy and Immunology fellowship hoping Dr. Bukantz had by then forgotten about that little shipping bill incident. I interviewed with Dr. Richard Lockey at the "Brass Monkey Tavern". A few beers must have been just enough to improve my chances.

It was during my fellowship that I met the most unforgettable person, John J. Stablein, MD. He was a relentless reader. I mean he read everything from the *New England Journal of Medicine* to the *Ladies Home Journal* to the *Journal of Non-reproducible Results*. I think he made the latter up. The rumor was he would slip some controversial article, usually from the *Ladies Home Journal*, under Dr. Lockey's door just about the time John was nearing a deadline. In five, and no more than ten minutes, the door would fly open and Dr. Lockey would run down the hall yelling "We have to respond to this, quick, send a letter to the editor!"

Part of being a fellow is doing research, something I had never done before. It was Dr. Stablein who gave me the idea and the half-written proposal to study the bald cypress pollen as an aeroallergen. I polished it up a little (17 drafts) and to my surprise it was approved and funded. Then I had to do it, the completion of which led to other aeroallergen studies including the Australian Pine pollen study by Dr. Al Hensel and bayberry pollen study by Dr. Robert Nelson. We did get more sophisticated including measurement of nasal resistance with the use of a modified fireman's mask. Not everyone could perform the nasal resistance maneuver. Dr. Nelson recovered with little ill effect after nearly aspirating the nasal oropharyngeal tube. My only regret is that we did not get funding for what I believe would have been the most informative study, the longleaf pine pollen. My suspicions were that the longleaf pine pollen may be an aeroallergen, but its extract was missing an important aeroallergen that may have been removed by ether in the extraction process. I had the opportunity to write "The Three-Year Aeroallergen Survey of Tampa Bay Area". The real credit goes to all the people who compiled the data and the editorial help and patience of Dr. Bukantz, who after the 16th revision threw his hands up in the air and said, "Please just submit the damn thing."

I am eternally in debt to Peggy Hales for her uncomplaining perseverance in the seemingly never-ending revisions. I remember one day I was in the secretary's office going over one such revision with Peggy's predecessor, Ginger Montuoro. An allergy fellow candidate came in asking Ginger, "I heard Dr. Lockey is pretty hard on the fellows?". Ginger replied, "Not really, but do you see that fellow over there", as she pointed to Dr. Steve Louie, "when he started, he was as big as that fellow", as she pointed to

Dr. Al Hensel. There were black tire marks leaving the parking lot.

The Allergy and Immunology Division had a number of social events, one of which was sponsored by yours truly on Lake Keystone. I was water skiing before I thought anyone would arrive, and, lo and behold, almost the entire Division was lined up on the dock like sparrows on a wire. I couldn't resist it and skied by the dock, not thinking the spray would go that far. Dr. Bukantz saw the humor in it and said, "Well done". Mrs. Bukantz said something else, referring to her new hairdo. One notable person who was not there for the water fun was Dr. Al Hensel, but he did show up later with 5 gallons of gumbo.

As an attending, I had the pleasure of learning and working with gifted trainees such as Dr. Dennis K. Ledford. He would ponder questions overnight or over the weekend and put it to me on the next day, often a Monday. After a while, I realized this was a trap, the "Ledford Trap", because the answer to the second question would make any answer to the first question implausible. He clearly had been thinking about it a lot.

I truly enjoyed my time in the Division and will always feel a part of the USF Division of Allergy and Immunology.

Fellowship

The first fellows in training, accepted in 1976, were Jack Parrino, MD and J. Wayne Phillips, MD. Since that time, the prestigious program has graduated 69 fellows as of 2020 from the Division's program. Program accreditation was received in 1976 from the American Council of Graduate Medical Education (ACGME) and has since remained accredited without interruption. This two-to-three year fellowship program accepts two or three fellows into the program each year.

Today, the USF Department of Internal Medicine's Division of Allergy and Immunology in collaboration with the Division of Allergy and Immunology at All Children's Hospital, offers a broad-based training program in allergy and immunology. Built on a foundation of financial security and balanced education, these allergy and immunology training programs strive to be "the best they can be" in training allergists/immunologists, internal medicine and pediatric residents, and medical students. During the two-to-three year training period, fellows participate in the treatment of patients with allergic or immunological diseases and conduct mentored projects in basic or clinical research.

It is the faculty's goal to train academicians as well as clinicians. Academic medicine involves practicing in a medical school with abundant opportunities for teaching, learning through seminars and symposia, stimulating interaction with diverse colleagues, and engaging in research. These unique benefits provide the fellows with a well-rounded educational and clinical experience.

The success of the USF Allergy and Immunology fellowship program is rooted in its balance and diversity. The Division's strengths are in the education of fellows, medical students, internists, and pediatricians. All fellows study under 26 academic and clinical faculty. Four of the faculty also operate a clinical practice near USF. Physician faculty teach fellows the "ins and outs" of running a clinic during the approximately 25 to 30 hours per week each member spends in the clinic. The Division's faculty also supervise training and patient care in several USF clinics, including a world-renowned immune-deficiency clinic at All Children's Hospital, St. Petersburg, Florida. Clinical and basic faculty members participate in clinical and basic research at the Joy McCann Culverhouse Airway Disease Research Center. This allows fellows to have a very broad-based opportunity to participate in a variety of basic and clinical research. The experience includes a rotation through an active clinical research unit where clinical research projects instituted by faculty, fellows, as well as pharmaceutical firms, are carried forward.

Faculty members have diverse interests. Some are focused on allergic diseases while others are interested in immunologic disorders. All have an interest in both arms of the specialty, i.e., allergy and immunology. The Pediatric Program participates in an active bone marrow transplantation service for primary immunodeficiency patients. Therefore, the USF Allergy and Immunology training program experience provides a unique opportunity for patient contact and "hands-on" experience in both pediatric and adult allergy and immunology research, teaching, and patient care, giving the program a "big" A (Allergy), " big" I (Immunology) identification, unique in the field of allergy and immunology training programs.

Both the Department of Internal Medicine Division of Allergy and Immunology and the Department of Pediatrics Division of Allergy and Immunology have an ongoing cooperative program whereby the residents from the pediatric program rotate at least one day per week through the internal medicine program and vice-versa. Individuals from the Department of Internal Medicine program rotate each Tuesday at All Children's Hospital, located approximately 45 minutes from the USF Tampa campus, where they participate in a primary and secondary immunodeficiency clinic, one of the best in the world. The pediatric fellows rotate on Mondays at the Tampa Campus, where they are exposed to one of the most diverse patient population with allergic, immunologic, and immunodeficiency diseases.

Approximately 30% of former trainees are in academic medicine and 70% in clinical practice. The Director, Richard F. Lockey, MD, MS, and faculty remain in contact with trainees, all of whom have gone on to acquire excellent reputations in the medical schools and/or communities in which they practice. The faculty are all members of the Division of Allergy and Immunology in the USF Department of Internal Medicine as well as the Division of Allergy and Immunology in the USF Department of Pediatrics.

The USF Department of Internal Medicine, Division of Allergy and Immunology is committed to preparing and training specialists who will provide exemplary state-of-the-art care to patients with allergic and immunologic diseases. The faculty expect its graduates to share this vision, assume leadership positions, and advance the science of the field of allergy and immunology. All fellows who have graduated from the program in the past fifteen years have passed Boards and many have now assumed leadership positions, either in medical schools or clinical practice.

Allergy/Immunology Internal Medicine Fellows

Jack Parrino, MD	1977 – 1979
J. Wayne Phillips, MD	1977 - 1979
Roger W. Fox, MD	1978 - 1980
Linn R. Klotz, MD	1979 - 1981
John J. Stablein, MD *	1979 - 1981
Gerald A. Bucholtz, MD	1980 - 1982
Steven J. Louie, MD	1981 - 1983
Albert E. Hensel, MD	1982 - 1984
Dennis K. Ledford MD	1983 - 1985
Mark W. Minor, MD	1985 - 1987
Robert P. Nelson, MD	1985 - 1987
Joseph D. Diaz, MD	1986 - 1988
Donald W. Russell, MD	1987 - 1990
Richard P. Silton, MD	1988 - 1990
David N. Wright, MD	1988 - 1991
Thomas B. Edwards, MD	1990 - 1992
Carlos M. Jacinto, MD	1990 - 1992
G. Edward Stewart, MD	1991 - 1994
Brett E. Stanaland, MD	1992 - 1995
Jose Andrade, MD	1993 - 1995
Stephen F. Kemp, MD	1993 - 1996
Lizette S. Hernandez, MD	1994 - 1997
Kevin P. Rosenbach, MD	1995 - 1998
Giana L. Nicoara-Kasti, MD	1996 - 1998
Demetrios S. Theodoropoulos, MD	1997 - 2000
Thomas W. Luck, MD	1999 - 2001
Daniel A. Reichmuth, MD	1999 - 2002
Nina C. Ramirez, MD	2000 - 2002
Richard E. Crockett, MD	2000 - 2003
Jose R. Arias Jr., MD	2001 - 2003
A. Sean McKnight, MD	2002 - 2004
Patrick J. DeMarco, MD	2003 - 2005
John T. Ramey, MD	2003 - 2005
Alex T. Vu, MD	2004 - 2006
Denise M. Kearney, MD	2004 - 2006
Steven L. Cole, DO	2005 - 2007
Thomas Chacko, MD	2005 - 2007
Andrew Bagg, MD	2006 - 2008
Ronald Purcell, MD	2006 - 2008
Byol Shin, DO	2006 - 2008
Joshua Phillips, MD	2007 - 2009
Mathew Varghese, MD	2007 - 2009
Dennis Kim, MD	2008 - 2010
Efren Rael, MD	2008 - 2010
Robert Pesek, MD	2009 - 2011
Michel Alkhalil, MD	2009 - 2011
Ahmed Butt, MD	2010 - 2012
David Fitzhugh, MD	2010 - 2012
James Parkerson, DO	2010 - 2012
Salman Aljubran, MD	2010 - 2013
Susan Culverhouse, MD	2011 - 2013
Neetu Talreja, MD	2011 – 2013
Gregory M. Cowan, MD	2012 - 2014
Nauman Salim, MD	2012 - 2014
Michael C. Balduzzi, MD	2013 - 2015
Adam C. Udegraff, DO	2013 - 2015
Jennifer E. Fergeson, DO	2014 - 2016
Andrew J. Cooke, MD	2014 - 2016
Adeeb A. Bulkhi, MD	2014 - 2017
Peter Ricketti, DO	2015 - 2017
Sultan Alandijani, MD	2015 - 2017
Chen Lin, MD	2015 - 2017
Amber Pepper, MD	2016 - 2018
Emma Westermann–Clark, MD	2016 - 2018
Shiven S. Patel, MD	2017 - 2019
Tara V. Saco, MD	2017 - 2019
Kirk V. Shepard II, MD	2017 - 2019
Raul Sergio Villarreal, MD	2018 - 2020
Claudia Gaefke, MD	2018 - 2020
Nicholas Kolinsky, DO	2019 - 2021
David Gubernick, MD	2019 - 2021
Stephanie Hudey, MD	2019 - 2021
Natalie Diaz-Cabrera, MD	2020 - 2022
Donya Imanirad, MD	2020 - 2022

* Deceased

Clinical and Laboratory Immunology Fellowship

The Clinical Laboratory Immunology Fellowship began in the Division in 1986. It was an optional one-year fellowship following two years of training in the Allergy and Immunology Fellowship. The program focused on the laboratory aspect of clinical immunologic diseases. It offered experience in immunology laboratory techniques, their application to disease management, and detailed interpretation of laboratory tests. Dr. Dennis Ledford was the first fellow to train in the program in the Division and in the country. He also became one of the first directors of a clinical and laboratory immunology fellowship at USF. Fellows performed research in the clinical laboratory of Linda Bergen-Losee, MS. The lab was located on the Medical School campus in the MDC Building on the fourth floor. This program was discontinued by the American Council of Graduate Medical Education in 2000.

USF "Immunodeficiency Clinic"

Early 1980s ... the topic of human immunodeficiency virus (HIV) became an erupting and controversial topic. One of the Division's trainees, Robert P. Nelson, MD, who graduated in 1987, acquired a profound interest in the virus during his fellowship. Dr. Lockey, with Dr. Ledford's help and support, decided to establish a one-of-a-kind immunodeficiency clinic primarily to care for HIV patients. Great controversy arose from College of Medicine faculty members regarding the development of the clinic. After much opposition, and the continued prodding by Dr. Lockey, the clinic became a reality as Andor Szentivanyi, MD, DSc, Dean of the College of Medicine and courtesy faculty member of the Division, "indicated" that there would be an "immunodeficiency clinic", not an HIV or "AIDS" clinic. Despite the apprehension of the disease etiology and pathogenesis, the clinic was originally staffed by Drs. Richard F. Lockey, Dennis K. Ledford, Robert P. Nelson, and Division fellows-in-training. Quite an accomplishment and one of the first clinics in the country to care for AIDS.

Faculty, fellows and nurses who initially worked in the clinic, and their families, were extremely apprehensive about contracting this disease; its etiology and pathogenesis were unknown. Before caring for patients suspected of being infected, physicians and nurses masked, gowned, and gloved. Being interested in the pathogenesis of the disease, each patient was asked to complete an extensive questionnaire to learn how the disease was transmitted. Faculty were convinced that the disease was viral in etiology and the transmission was via bodily secretions, as the literature now indicates.

This was an incredible and unusual experience for the Division even though this was a difficult clinic to work in because of tragic outcomes. Each week patients would be asked not to return to clinic because there was nothing more to offer them. As the disease etiology was identified and medications became available, the epidemic came under control. The clinic was eventually turned over to the Division of Infectious Diseases and International Medicine following Dr. Robert P. Nelson's acceptance of a position at the University of Indiana to join their bone marrow transplantation program.

Animal Research

Another major controversy that arose was promoted by the "animal rightists" and occurred in Tampa in the mid-1980s. It concerned whether or not the College of Medicine would continue to obtain unwanted Hillsborough County pound dogs for basic research. The county commissioners did not want to address or vote on this issue, so they placed it on the Hillsborough County ballot for the public to decide. Dr. Lockey became the lead member at the College of Medicine to promote the idea that pound animals should not just be euthanized and wasted, but some of those ultimately to be destroyed should be available for research performed humanely at little or no cost to the College of Medicine. The "Committee on Animal Research" and Dr. Lockey raised approximately $50,000 to support the cause and publicize the importance of animal research. The election was won by 69% of the vote. During this controversy, Dr. Lockey's and other faculty members' lives were threatened. Faculty members were extremely pleased that the College of Medicine took a stand to educate the public about the importance of animal research. Animal research remains essential to the advancement of science and medicine to this day.

Endowments

With unending gratitude, the Division is indebted to Mrs. Joy McCann Culverhouse and to Mr. and Mrs. George Simmons for the gracious gifts of two endowments, The Joy McCann Culverhouse Endowment ($4,557,200 and matched by the State) in April 1997 was solicited by Dr. Lockey and the Mabel and Ellsworth Simmons Endowment ($1,238,924 and $929,193 matched by the State) by Alan Goldman, MD, Chief of Internal Medicine at that time, and Dr. Lockey, in October 1998. These two endowments resulted in the Joy McCann Culverhouse Chair in Allergy and Immunology, occupied by Richard F. Lockey, MD, MS, and the Mabel and Ellsworth Simmons Professorship in Allergy and Immunology, originally occupied by Shyam S. Mohapatra, PhD and subsequently awarded to Dennis K. Ledford, MD. As a result of the Joy McCann Culverhouse Endowment, The Joy McCann Culverhouse Airway Disease Research Center was instituted in 1998 where multi-disciplinary state-of-the-art research has been ongoing.

Both endowments support salaries, equipment, and expenses to assist in underwriting the cost of Division research and teaching. Undergraduate and graduate students and post-doctoral researchers have been awarded unique opportunities to train and acquire scholarly research experience. A diverse group of researchers have studied in the Division including students from USF and other universities in the United States and researchers and physicians from foreign countries. In addition to supporting research, the endowments have enabled the Division to invite world-renown researchers to the University. Current values (2020) of the endowments are $12,475,172 for the Joy McCann Culverhouse Endowment and $2,683,905 for the Mabel and Ellsworth Simmons Professorship.

The Joy McCann Culverhouse Airway Disease Research Center

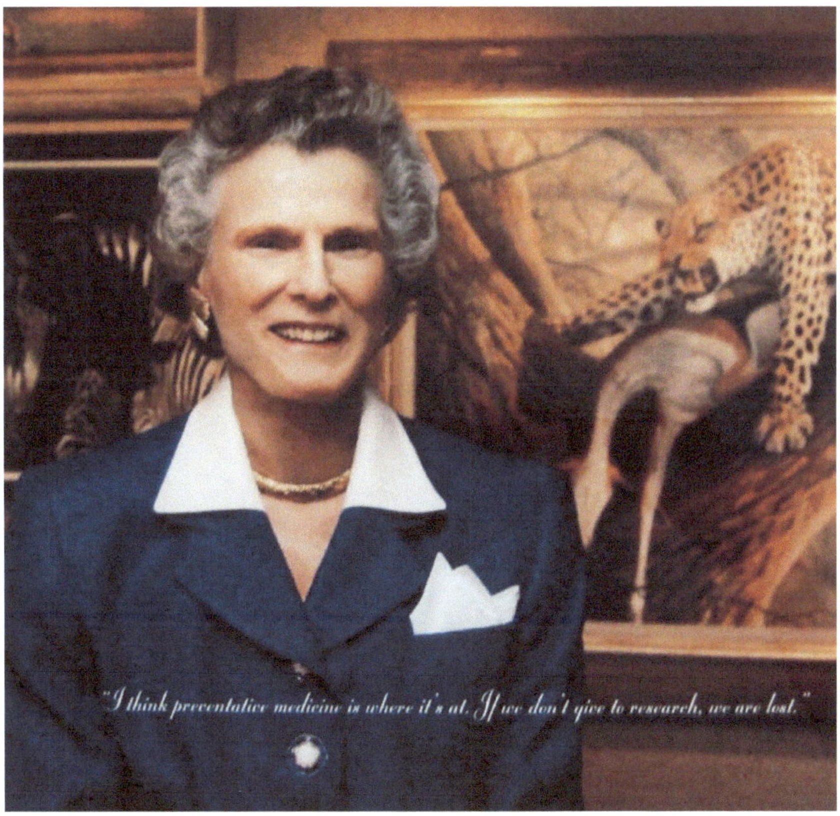
"I think preventative medicine is where it's at. If we don't give to research, we are lost."

The Joy McCann Culverhouse Airway Disease Research Center was dedicated in 1998.

Mabel and Ellsworth Simmons Professorship in Allergy and Immunology Basic Research

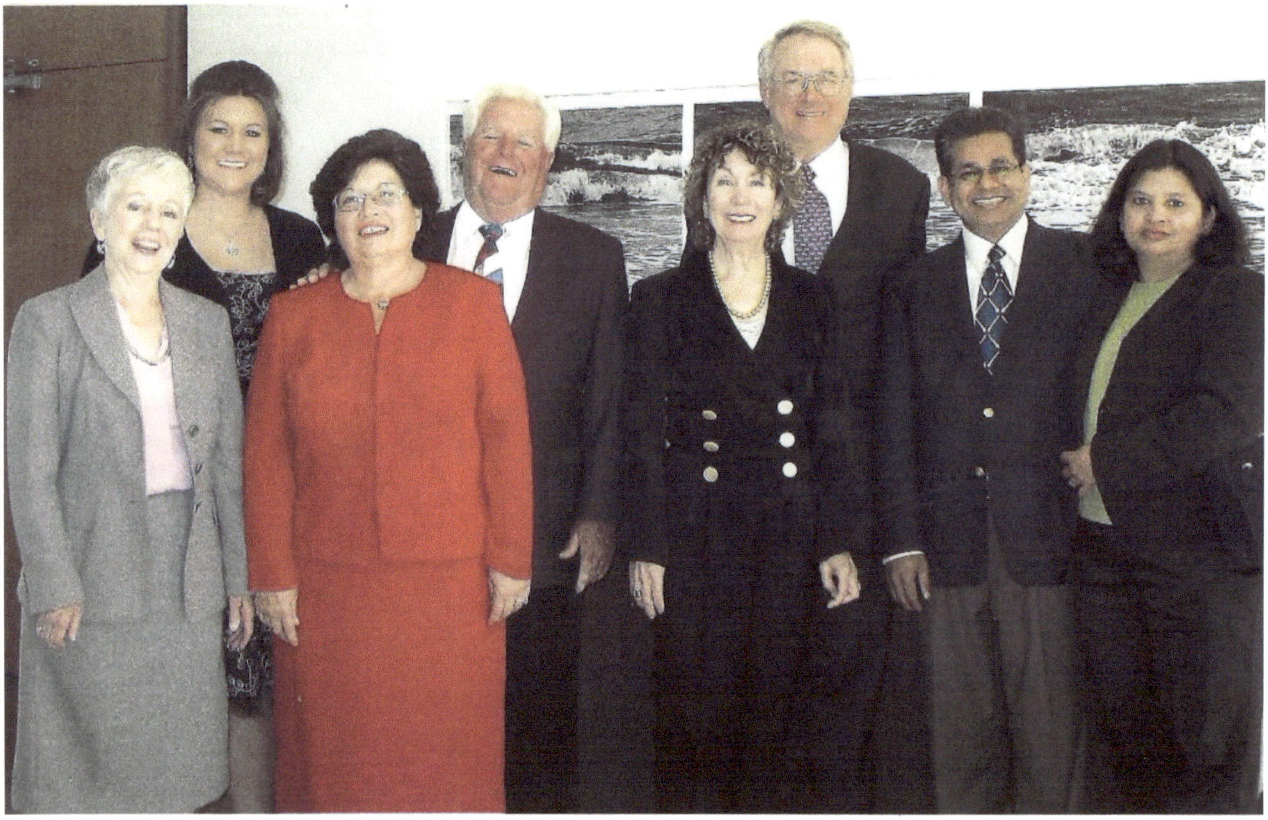

Front row (left to right): name unknown, Sandy Simmons; Carol Lee Lockey; Shyam S. Mohapatra, PhD; Subhra Mohapatra, PhD.
Back row (left to right): name unknown; George Simmons; Richard F. Lockey, MD, MS.

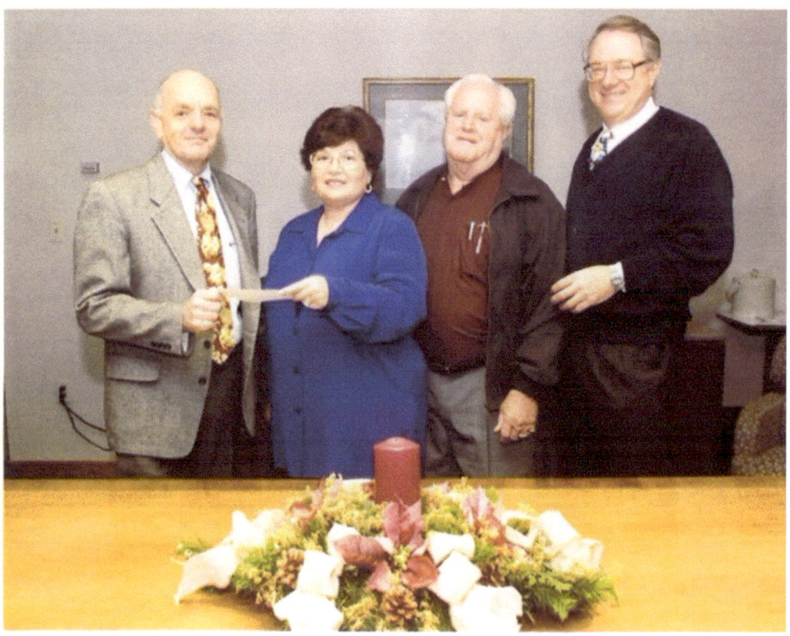

Awarding the Mabel and Ellsworth Simmons endowment to the Division of Allergy and Immunology in 2001. Left to right: Dean Martin Silbiger, MD; Sandy Simmons; George Simmons; and Richard F. Lockey, MD, MS.

Basic Research

In 1997, the Division of Allergy and Immunology established a multi-disciplinary basic research lab facility at the University of South Florida Morsani College of Medicine to promote and conduct basic research in allergy, immunology, airway disease, and pulmonary medicine.

The basic research program consists of six faculty researchers. Drs. Camoretti-Mercado, Cardet, Cho, Galam, Kolliputi and Teng maintain multidisciplinary laboratories as part of the Joy McCann Culverhouse Airway Disease Research Center located at the Morsani College of Medicine. The Center was dedicated in 1998. The goals of the Joy McCann Culverhouse Airway Disease Research Center are to: 1) promote and conduct research in the area of airway disease and pulmonary medicine at the USF Health Morsani College of Medicine, 2) conduct research seminars and conferences related to respiratory disease, 3) bring together basic and clinical scientists who translate bench and clinical research into improved treatment of patients who suffer from asthma, allergic and immunologic diseases, and 4) encourage all faculty and fellows to participate in the Center's research opportunities.

The scientific programs in the Division are supported by the Joy McCann Culverhouse and Mabel and Ellsworth Simmons Endowments. Funds are utilized to support salaries, equipment, and expenses to help underwrite Division costs. Research has also been supported by grants from the American Academy of Allergy Asthma & Immunology ARTrust; American Heart Association; American Lung Association; Florida Department of Health; National Heart, Lung and Blood Institute; National Institute of Allergy and Infectious Diseases; National Institutes of Health; Patient-Centered Outcomes Research Institute; and the Food Allergy Network.

Research interests (2020) include chronic rhinosinusitis, nasal polyps, mast cell biology, pollen identification, the role of RNA-editing in Acute Respiratory Diseases (ARDS), development of a mouse model that will recapitulate age-associate Idiopathic Pulmonary Fibrosis (IPF) in humans, translational strategies to attenuate oxidative stress-mediated acute lung injury (ALI), pulmonary fibrosis and pulmonary arterial hypertension, host virus interactions for RSV pathogenesis, interactions between cellular signal transduction machinery and viral proteins, genomic determinants of lung dysfunction, and mechanisms of oxidative stress with respect to SOCS-1 protection against hyperoxic acute lung injury.

Shyam S. Mohapatra, PhD was recruited from the University of Manitoba, Winnipeg, Canada, in 1996. Drs. Mohapatra and Lockey met serendipitously at the American Academy of Allergy Asthma & Immunology Annual Meeting that year. Dr. Mohapatra was receptive to a career relocation and was recruited to the Division. He worked in the Division for 15 years before leaving to form his own basic research entity, the Division of Translational Medicine, which has prospered at the University. Drs. Mohapatra and Lockey recruited a multitude of basic researchers, many of whom are still at the University. Dr. Mohapatra has been highly successful as a basic research investigator.

Dr. Subhra Mohapatra was also an integral part of Dr. Mohapatra's lab in the Division's Joy McCann Culverhouse Airway Diseases Research Center. She was a fundamental part of the lab's extensive research program in respiratory diseases and in the training of postdoctoral and graduate students. Additionally, Srinivas Nagaraj, PhD joined Dr. Shyam Mohapatra's lab to conduct research in his area of expertise, tumor immunology and immunotherapy. Both Drs. Subhra Mohapatra and Srinivas Nagaraj joined Dr. Shyam Mohapatra when he established the Division of Translational Medicine.

Over the years, the Division has trained more than 150 basic researchers including both national and international undergraduate students, graduate students, post-doctoral fellows, exchange students, and visiting faculty scholars. Many of these individuals are now faculty members, and some leaders in academic centers and the pharmaceutical industry throughout the world. Overall goals of the researchers are to understand the basic mechanisms of asthma and allergic and immunologic diseases to provide therapeutic options for patients suffering with these critical diseases.

Resulting from excellence in research, numerous patents and invention disclosures have resulted from Division research. According to a USF newsfeed of June 2, 2020, "The inventive efforts of University of South Florida researchers continue to place the institution in the top ranks of global universities in producing new U.S. utility patents in 2019, according to a new ranking released today by the National Academy of Inventors and the Intellectual Property Owners Association."

(https://www.usf.edu/news/2020/usf-ranks-among-academic-world-leaders-in-us-patent-production.aspx, accessed September 6, 2020)

Patents
Division of Allergy and Immunology, Department of Internal Medicine

INTERNAL ID	PATENT TITLE	LEAD INVENTOR	WORKING FOR COMPANY	WORKING FOR DEPT	PATENT NO	ISSUE DATE	COUNTRY
15B170PRC	Rodent Immobilization Apparatus and Method of Use Thereof	Fukumoto, Jutaro	College of Medicine	Internal Medicine (COM)	9,622,842	4/18/2017	United States
13A010PRC	Inflammatory Disease Diagnosis and Methods of Treatment Using Lipopolysaccharides-responsive Beige-like Anchor	Wang, JiaQi; Lockey, Richard	College of Medicine	Internal Medicine (COM)	9,738,706	8/22/2017	United States
14B153PRC	Animal Model and Method for Studying Gene-Gene Interactions	Wang, JiaQi; Lockey, Richard	College of Medicine	Internal Medicine (COM)	9,974,290	5/22/2018	United States
13B164PRC	Multiplexed RNA qPCR Assay	Wang, JiaQi; Lockey, Richard	College of Medicine	Internal Medicine (COM)	10,030,263	7/24/2018	United States
13A010PRCDV	Inflammatory Disease Diagnosis and Methods of Treatment Using Lipopolysaccharides-responsive Beige-like Anchor	Wang, JiaQi; Lockey, Richard	College of Medicine	Internal Medicine (COM)	10,654,918	5/19/2020	United States
13A010PRCDV	Inflammatory Disease Diagnosis and Methods of Treatment Using Lipopolysaccharides-responsive Beige-like Anchor	Wang, JiaQi	College of Medicine	Internal Medicine (COM)	10,654,918	5/19/2020	United States
18A048PRC	Aldh-1 Shields Endothelial cells against oxidative stress via activation of ALDH2	Kolliputi, Narasaiah; Lockey, Richard; Galam, Lakshmi	College of Medicine	Internal Medicine (COM)	10,660,873	5/26/2020	United States

Clinical Research

Roger W. Fox, MD, fellow 1978 - 1980, joined the faculty following completion of his fellowship. Dr. Lockey purchased space at 13801 Bruce B. Downs Blvd in 1979 to move his clinical practice from 3000 Medical Park Drive to the fifth floor of the new building. Dr. Fox joined the faculty and the clinical practice which permitted it to become an integral and essential part of the Division's teaching and research program. During this time, Ms. Lolita R. F. Binford served as clinical research coordinator.

The Division's research program was augmented by the arrival of Saber Samaan, PhD, a pharmacologist who was born and raised in Egypt and was a Division member from approximately 1982 to 1984. Studies involving pharmacokinetics took place on weekends at the now Clarion Hotel on Fowler Avenue with student volunteers from the College of Engineering. Drs. Bukantz, Fox, Lockey and Samaan and Irene Baird-Warren, clinical research coordinator, spent the weekends doing research. Many Division papers published in the early 1980s were pharmacokinetic studies which were the result of the weekend research which took place at the Hotel with appropriate IRB-approval and precautions taken.

Clinical Research Unit

The Division's Clinical Research Unit (CRU) was established in 1977 to improve the treatment of patients who suffer from asthma and allergic and immunologic diseases. The CRU provides quality research in a variety of clinical areas which include: allergic conjunctivitis; allergen immunotherapy; allergen skin testing; allergic rhinitis; asthma; atopic eczema; bronchitis, acute and chronic; contact dermatitis; chronic obstructive pulmonary disease; exercise-induced asthma; headache (temporomandibular joint dysfunction and tension); hereditary angioedema; immunodeficiency diseases; insect allergy; intravenous immunoglobulin; nasal polyps; sinusitis, acute and chronic; temporomandibular joint disease; urticaria; and vasomotor rhinitis.

The CRU has conducted over 400 Phase II, III, IV clinical trials and has established a working relationship with more than 50 pharmaceutical sponsors. The CRU was an American Lung Association Airways Clinical Research Center from 2000 until 2019, one of 20 centers in the U.S., comprised of a network of academic asthma research centers funded to conduct multicenter clinical research trials in asthma relating to treatment. Activities have been augmented by the arrival of Thomas B. Casale, MD, who assumed the responsibility of Director of the CRU from Dr. Lockey in 2014. It is now one of the largest clinical research units within the University of South Florida Morsani College of Medicine and the largest in the Department of Internal Medicine.

The CRU is currently located immediately adjacent to the clinical practice of Drs. Lockey, Fox (retired), Ledford (retired only from practice; full-time academician and clinician at the James A. Haley VA Hospital), Glaum, Cho, and Pepper at 13801 Bruce B. Downs Blvd., Suite 505. It is University-affiliated and all monies generated by the Unit go to the Division and College of Medicine. As part of their USF responsibilities, the faculty members staff the CRU for patient care.

Present Clinical Research Unit Personnel

Tiffani Kaage | Catherine Renee Smith | Michelle Twitmyer

Former Clinical Research Unit Personnel

Jeaneen Ahmad	Irene Baird-Warren	Menayra Caro
Wendy Allota	Matt Baker	Sara Croker
Shawna Atha	Lolita Binford	Alisa Deicidue

Brooke Fimbel	Rebecca Dawn McCrery	Ivonne Pena
Michelle Grandstaff-Singleton	Shirley McCullough	Rikesh Patel
Michelle Hernandez	Stephanie Merrell	Cindy Reichart
Ray Heromin	Yvette Meunier	Carlotta Riner
Rita Johnson	Diana Miller	Sharon Siegel
Sarah Lewis	Pam Neu	Nadira Sultana

Presidents

The presidents!!! Throughout the Divisions history, several faculty have held prestigious presidential offices in specialty organizations. The American Academy of Allergy Asthma & Immunology (AAAAI) is the premier allergy and immunology organization with greater than 7,000 members in the United States, Canada and 72 other countries. Members include medical professionals from the field of allergy and immunology, specialists from related medical fields, allied health professionals, and related healthcare professionals, all with an interest in advancing the knowledge and practice of research and the treatment of allergic and immunologic diseases.

The evolution of the American Academy of Allergy Asthma & Immunology (AAAAI) dates back to the early 1920s with the founding of two professional organizations: the Society for the Study of Asthma and Allied Conditions (on the East Coast) and the American Association for the Study of Allergy (on the West Coast). In 1943, these two entities joined forces to become one stronger, integrated professional society, the American Academy of Allergy, as it was called from 1982 to approximately 1993. Thereafter, the name was changed to the American Academy of Allergy Asthma & Immunology. Although its name has changed, the Academy's mission has remained the same: the advancement of the knowledge of allergy, asthma, and immunology for optimal patient care.

Esteemed faculty who have been president of the AAAAI include Richard F. Lockey, MD, MS, 1992-1993; Thomas B. Casale, MD, 2007-2008; Mark M. Ballow, MD, 2010-2011; and Dennis K. Ledford, MD, 2011-2012. Likewise, Dr. Bukantz was honored as being elected Vice-President of the AAAAI. Dr. Ballow's core faculty appointment is in the USF Pediatric Division of Allergy and Immunology. There is no other university in the country which has four Academy past-presidents on their faculty. Because of their abounding integrity, their presidential terms promoted positive growth and advancement of the organization.

American Academy of Allergy Asthma & Immunology Foundation

The establishment of AAAAI lectureships has enabled the Academy to continue its mission of supporting the training of physicians and research in the specialty leading to advancement in optimal patient care.

AAAAI Foundation and Richard F. Lockey, MD MS FAAAAI & University of South Florida Lectureship ($250,000)

Initiated by Dennis K. Ledford, MD, former fellow and faculty member since 1985, and Joseph D. Diaz, MD (1986-1988), the AAAAI Foundation announced the establishment of the Richard F. Lockey, MD, MS, FAAAAI & University of South Florida A/I Program 15-Year Lectureship and Faculty Development Award in 2019. The award reached the goal of $250,000 in one year.

Dennis K. Ledford, MD, FAAAAI and University of South Florida Allergy & Immunology Division Lectureship ($100,000)

During the 2018 AAAAI/WAO Joint Congress in Orlando, the Dennis K. Ledford, MD, FAAAAI and University of South Florida Allergy & Immunology Division Lectureship was announced. The inaugural presentation was at the 2019 AAAAI Annual Meeting.

Stephen D. Lockey, Jr., MD Lectureship: Investing Together in Our Future ($100,000)

In 2013, Richard F. Lockey, MD, MS, FAAAAI and his immediate family established the ARTrust and Stephen D. Lockey, Jr., MD lectureship in loving honor of Dr. Lockey's father and mother, Stephen D. Lockey, Jr., MD and Anna Funk Lockey. Dr. Stephen D. Lockey, Jr. practiced in Lancaster, Pennsylvania and was a pioneer in the field of allergy and immunology. Proceeds from the five-year Lectureship helped to support young investigators in researching the prevention and cure of asthma and allergic and immunologic disease. The Lectureship was retired in 2018.

American Academy of Allergy Asthma & Immunology Pollen Counting Station

The Division has been collecting pollen counts through pollen counting stations located at the VA Hospital or the USF College of Medicine since the 1970s. Pollen counts were originally collected by Lolita Binford, Irene Baird-Warren, and Debbie Serbousek in the 1970s and 1980s.

The National Allergy Bureau™ (NAB™) is the section of the Academy's Aeroallergen Network responsible for reporting current pollen and mold spore levels. The Division is one of approximately 84 counting stations in the United States. Mark C. Glaum, MD, PhD and Rosa Codina, PhD are certified to read the air samples collected from the Burkard Manufacturing Company (Rickmansworth, Hertfordshire, England) volumetric air sampler. Certification is administered through the Academy's Aerobiology Committee.

Alumni Dinner

One of the highly anticipated events at the annual AAAAI meeting is the Division's Alumni Dinner. The first alumni dinner was held approximately 20 years ago and was received with great accolades. The dinner has become an annual event and gives the alumni and current members of the Division the opportunity to meet, reminisce, and share stories from the past while becoming acquainted with alumni who have graduated prior and subsequent to their graduate year. This evening of camaraderie always provides fascinating and amusing accounts of the fellows' training. Attending the dinner assuredly provides an evening filled with laughter and friendship.

World Allergy Organization

Another prestigious organization known in the specialty is the World Allergy Organization (WAO). The WAO is an international umbrella organization consisting of 103 regional and national allergology and clinical immunology societies throughout the world providing educational outreach programs, conferences and lectureships to members. Dedicated to his presidency in 2010 - 2011, Dr. Lockey inspired the growth of the WAO, democratized the Organization, and created the official journal of the WAO, the *World Allergy Organization Journal*. The *Journal* provides up-to-date, quality content focusing on the epidemiology of allergy, asthma, and clinical immunology.

"History of the World Allergy Organization: Reflective Recollections of the WAO Presidency, 2010-2011" is a personal account of Dr. Lockey's term as WAO president and can be viewed at the website

"https://waojournal.biomedcentral.com/track/pdf/10.1097/WOX.0b013e318249715a".

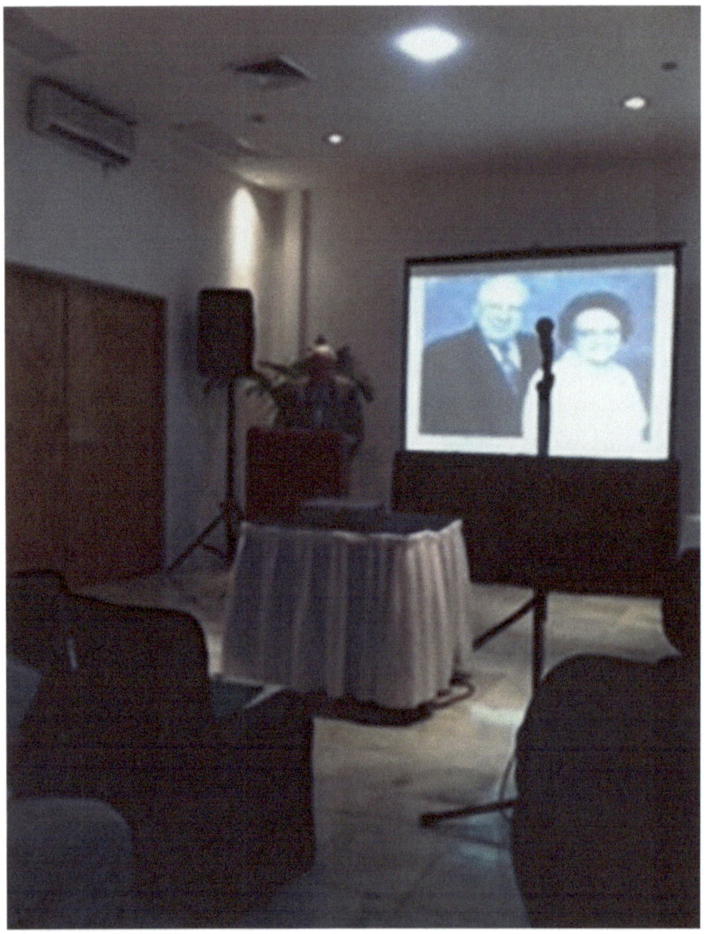

Dr. Lockey's World Allergy Organization Presidential Address, dedicated to his father and mother, Stephen D. Lockey, Jr., MD and Anna Funk Lockey, 2011.

Informative and detailed articles regarding the history of the WAO, authored by WAO past and present leaders, can be found at the website "https://www.worldallergy.org/about-wao/wao-history-project". The articles were published in the *WAO Journal*.

World Allergy Organization (WAO) Center of Excellence

The Division was honored to be chosen as one of three North American WAO Centers of Excellence from 2016 to 2019. It was renamed as a Center of Excellence from 2020 to 2026. WAO Centers of Excellence intensify and accelerate multidisciplinary scientific and clinical innovation, education, and advocacy worldwide providing excellence in education, research, and training in allergy, asthma, and clinical immunology. The Division was selected because of proficiency in research, clinical care, education and training, and networking and advocacy.

Florida Allergy, Asthma & Immunology Society

The Florida Allergy Asthma & Immunology Society (FAAIS) promotes the advancement of the specialty in the State of Florida. The Internal Medicine and Pediatric Divisions have been honored to have the following faculty and fellowship graduates serve as presidents of the FAAIS.

FAAIS Past-Presidents: Graduates or Faculty of USF Divisions of Allergy and Immunology

President	Year of Presidency	Position and A/I Core Division
Samuel C. Bukantz MD	1978	Emeritus Professor (Int Med)
Richard F. Lockey, MD	1981	Distinguished University Health Professor (Int Med)
Roger W. Fox, MD	1985	Fellow (1978-1980 Int Med); Professor (Int Med)
John J. Stablein, MD	1988	Associate Professor (Int Med)
Dennis K. Ledford, MD	1991	Fellow (1983-1985 Int Med); Professor (Int Med)
Dennis K. Ledford, MD	1992	Fellow (1983-1985 Int Med): Professor (Int Med)
Mandel R. Sher, MD	1997	Professor (Pediatrics)
Hugh H. Windom, MD	1998	Clinical Professor (Int Med)
Mark W. Minor, MD	1999	Fellow (1985-1987 Int Med)
G. Edward Stewart II, MD	2002	Fellow (1991-1994 Int Med); Clinical Professor (Int Med)
Samuel Gubernick, DO	2005	Fellow (1991-1993 Pediatrics); Assistant Professor (Pediatrics)
Steven Louie, MD	2006	Fellow (1981-1983 Int Med)
Samuel Gubernick, DO	2007	Fellow (1991-1993 Pediatrics); Assistant Professor (Pediatrics)
Bernard Zeffren, MD	2009	Fellow (1994-1996 Pediatrics)
Patrick DeMarco, MD	2012	Fellow (2003-2005 Int Med)
Andrew Bagg, MD	2014	Fellow (2006-2008 Int Med)
Nina Ramirez, MD	2018	Fellow (2000-2002 Int Med)
Samuel Gubernick, DO	2020	Fellow (1991-1993 Pediatrics); Assistant Professor (Pediatrics)

Annual Christmas / New Year's Celebration

A unique aspect of the early Division's activities was the annual Christmas / New Year's party at which time Division members and guests from the James A. Haley Veterans' Hospital and the USF Morsani College of Medicine joined us in the hallway of the VA Research Building, commonly referred to as Building 2, for a three- or four-hour celebration. A unique aspect of the party was to have a champagne "cork popping" contest. Unexpected and funny prizes were awarded to individuals whose popped cork flew the furthest or the shortest distance down the hallway of the Research Building. Names for a gift exchange were also chosen prior to the party. Gag gifts were sometimes given such as a pair of underwear to Dr. Lockey, from Dr. Fox, with the inscription "GO Michigan" on the back. The party brought everyone together for a wonderful celebration at the end of the year. The Division's staff and faculty were always extraordinarily close in their social and professional activities, something dearly lacking in this more "politically correct" day and age.

In 2015, the Division was relocated on the VA campus to the second floor of a manufactured two-story building, Building 41, or commonly referred to as the "HR Building". Division parties have since been held at the Division's Clinical Research Unit on the fifth floor at 13801 Bruce B. Downs Blvd. Parties have become smaller but still maintain the personable and entertaining atmosphere of the previous location.

Core Faculty
Division of Allergy and Immunology (Department of Internal Medicine)

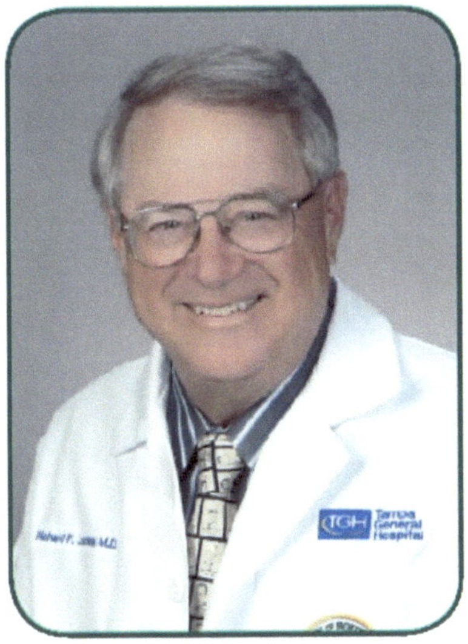

Richard F. Lockey, MD, MS
(1973-present)
Distinguished University Health Professor
Professor of Medicine, Pediatrics, & Public Health
Director, Division of Allergy and Immunology
Joy McCann Culverhouse Chair in Allergy and Immunology

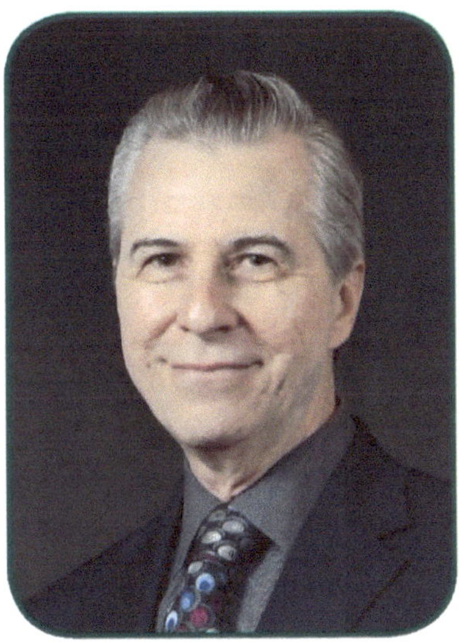

Thomas B. Casale, MD
(2013-present)
Professor of Medicine & Pediatrics

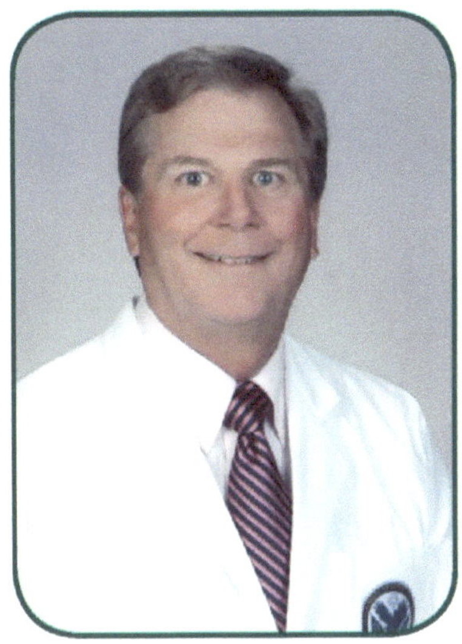

Roger W. Fox, MD
(1980-present)
Professor of Medicine, Pediatrics,
& Public Health

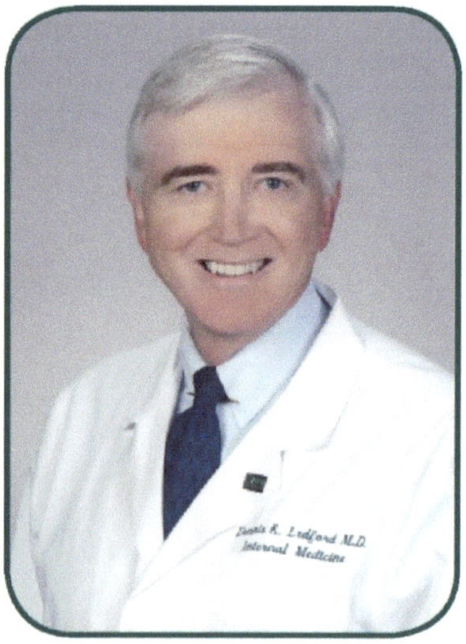

Dennis K. Ledford, MD
(1985-present)
Professor of Medicine & Pediatrics
Mabel & Ellsworth Simmons Professor
of Allergy and Immunology

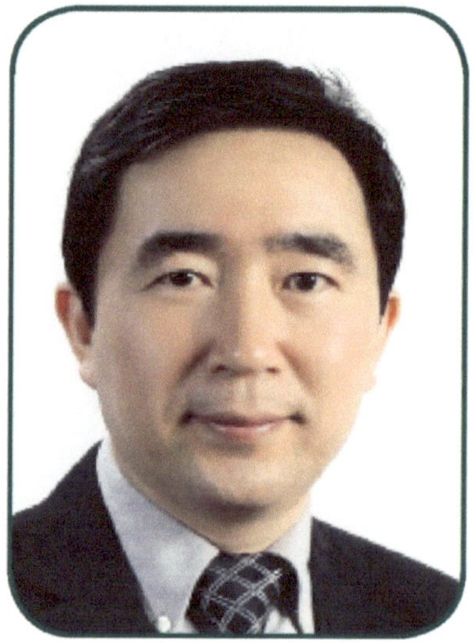

Seong Cho, MD
(2015-present)
Associate Professor of Medicine &
Pediatrics

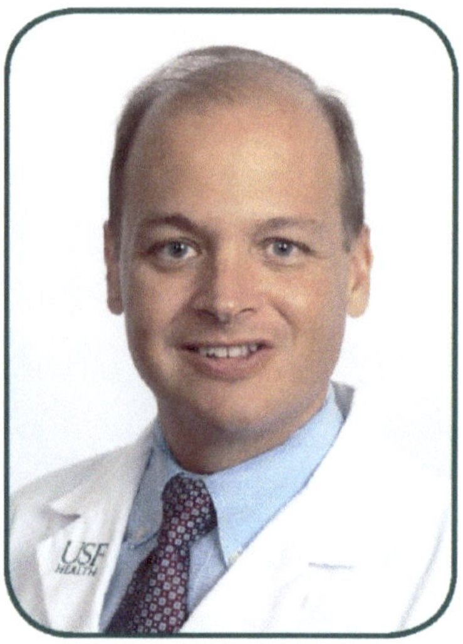

Mark C. Glaum, MD, PhD
(2004-present)
Associate Professor of Medicine & Pediatrics
Training Program Director

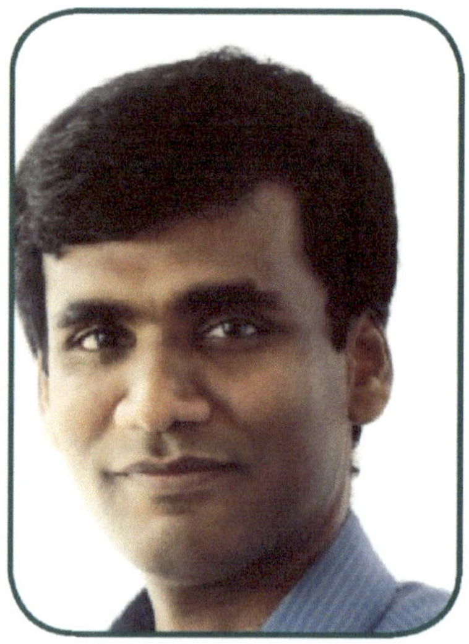

Narasaiah Kolliputi, PhD
(2010-present)
Associate Professor of Medicine, Molecular
Medicine, & Pediatrics

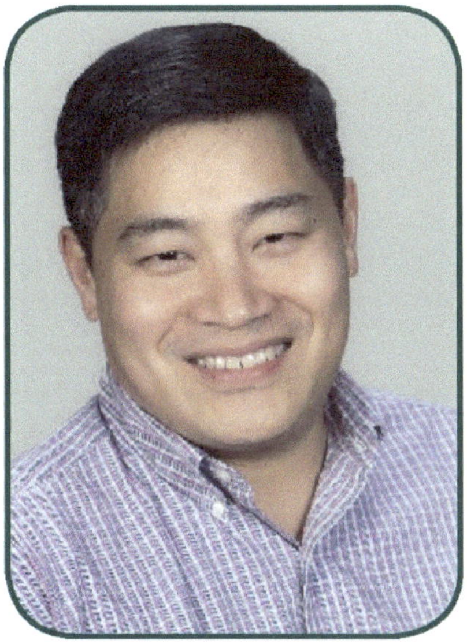

Michael Teng, PhD
(2010-present)
Associate Professor of Medicine, Pediatrics, Molecular Medicine, & Pharmaceutical Sciences

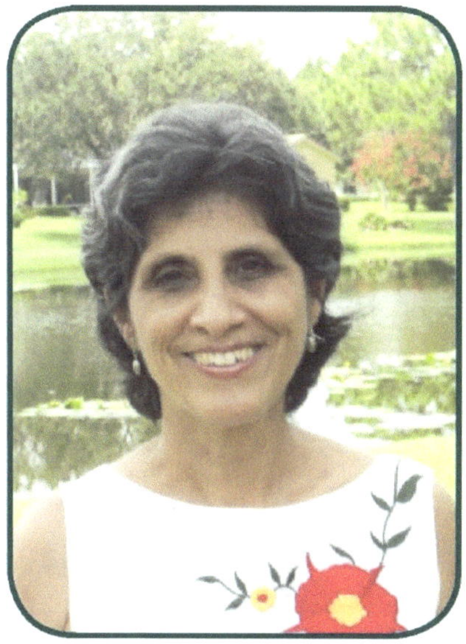

Blanca Camoretti-Mercado, PhD
(2012-present)
Assistant Professor of Medicine & Pediatrics

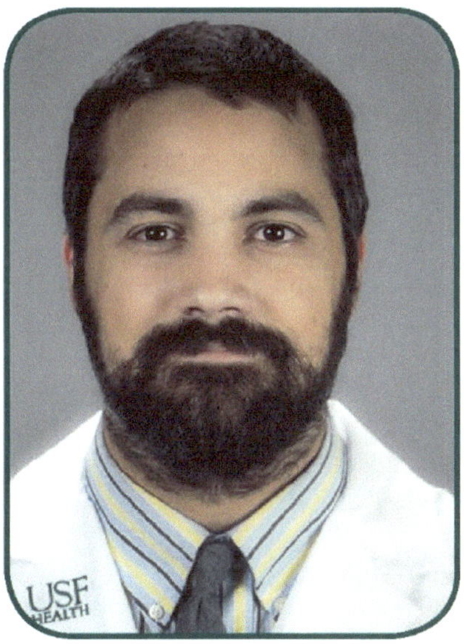

Juan Carlos Cardet, MD, MPH
(2017-present)
Assistant Professor of Medicine & Pediatrics

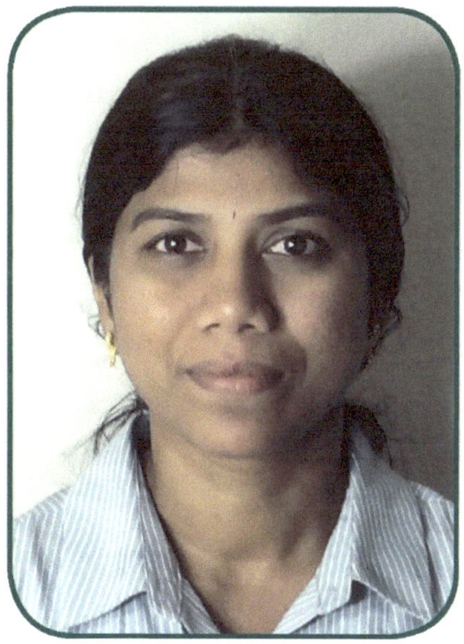

Lakshmi Galam, PhD
(2016-present)
Assistant Professor of Medicine

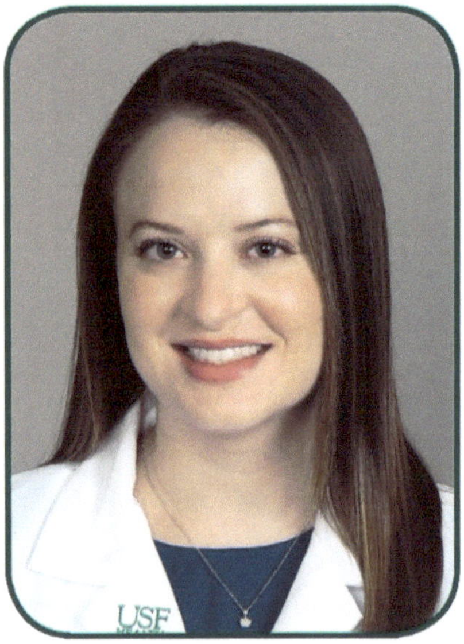

Amber Pepper, MD
(2018-present)
Assistant Professor of Medicine & Pediatrics

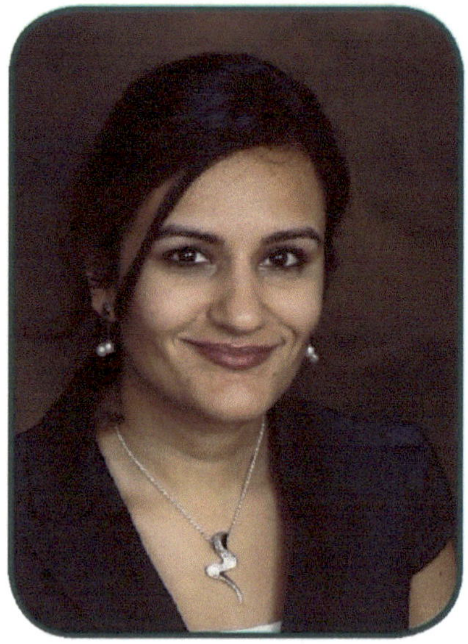

Farnaz Tabatabaian, MD
(2015-present)
Assistant Professor of Medicine & Pediatrics

Joint Faculty

Jolan Walter, MD, PhD
(2016-present)
Robert A. Good Endowed Chair in Immunology
Associate Professor of Pediatrics & Medicine
Chief, Pediatric Division of Allergy and Immunology

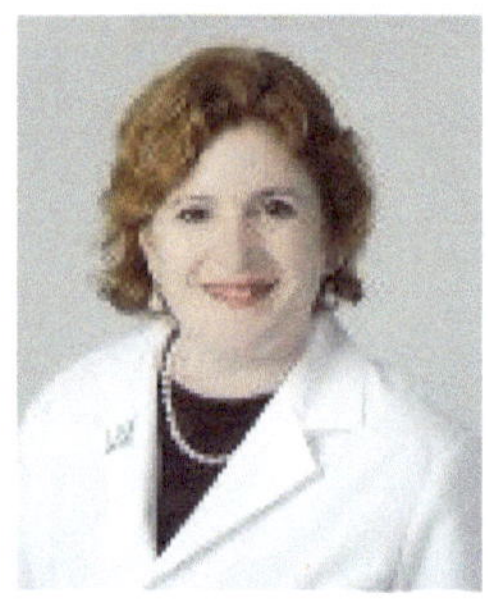

Mark Ballow, MD
(2013-present)
Professor of Pediatrics & Medicine

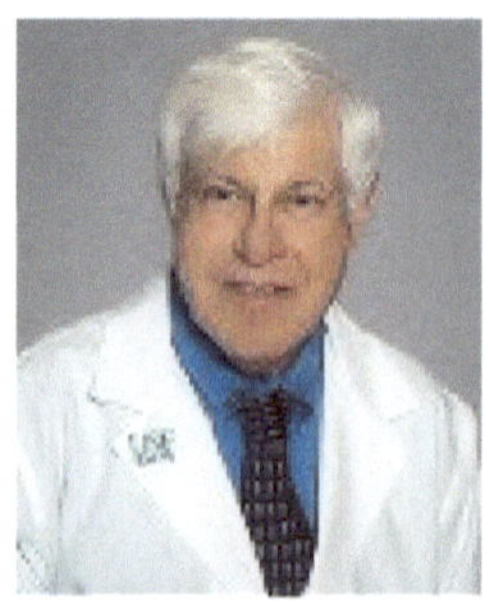

Mandel Sher, MD
(1985-present)
Professor of Pediatrics & Medicine

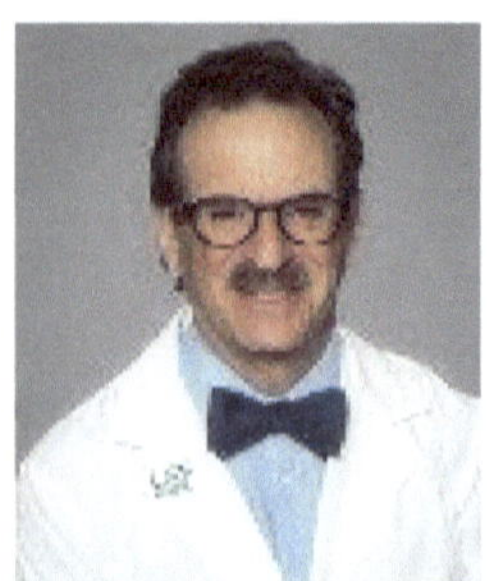

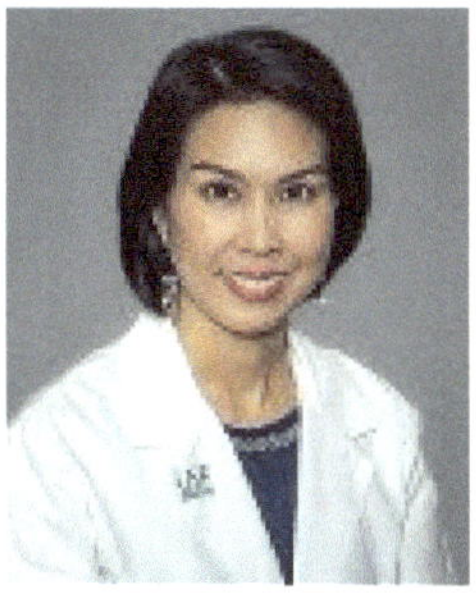

Panida Sriaroon, MD
(2009-present)
Associate Professor of Pediatrics & Medicine

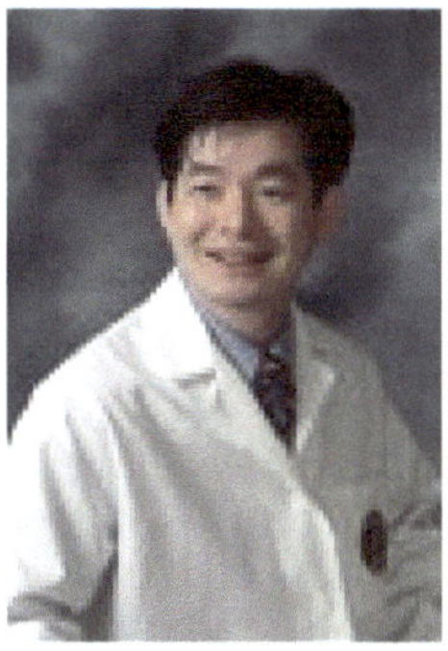

Nathan Tang, MD
(2000-present)
Associate Professor of Pediatrics & Medicine

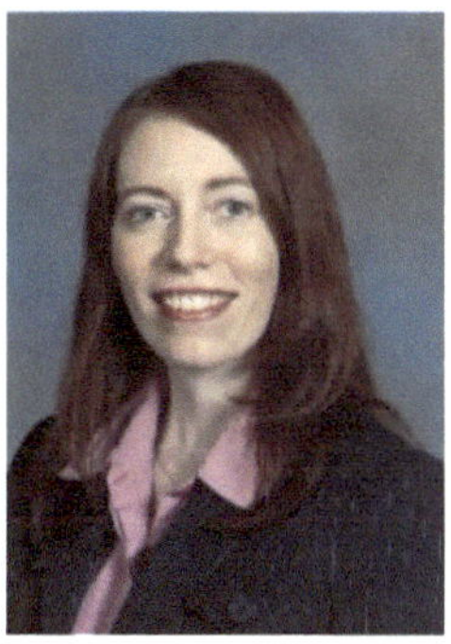

Emma Westermann-Clark, MD
(2019-present)
Assistant Professor of Pediatrics & Medicine

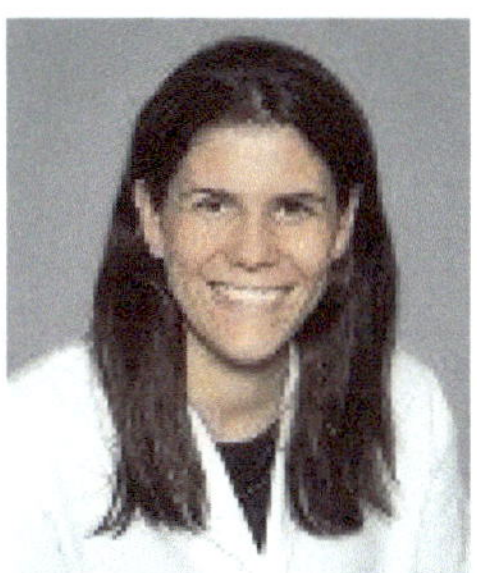

Jennifer Leiding, MD
(2012-present)
Associate Professor of Pediatrics & Medicine

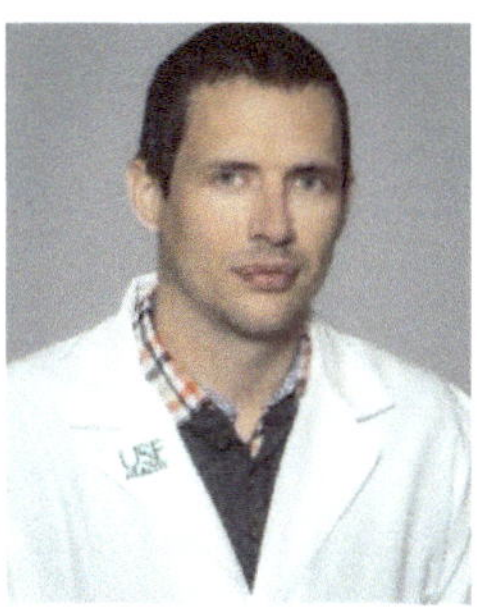

Krisztian Csomos, PhD
(2018-present)
Research Associate

Affiliate Faculty
Division of Allergy and Immunology, Department of Internal Medicine

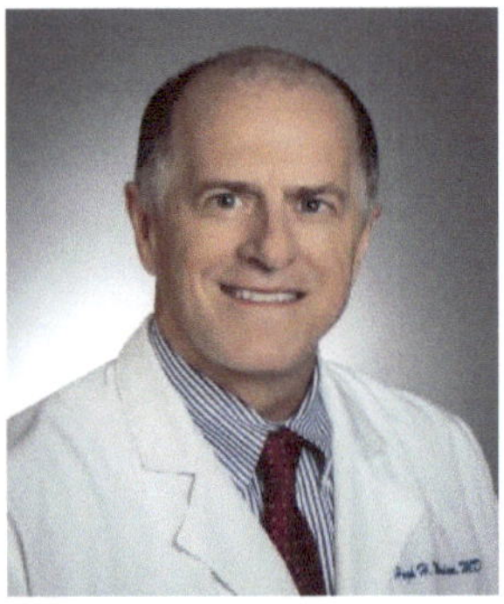

Hugh H. Windom, MD
(1992-present)
Clinical Professor of Medicine

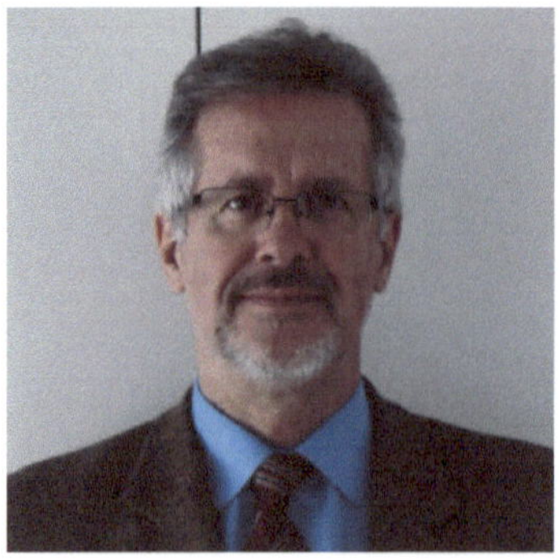

Enrique Fernandez-Caldas, PhD
(2010-present)
Clinical Professor of Medicine
Associate Professor of Medicine (1986-1995)

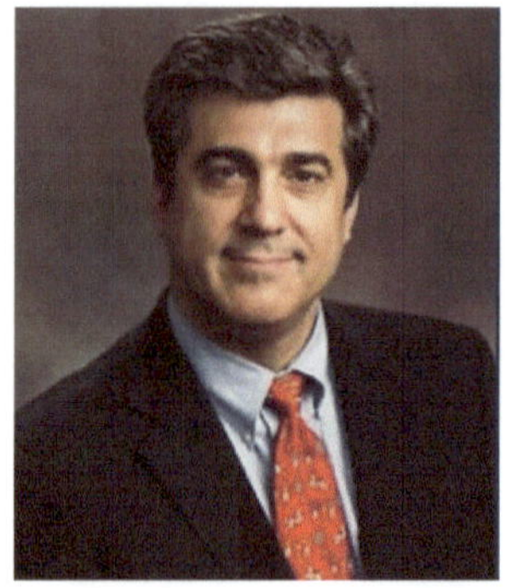

Donald C. Lanza, MD
(2016-present)
Clinical Professor of Medicine

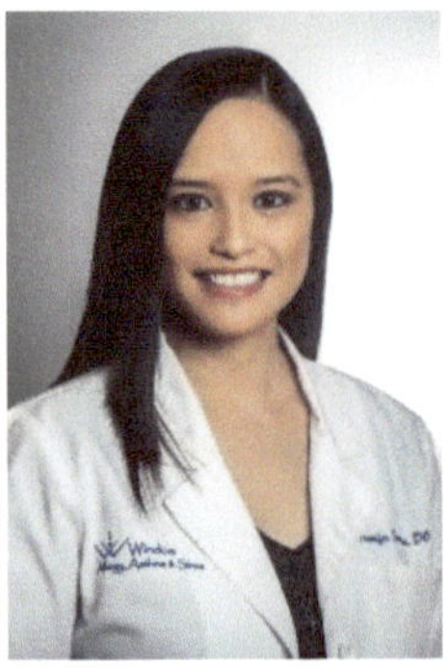

Jennifer Fergeson, DO
(2016-present)
Clinical Assistant
Professor of Medicine

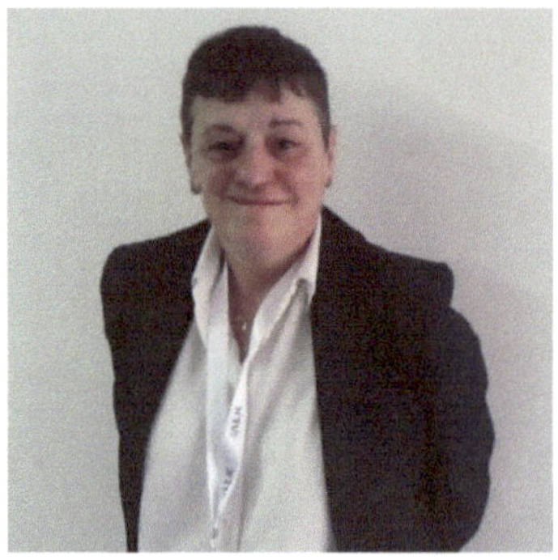

Rosa Codina, PhD
(2003-present)
Clinical Associate Professor of Medicine
Assistant Professor of Medicine (2000-2002)
Instructor of Medicine (1999-2000)
Assistant of Medicine (1996-1999)
Research Assistant (1994-1996)

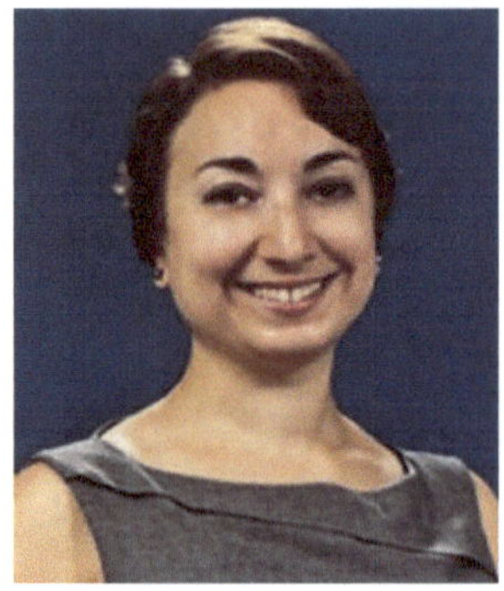

Alla Solyar, MD
(2016-present)
Clinical Assistant
Professor of Medicine

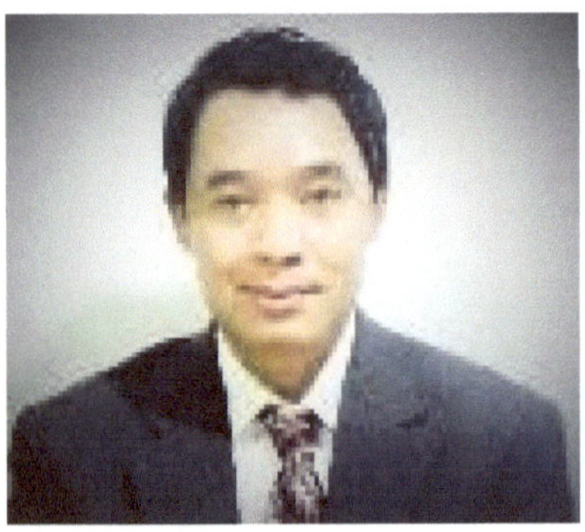

Jia-Wang Wang, PhD
(2016-present)
Clinical Assistant
Professor of Medicine
Assistant Professor of
Medicine (2013-2016)

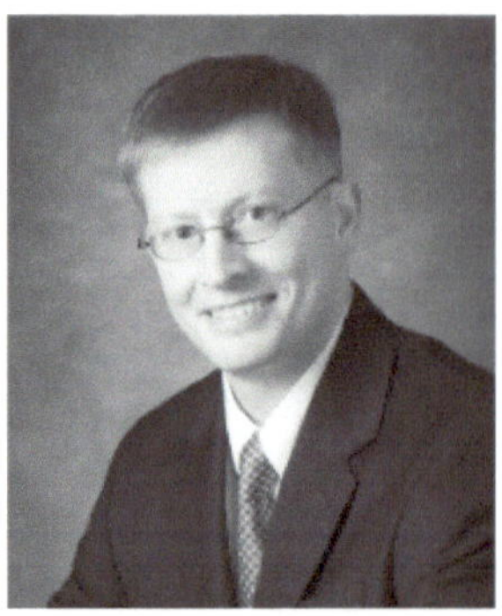

Thomas L. Johnson II, MD
(2015-present)
Clinical Assistant Professor of
Medicine

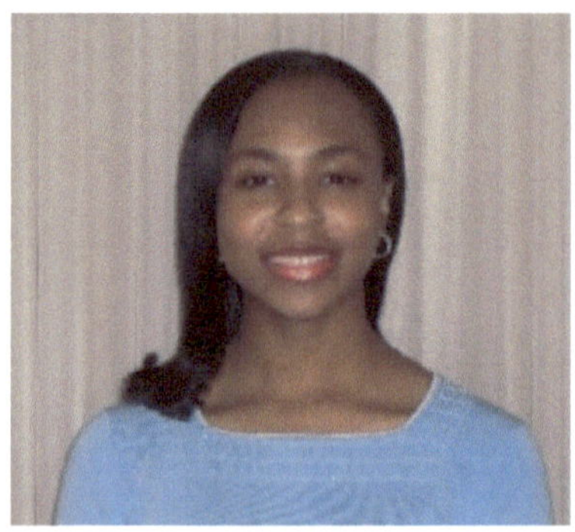

Andrea Nicole McCray, PhD
(2015-present)
Clinical Assistant Professor of
Medicine

Pediatrics

The USF Tampa Division of Allergy and Immunology is under the auspices of the Department of Internal Medicine. The Division has a close affiliation with the USF Department of Pediatrics, Division of Allergy and Immunology, founded in 1987 and first chaired by Robert A. Good, MD, PhD, DSc. Dr. Good was a world-renowned transplant pioneer and performed the first successful human bone marrow transplantation. He is regarded as the founder of modern immunology. Dr. Good's wife, Noorbibi Day-Good, PhD, a recognized expert in complement and complement deficiencies, joined the Pediatric Division with Dr. Good. The program is located in St. Petersburg at Johns Hopkins All Children's Hospital. Dr. Good dignified the March 19, 1973 cover of *Time Magazine* which also included the scholarly article "Toward Control of Cancer", reviewing Dr. Good's pioneering cancer research. Both programs are accredited to train board-eligible allergists/immunologists. In 2002, John Sleasman, MD, from the University of Florida, assumed Dr. Good's position where he was chair of the Pediatric Division from 2002 to 2013. Dr. Sleasman thereafter assumed a position at Duke University where he currently chairs the Pediatric Division of Allergy and Immunology. In 2016, Jolan Walter, MD, PhD, assumed the position of chief of the Pediatric Division and the Robert A. Good, MD, PhD, DSc Chair. Dr. Walter is an international expert in primary immunodeficiencies and immune dysregulation. Her research interest is to better understand diseases associated with the under- and overactive immune system. Dr. Walter and the Division are dedicated to the delivery and ongoing development of interdisciplinary clinical care, research, and educating future physicians in the specialty.

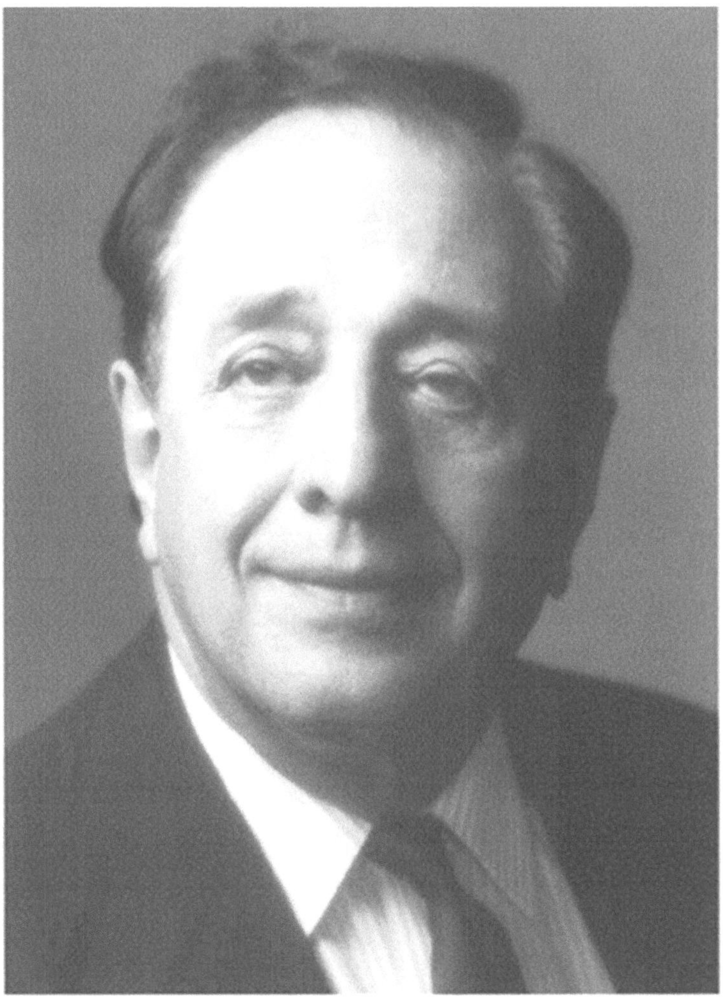

A Tribute to Robert A. Good, MD, PhD, DSc

May 21, 1922 – June 13, 2003

By Richard F. Lockey, MD, MS

Robert A. Good, MD, PhD, DSc, the father of modern clinical immunology, passed away on June 13, 2003. Dr. Good was a "compleat" physician (as in *The Compleat Angler,* 1653, by Issac Walton), inspiring academician and a renowned researcher. He began his work more than 50 years prior to his death. In 1944 he defined experimentally the immunologic function of the plasma cell as the antibody reproducing cell. His research achievements include discovery of the function of the thymus and definition of two distinct major cellular components of the immune system. He performed the first successful bone marrow transplant in the world in 1968 at the University of Minnesota. Everyone who associated with Dr. Good learned about "experiments of nature", and much of his work was designed to imitate what nature, by intent or default, has done.

In 1973, Dr. Good became President and Director of the Sloan-Kettering Institute for Cancer Research and Director of Research at Memorial Hospital in New York where he committed 10 years to these institutions. He developed the first bone marrow transplantation program at Memorial Hospital. The cover story of the March 19, 1973 edition of *TIME Magazine* honored Dr. Good and featured the article "Toward Control of Cancer." In 1982, he joined the Oklahoma Health Sciences Center as a member and the Head of the Cancer Research Program, Professor of Pediatrics, Research Professor of Medicine and Professor of Microbiology and Immunology. Dr. Good joined All Children's Hospital and the University of South Florida College of Medicine as Physician-in-Chief in 1985 and directed the Hospital's Division of Allergy and Immunology. He developed the Hospital's first Bone Marrow Transplantation Unit and clinical programs in pediatric allergy and immunology, pediatric rheumatology and pediatric HIV. In his 18 years of service to All Children's Hospital, Dr. Good and his research teams received millions of dollars in federal and private research grants. More than 300 physicians and scientists were trained or mentored over the past 50 years under his guidance, of which greater than 200 are now professors or department chairs at institutions throughout the world.

Dr. Good held the title of Distinguished University Professor of Pediatrics, Medical Microbiology and Immunology, and Medicine at the University of South Florida, College of Medicine. He also served as President of the St. Petersburg-based Children's Research Institute. Through the Eleanor Dana Charitable Trust, an endowed chair in pediatric immunology was created in honor of Dr. Good at the University and All Children's Hospital. His research included the influence of nutrition on longevity, immunity, health span and disease of aging, fundamental and practical aspects of bone marrow and stem cell transplantation, and other forms of cellular engineering. Dr. Good's work with immunology is only one aspect of his lifetime devotion to research. He received 13 honorary degrees from academic institutions throughout the world and over 100 awards. The latter included the Albert Lasker Clinical Medical Research Award, The Gairdner Foundation Award in 1970, and the Order of the Sacred Treasure Gold and Silver Star conferred by his Excellency the Emperor of Japan. Dr. Good was also a member of the National Academy of Sciences and Charter Member of the Institute of Medicine, National Academy of Sciences. He was President of many distinguished and learned societies including the American Association of Immunologists and American Society for Investigative Pathology (formerly The American Society for Investigative Pathology). He authored or coauthored more than 2,000 publications and wrote or edited 50 books.

Dr. Good's legacy lives on in his innovative research, the patients who live because of such research, and most importantly, in his trainees, colleagues, and collaborators. Several things stand out in my mind about Dr. Good: first, he was a scholar and a gentleman; second, he was one of the few individuals who truly understood the great spectrum of molecular biology, basic immunology, and clinical medicine and immunology; third, I will never forget all his wonderful summaries of conferences that I attended with him. I always told the students and the residents, if you listen to Dr. Good's summary, you will understand the nuts-and-bolts of what is the most important information presented during the conference.

When Dr. Good came to the University of South Florida and All Children's' Hospital in 1985, one of my colleagues asked how that would influence my stature at the University. I replied, "What do you do when God is gracing you with the presence of a world-renowned genius? I will do whatever he asks me to do". Our relationship was one of mutual admiration, collaboration, collegiality and friendship. He was a great friend and I truly miss him.

Dr. Robert Good's inspirational guidance and contributions can be found at the University of South Florida and the many Universities and conferences at which he spoke and received distinguished honorary degrees and worked. It is living in the innumerable children and adults who are alive because of his research and all those whom he taught, influenced and those who continue the quest to cure primary and secondary immunodeficiency diseases.

I would be extremely laxed if I also did not mention my good friend, Dr. Noorbibi Day-Good, Bob's wife. Dr. Day-Good was an outstanding renowned scientist in her own right, especially in complement and immunodeficiency diseases. Behind every great woman is a great man. That was Robert Good. Behind every great man is a great woman. That was Bibi Day. Bibi served in many ways as the gray eminence for my dear friend and colleague as he grew older. Bibi is appreciated for all of her great accomplishments and all that she did for medicine and as Bob's loving wife and friend. Regrettably, Noorbibi K. Day-Good, PhD, passed away on December 16, 2018. They are survived by Dr. Good's five children, Dr. Day's two children, and 17 grandchildren.

Dr. Bob Good was born on May 21, 1922, in Crosby, Minnesota. He vowed to become a doctor at age six when his father died of cancer. He attended the University of Minnesota, overcoming a polio-like disease in his junior year, and continued his career at the University's Medical School. He received his bachelor's degree in 1944, MB in 1946, and was awarded his PhD and MD in 1947, the first time the University awarded dual degrees in a single ceremony.

Dr. Good was a true intellectual giant who influenced and led the field of clinical immunology into the 21st century. He was an inspiration to all of us who worked with him and is missed by all of us.

The Robert A. Good Honor Society (RGHS) was introduced by the University of South Florida Morsani College of Medicine April 19, 2017, as an initiative to recognize medical students, faculty and alumni who have been notably successful in scholarly endeavors. The following is a link which provides more information about the Society: https://health.usf.edu/medicine/mdprogram/ rise/rghs.

The Robert A. Good Endowed Lecture Series was established in October 2000 to support a lecture series in immunology in Dr. Good 's honor. The Lecture Series has been used to support attendance at the Federation of Clinical Immunology Societies (FOCIS) Annual Meeting and in 2020 a plenary session entitled: "Cell and Gene Therapy", at the San Francisco meeting, October 28 – 31, 2020. It is anticipated that the Robert A. Good Endowed Lecture Series will also support the 2021 annual meeting in a similar manner.

Pictured below is Robert A. Good, MD, PhD, DSc and his wife, Noorbibi Day, PhD, circa 2002, at the Annual Division of Allergy and Immunology, Department of Internal Medicine, Christmas/Holiday party. Both Drs. Day and Good were world renowned experts in their respective areas of academic medicine, and both were members of the Division of Allergy and Immunology, Departments of Pediatrics & Internal Medicine, for over twenty years.

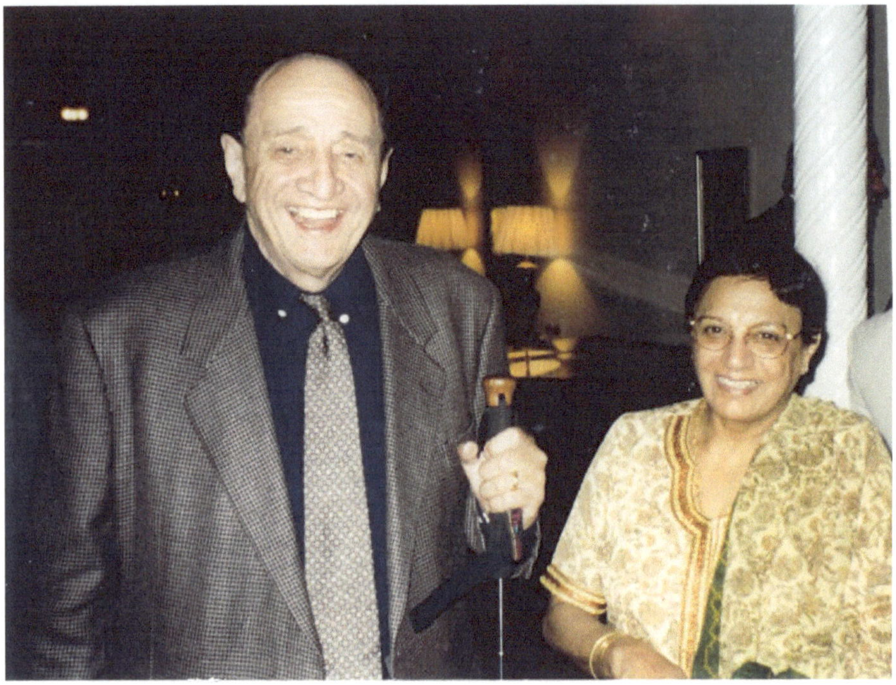

Robert A. Good, MD, PhD, DSc and Noorbibi Day, PhD

Comments from Jolan Walter, MD, PhD

Dr. Robert A. Good is regarded as the founder of modern immunology. His career started in his home state, Minnesota, where he published several seminal papers in the field of clinical immunology. In 1962, he documented the importance of the thymus gland, the role of which was elusive at that time. In 1965, along with Max D. Cooper, MD, he published the first paper describing the thymus and bursal lymphoid system in chicken in the journal *Nature*. This work served as a foundation for distinguishing the development sites of the adaptive immune system (T and B cells). In 1968, Dr. Good performed the first successful human bone marrow transplant between persons who were not identical twins. The recipient was a 4-month-old boy from a family where 11 children had died secondary to severe combined immunodeficiency.

Dr. Good aspired to cure cancer by understanding the immune system. In 1972 he moved to NYC and became resident of the Sloan-Kettering Institute for Cancer Research and by 1973, he was on the cover of *TIME Magazine* with the heading: "Toward control of CANCER". His work on immune therapy for cancer, entitled "Conquest of Cancer Program", was part of the War on Cancer endorsed by President Nixon. His continued research on the human immune system has resulted with 2,136 papers 1945-2005 (60 years) along with numerous awards including the Albert Lasker Award for Clinical Medical Research. Later in his career in 1985, he was invited by Dr. Andor Szentivanyi, Dean at USF and an internationally known asthma researcher, to join the USF faculty.

Dr. Good became the Physician-in-Chief at the All Children's Hospital in St. Petersburg, Florida and was an active leader in the Department of Pediatrics at the USF Morsani College of Medicine. He placed Florida and USF on the map in the rapidly evolving translational science of immunology. Quoting his wife, Professor Bibi Day: "Dr. Good saw the best in people, empowered them, and stimulated them to give their best and gave credit where it was due. He was a magnificent and indefatigable professor, scientist, mentor, role model, humanitarian and friend and he is sorely missed, but not forgotten."

Jolan Walter, MD, PhD
Robert A. Good Endowed Chair in Immunology
Associate Professor of Pediatrics and Medicine
Chief, Pediatric Allergy and Immunology
Department of Pediatrics
University of South Florida
Morsani College of Medicine

Allergy/Immunology Pediatric Fellows

Ragab Salem Aoun, MD	1986 – 1988
Lionel Bonini, MD	1986 – 1988
Harumi Jyonouchi, MD	1987 – 1989
Ranjith M. Shetty, MD	1988 – 1990
Michael McCann, MD	1988 – 1990
Krishna Urval, MD	1988 – 1990
Roberto DiNicolo, MD	1989 – 1991
Shivasundara Krishna, MD	1989 – 1991
Harry Lee, MD	1989 – 1991
Cleveland Moore, MD	1990 – 1992
Samuel Gubernick, DO	1991 – 1993
Craig Kalik, MD	1991 – 1993
Maria Teresa de la Morena, MD	1991 – 1995
Jose Carro, MD	1990 – 1992
Sai Karlapudi, MD	1990 – 1992
Jeanette Warner, MD	1992 – 1994
Maria Macias, MD	1992 – 1994
Jocelyn Celestin, MD	1993 – 1994
Maria Olivero, MD	1993 – 1995
Angelos Koutsonikolis, MD	1993 – 1996
Margaret Kelleher, MD	1994 – 1995
Jamie Kratz, MD	1992 – 1994
Bernard Zeffren, MD	1994 – 1996
Ramarathinam Nagarajan, MD	1994 – 1996
Emerita Brigino-Buenaventura, MD	1994 – 1997
Duygu Uckan, MD	1994 – 1997
Maria J. Pochcial, MD	1995 – 1997
John Duplantier, MD	1995 – 1997
Jada L. Armstrong, MD	1995 – 1997
Shafqat Sayeed, MD	1996 – 1998
Nathan Tang, MD	1996 – 1999
Chris Christodoulou, MD	1997 – 1999
Latha Chamarthy, MD	1997 – 1999
Shahid Iqbal, MD	1997 – 2000
Belen Tan, MD	1998 – 2000
Voravich Luangwedchakarn, MD	1998 – 2001
Stuart White, MD	1998 – 2001
Suwannee Uthaisangsook, MD	1999 – 2000
Dave Provencher, MD	1999 – 2001
Roberto Rivera, MD	1999 – 2001
Roselyn M. Hicks, MD	2000 – 2002
Hyder Ali Khan, MD	2000 – 2002
Michael J. Palumbo, MD	2001 – 2003
Diana P. Jerez-Martin, MD	2001 – 2003
Rajivi Pothiraj Rucker, MD	2001 – 2004
Dawn M. Zacharias, MD	2002 – 2004
Dareen Siri, MD	2003 – 2005
Albert S. Hartel, MD	2004 – 2006
Richard F. Lavi, MD	2004 – 2006
Madhurima Sanka, DO	2005 – 2007
Adriana S. McCubbin, MD	2005 – 2007
Panida Sriaroon, MD	2006 – 2009
Jason Caldwell, DO	2007 – 2009
Loren Isakson, MD	2008 – 2010
Woei Yeang Gary Eng, MD	2008 – 2010
Maliena Longley, MD	2009 – 2011
Doanh Nguyen, MD	2010 – 2012
Araceli Elizalde, MD	2010 – 2012
Jean Marie Brown Ly, MD	2011 – 2013
Hava Tillipman Ladinsky, MD	2011 – 2013
Hana Niebur, MD	2012 – 2014
Farnaz Tabatabaian, MD	2013 – 2015
Catherine Kubiak, MD	2013 – 2015
Sheila Bina, MD	2014 – 2016
Jenni Yoon, MD	2014 – 2016
Bhumika Patel, MD	2015 – 2017
Johana Castro-Wagner, MD	2015 – 2017
Sonia Joychan, MD	2016 – 2018
David Lindsay, MD	2016 – 2018
Warit Jithpratuck, MD	2017 – 2019
Fatima Khan, MD	2017 – 2019
Jacqueline Squire, MD	2018 – 2020
Irina Dawson, MD	2018 – 2020
Maria Chitty-Lopez, MD	2019 – 2021
Mary Ann Miranda, MD	2020 – 2022
Priyank Timothy, MD	2020 – 2022

Former Core, Joint, and Affiliate Faculty, Researchers, Students, Research Scholars, and Office Personnel

The Division has been privileged to include on the faculty physicians, researchers, and academicians who have had core, joint, or affiliate appointments in the Division and have relocated, retired, are solely practicing clinical medicine, or have accepted appointments at other universities.

Former Core Faculty

- Samuel C. Bukantz, MD†; Professor Emeritus; Professor of Medicine and Medical Microbiology
- Gerald A. Bucholtz, MD; Assistant Professor of Medicine and Pediatrics
- Rosa Codina, PhD; Assistant Professor of Medicine
- Rama Ganguly, PhD, MPH; Professor of Medicine
- Prasanna Kumar Jena, PhD; Research Assistant Professor of Medicine
- Arun Kumar, PhD; Research Assistant Professor of Medicine
- Shyam S. Mohapatra, PhD; Professor of Medicine and Pediatrics
- Subhra Mohapatra, PhD; Associate Professor of Medicine
- Srinivas Nagaraj, PhD; Research Assistant Professor of Medicine
- Robert P. Nelson, MD; Associate Professor of Medicine and Pediatrics
- Saber Samaan, PhD; Assistant Professor of Medicine
- R. Lawrence Siegel, MD, PhD; Assistant Professor of Medicine
- John J. Stablein, MD†; Assistant Professor of Medicine
- Homero San Juan Vergara, MD, PhD; Research Assistant Professor of Medicine
- Jia-Wang Wang, PhD; Assistant Professor of Medicine
- Weidong (Wilson) Xu, PhD; Research Assistant Professor of Medicine
- Weidong Zhang, MD, PhD; Research Assistant Professor of Medicine

† Deceased

Former Joint Faculty

- Sami L. Bahna, MD, Dr. PH; Professor of Pediatrics and Medicine
- Stuart M. Brooks, MD; Professor of Public Health and Medicine
- Latha M. Chamarthy, MD, Associate Professor of Pediatrics and Medicine
- My Lien Dao, PhD; Associate Professor of Biology and Medicine
- Noorbibi Day, PhD† Professor of Pediatrics and Medicine
- Morna Dorsey, MD, MMSc; Assistant Professor of Pediatrics and Medicine
- Sandra G. Gompf, MD; Assistant Professor of Medicine
- Robert A. Good, MD, DSc†; Professor of Pediatrics and Medicine
- Samuel Gubernick, DO; Assistant Professor of Pediatrics and Medicine
- John W. Hadden, MD, Professor of Medicine; Division of Immunopharmacology
- Soichi Haraguchi, PhD; Assistant Professor of Pediatrics and Medicine
- Martin R. Klemperer, MD†; Professor of Pediatrics and Medicine
- Stephen Kornfeld, MD; Associate Professor of Pediatrics and Medicine
- Gary W. Litman, PhD; Hines Professor of Pediatrics and Medicine
- Michael Nieder, MD; Affiliate Associate Professor of Pediatrics and Medicine; Director, Blood and Marrow Transplant Program

- Robert Nickeson Jr., MD; Assistant Professor of Pediatrics and Medicine
- Elena E. Perez, MD, PhD; Assistant Professor of Pediatrics and Medicine
- Aleksandra Petrovic, MD; Affiliate Assistant Professor of Pediatrics and Medicine
- Mitchel J. Seleznick, MD; Associate Professor of Medicine, Division of General Internal Medicine
- Lawrence Siegel, MD, PhD, Assistant Professor of Pediatrics and Medicine
- John W. Sleasman, MD; Professor of Pediatrics and Medicine; Robert A. Good Professor of Immunology; Chief, Division of Allergy and Immunology
- Andor Szentivanyi, MD, DSc†; University Distinguished Professor of Medicine and Pharmacology

† Deceased

Former Affiliate Faculty

- Michel Alkhalil, MD; Clinical Assistant Professor of Medicine
- Phillip W. Devoe, MD; Clinical Assistant Professor of Medicine
- Elliot Ellis, MD†; Clinical Professor of Medicine
- Lawrence A. Holfelder, MD; Clinical Assistant Professor of Medicine
- Mary L. Jelks, MD†, Clinical Assistant Professor of Medicine
- Dennis Kim, MD; Clinical Assistant Professor of Medicine
- Monroe J. King, DO; Clinical Associate Professor of Medicine
- German F. LeParc, MD; Clinical Professor of Medicine
- Ronald Purcell, MD, Clinical Assistant Professor of Medicine
- Brett E. Stanaland, MD, Clinical Professor of Medicine
- Mark R. Stein, MD; Clinical Associate Professor of Medicine
- G. Edward Stewart II, MD, Clinical Professor of Medicine
- Glenn Whelan, PharmD; Clinical Assistant Professor of Medicine
- Robert E. Windom, MD†, Clinical Professor of Medicine

† Deceased

Former Research Staff

- Mahesh Kumar Abbengula, MS, MD
- Matthew D. Alleyn, BS
- Irene Baird-Warren
- Donnie Banerji, MD
- Aruna Behera, PhD
- Linda Bergen-Losee, MS
- Lolita R.F. Binford
- Sandhya Boyapalle, PhD
- Mason T. Breitzig, BS
- Eduardo Calderon, MD
- Marcia Cubillos, BS
- Mahasweta Das, PhD
- Runa Diwadkar
- Cayla Fezzie, BS, MS
- Jutaro Fukumoto, MD, PhD
- Lakshmi Galam, PhD
- Julio Garay, PhD
- Gary Hellermann Sr, PhD
- Cristina Jaen, BS
- Battula Kiran, PhD
- Xiaoyuan (Sonya) Kong, MD
- Nicole Kuderer
- Mukesh Kumar, PhD
- Kunyu Li
- Guoqing Liu, PhD
- Silvia Montalvo
- Allison Nelson
- Sonali Nimal
- S.J. Park
- Juan Carlos Pena
- Jian Qin, PhD
- Saniya Rangooni, MS,

- Sowndharya Ravi, MD, MPhil
- Michelle Reiser, MS
- Eileen Rifkin
- Debbie Serbousek, BS
- Hassan Syed, MD
- Walter Trudeau III, MS†
- Jia-Wang Wang, PhD
- Weidong Xu, PhD
- Weidong Zhang, MD

† Deceased

Former Students and Research Scholars

- Sadahiro Asai, MD (Japanese Postgraduate Fellow); November, 1979 - October, 1981.
- Yuji Sakamoto, MD (Japanese Postgraduate Fellow); November, 1982 - September, 1984.
- Terufumi Shimoda, MD (Japanese Postgraduate Fellow); July, 1985 - November, 1986.
- Takashi Watanabe, MD (Japanese Postgraduate Fellow); November, 1986 - July, 1988.
- David Aronoff (USF Medical Student); 1988 Summer Fellowship, American Academy of Allergy & Immunology.
- Eduardo G. Calderon, MD (Visiting Resident & Research Scholar); August, 1988 - August, 1989
- Gustavo Cuadros, MS, (Master in Biology and Research Specialist); September, 1988 - November, 1988
- Eduardo Alonso Garcia-Ramos, MD (Research Scholar); January 10, 1990 - December 20, 1990
- Mohammed Askar, MD (Research Scholar); February, 1990 - February, 1992
- Dong Keun Lee, MD (Research Scholar); March 3, 1991 - February, 1992.
- Rafael Jinete, MD (Research Scholar), August 22, 1991 - December 1, 1991.
- Khalid Ali, MD (Research Scholar); 1991.
- Ingrid and Eduardo Lima, MDs (Research Scholars); January 1993 - March 1993
- Leonardo Puerta, MS (Research Scholar, PhD Candidate); University of Cartagena, 1993 - 1995.
- Rosa Codina, PhD (Post-Graduate Biologist); September, 1994 - March, 1997.
- Zhaoming Wen, MD (Research Scholar); August, 1994 - November, 1994
- Carina Gabriela Uasuf, MD (Research Scholar); February, 1995 - April, 1995.
- Adriana Rodriguez Ciodaro, MS (Research Scholar); April, 1995 - May, 1995
- Albert Oehling, MD, (Research Scholar); February, 1996 – December, 1996
- Isabel Ojeda Fernandez, MD, (Research Scholar); April, 1996 - May, 1996
- Hiroto Matsuse, MD, (Research Scholar); May 1997 - May 1999
- Jianan Hu, MD (Research Scholar); 1999
- Jianan Zhang, MD (Research Scholar); 1999
- Cristina Jaen, MS, (Research Scholar); September 1998 - September 1999.
- Homero San Juan, MD, (Research Scholar); August 1999 – August 2004
- Szilvia Nagy, MD, PhD, (Research Scholar); 1999 - 2002
- Mukesh Kumar, PhD, (Research Scholar); December 1996 - June 2002
- Aruna Behera, PhD, (Research Scholar); February 1997 - June 2002
- Gary Hellermann, PhD (Research Scholar); 1999 – 2005
- Shawna Shirley (PhD Student); 2003 – 2008
- Elena Hernandez, MD (Research Scholar); October 2004 – January 2005
- Alison Jones (PhD Student); 2004 - 2008
- Weidong Zhang, MD (Research Associate); 2004 - 2005
- Arun Kumar, PhD (Research Associate); 2004 - 2005
- Bishwabhusan Sahoo (Research Associate); 2004 - 2005
- Dong-Keun Lee (Post-Doctoral Fellow); 2005 - 2006

- Weidong Xu (Research Scientist); 2005 - 2009
- Xiaoqin Wang (Graduate Student); 2005 - 2008
- Dongqing Chen, MD (Research Assistant); 2006
- Sang-Joon Park, MD (Research Scholar); 2006 - 2008
- Hongyu Zheng (Research); 2007 – 2008
- Murali Kanakanalli (Research); 2007 – 2008
- Leigh Nattkemper (Research); 2007 – 2008
- Brittany Caddick (Research); 2007 – 2008
- Wilson Xu, PhD (Postdoctoral Fellow); 2007 – 2008
- Liotta Dowdy (Undergraduate Student); 2007 – 2008
- Ruckmani Kandasamy, PhD (Research Scholar); 2007 - 2008
- Yvonne Davis (Graduate Student); 2007- 2013
- Terianne Wong (Graduate Student); 2009 - 2013
- Jordan Heft (Graduate Student); June, 2010 – December, 2011
- Michael Cheung (Graduate Student); 2010 – present
- Rhonda Wilbur (Graduate Student); 2010 – 2012
- Amos Ben Zvi, MD (Visiting Professor); September, 2012 – August, 2013
- Xinjian Xiaoyin, PhD (Research Scholar); 2010 – present
- Asfiya Yunus (Undergraduate Honor's Student); 2011
- Jamileh Ahmed (Master's Student); 2011
- Beth Coughlin (Research Assistant); 2011
- Tran (Graduate Student); 2011 - 2012
- Sara Garcia, (Undergraduate Honor's Student); 2011 - 2012
- Bao Huynh (Research Assistant/Student); 2011 - 2012
- Gurukumar Ramanathan, PhD (Postdoctoral Fellow); 2011 – 2012
- Kumar Praveen, PhD (Postdoctoral Fellow), 2011 – 2012
- Sam Jalali (Undergraduate Honor's Student); 2011 – 2012
- Venugopal Rajanbabu, PhD (Postdoctoral Fellow); 2011-2013
- Matthew Ho (Research Student); 2011 - 2014
- Amanda Hodgkins (Assistant/Student); 2011 - 2014
- Jutaro Fukumoto, PhD (Postdoctoral Fellow), May 2011 – 2015
- Ruan J. Cox (PhD Student); 2011 – 2015
- Jillian Whelan (Graduate Student); 2011 - 2015
- Osvaldo Martinez, (Master's Student); 2012
- Tucker Maute (Research Student); 2012
- Omar Qazi, (Medical Student); 2012-2013
- Salman Aljubran, MD (Postdoctoral Fellow); 2012-2013
- Troy Lane, (Master's Student); 2012 - 2014
- Anu Stephen (Research Student); 2012 - 2014
- Olivia Smith (Volunteer Research Student); 2012 - 2014
- Rebekah Cook (Volunteer Research Student); 2012 - 2014
- Karnisha Woolery, (PhD Student); May 2012 – 2015
- Oluwakemi Phillips, (Master's Student); 2012 – 2015
- Bangmei Wang (Volunteer Research Student); 2012 - 2015

- Prasanna Tamarapu Parthasarathy, (Master's Student); 2012 - 2016
- Dalgys Martínez, MSc (Research Scholar); October 2013 – December 2013
- Sayantani Bandyopadhyay (Master's Student); 2013 - 2015
- Adrien Marziale (Visiting Student); July 3, 2014 – August 28, 2014
- Venu Lagishetty, PhD (Postdoctoral Fellow); 2014 – 2015
- Emma Westermann-Clark, MD (Postdoctoral Fellow); 2014 – 2016
- Christina Turn, (Medical Student); 2014-2016
- Tara Saco, (Medical Student); 2014
- Grant Wallenfelsz (Research Student); 2014 - 2015
- A. Ra Jo, PhD (Postdoctoral Fellow); May 2015 - present
- Dae Woo Kim, MD, PhD (Visiting Research Scholar); 2015 – 2016
- John Canfield (Graduate Student); 2015
- Jianjin Chen, MD (Visiting Research Scholar); 2015
- Lashea Johnson (Research Student); 2015
- Michelle Kaminsky (Research Assistant/Student); 2014 - 2016
- Amy Wang (Volunteer Research Student); 2015
- Bangmei Wang (Volunteer Research Student); 2015
- Andrew Cooke, MD (Postdoctoral Fellow); 2015 - 2016
- Priyanshi Patel (Undergraduate Honor's Student); 2015 - 2016
- Nima Hosseinian (Undergraduate Honor's Student); 2015 - 2017
- Jeong Song (Visiting Student); July 18, 2016 – July 29, 2016
- Seo Hong (Visiting Student); July 18, 2016 – July 29, 2016
- Venkata Narla, PhD (Postdoctoral Fellow); 2016 - 2017
- Adeeb Bulkhi, MD (Postdoctoral Fellow); July 2016 – June 2017
- Jianjun Chen, MD (Visiting Research Scholar); October 2015 – September 2016.
- Wenjing Li, MD (Visiting Research Scholar); October, 2016 – September 2017
- Venkata R. Narala, PhD (Visiting Research Scholar); 2016 – 2017
- Pawel Bigos (Undergraduate Student); 2016
- Andrew McGill (Graduate Student); 2016 - 2017
- Bryann Tan (Undergraduate Student); 2016 - 2017
- Helena Hernández-Cuervo, (PhD Student); 2016 – 2018
- Luis Caraballo, MD, PhD (Visiting Research Scholar); 2017
- Isabelle Puppa (Undergraduate Student); 2017
- Sahebgowda Patil (Graduate Student); 2017
- Irene John (Undergraduate Student); 2017
- Sudarshan Krishnamurthy (Undergraduate Student); 2017 - 2018
- Sngri Ross (Undergraduate Student); 2017
- Smita Saji (Undergraduate Student); 2017
- Sriraja Srinivas (Undergraduate Student); 2017
- Michael Carroll (Medical Student); 2017-2018
- Sai Manasa Jandhyala (Volunteer Student); 2018
- Doo-Hee Han, MD, PhD (Visiting Research Scholar); March 2019 – February 2020
- Sun-Hee Choi, MD, PhD (Visiting Research Scholar); March 2019 – February 2020
- Kate Lee (Visiting Student); July 1, 2019 – July 12, 2019

- Yoo-Jin Kim (Visiting Student); July 1, 2019 – July 12, 2019

Former Office Staff

Tampa Office:

- Judy Bien
- Rebecca Carter-Muncey
- Karen Collins
- Deborah Martinez
- Rebecca McCrery (JMC Airway Disease Research Center)
- Stephanie Medley (JMC Airway Disease Research Center)
- Ginger Montuoro
- Sandra Rocha
- Patricia Walsh

Johns Hopkins All Children's Hospital:

- Amy Baldwin
- Linda Baxter
- Linda Callahan
- Marjorie Peak
- Tazim Verjee

Current Division Personnel

Research Associates:

Research Staff

- Matthew D. Alleyn, BS
- Jutaro Fukumoto, MD, PhD
- M. Helena Hernandez Cuervo, MD
- A. Ra Jo, PhD
- Hannah Lee, BS
- Ramani Soundararajan, PhD
- Kim-Li Teng, MS

Research Students

- Emily Chan
- Kevin Duan
- Sandy Hornung
- Muling Lin
- Smita Saji
- Sahebgowda Sidramagowda Patil

IMpact:

- Jennifer Newcomb, MS

Tampa USF Office:

- Geeta Gehi
- Peggy Hales
- Earle Trott

Johns Hopkins All Children's Hospital:

- Yolanda Alexander
- Daniela Sredkova

Division CME Conferences

What better place to hold annual conferences than Lake Buena Vista, located on the Disney property? The first Division allergy and immunology conference was held in December 1981 and was well-received by approximately 100 attendees. Division faculty and trainees presented a state-of-the-art conference to invited physicians and health professionals from throughout the country. Conference registration and check-in began on Thursday evening with the conference presentations taking place on Friday, Saturday, and Sunday mornings. This schedule allowed attendees to explore and enjoy Orlando and Disney attractions for the remainder of the day. For the majority of years, the conference was held at the lavish Buena Vista Palace before a postponement of the conference occurred.

One of the favorite conference events attended by Division faculty and spouses and Division staff, who were able to arrive at the hotel on Thursday evening, was a relaxing dinner held at one of the restaurants in the Buena Vista Palace. It was always a welcomed highlight for Founding Director, Samuel C. Bukantz, MD, and Richard F. Lockey, MD, MS, to be able to enjoy the company of the Division faculty and staff in this pleasant setting.

In 2014, the conference resumed but the venue was changed to the USF Health Center for Advanced Medical Learning and Simulation (CAMLS) in downtown Tampa. The format of the conference includes scholarly lectures and conversations between conference faculty and attendees on Friday morning and afternoon and Saturday in the morning. A state-of-the-art rhinoscopy course, under the direction of faculty member, Mark C. Glaum, MD, PhD, has become a focal point of the conference. The conference has been held several times in January on the weekend of the Gasparilla Children's Parade, allowing attendees and their families to attend and enjoy the festivities.

IMpact:

In 2017, Dr. Lockey's idea to initiate a USF Morsani College of Medicine website, which was to become a one-stop writing resource available to professionals at USF-affiliated institutions, became a reality. *IMpact* is designed as a writing resource for scientific abstracts, posters, literature reviews, research articles, case reports and book chapters. Physicians, healthcare professionals, and researchers can gain valuable insight to become successful authors of scientific literature from this resource. Materials and needed information to write and publish in the scientific literature are available in an easy to navigate centralized website. *IMpact's* faculty editorial board provide feedback on the quality, clarity of presentation, structure, language and content.

IMpact now serves USF Health Morsani College of Medicine, College of Nursing, College of Pharmacy, James A. Haley Veterans' Hospital, Johns Hopkins All Children's Hospital, Lehigh Valley Health Network, and Moffitt Cancer Center.

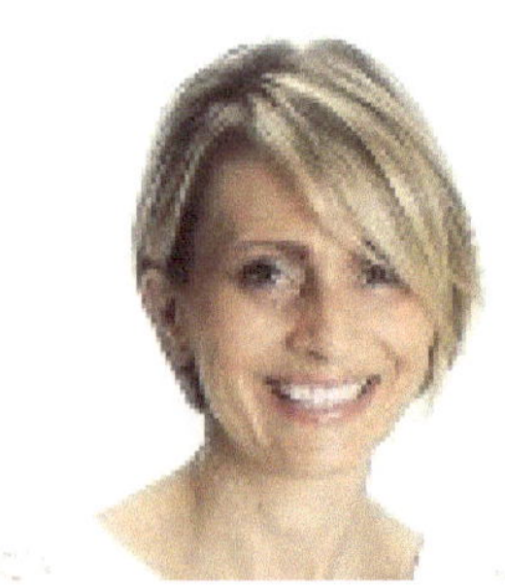

Jennifer Newcomb, MS
Managing Editor

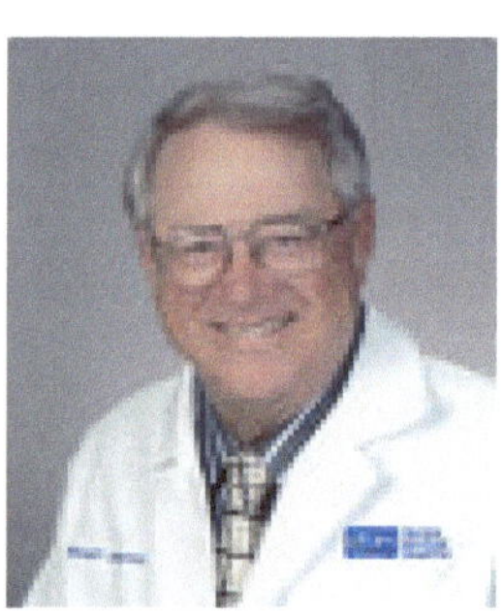

Richard F. Lockey, MD, MS
Editor-in-Chief

Biographical Sketches of Division of Allergy and Immunology, Department of Internal Medicine, Core Faculty

Richard F. Lockey, MD, MS

Professor Richard F. Lockey, MD, MS, received his BS degree from Haverford College, Haverford, Pennsylvania; M.D. from Temple University, Philadelphia, Pennsylvania (Alpha Omega Alpha); MS from the University of Michigan in Ann Arbor, Michigan, where he trained in Internal Medicine and Allergy/Immunology (A/I), and was a Major in the US Air Force and Chief of A/I at Carswell Air Force Base, Fort Worth, Texas, from 1970-1972. He is a Distinguished University Health Professor; the Joy McCann Culverhouse Chair of Allergy and Immunology; Professor of Medicine, Pediatrics and Public Health; and Director, Division of Allergy and Immunology, Department of Internal Medicine, University of South Florida Morsani College of Medicine.

In 2000, he received the Florida Academy of Sciences Medal for his dedication and work to improve the health and well-being of the community and citizens of Florida. The Dr. Robert D. and Alma W. Moreton Original Research Award from the Southern Medical Society was granted in 2012. The American Academy of Allergy Asthma and Immunology presented him with a Special Recognition Award in 1993, Distinguished Service Award in 1999, and Distinguished Clinician Award in 2008. The World Allergy Organization Gold Medal Award was presented to him in 2015, and the Boy Scouts of America Distinguished Eagle Scout Award, 2018.

He is the recipient of the Lifetime Achievement Award, Florida Allergy, Asthma & Immunology Society, July 9, 2011. In addition, in 2019 the American Academy of Allergy Asthma and Immunology Foundation established the 15-year Richard F. Lockey, MD, MS, FAAAAI & University of South Florida Lectureship and Faculty Development Award. Dr. Lockey became a member of the USF Chapter of the National Academy of Inventors (NAI) in 2020.

Professional honors include President of the American Academy of Allergy Asthma and Immunology (1992), past Director of the American Board of Allergy and Immunology (1993- 1998), and President of the World Allergy Organization (2010-2012). He has also served as co- editor or participant of two World Health Organization reports, the most important of which is the 1998-1999 WHO Position Paper – *Allergen Immunotherapy: Therapeutic Vaccines for Allergic Diseases*. He serves or has served on a variety of different journal editorial boards and was instrumental in democratizing the American Academy of Allergy Asthma and Immunology and the World Allergy Organization. Under his leadership, the Division of Allergy and Immunology, Department of Internal Medicine, was selected as a World Allergy Organization (WAO) Center of Excellence for the 2016- 2019 term.

He has the honor of authoring or co-authoring over 800 publications, has edited or co-edited 20 monographs and 19 books, and has lectured on numerous occasions both nationally and internationally. He is the co-editor, with Dennis K. Ledford, MD, of the 6th edition of *Allergens and Allergen Immunotherapy: Subcutaneous, Sublingual and Oral*, published in 2020 by the CRC Press/Taylor & Francis Group.

Over 100 physician specialists and 55 international post-graduate PhDs or MDs in basic and clinical research and medicine, many of whom have assumed leadership positions throughout the world, have been trained in the Division. The Division's staff consists of 7 clinicians, 4 basic scientists, and approximately 60 other healthcare professionals including physicians and support and laboratory personnel. Areas of expertise and research: insect allergy, allergen immunotherapy, asthma, inflammatory lung diseases, pulmonary fibrosis, co-morbid conditions of asthma, sleep apnea, food allergy, hereditary angioedema, atopic eczema, finding better ways to administer epinephrine, and idiopathic urticaria and angioedema.

Some of the contributions in the medical literature made by Dr. Lockey and colleagues include: the largest demographic skin test and immunotherapy study on Hymenoptera hypersensitivity; the refractory period in aspirin-exacerbated respiratory disease; the allergens responsible for imported fire ant hypersensitivity are contained in imported fire ant whole body extract; sentinel information on anaphylactic deaths secondary to allergen immunotherapy; why red tide toxin causes cough and exacerbations of asthma; the first national paper on ant hypersensitivity caused by various species of stinging ants; venom allergen immunotherapy to Hymenoptera insects is safe; intranasal oxymetazoline can be safely administered with concurrent inhalation of glucocorticosteroids; familial occurrence of aspirin exacerbated respiratory disease; Hymenoptera venoms are safe in pregnancy; neurologic sequelae from imported fire ant stings; major allergens which cause allergic diseases in Florida; *Blomia tropicalis* is an important allergen in Florida and South America; many different dust mites cause allergic disease; IgE levels are elevated in children with the human immunodeficiency virus (HIV); soy beans contain different allergens depending on the environmental exposure; unique allergens which cause anaphylaxis including benzocaine, ferret dander, food allergens contaminated with dust mites, the Tine test, and others. In addition, research about HIV infected subjects who develop various forms of arthritis and discoveries about interstitial pulmonary fibrosis, HIV disease, asthma, rhinitis, chronic rhinosinusitis, and COVID-19.

Thomas B. Casale, MD

Before joining USF in October 2013, as Professor of Medicine and Chief of Clinical and Translational Research, Dr. Thomas Casale was Professor of Medicine and Medical Microbiology and Immunology and Chief of Allergy and Immunology at Creighton University, Omaha, Nebraska. He did an allergy and immunology fellowship at the National Institutes of Health, Bethesda, MD, where he was chief medical staff fellow. From 1984 to 1996, he was at the University of Iowa where he attained the rank of Professor of Medicine and Director of Allergy and Immunology.

Dr. Casale is a member of the American Thoracic Society and served on their Board of Directors; American Society for Clinical Investigation; and a Fellow of the American College of Physicians and both the American College and American Academy of Allergy Asthma & Immunology. He is a Past President of the American Academy of Allergy Asthma & Immunology and was the Executive Vice President for ten years until 2018. He is a past member of the Board of Directors of the World Allergy Organization, served on the American Board of Allergy and Immunology and was Chair from 2005-2006, and now is the Chief Medical Advisor for Food Allergy Research and Education (FARE).

Dr. Casale is Director, Division of Allergy and Immunology, Department of Internal Medicine, Joy McCann Culverhouse Clinical Research Center. His clinical and basic research interests are directed toward the determination and treatment of the pathophysiologic mechanisms involved in respiratory and allergic diseases. He has published over 435 scientific papers, reviews and chapters on these topics. He is the principal investigator of USF's American Lung Association Airways Clinical Research Center. His research is funded by the National Institutes of Health, the American Lung Association, the Patient Centered Outcomes Research Institute, and various industry sources.

Roger W. Fox, MD

Roger Fox, MD FAAAAI, received his medical degree at St. Louis University School of Medicine. He completed three years of Internal Medicine and two years of Allergy and Immunology at the University of South Florida Morsani College of Medicine in Tampa, Florida. He is board certified in Internal Medicine and Pediatric and Adult Allergy and Immunology.

He has been elected to "The Best Doctors in America" for the past two decades and was involved in training over 100 physicians in the specialty. He was the USF Training Program Director for 20 years. He has published extensively and lectured locally, nationally, and internationally and served on various boards, including the Hillsborough County Medical Association, the Florida Allergy, Asthma & Immunology Society, of which he is a past-president, and numerous committees of the American Academy of Allergy Asthma & Immunology. He was elected to fellowships in American College of Physicians and the American Academy of Allergy Asthma & Immunology.

Dr. Fox has practiced medicine in the Allergy and Immunology Clinics and has served as a USF Health and JAH VA Hospital attending physician for 40 years. He was Director of the James A. Haley Veteran's Administration Hospital Allergy and Immunology Clinics for 30 years. He enjoyed being a clinician and mentor. Dr. Fox participated in clinical research in the USF Clinical Research Unit. He is USF Professor of Medicine and Pediatrics in the Division of Allergy and Immunology. He performed in-hospital consults at Tampa General Hospital, Moffitt Cancer Hospital, and James A. Haley Veterans' Hospital. His clinical interests included vocal cord dysfunction, chronic cough, acute and chronic urticaria and angioedema, allergic drug reactions, food allergy eosinophilic GI disorders, atopic eczema, chronic pruritus, allergic respiratory allergies, and sinusitis.

Dennis K. Ledford, MD

Dr. Dennis Ledford received his medical degree from the University of Tennessee Center for Health Sciences, Nashville, Tennessee. He completed his internal medicine residency there and served as chief medical resident for Dr. Gene Stollerman, MD, Chairman of Internal Medicine, at this same university. A fellowship in rheumatology and immunology followed at New York University and Bellevue Hospital in New York as well as a fellowship in allergy and immunology at the University of South Florida. In 2000, he joined the faculty at USF Morsani College of Medicine and achieved the rank of professor of medicine.

Local and regional activities include past service as President of the USF Medical Faculty of the Morsani College of Medicine and President of the Florida Allergy, Asthma and Immunology Society. He is current Head of the Allergy and Immunology Section, Florida Hospital, and the James A. Haley VA Hospital, Tampa, FL. National contributions include prior service as President of the American Academy of Allergy Asthma & Immunology, Associate Editor of the Journal of Allergy and Clinical Immunology, and Chair of the Steering Committee for the American Academy of Allergy Asthma & Immunology Education and Research Trust Fund (AAAAI Foundation). He also served as Co-Chair of the American Council of Graduate Medical Education (ACGME), Allergy and Immunology Residency Review Committee and Director of the American Board of Allergy and Immunology. He currently serves on the editorial board of the Annals of Allergy Asthma and Immunology. Dr. Ledford received the Distinguished Service Award from the University of South Florida, 2018, and Distinguished Clinician Award from the American Academy of Allergy Asthma & Immunology and the World Allergy Organization, 2014-2015.

Clinical responsibilities and student and resident teaching are combined with research interests in severe glucocorticoid-dependent asthma and biologic therapy of allergic disease.

Seong Cho, MD

Dr. Cho received his medical degree from Kyung-Hee University of Seoul, Korea, in February 1989. He pursued post-doctoral research in the Division of Pediatric Allergy and Immunology, University of California Los Angeles (UCLA), California, 1997, after completing his ear, nose, and throat residency at the University Medical Center, Seoul Korea. After he completed his residency training in internal medicine in Tennessee, and fellowship in the specialty of allergy and immunology, Department of Medicine, Northwestern University, Chicago, Illinois, he became an assistant professor at Northwestern University to further enhance his goal of becoming a physician/scientist in this specialty in the USA. He joined the Division of Allergy and Immunology, Department of Internal Medicine, University of South Florida College of Medicine in February 2015, where he was promoted to associate professor in August 2016.

Dr. Cho is board certified in internal medicine and allergy and immunology in the USA and otolaryngology in Korea. He received the American College of Allergy, Asthma & Immunology First Place Clemens von Pirquet Award, 2008, and the American Academy of Allergy Asthma & Immunology GSK Fellow Career Development Award, 2009, during his fellowship in allergy and immunology. Other research awards include awards from the American Heart Association and the National Institute of Health (NIH). His research interest includes the pathogenesis of asthma and chronic rhinosinusitis/nasal polyps and the role of mast cells in airway remodeling and other mast cell-related disorders.

He has published more than 50 original papers. He and his colleagues discovered that human mast cells are a novel and major source of plasminogen activator and inhibitor-1 (PAI-1), and that mast cell-derived PAI-1 plays an essential role in asthma and viral-induced asthma exacerbation. Furthermore, his research team found that PAI-1 inhibition by a specific inhibitor or soy isoflavones reduces airway inflammation and remodeling. It is hoped that this research on PAI-1 will lead to the discovery of a novel biomarker of airway remodeling and cell- or gene-specific personalized therapeutic invention for severe asthma.

Another area of investigation is the age-related differences in the pathogenesis of chronic sinusitis and nasal polyps, for which he has an NIH K23 grant. His laboratory discovered that the mitochondrial oxidative stress is related to nasal polyp formation, especially in the elderly, and blocking this pathway would be a novel and innovative treatment options for chronic sinusitis and nasal polyposis.

Mark C. Glaum, MD, PhD

Dr. Mark Glaum received a BA in psychology from Fordham University in New York, NY and a Master of Science in physiology from the School of Graduate Studies at Hahnemann University. Dr. Glaum continued on at Hahnemann, where he was awarded an MD degree and a PhD in immunology. He completed internship and residency in internal medicine at Hahnemann Hospital and then pursued fellowship training in allergy and immunology at the University of Pennsylvania where he received the Stanley E. Bradley Award for Bench Research in Internal Medicine. Dr. Glaum holds the rank of Associate Professor of Medicine and Pediatrics at the Morsani College of Medicine.

Dr. Glaum is board certified in internal medicine, and allergy and immunology. He became the Division's Fellowship Program Director in 2018. He is a fellow of the American Academy of Allergy Asthma & Immunology. He has been elected to "Top Doctors in America" for the last twelve years and enjoys teaching medical students, internal medicine residents and allergy and immunology fellows. He became a staff member of the James A. Haley Veterans' Hospital in 2016 where he sees patients. He also has staff privileges at Tampa General Hospital and Moffitt Cancer Center. He has served on the boards of the Allergy and Asthma Foundation of America and Hillsborough County Medical Society and is a past-chair of the Rhinosinusitis and Ocular Allergy Interest Section of the American Academy of Allergy Asthma & Immunology. Dr. Glaum is the Director and Co-PI of the USF Food Allergy Research and Education Foundation Clinical Center of Excellence.

Dr. Glaum's research interests include food allergy, chronic rhinosinusitis, nasal polyps, mast cell biology, and pollen identification.

Narasaiah Kolliputi, PhD

Dr. Narasaiah Kolliputi is Associate Professor and Division Director of Research Education for the Division of Allergy and Immunology, Department of Internal Medicine, USF Morsani College of Medicine, Tampa, FL. He received his postdoctoral training at Massachusetts General Hospital, Harvard Medical School, Boston, MA. Prior to that time, he received his BS in biology and chemistry in 1997, followed by an MS in biochemistry in 1999 at Sri Venkateswara University, Tirupati, India. He then completed his PhD in 2004 in biochemistry at Osmania University, Hyderabad, India.

Dr. Kolliputi has published 70 papers including papers in the journals *Circulation Research*, *Immunology*, and *Thorax*. He serves as a grant reviewer for the National Institutes of Health, VA Merit Grants, USA Department of Defense, and the American Heart Association. He is an associate editor for *Frontiers in Pharmacology*, *Frontiers in Physiology*, *Frontiers in Genetics*, and *Frontiers in Mitochondrial Physiology*, and is a guest associate editor for *Frontiers in Mitochondrial Physiology*. He is an editorial board member for *Translational Medicine*, and *Journal of Biocatalysis & Biotransformation*. Dr. Kolliputi's past and present research has been funded through several National Institutes of Health and American Heart Association grants as well as local USF grants. The USF Research Council selected Dr. Kolliputi for the 2017 Faculty

Outstanding Research Achievement Award. Dr. Kolliputi also received the 2018 Askounes-Ashford Distinguished Scholar Award from USF.

Dr. Kolliputi's research is focused on exploring the molecular mechanisms that drive pulmonary diseases. Specifically, his research explores the role of RNA-editing in Acute Respiratory Diseases (ARDS) as well as developing a mouse model that will recapitulate age-associated Idiopathic Pulmonary Fibrosis (IPF) in humans. Obtaining a greater understanding of these two subjects will inevitably lead to more and better therapeutic options for those suffering with these critical diseases.

He is working on translational strategies to attenuate oxidative stress mediated acute lung injury (ALI), pulmonary fibrosis and pulmonary arterial hypertension.

Michael N. Teng, PhD

Dr. Michael N. Teng received his PhD in immunology from the University of Chicago in 1993. He trained as a postdoctoral fellow studying viral pathogenesis at The Scripps Research Institute in La Jolla, CA. Subsequently, he became a research fellow at the National Institute of Allergy and Infectious Diseases, investigating the molecular biology of respiratory syncytial virus (RSV) and RSV vaccine development. In 2002, he accepted a faculty appointment in the Department of Biochemistry and Molecular Biology at Pennsylvania State University, University Park, PA, where his laboratory continued studies on RSV pathogenesis.

Dr. Teng joined the faculty of the Division of Allergy and Immunology at USF Morsani College of Medicine (MCOM) in 2010 and is Director of Basic Research in the Division. He holds joint appointments in the Departments of Pediatrics, Molecular Medicine, and Pharmaceutical Sciences (College of Pharmacy). Dr. Teng is currently Associate Dean of PhD and Postdoctoral Programs at the MCOM. He serves as a grant reviewer for the National Institutes of Health and the American Heart Association. His past and present research funding includes grants from the National Institutes of Health, American Heart Association, Florida Department of Health, and contracts with pharmaceutical companies.

Dr. Teng's research focuses on the host-virus interactions important for RSV pathogenesis. In particular, he is interested in the mechanisms by which RSV inhibits innate immune responses to enhance viral replication. Understanding the interplay between RSV proteins and innate immunity may lead to the development of more immunogenic RSV vaccine candidates. Additionally, Dr. Teng studies the interactions between cellular signal transduction machinery and viral proteins, with a view to discovering potential targets for antiviral therapy.

Blanca Camoretti-Mercado, PhD

Dr. Blanca Camoretti-Mercado received her BS and PhD degrees from the University of Buenos Aires, Argentina and her MS degree in Business Analytics and Information Systems from the University of South Florida in 2019. She trained as post-doctoral fellow at the University of Chicago where she later joined the faculty of the Section of Cardiology and ultimately the Section of Pulmonary and Critical Care in the Department of Medicine. In November 2012, she was recruited to the University of South Florida. A recipient of diversity, mentor, and teacher awards, she is an active member of the American Thoracic Society (ATS), and the 2016-2018 chair of the Assembly on Respiratory Structure and Function (RSF). Dr. Camoretti-Mercado has served on the ATS Board of Directors and the Finance Committee and was the founder and inaugural chair of the ATS PhD and Basic and Translational Scientists Working Group as well as a member of the Governance Task Force, the Planning and Evaluation Committee, and the Program Review Subcommittee. She has served as chair of the Program and Nominating committees, as a member of both the International Lung Health and the Members in Training and Transition Committees and was the founding member of the ATS Science and Innovation Center. She organized and chaired numerous ATS symposia and poster discussions and has presented her studies in academic and non-academic institutions worldwide. Dr. Camoretti-Mercado chaired the Women's Lung Conference of the American Lung Association (ALA-Chicago, ATS Chapter) and serves as reviewer for the National Institutes of Health (NIH) and American Heart Association (AHA) Study Sections. She is on the editorial board of several journals.

Dr. Camoretti-Mercado has published over 50 original scientific articles, reviews, and editorials and book chapters. Her research has been funded by the NIH, AHA, ALA, the LAM Foundation, and the Blowitz-Bridgeway Foundation. She also received the inaugural award from the ATS Research Foundation. Her translational investigations focus on the molecular bases, cellular signaling, and genetic determinants of lung dysfunction, applying state-of-the-art methodologies, bioinformatics and machine learning approaches. Dr. Camoretti-Mercado focuses on the airway smooth muscle (ASM), the key effector of contraction and relaxation and the source of inflammatory mediators that contribute to asthma, COPD and LAM diseases, and the target for drug discovery. She has cloned several genes involved in contractile responses of the skeletal and ASM, established the role and pathways of TGF action on gene expression and growth in ASM, created pre-clinical models of airway remodeling and hyperresponsiveness, and discovered an efficient relaxing mechanism of bitter taste receptor action in ASM.

Juan Carlos Cardet, MD, MPH

Juan Carlos Cardet, MD, MPH received his BS degree from Harvard University, Cambridge, Massachusetts, in 2004; medical degree from the University of Puerto Rico, San Juan, Puerto Rico in 2008; and master's in public health degree from Harvard University, Boston, Massachusetts, in 2017. He completed his internal medicine training at the University of Connecticut in 2011, where he was given the Maxwell O. Phelps, MD award for scholarship and the Hartford Hospital Outpatient Clinic Resident of the Year Award. He completed his allergy and immunology training at Brigham and Women's Hospital/Harvard University in 2014. He served as an instructor in medicine at Harvard Medical School and as the assistant director of the Asthma Research Center at Brigham and Women's Hospital from July 2014 until June 2017.

Dr. Cardet is an assistant professor in the USF Department of Internal Medicine. He specializes in the treatment of patients with asthma, chronic urticaria, chronic rhinitis, and other allergic and immunologic diseases. He is board certified in internal medicine and in A/I, and a fellow in the American Academy of Allergy Asthma & Immunology. He enjoys working with medical students, residents, and allergy and immunology fellows. His translational research focuses on understanding the pathophysiology of severe asthma with the aim of identifying novel therapies. In 2017, he was awarded a K23 grant by the National Institute of Allergy and Infectious Diseases (NIAID) so that he could pursue this endeavor. He is an investigator with the AsthmaNet, Severe Asthma Research Program (SARP), and PRECISE NHLBI research networks. He is the co-chair of the executive, publications, and data sharing committees of the Patient Centered Outcomes Research Institute (PCORI)-funded PRECISE trial.

Lakshmi Galam, PhD

Dr. Lakshmi Galam is an assistant professor in the Division of Allergy and Immunology, Department of Internal Medicine, at the USF Morsani College of Medicine, Tampa, FL. She completed her postdoctoral training at Oklahoma State University, Stillwater, OK. Prior to that, she received her BS in biology and chemistry in 1996, followed by an MS in biotechnology in 1998 at Andhra University, Vishakapatnam, India. She then completed her PhD in genetics at Osmania University, Hyderabad, India, in 2004.

Dr. Galam's research work is published in various prestigious scientific journals. She is highly experienced in the development and use of automated liquid handling systems integrated with high throughput analytical platforms. She also has extensive experience in high throughput screening and hit validation studies to identify small molecule inhibitors in drug discovery. She serves as Course Director for the Applied Bioinformatics Course.

Amber N. Pepper, MD

Dr. Amber N. Pepper received her BS degree in Integrative Biology from the University of Florida, Gainesville, FL and MD degree from the University of South Florida Morsani College of Medicine, Tampa, FL. She was inducted into the Alpha Omega Alpha Honor Medical Society during her third year of medical school. She completed her residency in internal medicine (chief resident) and fellowship in allergy and immunology (chief fellow) at the University of South Florida Morsani College of Medicine. She joined the University of South Florida, Division of Allergy and Immunology, Department of Internal Medicine, as Assistant Professor in August 2018.

Dr. Pepper is Associate Director of the Division of Allergy and Immunology, Department of Internal Medicine, Joy McCann Culverhouse Clinical Research Center. She was Co-Director of the USF Health Divisions of Allergy and Immunology 2020 Symposium Updates in Allergy and Immunology, January 17-18, 2020, Tampa, Florida. She is board certified in internal medicine and allergy and immunology. She is also a member of the American Academy of Allergy Asthma & Immunology and the American College of Allergy, Asthma & Immunology. She has authored abstracts and scientific review articles and enjoys teaching medical students, residents, and fellows.

Dr. Pepper's research interests include food allergy and oral immunotherapy, allergic rhinitis, asthma, atopic dermatitis, and urticaria.

Farnaz Tabatabaian, MD

Dr. Farnaz Tabatabaian received a BS in chemistry from Wright State University in Dayton, OH. Following graduation, she earned her Master of Science in Anatomy and Physiology at Wright State University where she had direct exposure to research in innate immunology and inflammation. She pursued an MD degree at Northeast Ohio University of Medicine, Akron, OH. She completed her internship and residency in internal medicine at the Wexner Medical Center, Ohio State University, and then did her fellowship training in allergy and immunology at the University of South Florida, Pediatric Division of Allergy and Immunology, Johns Hopkins All Children's Hospital, St. Petersburg, FL.

Dr. Tabatabaian is board certified in internal medicine and allergy and immunology. She directed the 2019 and 2020 Symposium Updates in Allergy and Immunology, January 18-19, 2019, and January 17-18, 2020, at the Center for Advanced Medical Learning and Simulation (CAMLS), University of South Florida, Tampa, Florida. She enjoys teaching medical students, internal medicine residents and allergy and immunology fellows. She sees patients in internal medicine and allergy and immunology at the University of South Florida Morsani College of Medicine. Dr. Tabatabaian is involved in implementing and creating a curriculum in high value education for residents to help devise a way to decrease healthcare costs while providing excellence in care.

Dr. Tabatabaian's research interests include adult immunology with a focus on common variable immunodeficiency, inflammation and asthma, and the impact of nicotine on the bronchi and epithelial cells.

Recollections of COVID 19
by Richard F. Lockey, MD, MS

August 5, 2021

The first inklings of a possible forthcoming pandemic were heard in early January 2020. Leaders from the USA Centers for Disease Control and Prevention (CDC) and National Institutes of Health (NIH) indicated that they did not think that COVID-19 would become a major pandemic. However, by mid-February 2020, I sensed that there was going to be a problem, a major problem. I immediately requested my family and associates to obtain N95 masks for potential use at the allergy/immunology USF-affiliated clinic at 13801 Bruce B. Downs Blvd. I, too, sought as many masks as possible for one week, even at hardware stores where the same masks are utilized for high-risk occupational exposure. N95 masks soon became unavailable even from medical supply sources. It was a perfectly logical step to take to protect the physicians and healthcare professionals in the clinic. On March 8, 2020, the Director of the National Institute of Allergy and Infectious Diseases at the NIH stated, "There's no reason to be walking around with a mask. When you're in the middle of an outbreak, wearing a mask might make people feel a little bit better and it might even block a droplet, but it's not providing the perfect protection that people think that it is. And, often, there are unintended consequences — people keep fiddling with the mask and they keep touching their face." This idea of the mask not being helpful was echoed by other national medical leaders.

Not being able to concur with the statements from national leaders regarding masks not being beneficial, I began wearing them in mid-February. Precautions needed to be taken. I recall that during my residency training, surgical masks were mandated on tuberculosis wards and periodic BCG tests indicated to assure that physicians and other healthcare personnel did not contract tuberculosis Likewise, in the early 1980s when the Division established the USF Human Immunodeficiency Virus (HIV) Clinic, healthcare professionals were required to wear masks, goggles, gowns, booties, as well as surgical caps, when we treated HIV patients because it was not yet recognized that the virus was almost exclusively transmitted sexually.

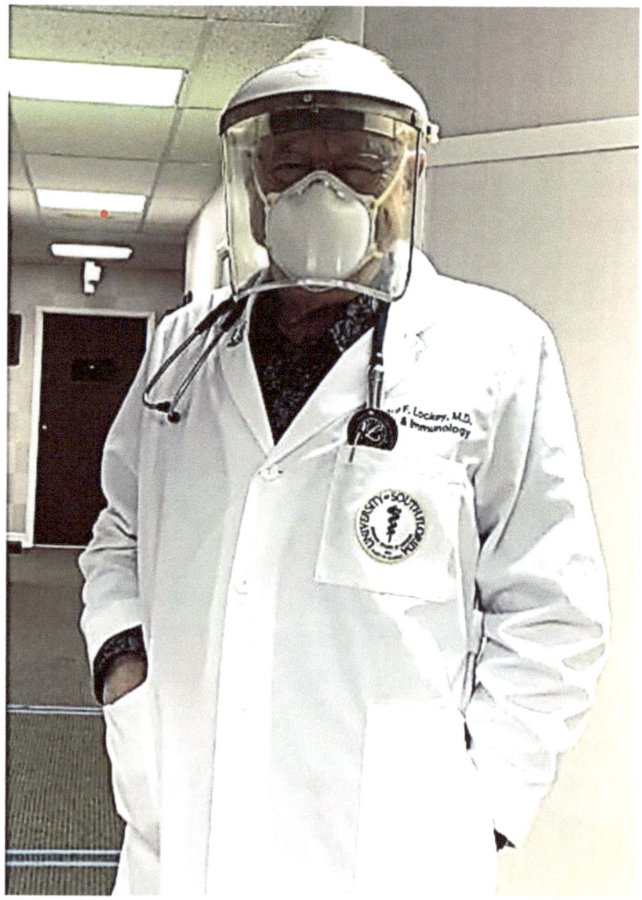

Richard F. Lockey, MD, MS

As the COVID-19 epidemic became more prevalent in early March, concerned physicians called and implored me to retire from practice because of the known risks to individuals over age 65. As with the HIV Clinic situation, I responded that as physicians, it is our responsibility to take a stand, do everything we can to protect ourselves, and continue seeing patients who need our care, especially during a potential epidemic. I did so. Quite honestly, when Drs. Robert P. Nelson, Dennis K. Ledford, and I established the HIV Clinic at the University of South Florida, it was a much more of a terrifying experience because HIV at that time was universally fatal. If you contracted it,you died. We were unsure about the ways it could possibly be transmitted. As the understanding of how HIV was transmitted, masks and gowns became unnecessary.

During the COVID-19 epidemic, masks and a face shield were worn by me in the clinics beginning sometime in February 2020. All staff gradually were required to wear at least a surgical mask, given the option of using an N95 mask, as well as using an eye shield. I am convinced that the use of masks were instrumental in protecting us throughout the epidemic. Overs the next year-and-a-half, those few clinic employees who did develop COVID-19 were able to trace their contact back to a family member, not to a patient.

Weekly conferences and meetings within the Division became electronic in the early spring 2020. On Monday morning of each week, a COVID-19 discussion was led by Michael Teng, PhD, Associate Professor of Medicine, an expert in viral-induced diseases. There were a variety of different treatments proposed, all of which lacked sufficient scientific evidence, the main one was the use of hydroxyzine hydrochloride to allegedly prevent or protect from the disease. Likewise, a host of over-the-counter remedies, sometimes proposed by physicians or other healthcare professionals, were equally ineffective. In the meantime, the number of deaths began to increase, particularly among those more susceptible to the disease, i.e., subjects over 65 and/or suffered from obesity, diabetes mellitus, kidney disease, cardiovascular disease, hypertension, or immunodeficiency problems.

COVID-19 shut down both personal and public communication within the Division of Allergy and Immunology as well as in the public domain. Hardly anyone met in person and when they did, they appropriately masked and shielded out of fear of transmitting or acquiring the disease. The James A. Haley Veterans' Hospital established a screening program in its main parking garage and faculty on consultation were required to be COVID tested several days before they became active consultants. Most of us worked at home, except when we were in clinic, but the clinics both at the USF-affiliated clinic located at 13801 Bruce B. Downs Blvd and USF Morsani Health continued to be active throughout 2020. As in all clinics, wipe-downs with Clorox and other disinfectants became the standard of care and patients were requested not to enter the clinic if they were suspected to have or had diagnosed COVID-19. Testing during the summer of 2020 became readily available and the public took advantage of this resource, at times on their own, to rule out the disease. If they did develop COVID-19 that required professional care, their primary care came through an emergency room and, when severely ill, a hospital. Because of the alleged risk, patients were not welcomed in most clinics. Press communication indicated that COVID-19 vaccines would be available first for physicians and other healthcare professionals by the end of the year. This was encouraging news!

News of potential effective treatment became available in September 2020 when scientific articles indicated that glucocorticosteroids, in particular, dexamethasone, was helpful for severe COVID-19 respiratory problems, the primary cause of death. This was one of the first major bona fide proven treatments for this disease primarily for patients hospitalized with COVID-19.

By late fall, data indicated the efficacy of different vaccines. This was good news for millions of people who were "hunkered down" and had been for months because of the fear of contracting the disease. The first immunizations were delivered both at Tampa General Hospital and the James A. Haley Veterans' Hospital to physicians and other healthcare professionals in December 2020. I received my first immunization in December and the second in January 2021. A month later I checked my antibody titers which were immunoprotective against COVID-19. By the end of the spring, most individuals who desired to be were immunized; however, there were many who did not want to be immunized and for the most part, it was impossible to convince them to do so. A variety of different reasons were given, primarily undue suspicion of the vaccine, an miRNA vaccine, considered experimental and not yet, as of August 2021, FDA-approved. By late spring, early summer 2021, masks were starting to come off, people were again going to restaurants and socializing without wearing masks. Individuals unvaccinated were encouraged to still wear a mask, but many did not. Additional good news was received during the summer 2021; another medication, ivermectin, was indicated as an effective therapy for hospitalized patients with severe COVID-19.

Then came the Delta variant July 2021. This caused a significant resurgence of the disease, particularly among the unvaccinated and youth. The Delta experience incentivized some individuals not yet immunized to become immunized, with the realistic possibility that about 20-25% would never agree to immunization. Of interest, I contracted the Delta variant in mid-July 2021 from an unknown source. I received monoclonal antibodies over two hours intravenously at Tampa General Hospital. The infusion of monoclonal antibodies against the virus has been life-saving to so many individuals in Tampa, Florida beginning in November 2020, when it was first administered at Tampa General Hospital to high-risk patients. I received it within 24-48 hours of onset of symptoms and felt markedly better within 24 hours. I am writing this essay on the fifth- or sixth-day post-infection and feel 100% back to normal.

Now, as we face the Delta variant, to take additional precautionary measures, the Division has reinstituted videoconferencing and masking to help prevent the transmission of the Delta COVID-19 variant. Hopefully, precautionary measures will only be needed for a few months. Those previously vaccinated have good protection to survive COVID-19, even those at high risk, although deaths are being reported even in COVID-19 vaccinated individuals. Where this will take us in the future, we know not. However, I believe that COVID-19 will become an endemic problem, and we will be immunizing individuals for COVID-19 just as we have for influenza for years to come. We are already hearing about a COVID booster shot.

COVID-19 has had and continues to have a profound impact on all our lives and the way we perceive the world. Most individuals know of someone who died from this disease or almost succumbed from it. Who would have thought it could affect the entire world and bring many of our lives to a standstill. It made society impersonal by no longer being able to greet one another, as smiles and other facial expressions, so important to humans, became indistinguishable through masks. People became more dependent on electronic media for communication, so much if it erroneous and self-serving. Likewise, many patients have delayed routine care, which is already having and will continue to have an effect on increased morbidity and mortality for years to come. I am also convinced that COVID-19 has led to much of the political disharmony that has occurred in the USA and throughout the world over the past year-and-a-half.

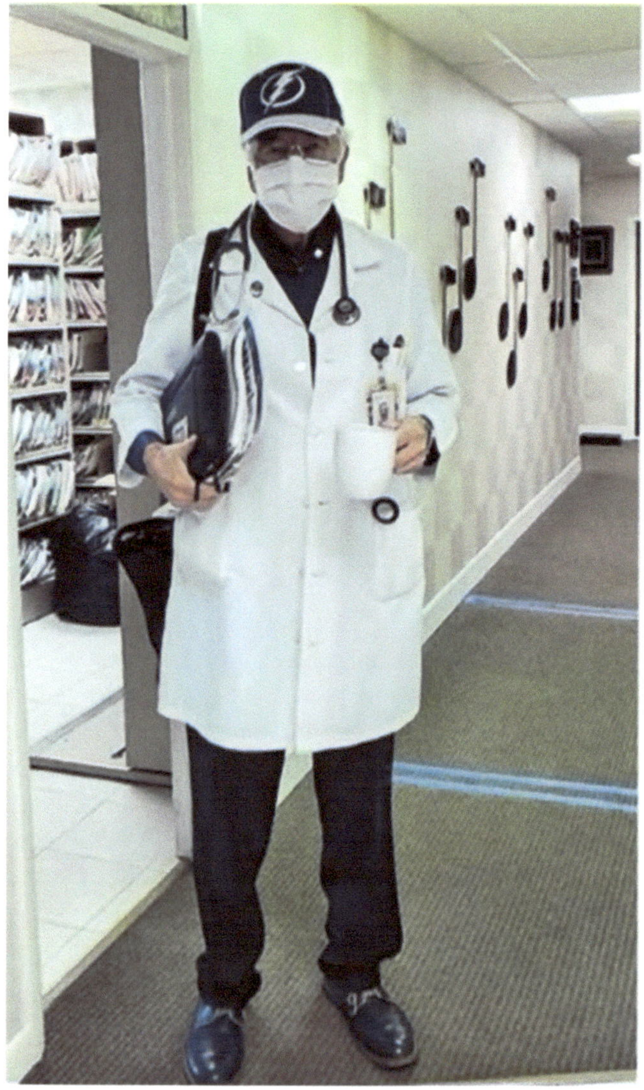

Dennis K. Ledford, MD

Herd immunity should gradually take place if COVID-19 variants continue to be susceptible to a previous infection or to the COVID-19 vaccines. If so, the epidemic should come to a halt. If not, the trauma from COVID-19 will continue well into the future until a better treatment or vaccine becomes available. COVID-19 has undoubtedly altered our lives and our personal memories of the COVID-19 epidemic are sure to be passed on from generation to generation.

"Facta duds vivent, operosague gloria rerum; Haec manet; hate avidos effugit una rogos."

—Ovid.

Translated:

"The leader's deeds and hard won glory live; This remains; this alone survives the funeral fires."

—Ovid.

Peggy L. Hales 9-1-21	Richard F. Lockey, MD, MS 9-1-21
Peggy L. Hales, AS Date	Richard F. Lockey, MD, MS Date

Chapter 2: Historical Overview as of 2006

Clinical Research Brochure circa 2006

University of South Florida

Department of Internal Medicine

Division of Allergy and Immunology

Clinical Research Unit

The Joy McCann Culverhouse Airway Disease Center

USF HEALTH

University of South Florida College of Medicine

CENTER OVERVIEW

The Division of Allergy and Immunology was established in the Department of Internal Medicine at the University of South Florida College of Medicine, Tampa, Florida in 1972.The University was established in 1956 and the College of medicine in 1971.

Professor Samuel C. Bukantz, M.D. founder of the Division, recruited Richard F. Lockey, M.D. in 1973, as a second faculty member. Drs. Bukantz and Lockey developed a clinical research and training program between 1973-1977, enabling trainees in internal medicine and other services to rotate at monthly intervals on the Allergy and Immunology Service. The first trainees in the speciality were selected in 1977 and graduated 2 years later. Initial accreditation was granted in 1983 by the Accreditation Council for Graduate Medical Education (ACGME) and the program has been accredited since that time.

Two separate but integrated programs in allergy and immunology currently exist at the University, one under the auspices of the Department of Internal Medicine, chaired by Professor Richard F. Lockey, and the second, in the Department of Pediatrics, chaired by Professor John Sleasman, M.D. Professor Sleasman succeeded the late Professor Robert A. Good, M.D., Ph.D., DSC, the "Father" of modern clinical immunology. He founded the USF Pediatric Allergy and Immunology Training Program in 1987. It was first ACGME accredited in June, 1988 and has been accredited since.

The Department of Internal Medicine program has 5 trainees, 2 or 3 each year, and the pediatric program has 3, one or two each year. The two programs have trained 90 allergists/immunologists, and both Divisions also have trained numerous American and foreign post-graduate and graduate research scholars. Many of these trainees are now faculty members in academic centers throughout the world.

Both USF Divisions have been endowed with funds donated for teaching, research, and patient care. There are three endowed positions in the two Divisions. Richard F. Lockey, M.D. occupies the Joy McCann Culverhouse Chair in Allergy and Immunology, John Sleasman, M.D. is the Robert A. Good Professor in Immunology and Shyam Mohapatra, PhD, is The Mabel and Ellsworth Simmons Professor in Allergy and Immunology. The Department of Internal Medicine's Division is located in Tampa at the University of South Florida College of Medicine and consists of five clinical faculty MDs, six PhDs, two research MDs and clinical research, administrative and volunteer support staff. The Pediatric Division has five clinical MDs, three PhDs, and a similar support staff and is located at All Children's Hospital in St. Petersburg, Florida, 45 minutes from the main campus located at 4202 E. Fowler Avenue, Tampa, Florida.

Both Divisions have extensive clinical and basic research programs and are funded by a variety of different institutions, including the National Institutes of Health, the Veteran's Administration, the American Lung Association and the American Heart Association. The two separate programs in Allergy and Immunology at the University of South Florida College of Medicine are extensively integrated for training, care of patients, and research. There are 72 ACGME accredited programs to train physicians in allergy and immunology in the United States. These are the only two in the State of Florida. Physician trainees in Allergy and Immunology must first be board qualified in internal medicine and or pediatrics. Both programs also train post- graduate and graduate, medical and nursing students.

Basic and clinical research interests for the two Divisions include indoor and outdoor allergens, primary and secondary immunodeficiency diseases, HIV research, bone marrow transplantation, insect hypersensitivity, allergen immunotherapy, the effect of gastroesophageal reflux disease on asthma, and the effect of viral respiratory tract infections on asthma and allergy in the elderly.

BASIC RESEARCH PROGRAM

From its inception, the Division has had a basic research program. However, the program expanded in the late 1990s when an endowment was donated by a grateful friend, Joy McCann Culverhouse. Because of this endowment, Shyam S. Mohapatra, Ph.D. was recruited in 1996 to the University of South Florida and now directs the Joy McCann Culverhouse Airway Disease Research Center. The basic research program at the Center aims to understand the molecular basis of allergic and viral diseases and to develop new strategies for protection from pathogenesis.

Research at the Center focuses on three areas: new strategies for prevention and treatment of respiratory syncytial virus infections, the use of nanoparticle-delivered interferon gamma for enhancing the immune response and applications of peptide therapy for asthma based on manipulation of the atrial natriuretic peptide hormone signaling system.

CLINICAL RESEARCH UNIT

The Department of Internal Medicine, Division of Allergy and Immunology Clinical Research Unit, is a 1,600 square foot facility, just off the main campus, in which pharmaceutical sponsored, divisional clinical research projects, and grant funded clinical research projects are conducted. It was established in 1977, the main goal of which is to improve the treatment of patients who suffer from asthma and allergic and immunologic diseases.

All studies performed are done under the supervision of the physicians and the staff and approved by the University's Human Research Committee. All trainees in allergy and immunology are required to participate in clinical research throughout their training. Trainees develop and carry out a clinical project on their own, with appropriate supervision of a faculty member. The fellow is responsible (with faculty guidance) for developing the protocol, preparing a budget, having it approved by the Institutional Review Board, and assisting with subject recruitment. For example, the Division is currently working on a study which compares skin test results in both sun exposed and non-exposed areas in allergic individuals in 2 age groups, 20 – 50 years and 60 years and over. A study just approved is one which will examine the effects of topical intranasal antibiotics to treat chronic sinusitis. A third project, also submitted by a trainee, is designed to determine whether or not the side-effects of intranasal oxymethazoline can be negated by the concurrent use of intranasal steroids.

Over the past 27 years, the Department of Internal Medicine's Allergy/Immunology Clinical Research Unit, has conducted over 300 Phase II, III, IV clinical trials and has established a working relationship with more than 30 pharmaceutical sponsors. Not only does the Clinical Research Unit provide trainees with the skills necessary to perform clinical research, but the funds generated from this Unit are also used to support the research and training programs.

The Clinical Research Unit has provided quality research for both children and adults in many areas including studies on acute sinusitis, allergen immunotherapy, allergen skin testing, allergic and non-allergic rhinitis, allergic conjunctivitis, acute and chronic urticaria, food allergy, contact dermatitis and atopic eczema. Pulmonary diseases such as asthma, acute and chronic bronchitis, COPD (chronic obstructive pulmonary disease), and exercise induced asthma have also been studied. The Unit has also conducted immunologic studies on HIV, intravenous immunoglobulin, common variable immunodeficiency, and hereditary angioedema. The pediatric division actively participates in basic and clinical research and the two divisions actively collaborate on a variety of projects.

Staffed by 5 professional medical personnel, the Division and the Clinical Research Unit are affiliated with various institutions in the Tampa Bay area including the H. Lee Moffitt Cancer Center, James A. Haley Veterans' Administration Hospital, Tampa General Hospital, the University of south Florida Medical Clinic, and All Children's Hospital.

State-of-the-art equipment is available for the staff to perform complete pulmonary function studies, methacholine and allergen challenge studies, rhinoscopy, and exercise challenge studies and exhaled nitric oxide testing. High-speed internet access, electronic data capture capabilities and a computerized patient database are available.

In June, 2000, the Clinical Research Unit was selected as one of the American Lung Association's Asthma Clinical Research Centers. There are 20 centers throughout the United States. The American Lung Association (ALA) centers are a network of academic asthma research centers funded to conduct multicenter clinical research trials in asthma that are relevant to practical questions about treatment. The ALA provides the infrastructure and direct research support for the center. Since June, 2000, four papers have been published and approximately 11 are on-going, in development, or in press.

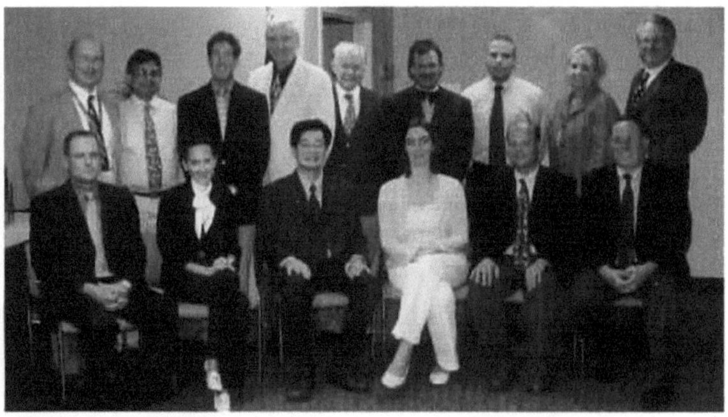

left to right- (back row)
John W. Sleasman, M.D., Shyam S. Mohapatra, Ph. D., Michael Nieder, M.D., Dennis K. Ledford, M.D., Monroe J. King, D.O., Mandel R. Sher, M.D., Glenn Whelan, Pharm. D., Michelle Grandstaff, LPN, Richard F. Lockey, M.D.
left to right- (top row)
Matthew Morrow, Morna Dorsey, M.D., MMSc, Nutthapong Tangsinmankong, M.D., Aleksandra Petrovic, M.D., Mark C. Glaum, M.D., Ph. D., Robert Nickeson, M.D.
Not pictured-
Samuel C. Bukantz, M.D., Rama Ganguly, Ph. D., M.P.H, Roger W. Fox, M.D., Prasanna Kumar Jena, Ph. D., Weidong Zhang, Ph. D., Stuart M. Brooks, M.D., Noorbibi Day, Ph. D., Gary W. Litman, Ph. D., Mitchel J. Seleznick, M.D., Sandra G. Gompf, M.D.

CORE FACULTY

Richard F. Lockey, M.D., Professor of Medicine, Pediatrics, and Public Health; Division Director; Joy McCann Culverhouse Chair of Allergy and Immunology

Samuel C. Bukantz, M.D., Professor Emeritus of Medicine and Medical Microbiology and Immunology; Director Emeritus

Rama Ganguly, Ph.D., M.P.H., Professor of Medicine

Dennis K. Ledford, M.D., Professor of Medicine and Pediatrics

Shyam S. Mohapatra, Ph.D., Professor of Medicine, Pediatrics and Molecular Medicine; Mabel and Ellsworth Simmons Professor of Allergy and Immunology; Director of Basic Research, Joy McCann Culverhouse Airway Disease Center, Director of Basic Sciences, USF Health Signature Program of Allergy, Immunology and Infectious Diseases

Roger W. Fox, M.D., Associate Professor of Medicine, Pediatrics and Public Health

Mark C. Glaum, M.D., Ph.D, Assistant Professor of Medicine and Pediatrics

Monroe J. King, D.O., Affiliate Associate Professor of Medicine and Pediatrics

Prasanna Kumar Jena, Ph.D., Research Instructor

Weidong Zhang, PhD., Research Instructor

JOINT FACULTY

Stuart M. Brooks, M.D., Professor of Public Health and Medicine

Noorbibi Day, Ph.D., Professor of Pediatrics and Medicine

John W. Sleasman, M.D., Professor of Pediatrics And Medicine, Robert A. Good Professor of Immunology; Chief, Division of Allergy, Immunology and Rheumatology, Department Of Pediatrics

Gary W. Litman, Ph.D., Hines Professor of Pediatrics And Medicine

Mitchel J. Seleznick, M.D., Associate Professor of Medicine

Nutthapong Tangsinmankong, M.D., Associate Professor of Pediatrics and Medicine

Morna Dorsey, M.D., MMSc Assistant Professor of Pediatrics and Medicine

Sandra G. Gompf, M.D., Assistant Professor of Medicine

Mandel R. Sher, M.D., Affiliate Professor of Pediatrics and Medicine

Matthew Morrow – Director, Flow Cytometry Services Children's Research Institute, USF

Michael Nieder, MD, Affiliate Associate Professor of Pediatrics, USF Director, Blood & Marrow Transplant Program, All Children's Hospital

Aleksandra Petrovic, MD, Affiliate Assistant Professor of Pediatrics, USF

Robert A. Nickeson Jr., MD, Assistant Professor of Pediatrics and Medicine, USF Director, Sub-division of Rheumatology, All Children's Hospital

CLINICAL AFFILIATE FACULTY

Robert E. Windom, M.D., Affiliate Professor of Medicine

G. Edward Stewart II, M.D., Affiliate Associate Professor of Medicine

Hugh H. Windom, M.D., Affiliate Associate Professor of Medicine

Rosa Codina, Ph.D., Affiliate Assistant Professor of Medicine

Mary L. Jelks, M.D., Affiliate Assistant Professor of Medicine

Brett E. Stanaland, M.D., Affiliate Assistant Professor of Medicine

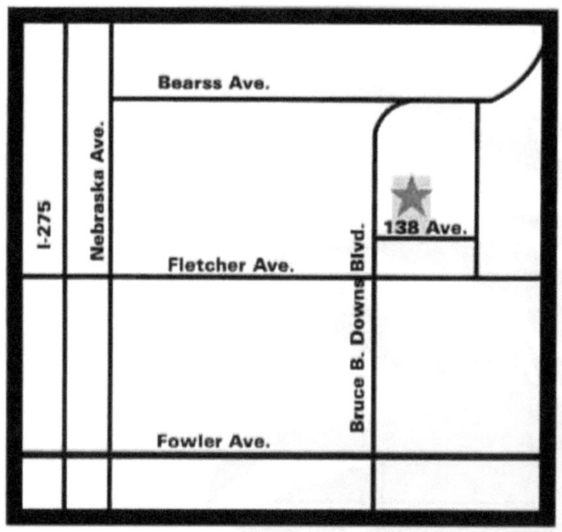

USF UNIVERSITY OF SOUTH FLORIDA

University of South Florida College of Medicine
Division of Allergy and Clinical Immunology
Care of the James A. Haley VA Hospital
Mail Code 111D
13000 Bruce B. Downs Boulevard
Tampa, Florida 33612
PHONE: 813-972-7631
FAX: 813-910-4041

If you are interested in making a tax deductible contribution to support research in Allergy and Immunology please contact Dr. Lockey or the Clinical Research Unit at 813-631-4024.

Chapter 3: Faculty Throughout the Years

Please note that years indicated in parentheses indicate the years of fellowship training in the Division.

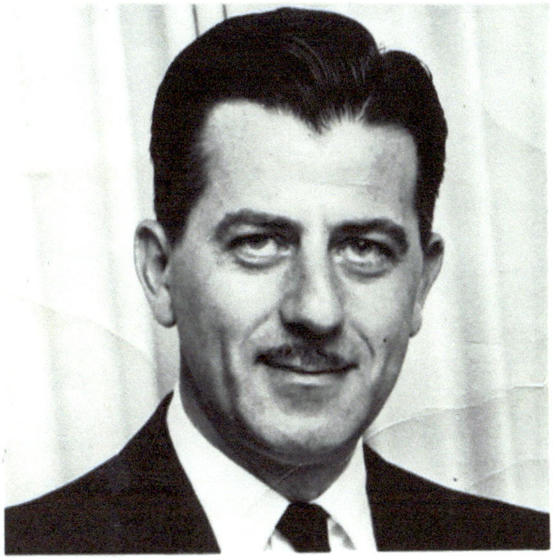

Samuel C. Bukantz, M.D., Founding Director, Division of Allergy and Immunology, Department of Internal Medicine; 1972.

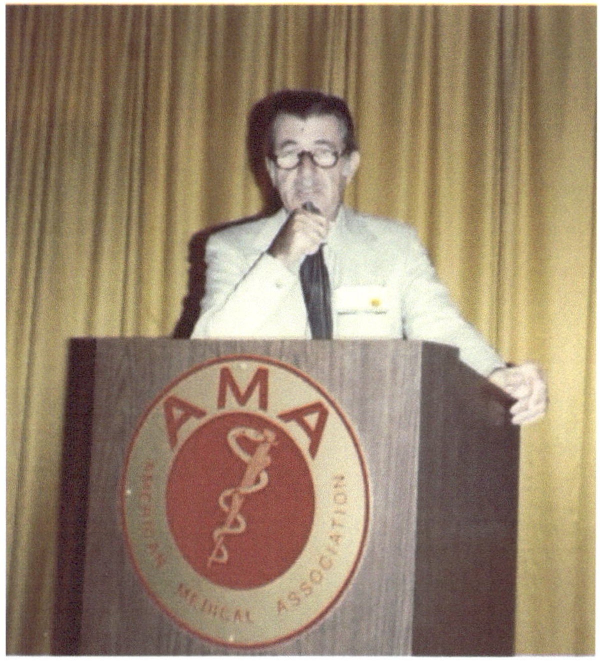

Samuel C. Bukantz MD, American Medical Association Meeting; circa 1975.

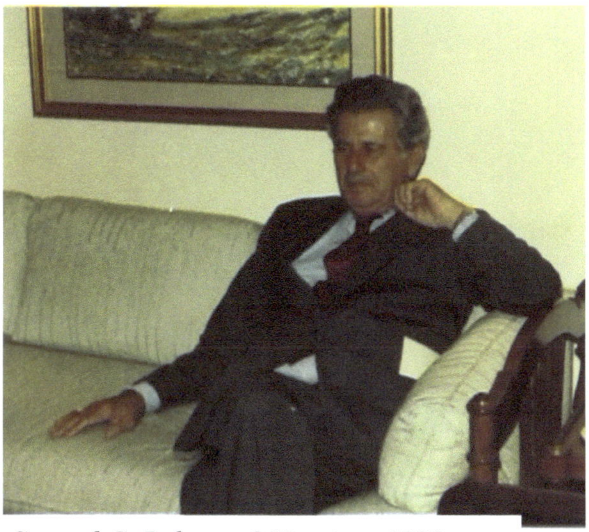

Samuel C. Bukantz, MD; circa 1980.

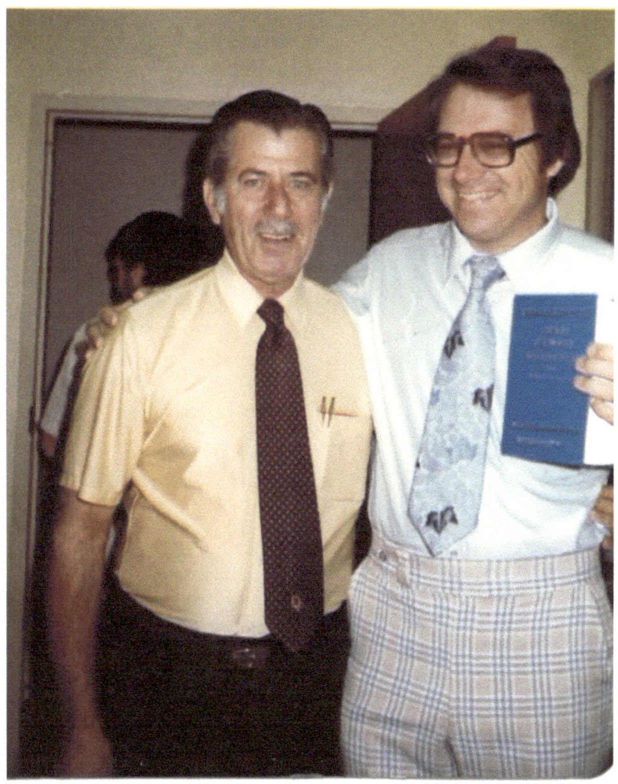

Left to right: Samuel C. Bukantz, MD and Richard F. Lockey, MD, MS. First book edited by Dr. Lockey; Lockey RF (ed): <u>Allergy and Clinical Immunology.</u> Medical Examination Publishing Co, Inc. Garden City, New York, 1980 (1193 pages). Also published by Hans Huber Publishers, Bern, Switzerland and Igaku-Shoin Ltd., Tokyo, Japan.

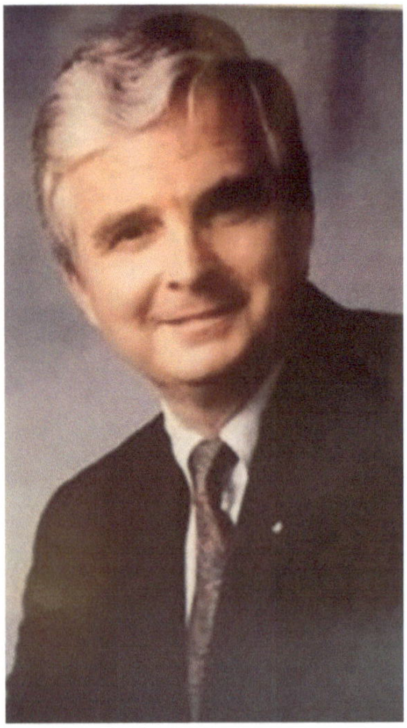

Lawrence A. Holfelder, MD; circa 1980.

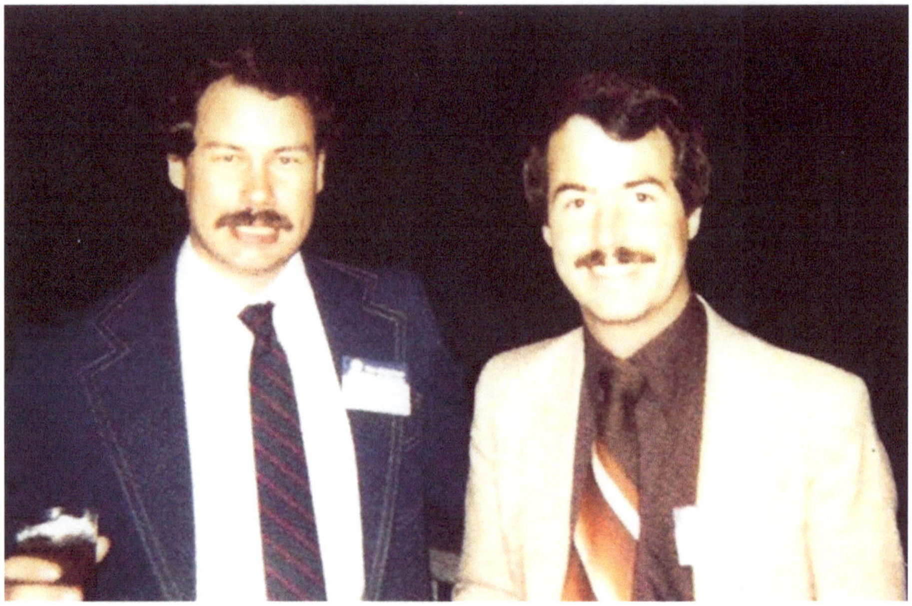

Left to right: Gerald A. Bucholtz, MD (1980-1982); John J. Stablein, MD (1979-1981); circa 1984.

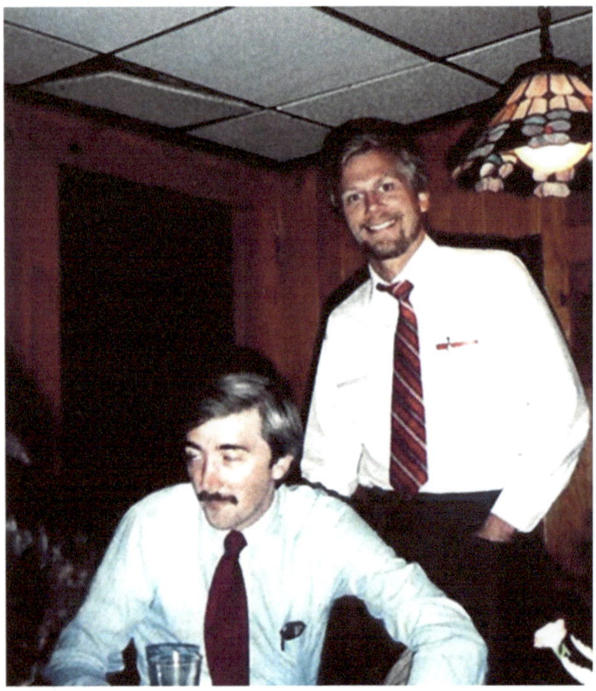

Dennis K. Ledford, MD (1983-1985), sitting; Roger W. Fox, MD (1978-1980), standing; circa 1986.

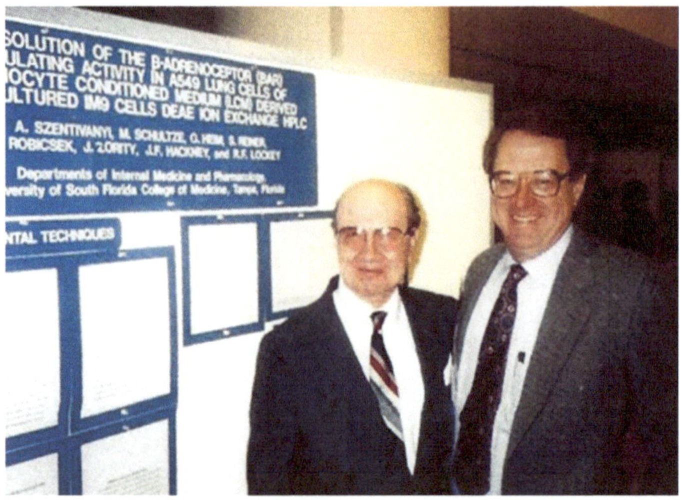

Left to right: Dean Andor Szentivanyi, MD, PhD and Richard F. Lockey, MD, MS; Abstract presentation – USF College of Medicine Research Day, 1991. Szentivanyi A, Schultze M, Heim O, Reiner S, Robicsek S, Zority J, Hackney JF, Lockey RF: "Resolution of the B-adrenoceptor (BAR) Regulating

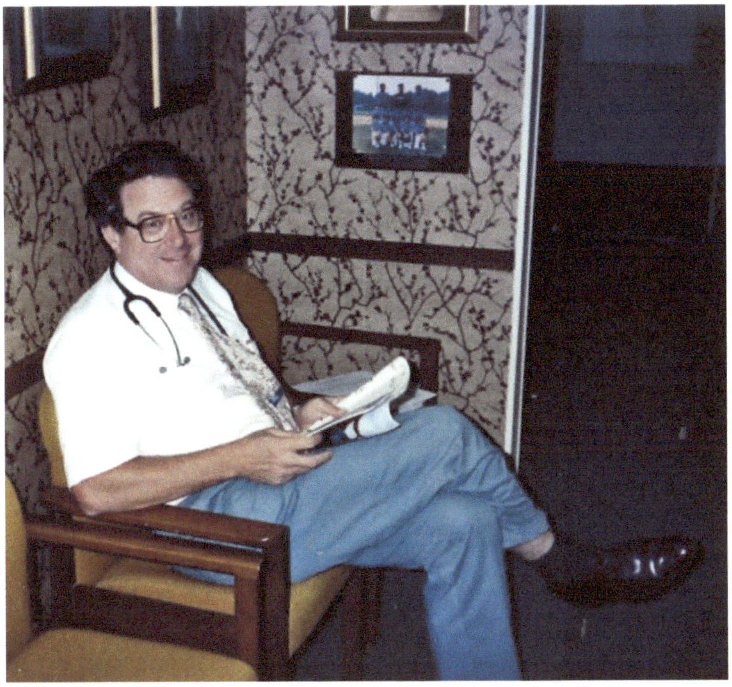

Richard F. Lockey, MD, MS; 1989.

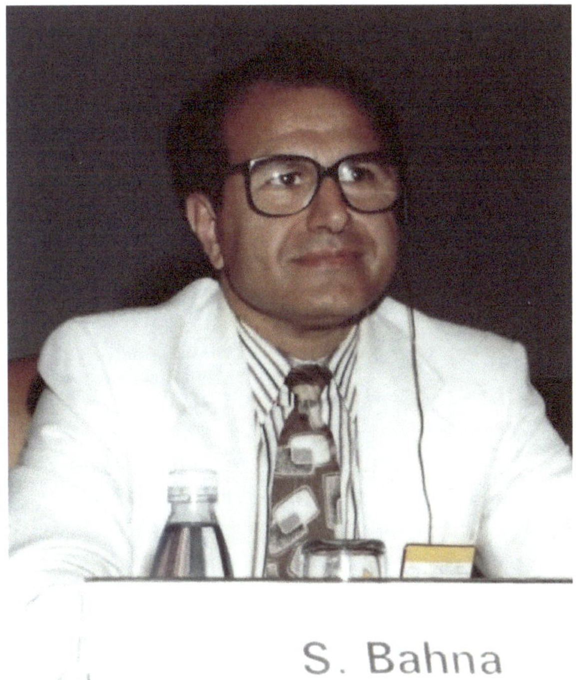

Sami L. Bahna, MD, DrPH; circa 1992.

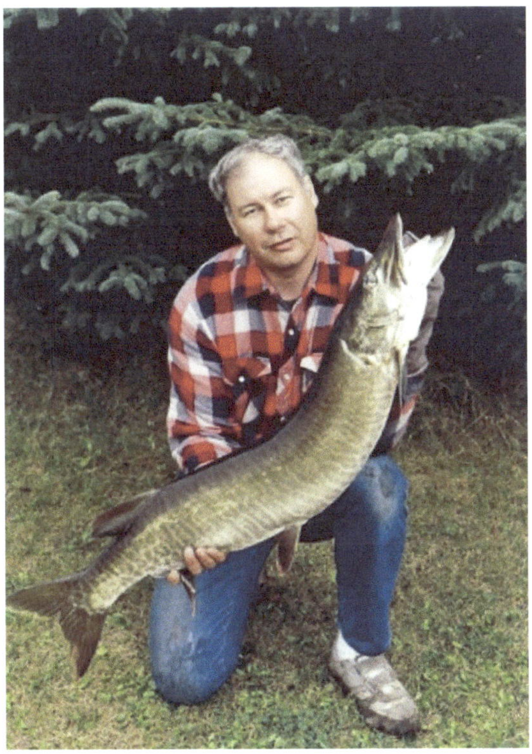

Gerald A. Bucholtz, MD; Wisconsin 1994; 44" muskie.

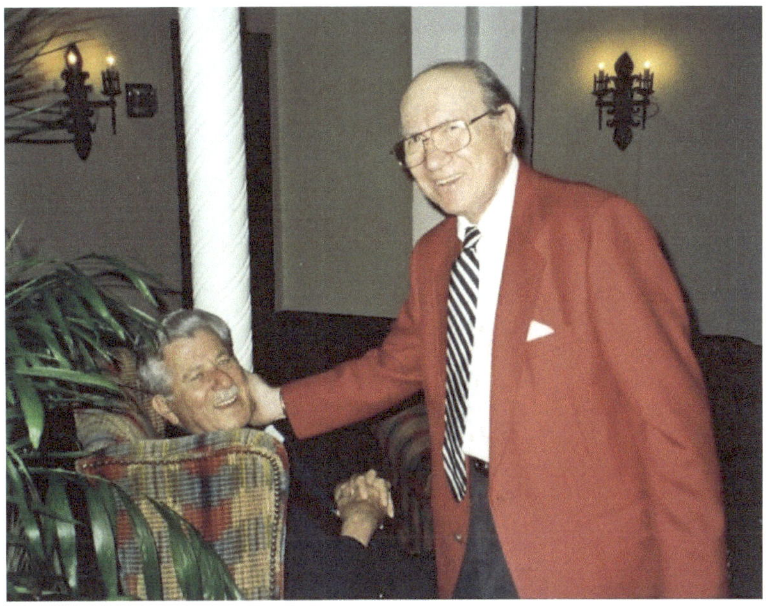

Left to right: Samuel C. Bukantz, MD; Andor Szentivanyi, MD (3rd Dean, USF College of Medicine; Distinguished University Professor); circa 1992.

Left to right: Samuel C. Bukantz, MD; Robert A. Good, MD, PhD, DSc; Richard F. Lockey, MD, MS; 1994.

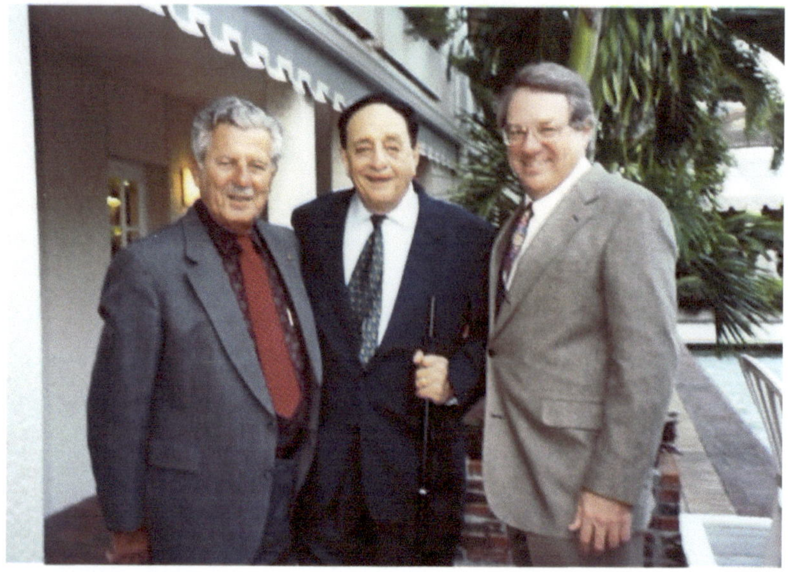

Left to right: Roger W. Fox, MD; Rosa Codina, PhD; Richard F. Lockey, MD, MS; circa 1995.

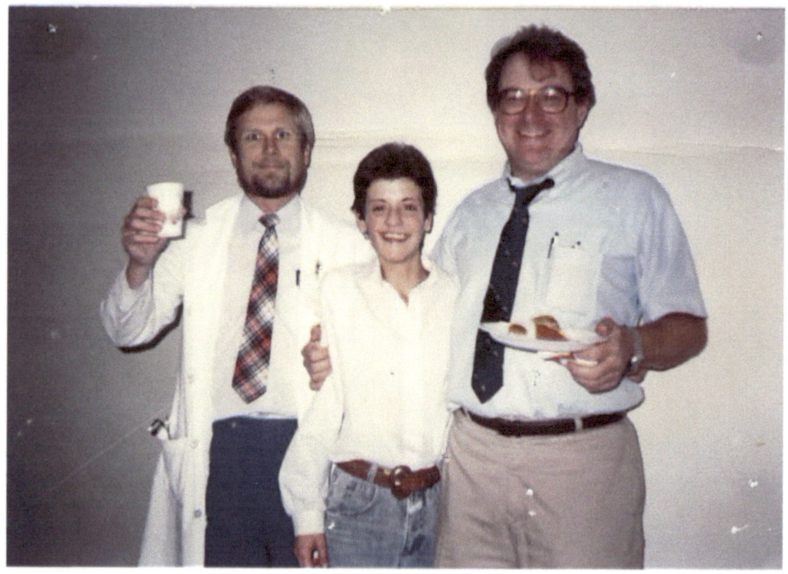

Left to right: Samuel C. Bukantz, MD and Richard F. Lockey, MD, MS; CDB Pizza, circa 1995.

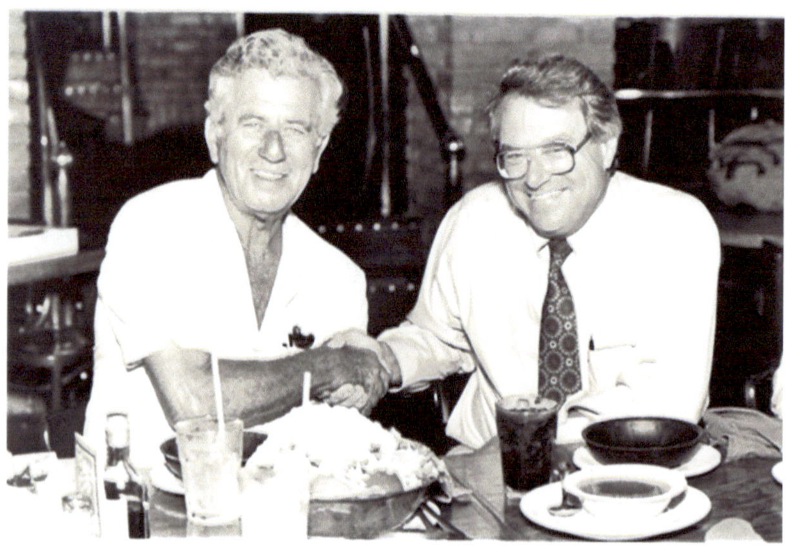

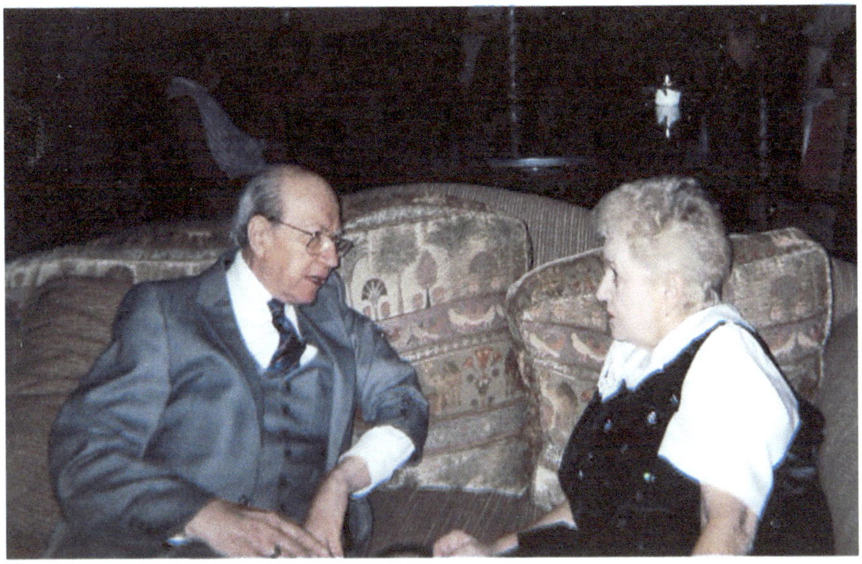

Drs. Andor and Judith Szentivanyi; circa 1995

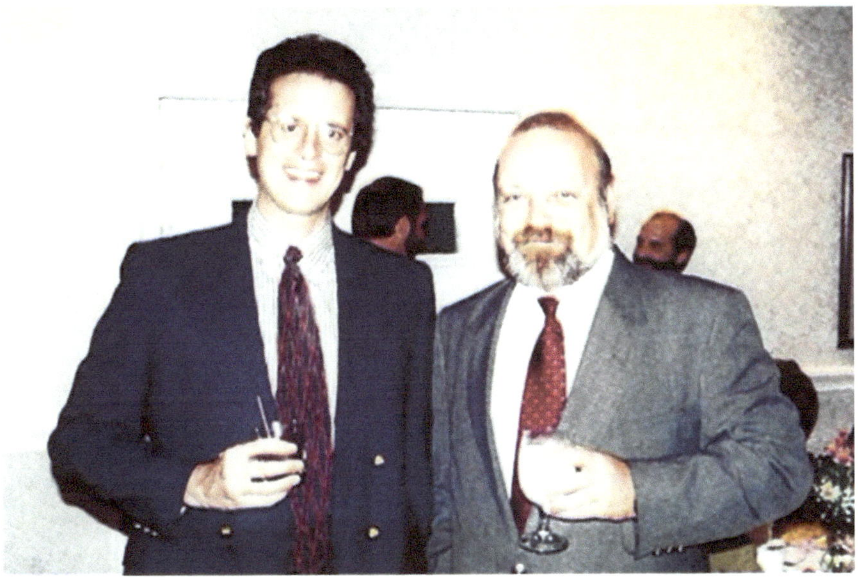

Left to right: Enrique Fernandez-Caldas, PhD and Walter Trudeau III, MS; circa 1995.

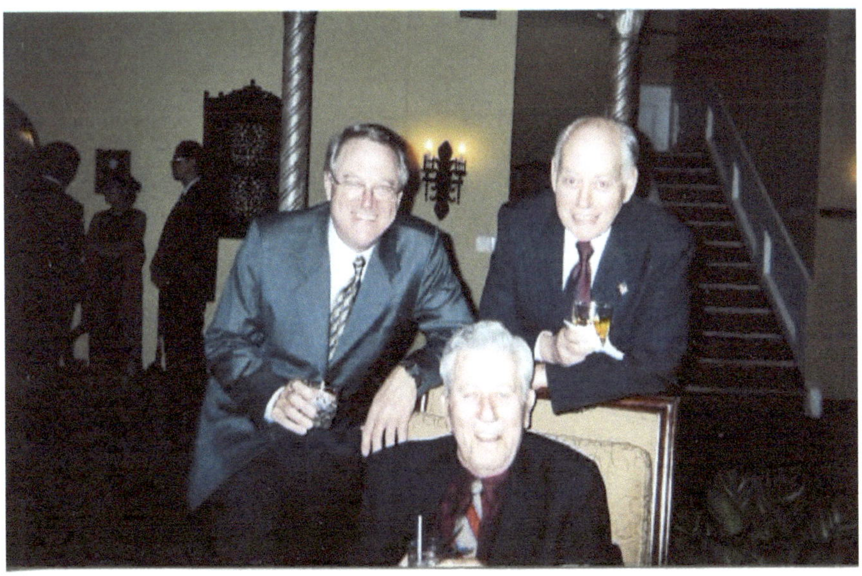

Samuel C. Bukantz, MD (sitting). Back (left to right): Richard F. Lockey, MD, MS; Monroe J. King, DO. Circa 1995.

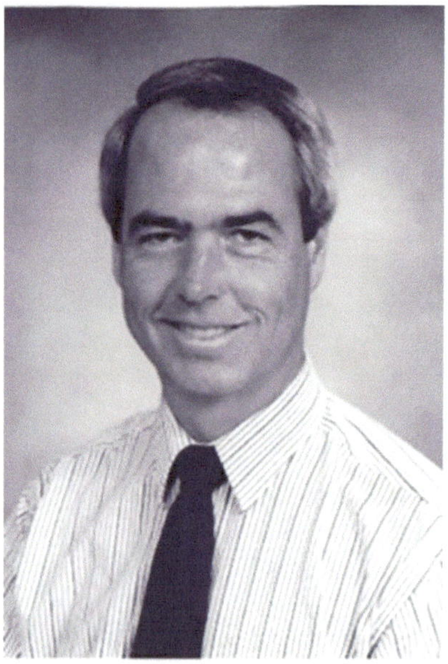

John J. Stablein, MD;
circa 1995.

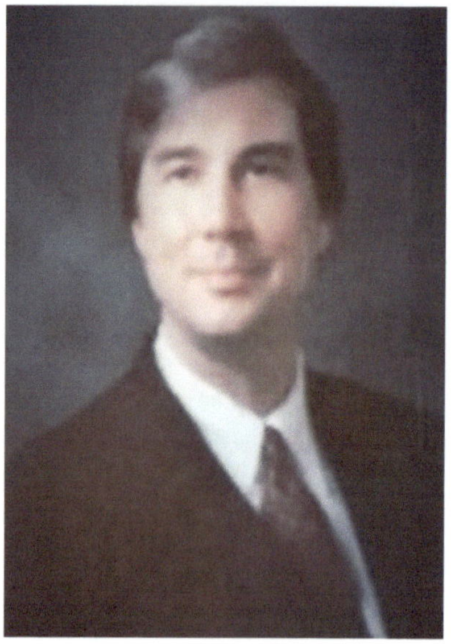

Robert P. Nelson, MD;
circa 1995.

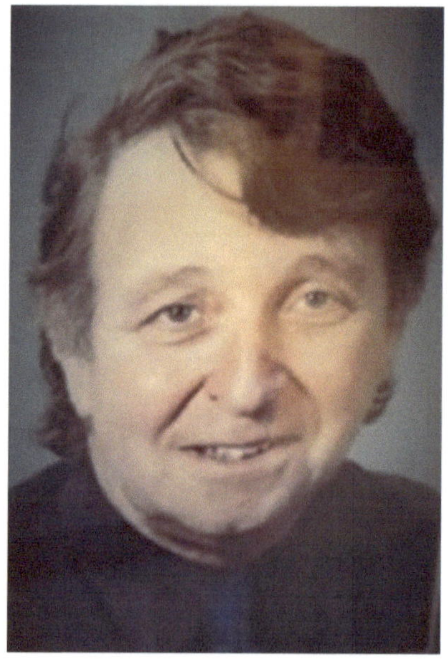

Stuart M. Brooks, MD;
circa 1995.

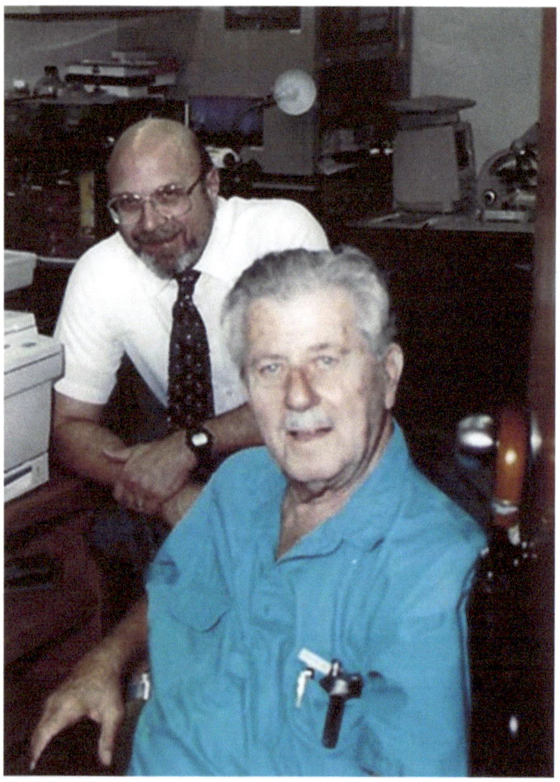

Samuel C. Bukantz, MD (front) and Joseph J. Krzanowski, PhD (Department of Pharmacology and Therapeutics); 1997.

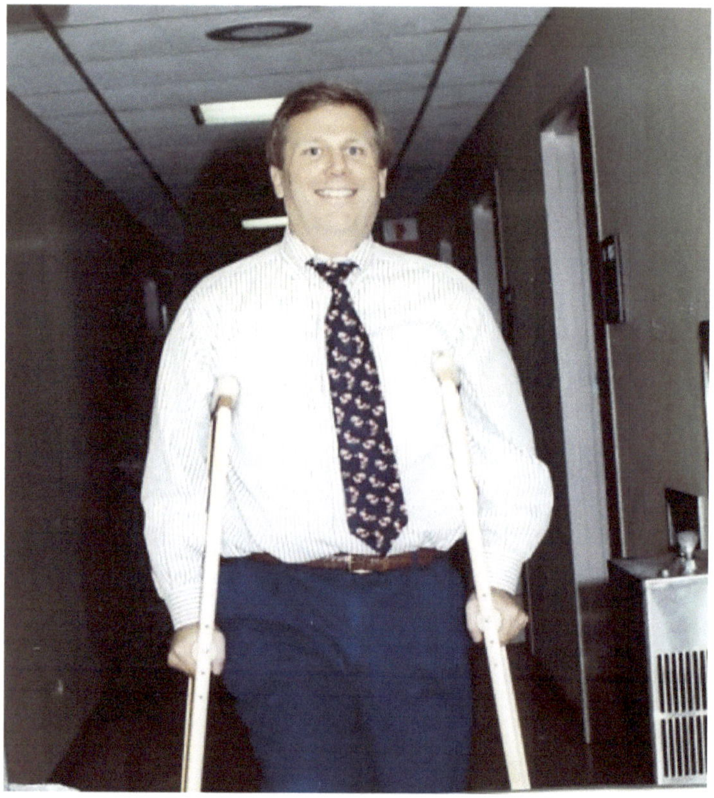

Roger W. Fox, MD; 1998.

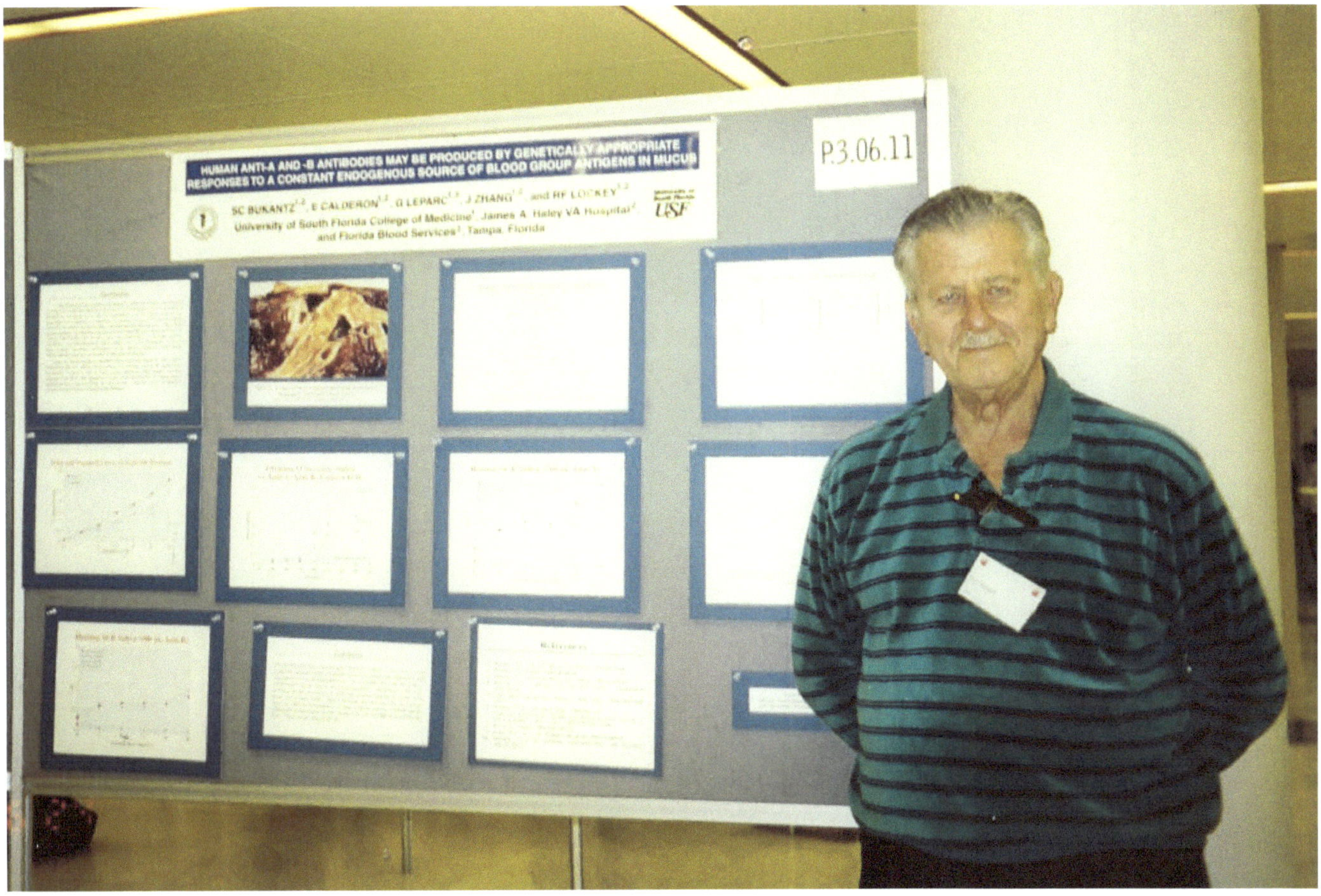

Samuel C. Bukantz, MD. Poster: Bukantz SC, Calderon E, Leparc G, Zhang J, Lockey RF: "Human anti-A and anti-B Antibodies may be Produced Genetically Appropriate Response to a Constant Endogenus Source of Blood Group Antigens in Mucus". 13th European Immunology Meeting. Amsterdam, Holland, June 22-25, 1997. 15th Aspen Allergy Conference. Aspen Colorado. July 22-25. 1997.

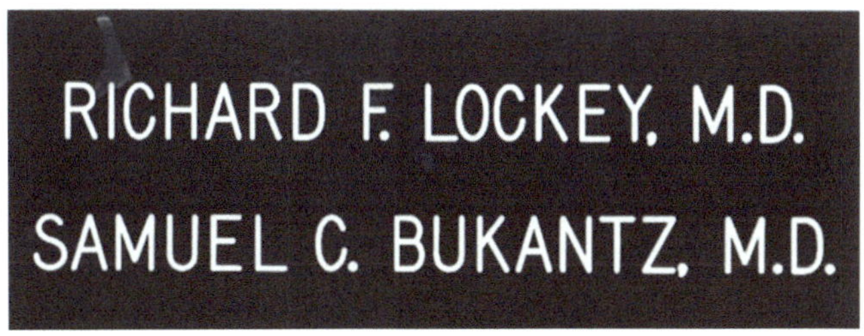

Wall plaque at the James A, Haley VA Research Building; circa 2000.

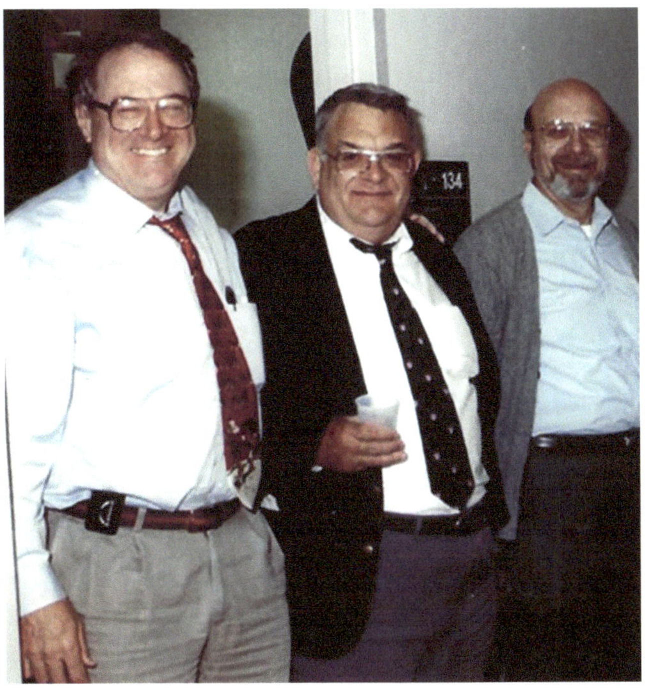

Left to right: Richard F. Lockey, MD, MS; John W. Hadden, MD (Division of Immunopharmacology); Joseph J. Krzanowski, PhD (Department of Pharmacology and Therapeutics); circa 1998.

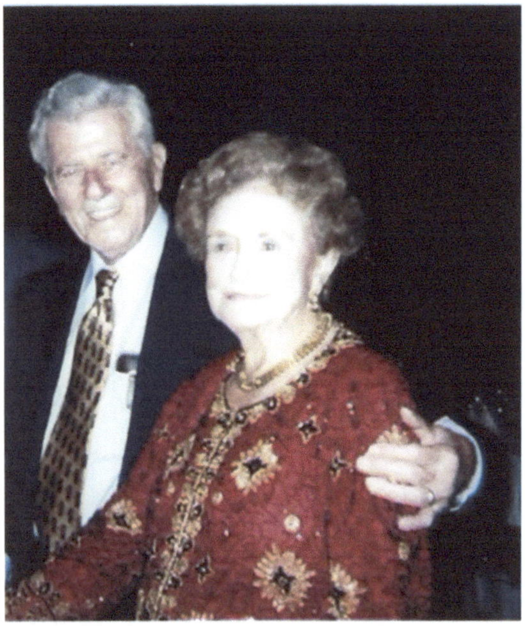

Samuel C. Bukantz, MD and Jewell Bukantz; Asthma & Allergy Foundation of America, Florida Chapter; Fundraising Dinner 2000.

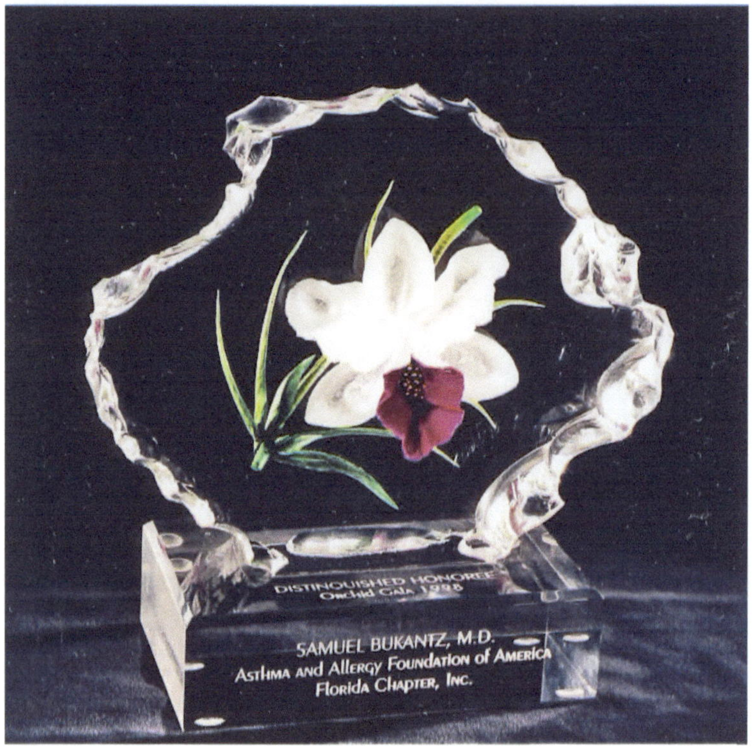

Samuel C. Bukantz, MD; Distinguished Honoree, Orchid Gala 1998; Asthma & Allergy Foundation of America, Florida Chapter.

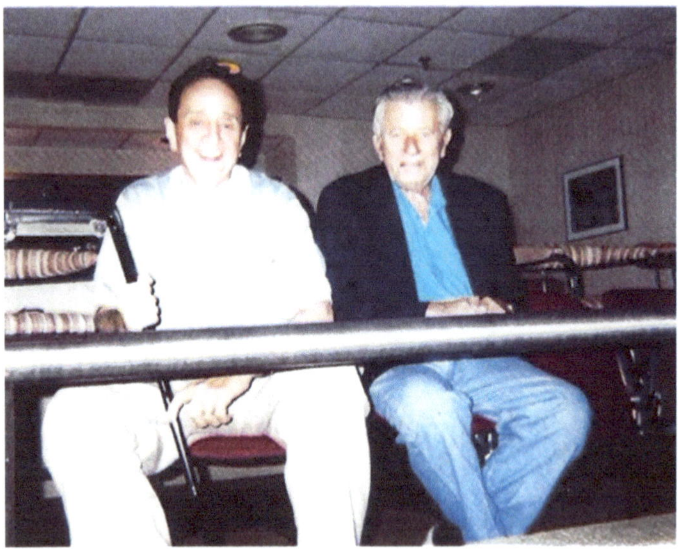

Left to right: Robert A. Good, MD, PhD, DSc and Samuel C. Buckhantz, MD; circa 2000.

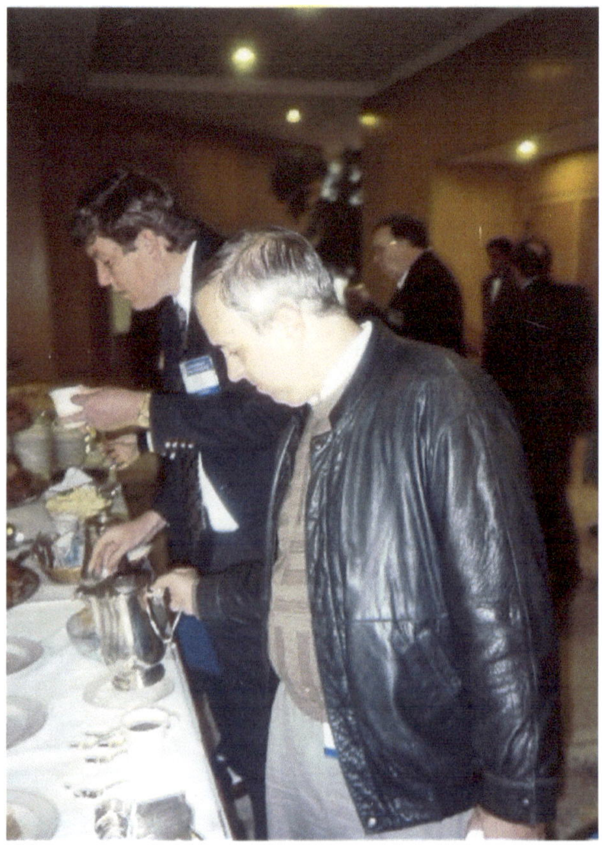

Mitchel J. Seleznick, MD; circa 2000.

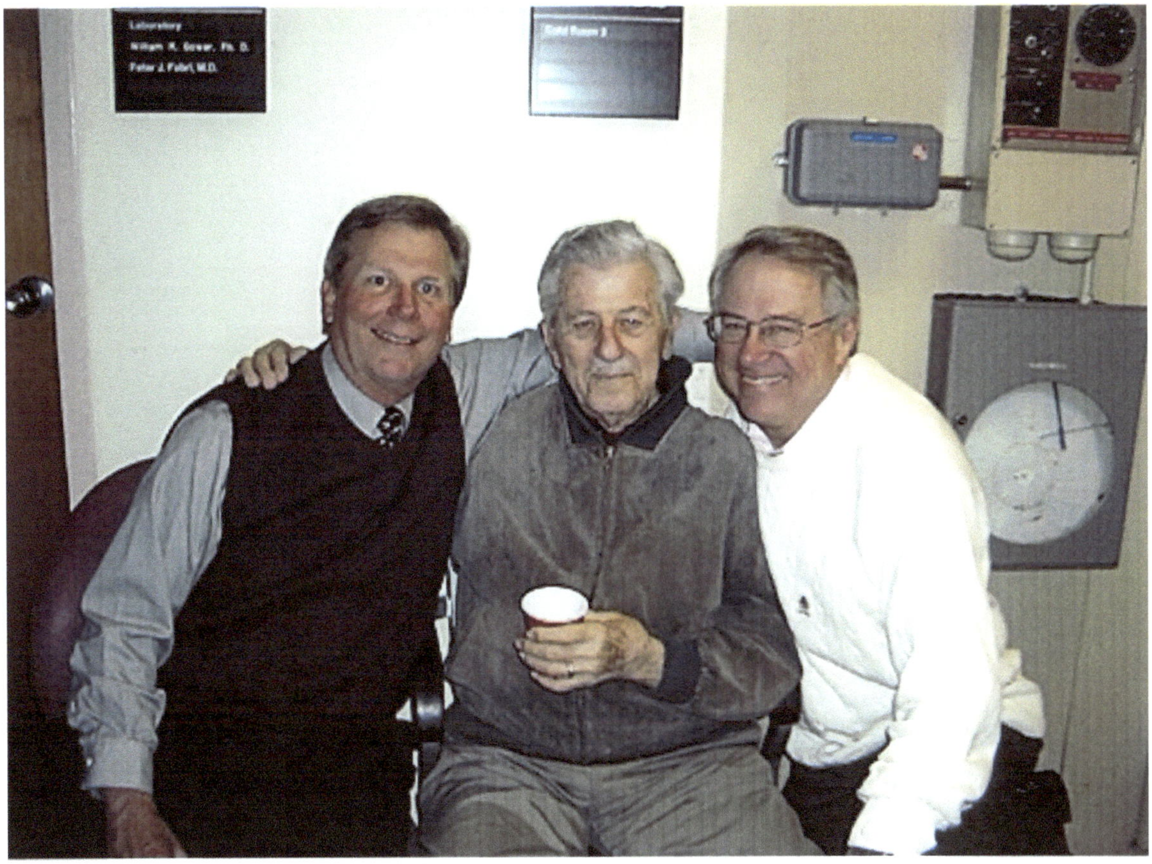

Left to right: Roger W. Fox, MD; Samuel C. Bukantz, MD; Richard F. Lockey, MD, MS; circa 2000.

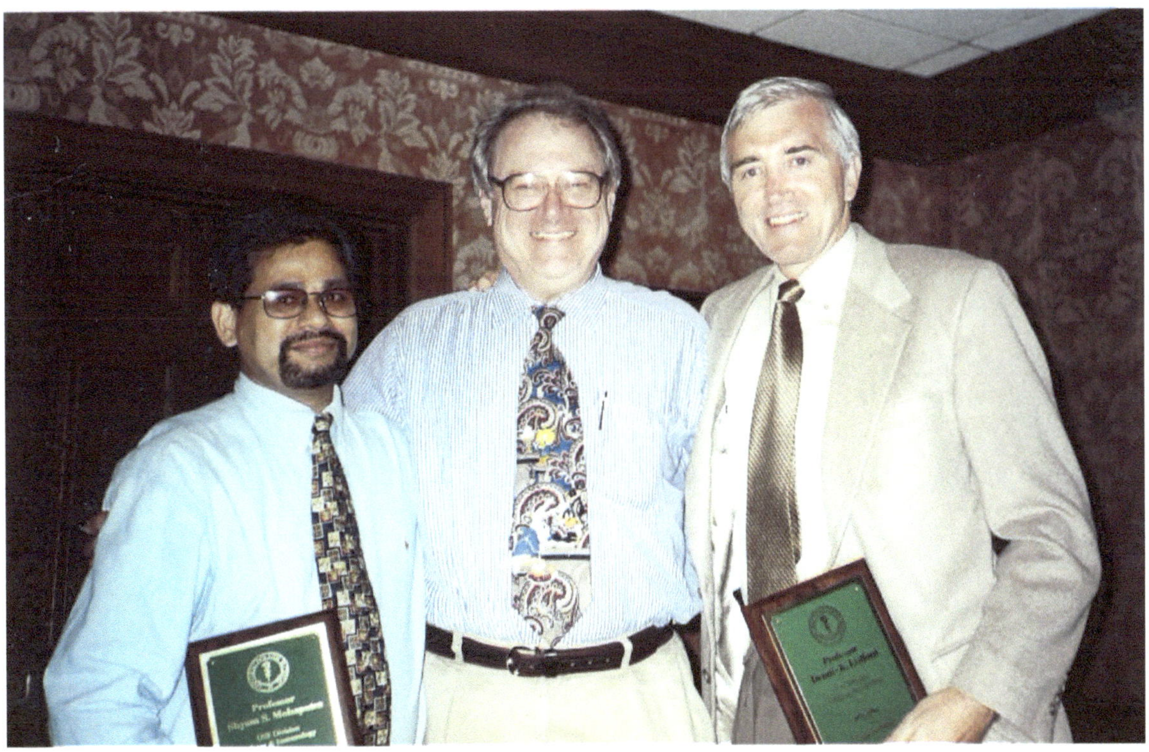

October 2000: Advancement to Professor: Drs. Ledford and Mohapatra. Left to right: Shyam S. Mohapatra, PhD; Richard F. Lockey, MD, MS; Dennis K. Ledford, MD.

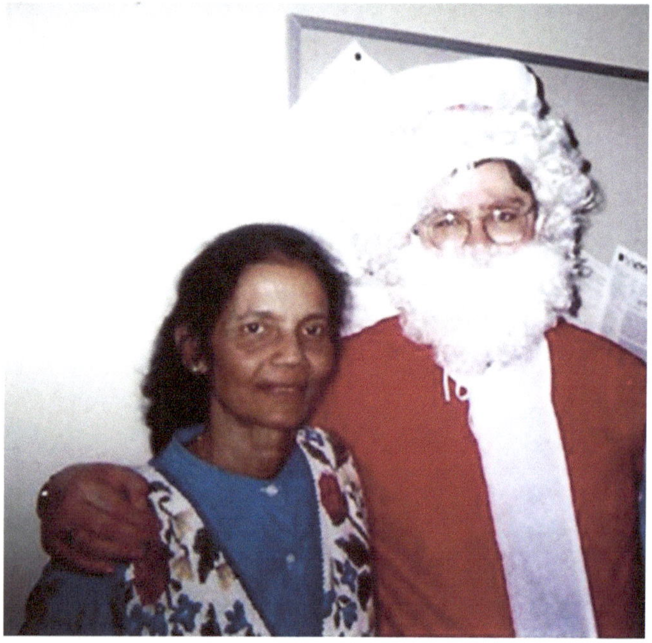

Rama Ganguly, PhD and Santa (Thomas Luck, MD 1999-2001); December 2000.

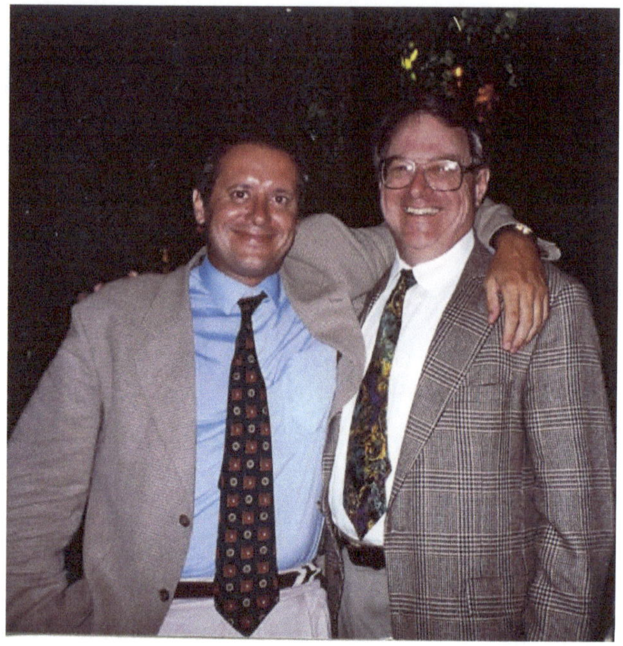

Left to right: Enrique Fernandez-Caldas, PhD and Richard F. Lockey, MD, MS; circa 2000.

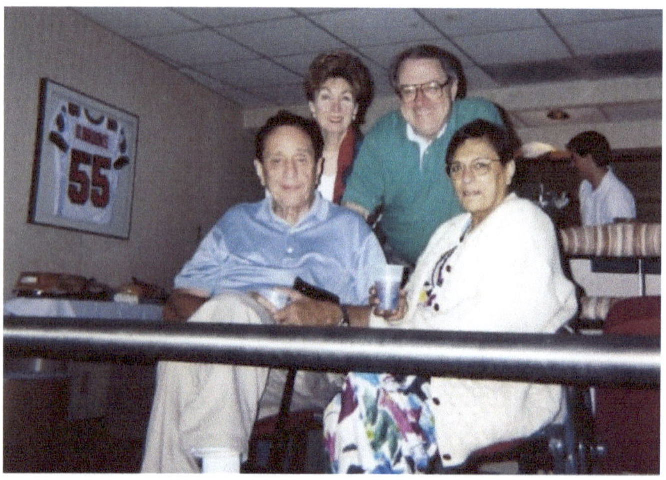

Front row: Robert A. Good, MD, PhD, DSc and Noorbibi Day, PhD.
Back row: Carol Lee Lockey and Richard F. Lockey, MD, MS. Circa 2001.

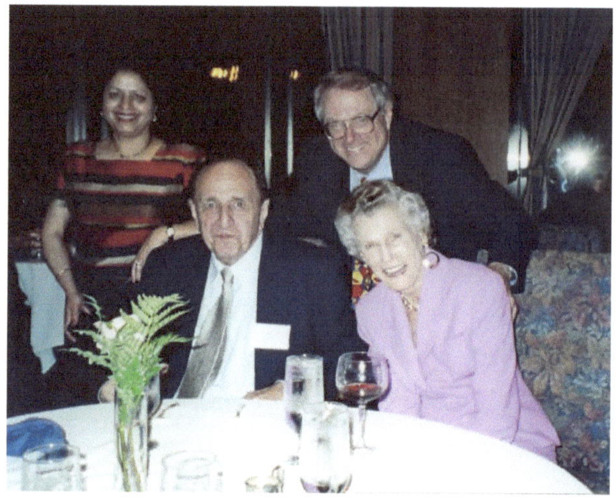

2001 Robert A. Good, MD, PhD, DSc Tribute.
Sitting (left to right): Robert A. Good, MD, PhD, DSc and Joy McCann Culverhouse.
Standing (left to right): name unknown; Richard F. Lockey, MD, MS.

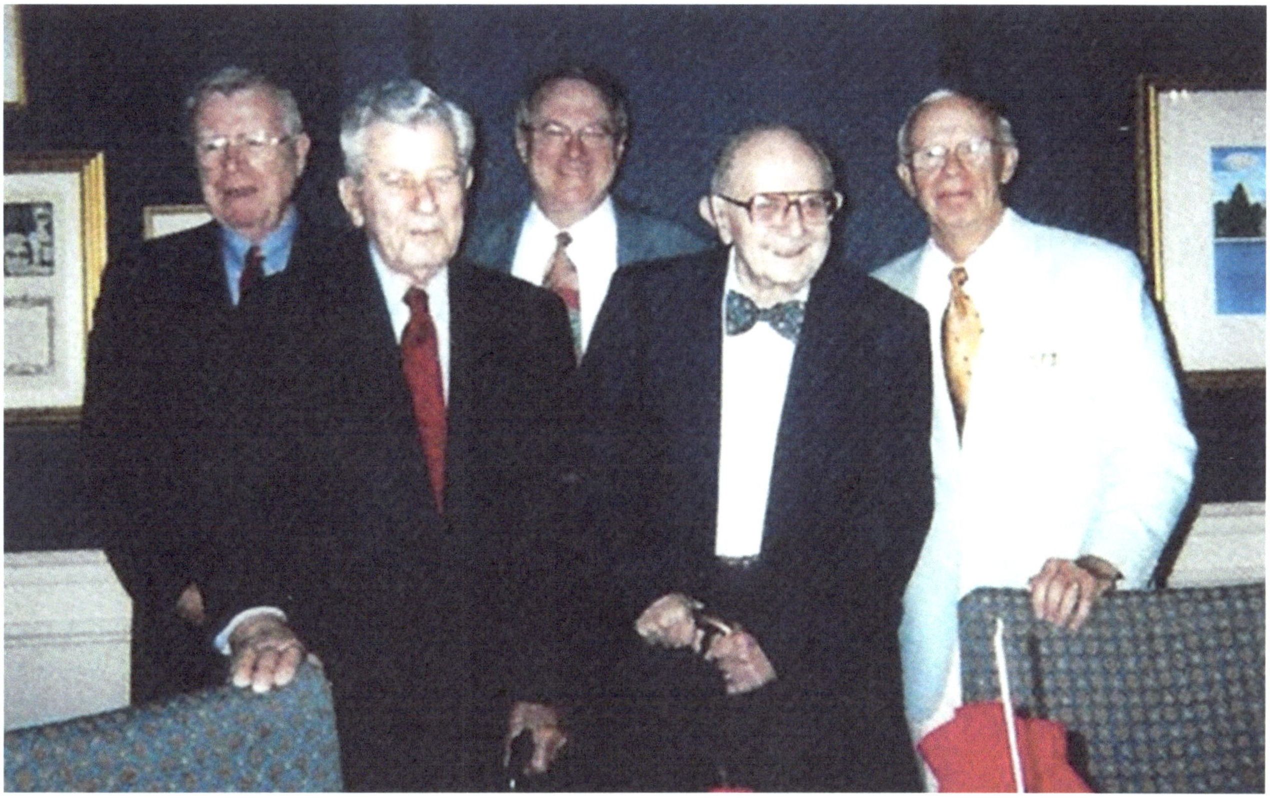

All College of Medicine charter faculty; celebration of Samuel C. Bukantz's retirement; June 2004. Front row (left to right): Samuel C. Bukantz, MD; Lewis A. Barness, MD; H. Worth Boyce, MD.Back row (left to right): Ray A. Olsson, MD; Richard F. Lockey, MD, MS.

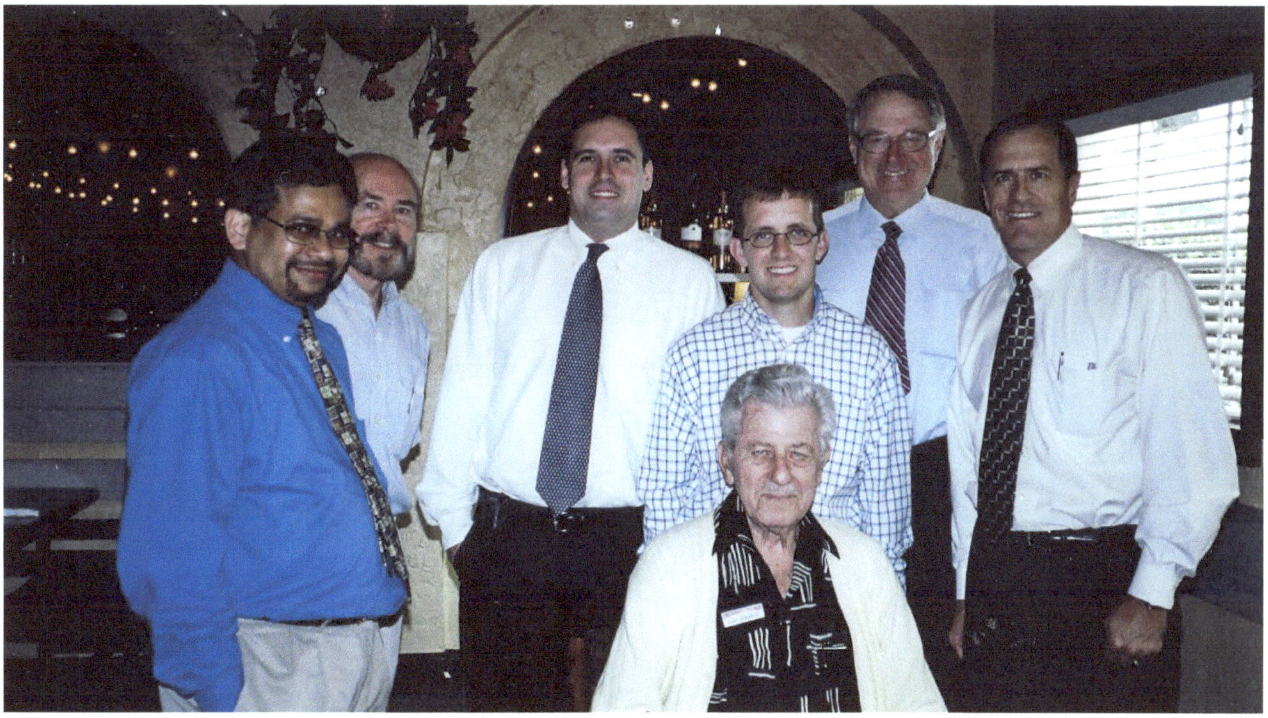

Samuel C. Bukantz, MD (sitting). Left to right: Shyam S. Mohapatra, PhD; Gary Hellermann, PhD; Patrick J. DeMarco, MD (2003-2005); John T. Ramey, MD (2003-2005); Richard F. Lockey, MD, MS; Hugh H. Windom, MD; circa 2004.

news
usf health sciences cen

Distinguished allergist and founding division chief Dr. Samuel Bukantz retires at 92

By Anne DeLotto Baier

Samuel C. Bukantz, MD, professor of medicine in the Division of Allergy and Immunology, retired June 30 following a distinguished career in academic medicine spanning more than 60 years. The Division has applied for Emeritus Professor status for Dr. Bukantz, 92, maintains an affiliate appointment with USF.

Dr. Bukantz joined the USF College of Medicine in 1972 as the first director of the Division of Allergy and Clinical Immunology in the Department of Internal Medicine at USF and chief of the Section of Allergy at James A. Haley Veterans' Hospital. He was among the handful of senior faculty who took night call at the newly opened Haley VA before the internal medicine residency program was filled.

Dr. Bukantz started the allergy and immunology clinic at the VA hospital, and his wife Jewell, a nurse, trained some of the earliest USF fellows in the art of preparing extracts for allergy skin testing.

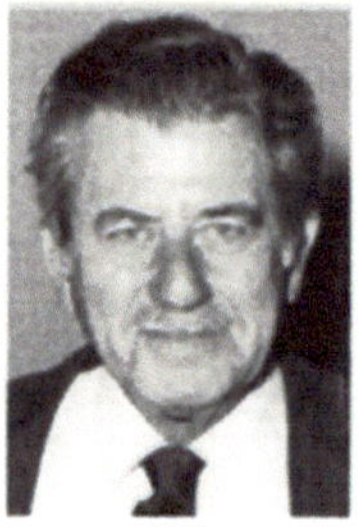

Dr. Bukantz

When Dr. Bukantz stepped down from clinical activities in 1983, he was succeeded by his protégé Richard Lockey, MD.

"He has been an excellent mentor, great physician and my best friend," said Dr. Lockey, professor and chair of Allergy and Clinical Immunology. "Dr. Bukantz is one of the brightest people I've had the pleasure to know and the best at teaching me how to write concisely for scientific publications. I still consult with him on research issues and he always offers invaluable feedback. I am delighted that he will remain active in the Division – it would not be the same without him."

Dr. Bukantz said one of his proudest accomplishments was helping build USF's fledgling allergy division into one of the largest and most well-respected in the country. "Our fellowship program has trained many physicians in the specialty of allergy and immunology who practice in Florida and are leaders in the field," he said.

Dr. Bukantz earned a lifetime of awards for his outstanding contributions to research in allergy and immunology, medical education and community service. In 1992, he was named Laureate of the Florida Chapter of the American College of Physicians — the state chapter's highest honor. Other awards include the Distinguished Clinician Award from the American Academy of Allergy and Immunology in 1991, the USF Distinguished Professor of Medicine Award, and the Henry Hyde Salter Award from the International College of Allergy and Clinical Immunology in 1979.

Dr. Bukantz has served on the editorial board of the *Journal of Allergy and Immunology* and as the editor of *Hospital Practice*. He has edited numerous books with Dr. Lockey, including *Fundamentals of Immunology and Allergy*, the *Primer on Allergic and Immunological Diseases* published by the *Journal of the American Medical Association*, and a recently published third edition of *Allergens and Allergen Immunotherapy*, a text used extensively by allergist training programs across the country.

He received his MD degree in 1934 from New York University College of Medicine.

Dr. Bukantz continues to study how the immune system maintains a lifelong ability to make antibodies to blood group antigens.

USF Health Sciences Center News, 2004.

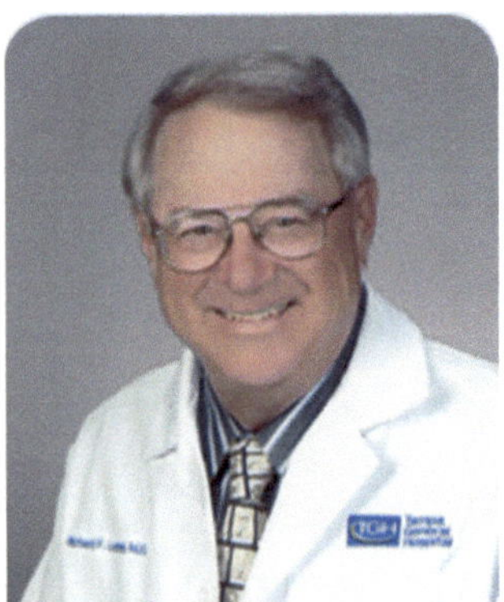

Richard F. Lockey, MD, MS; circa 2005.

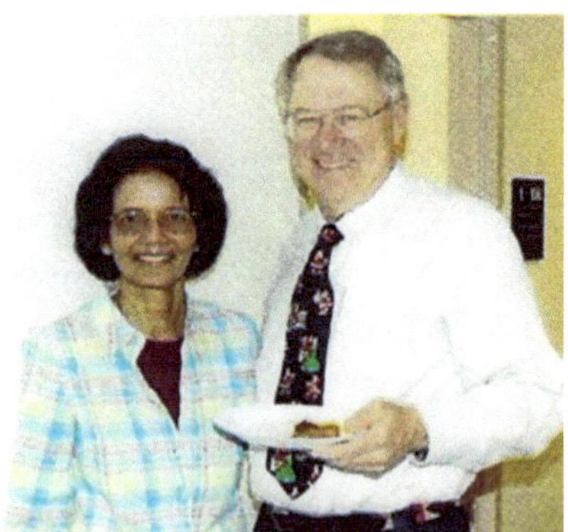

Left to right: Rama Ganguly, PhD; Richard F. Lockey, MD, MS; circa 2005.

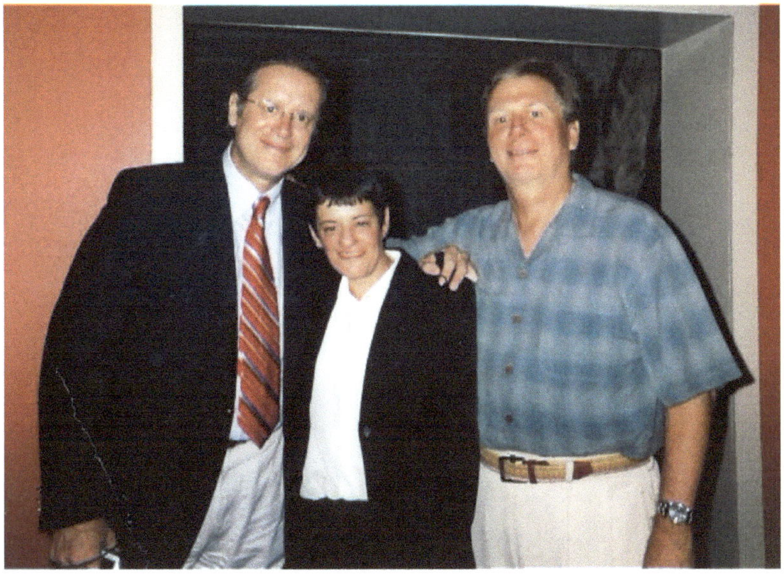

Left to right: Enrique Fernandez-Caldas, PhD; Rosa Codina, PhD; Roger W. Fox, MD

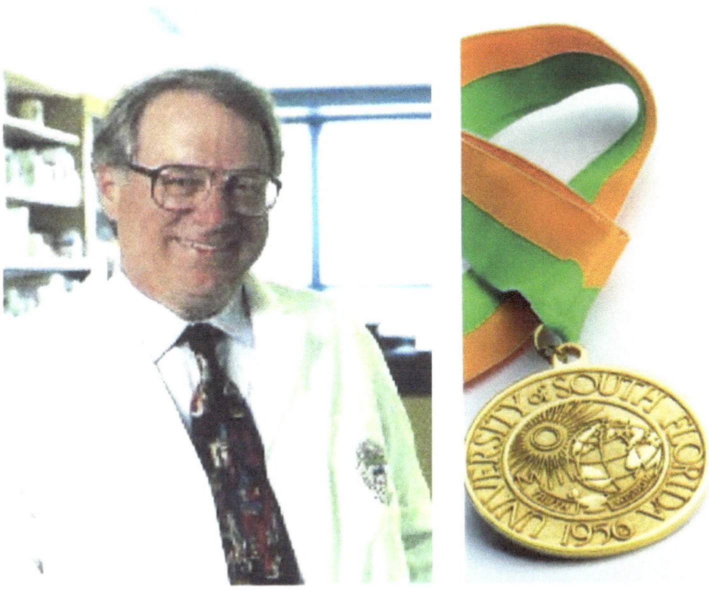

Richard F. Lockey, MD, MS; 2007; Charter member of USF Distinguished University Health Professors.
Dr. Lockey was recommended by his peers because of his significant achievements in research, teaching, and clinical care.

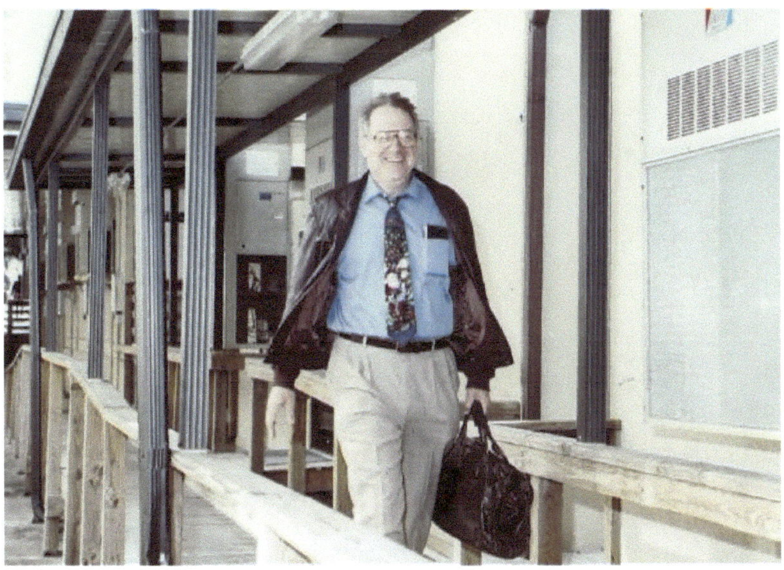

Richard F. Lockey, MD, MS; sidewalk construction outside VA Building 41, circa 2006.

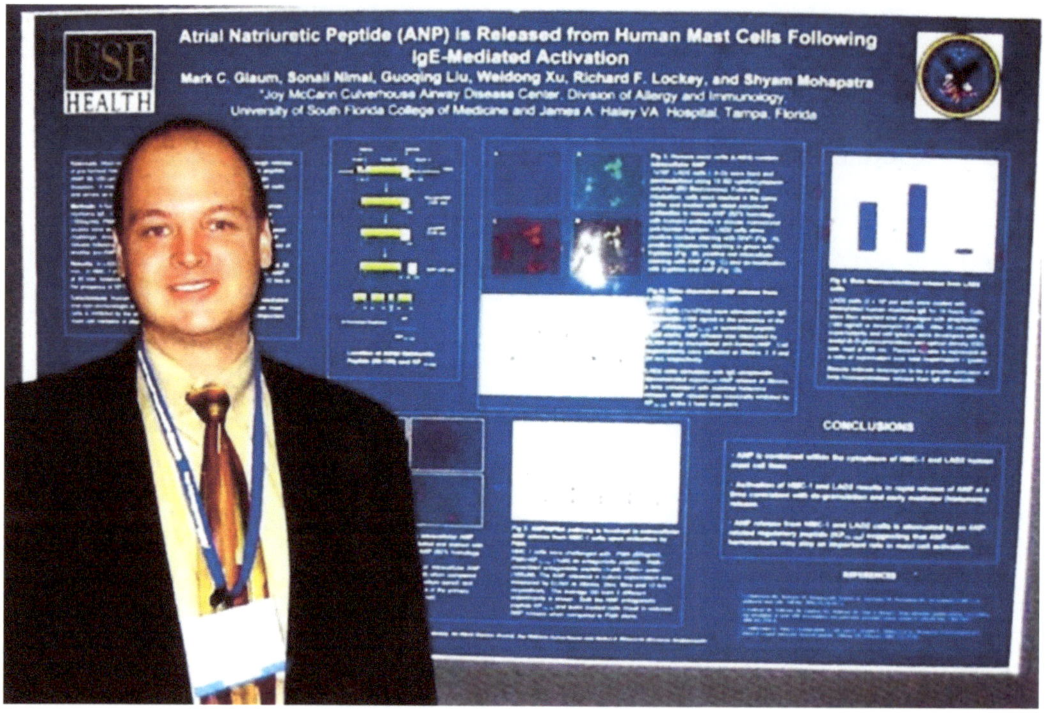

Mark C. Glaum, MD, PhD; 2007 American Academy of Allergy Asthma & Immunology Annual Meeting. Poster: "Atrial Natriuretic Peptide (ANP) is Released from Human Mast Cells Following IgE-Mediated Activation.

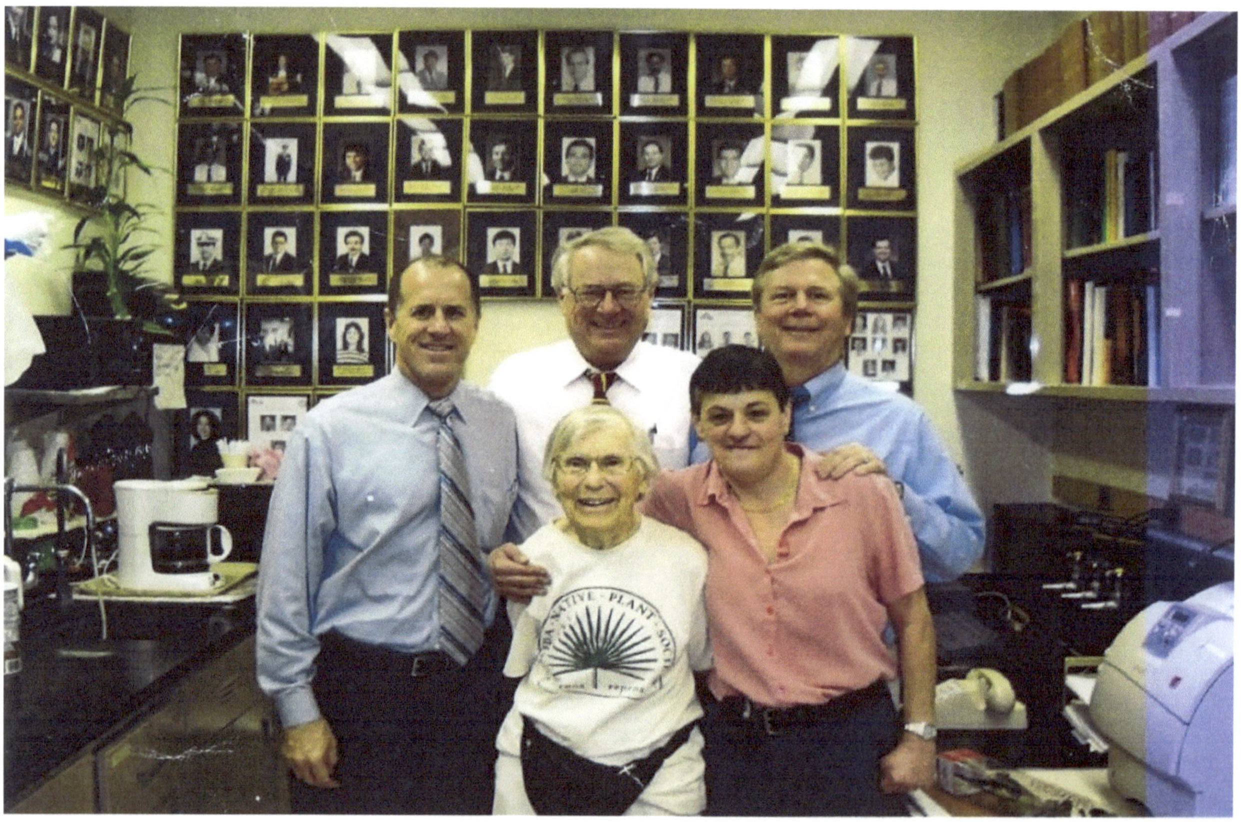

In the fellows' room in the VA Research Building (Building II) in 2010. Note the picture gallery of Division graduates in the background. Front row, left to right: Mary Jelks, MD, Rosa Codina, PhD. Back row, left to right: Hugh H. Windom, MD, Richard F. Lockey, MD, MS; Roger W. Fox, MD.

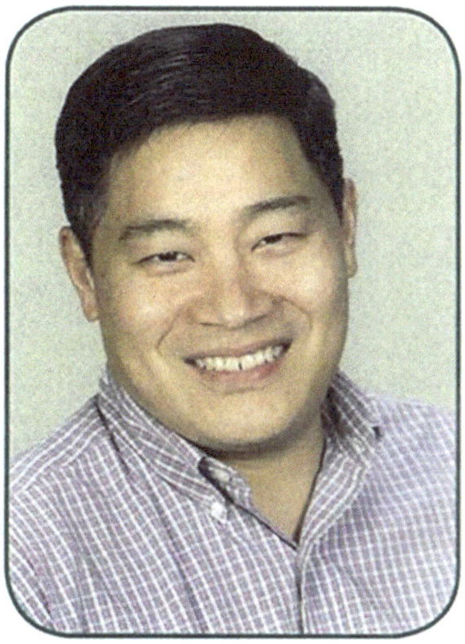

Michael N. Teng, PhD; 2010.

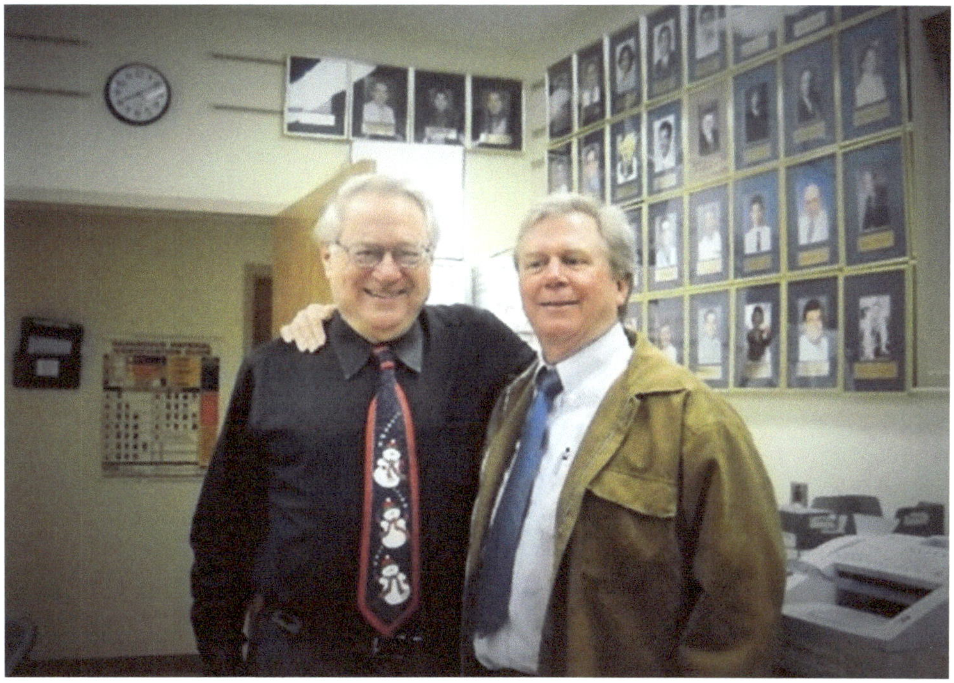

Richard F. Lockey, MD, MS and Roger W. Fox, MD (1978-1980); 2012.

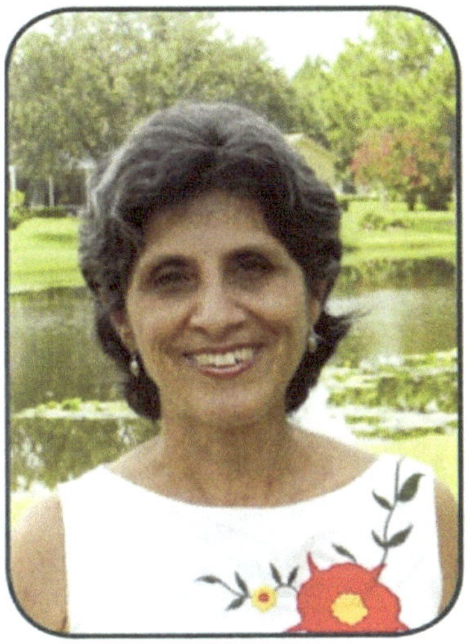

Blanca Camoretti-Mercado, PhD; 2012.

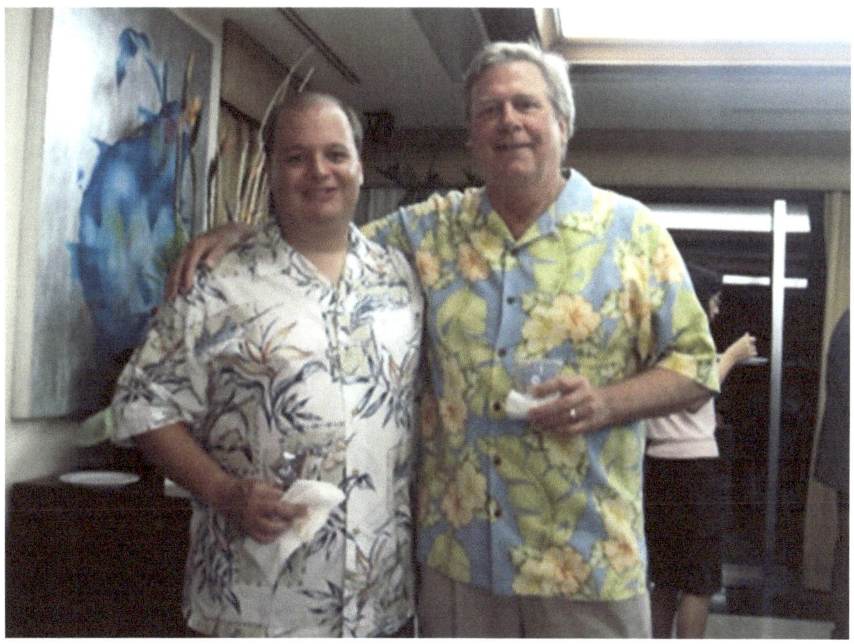

Mark C. Glaum, MD, PhD and Roger W. Fox, MD (1978-1980); circa 2011.

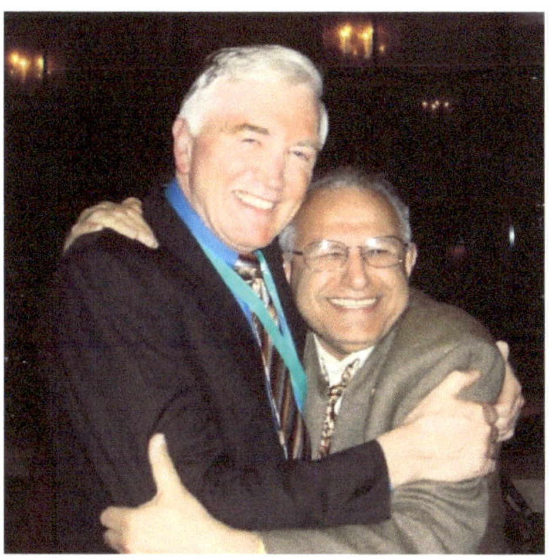

Dennis K. Ledford, MD and Sami Bahna, MD; circa 2010.

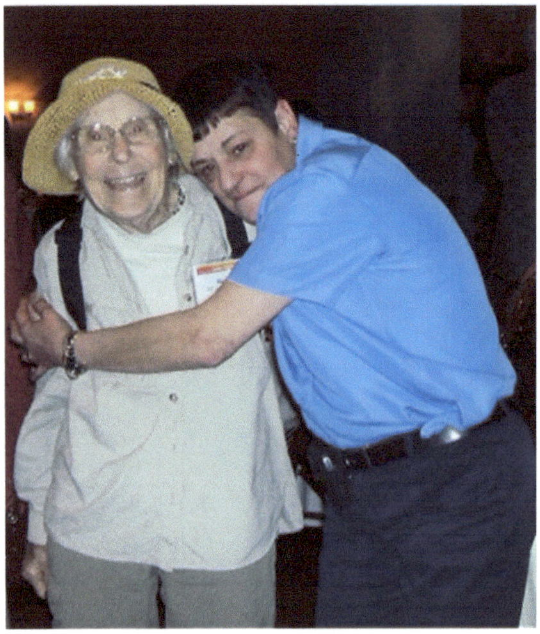

2012 American Academy of Allergy Asthma & Immunology Annual Meeting. Left to right: Mary Jelks, MD and Rosa Codina, PhD.

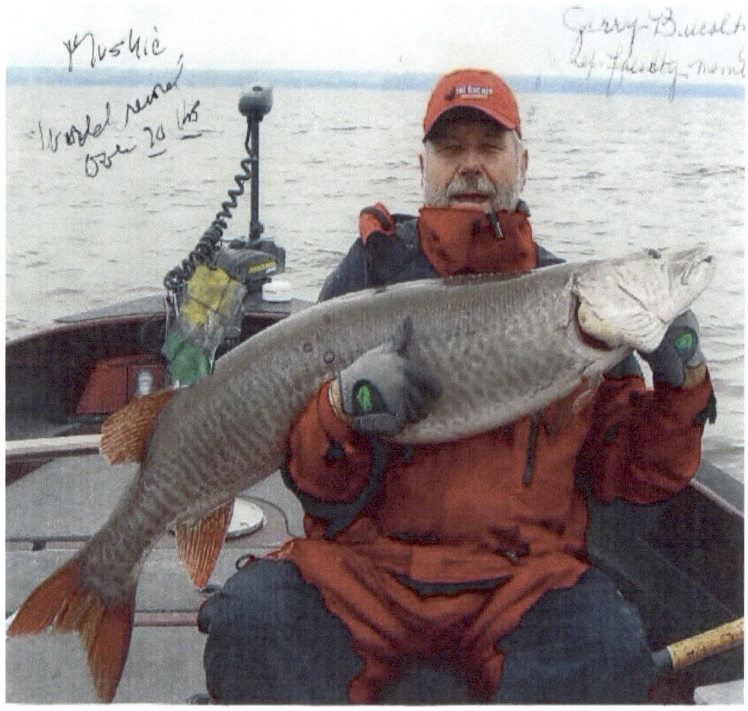

Gerald A. Bucholtz, MD; circa 2015.

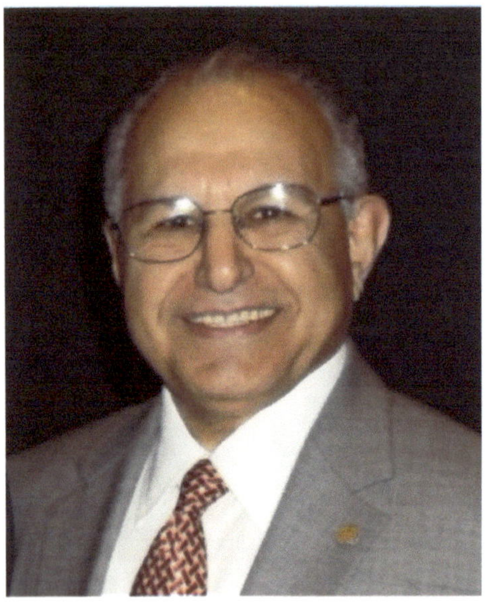

Sami Bahna, MD, DrPH; circa 2015.

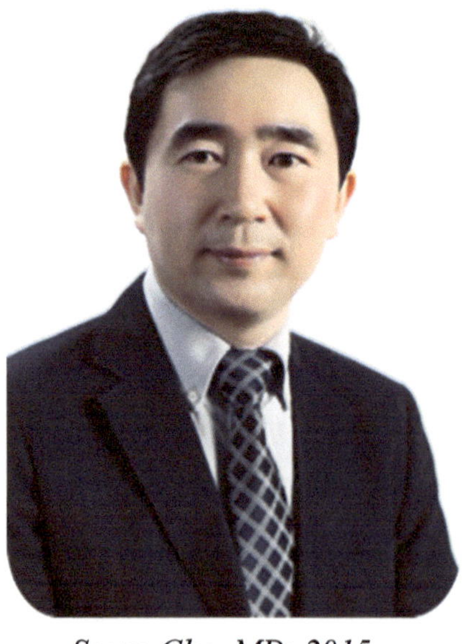

Seong Cho, MD; 2015.

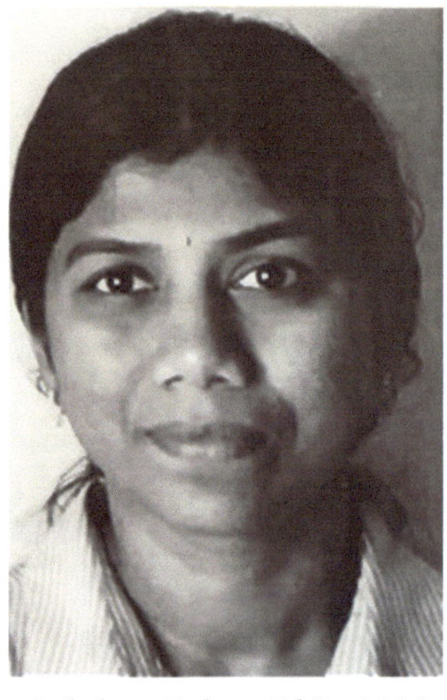

Lakshmi Galam, PhD; 2016.

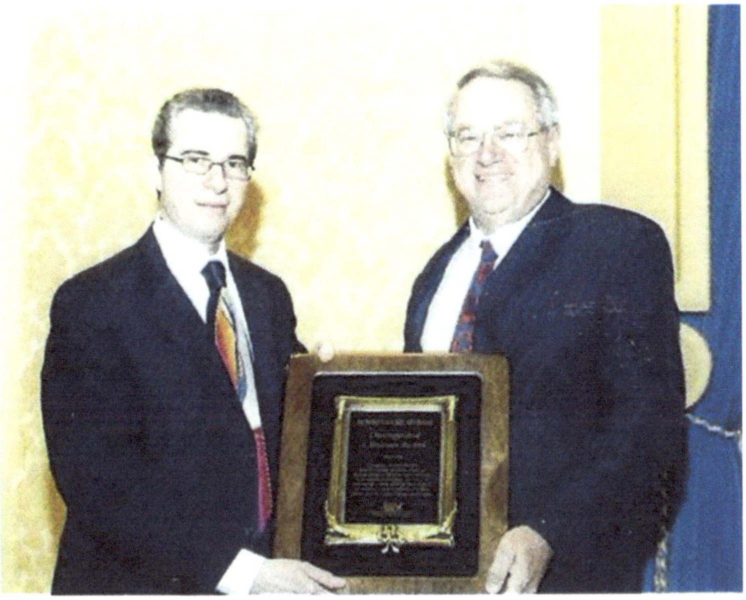

Richard F. Lockey, MD, MS receiving the Distinguished Service Award at the 2016 American Academy of Allergy Asthma & Immunology Annual Meeting. Left to right: Thomas B. Casale, MD and Richard F. Lockey, MD, MS.

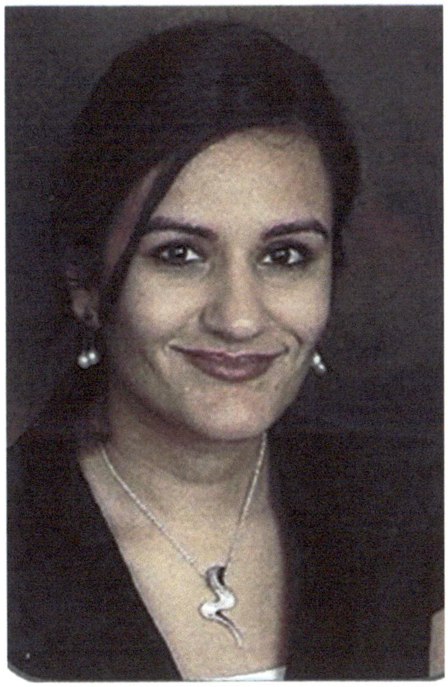

Farnaz Tabatabaian, MD; 2016.

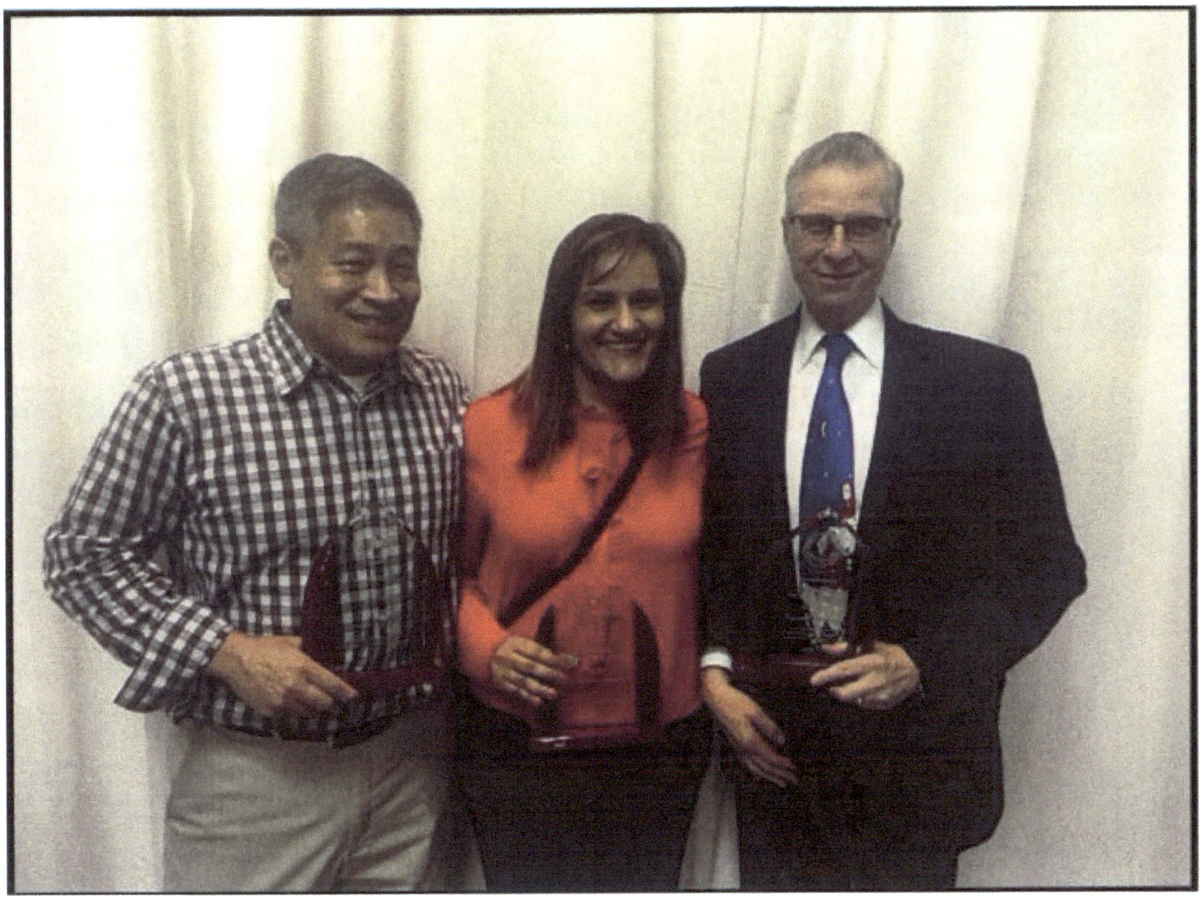

Left to right: Michael Teng, PhD (Excellence in Basic Research); Farnaz Tabatabaian, MD (Excellence in Patient Care); Thomas B. Casale, MD (Excellence in Clinical Research); awards from the USF Department of Internal Medicine; 2017.

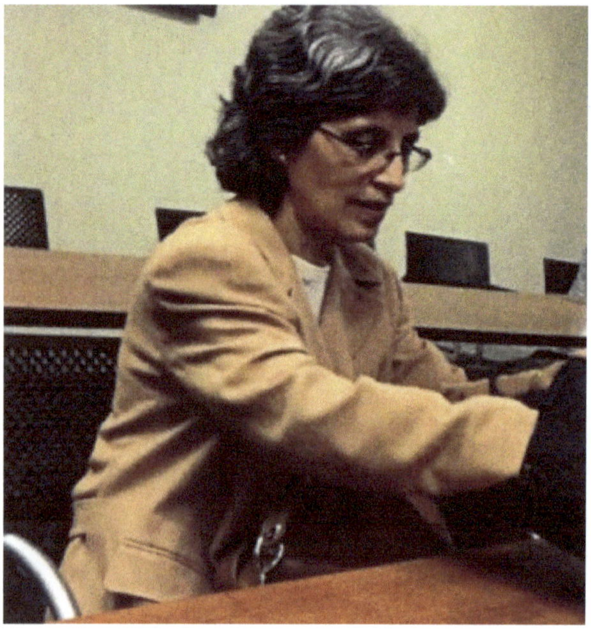

Blanca Camoretti-Mercado, PhD; 2016.

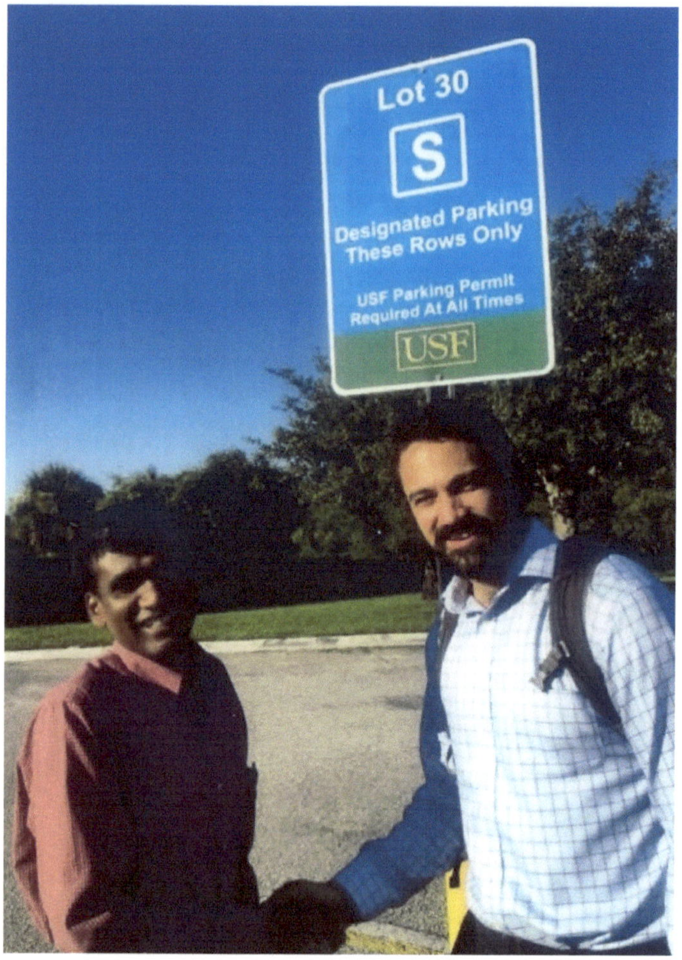

Lot 30
S
Designated Parking
These Rows Only
USF Parking Permit
Required At All Times
USF

Narasaiah Kolliputi, PhD welcoming new faculty member, Juan Carlos Cardet, MD, MPH; 2017.

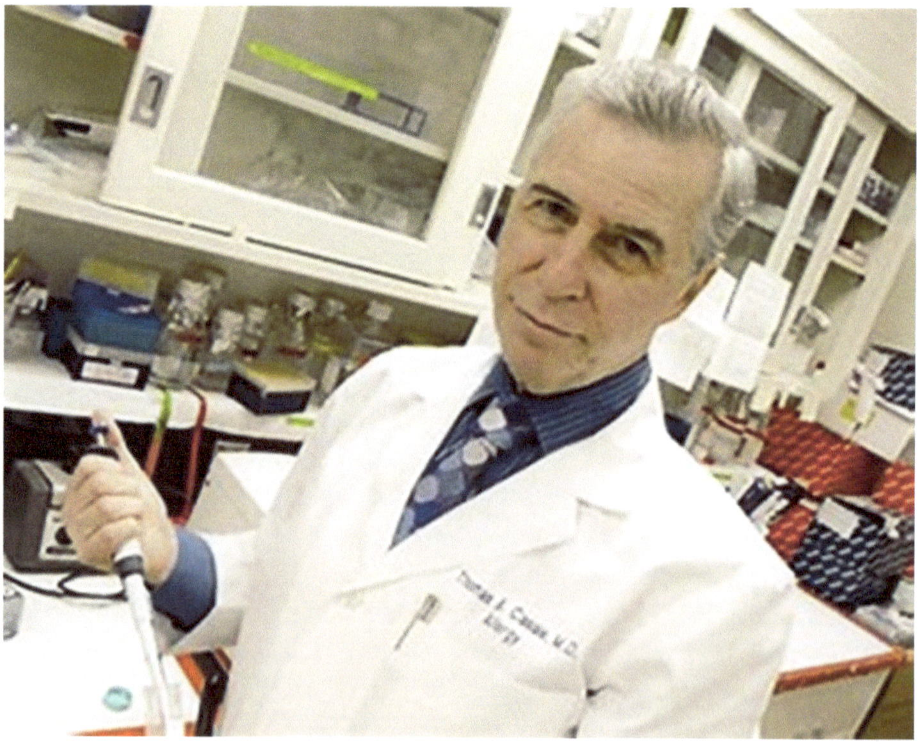

Thomas B. Casale, MD; 2017.

Chapter 4: Department of Internal Medicine, Allergy and Immunology Fellows

Please note that the years listed by the physician's name designate the years fellowship training occurred. Pictures were not necessarily taken during the years indicated.

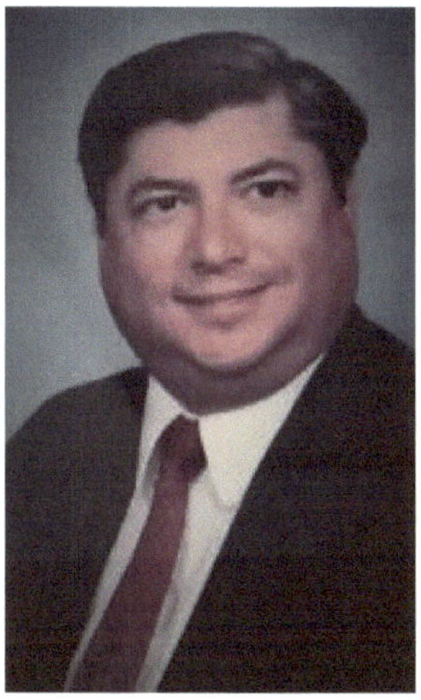

Jack Parrino, MD (1977-1979)

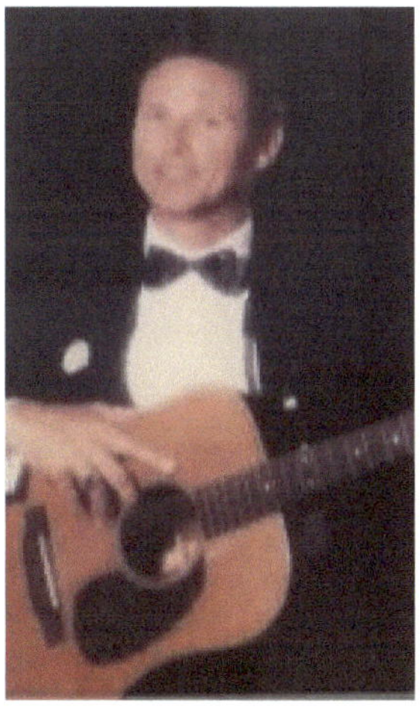

J. Wayne Phillips, MD (1977-1979)

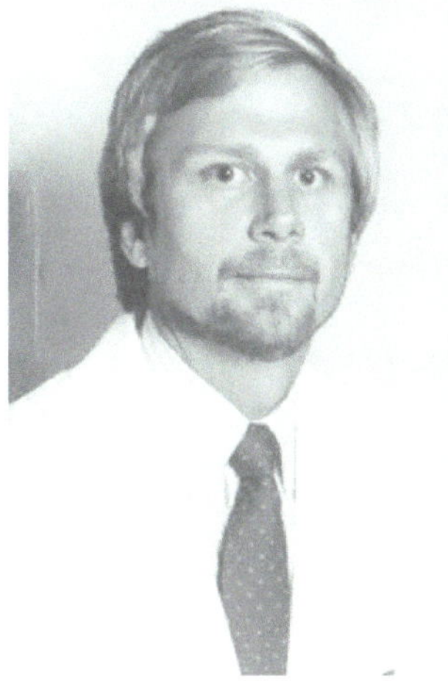

Roger W. Fox, MD (1978-1980)

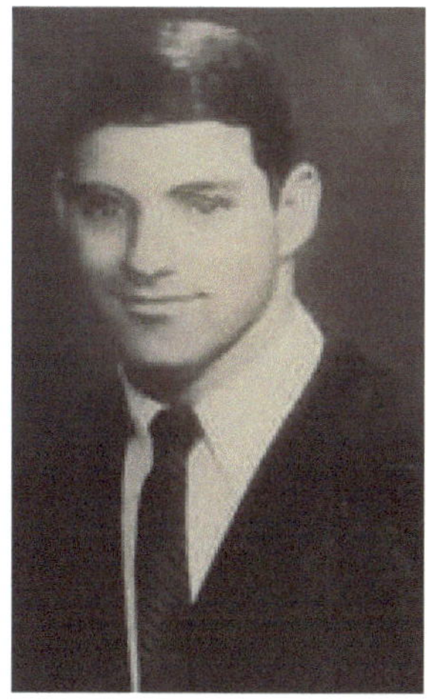

Linn R. Klotz, MD (1979-1981)

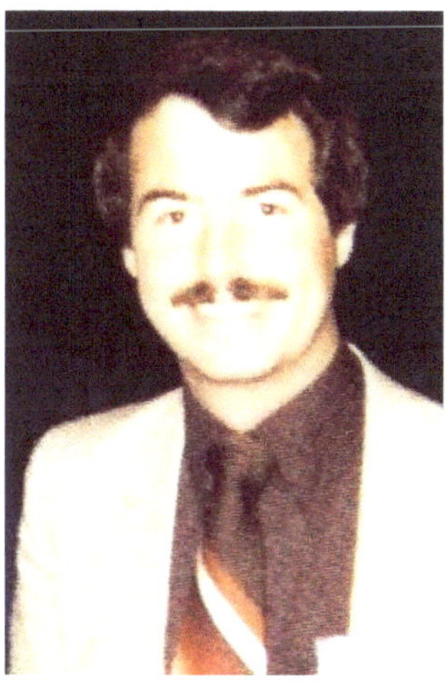

John J. Stablein, MD (1979-1981)

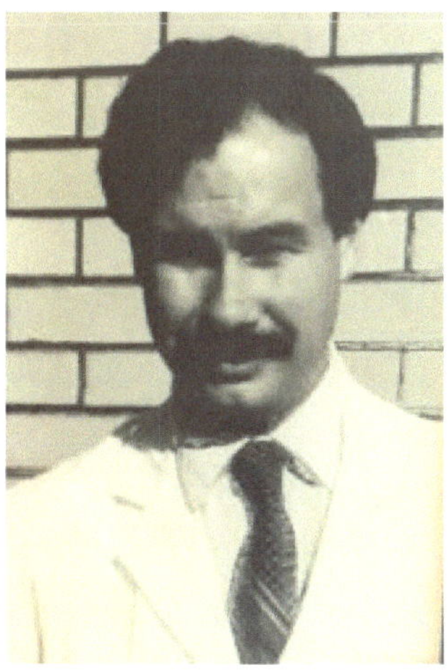

Gerald A. Bucholtz, MD (1980-1982)

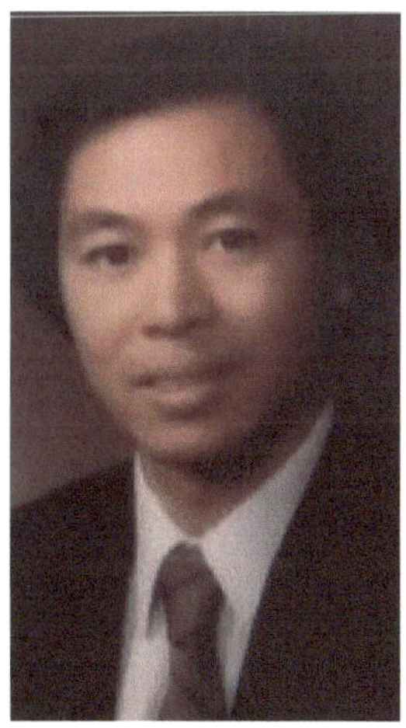

Steven J. Louie, MD (1981-1983)

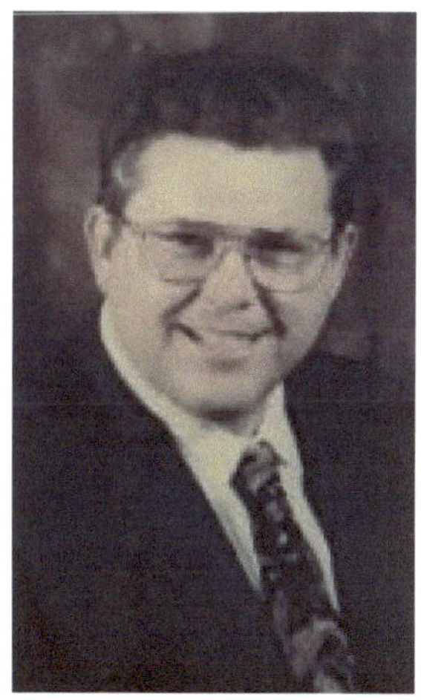

Albert E. Hensel, MD (1982-1984)

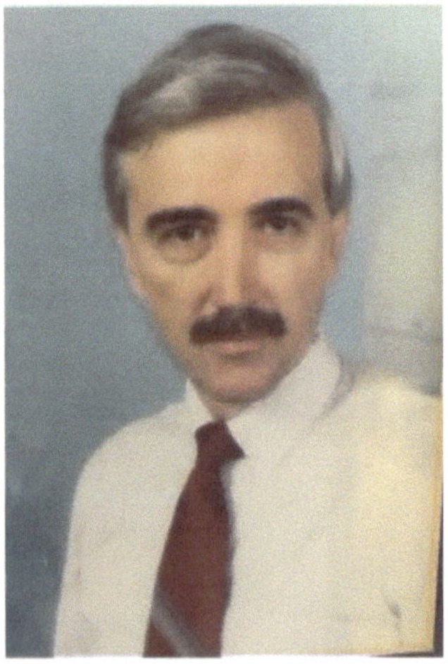

Dennis K. Ledford, MD (1983-1985)

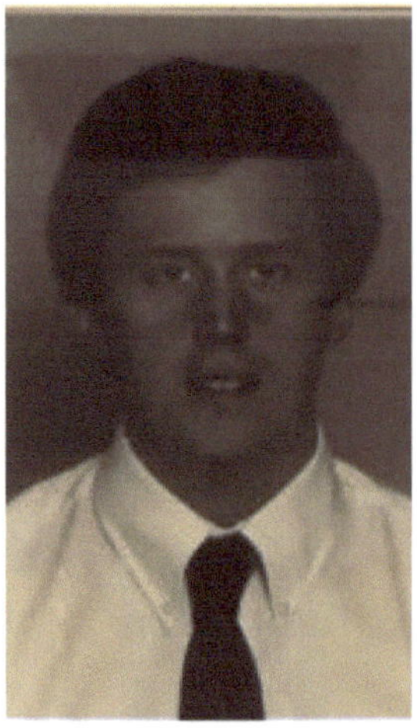

Mark W. Minor, MD (1985-1987)

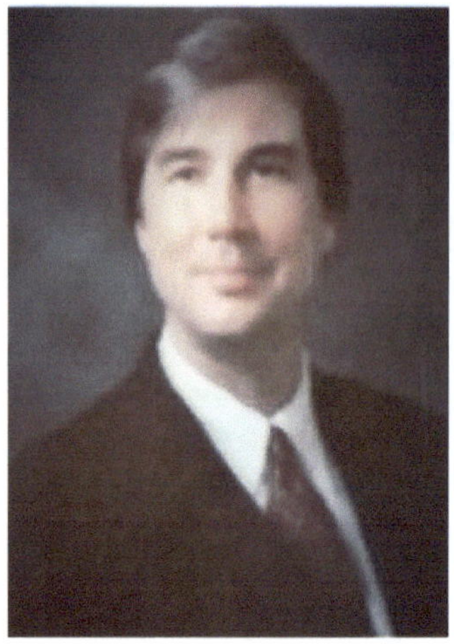

Robert P. Nelson, MD (1985-1987)

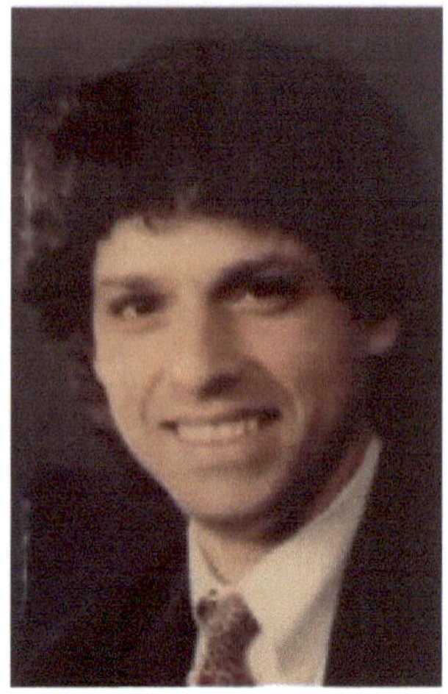

Joseph D. Diaz, MD (1986-1988)

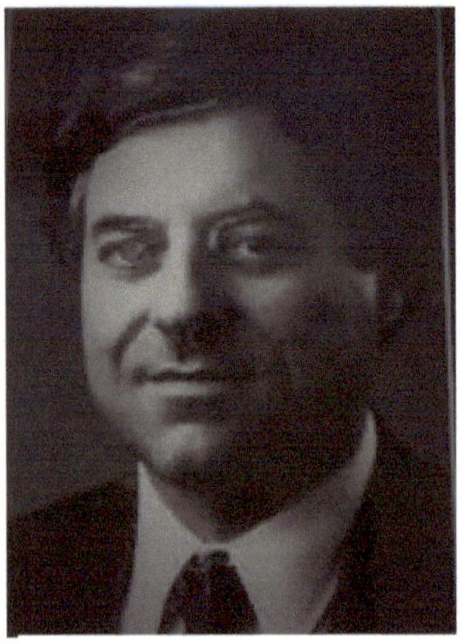

Donald W. Russell, MD (1987-1990)

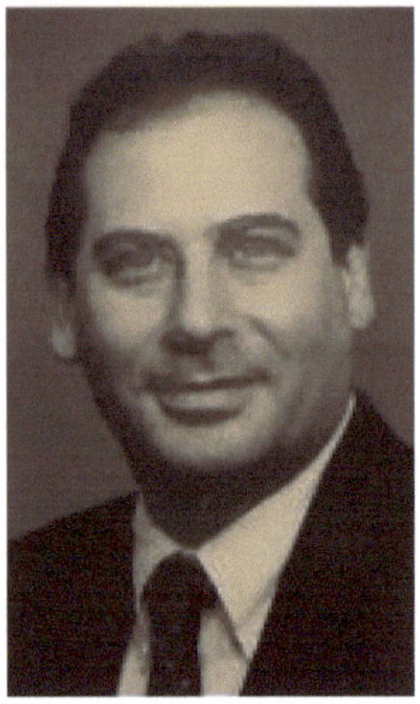

Richard P. Silton, MD (1988-1990)

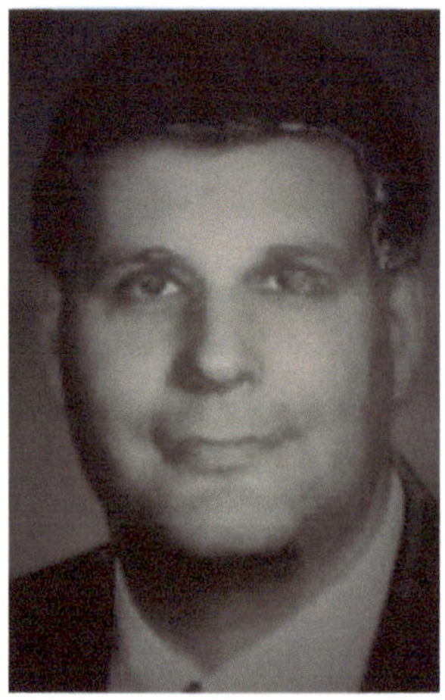

David N. Wright, MD (1988-1991)

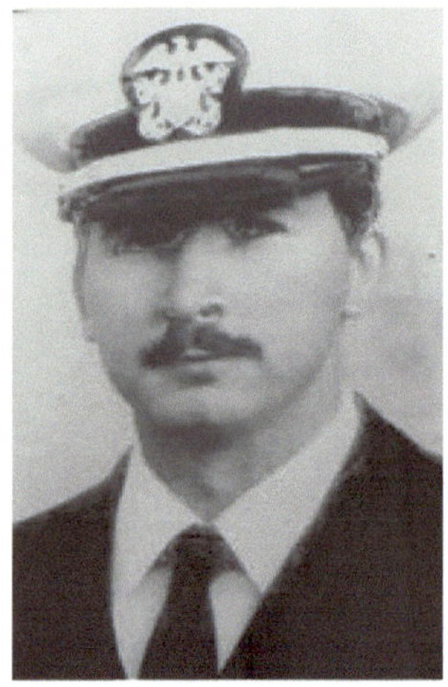

Thomas B. Edwards, MD (1990-1992)

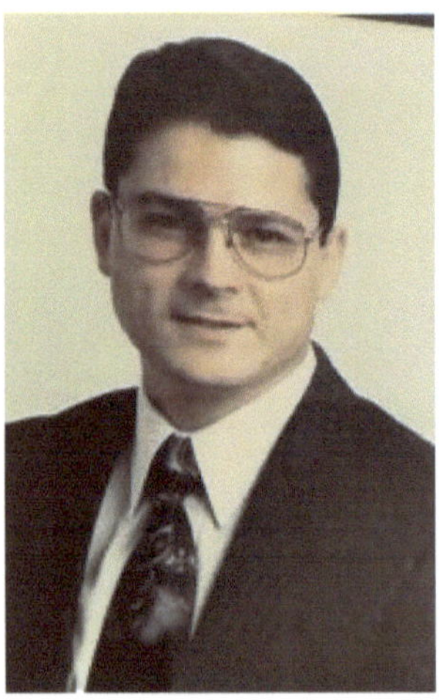

Carlos M. Jacinto, MD (1990-1992)

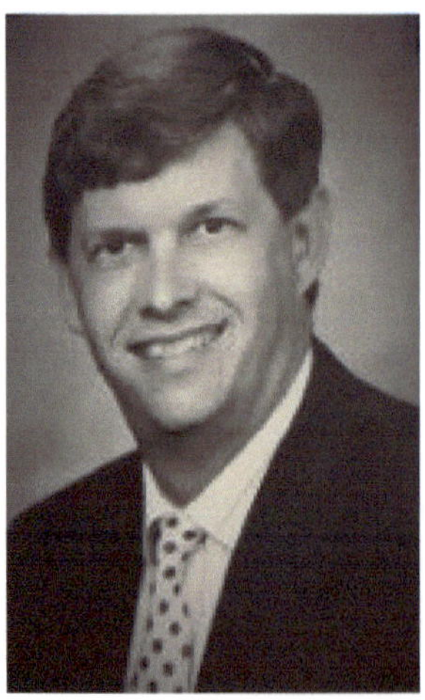

G. Edward Stewart, MD (1991-1994)

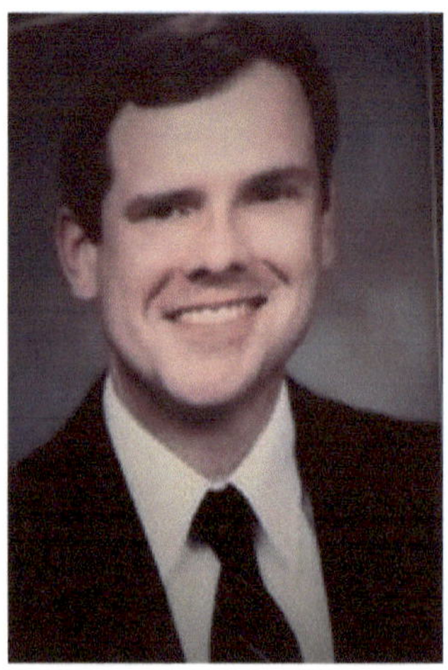

Stephen F. Kemp, MD (1993-1996)

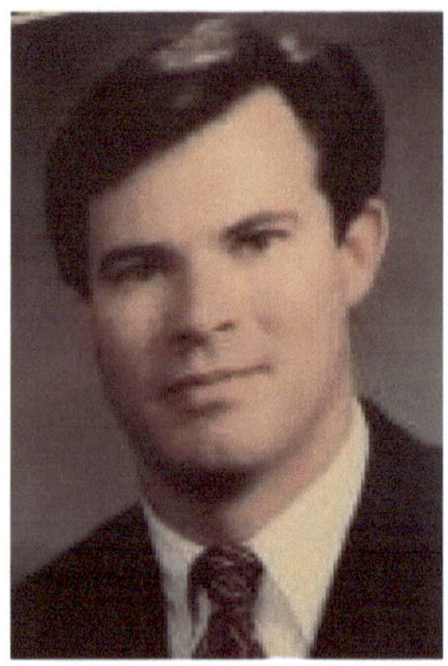

Brett E. Stanaland, MD (1992-1995)

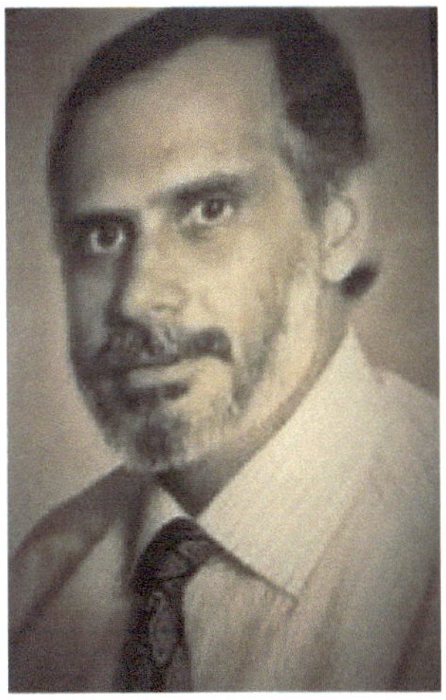

Jose Andrade, MD (1993-1995)

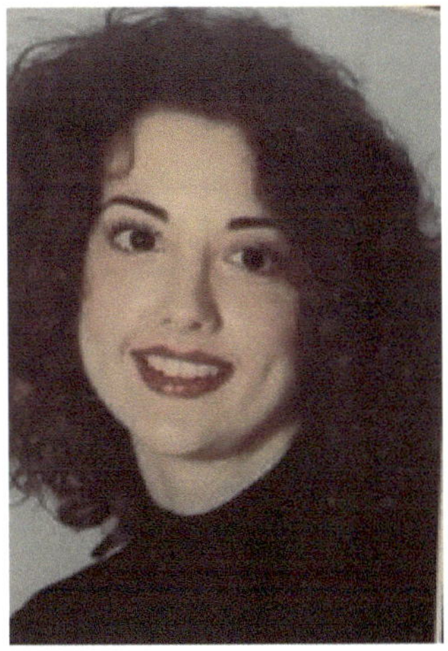

Lizette S. Hernandez, MD (1994-1997)

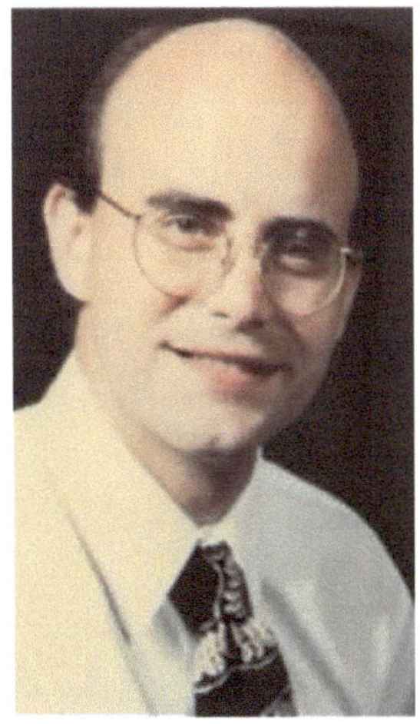

Kevin P. Rosenbach, MD (1995-1998)

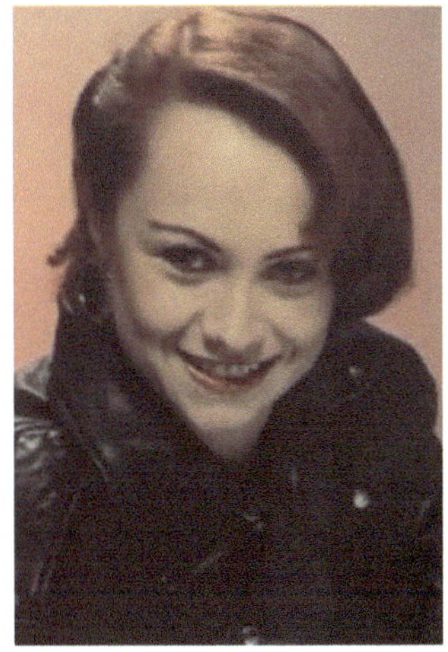

Giana L. Nicoara-Kasti, MD (1996-1998).

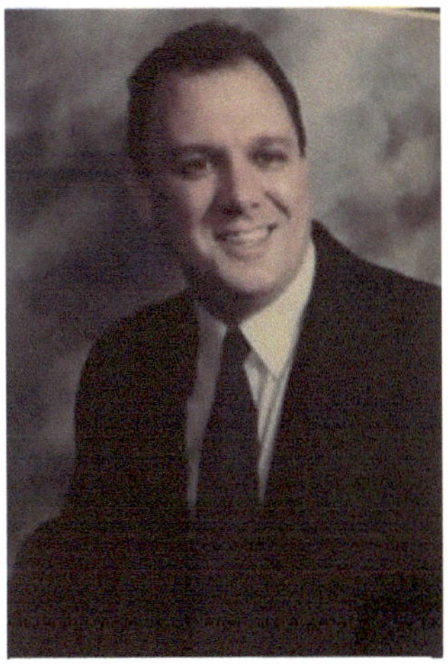

Demetrios S. Theodoropoulos, MD (1997-2000)

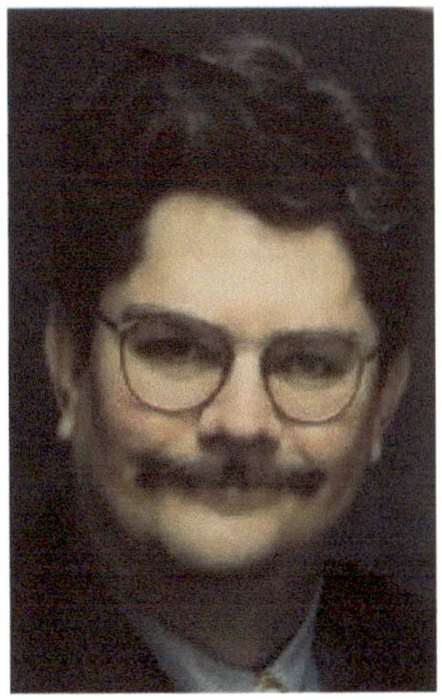

Thomas W. Luck, MD (1999-2001)

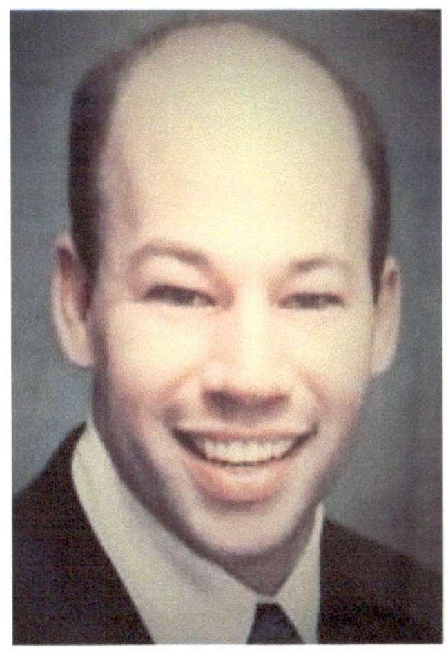

Daniel A. Reichmuth, MD (1999-2002)

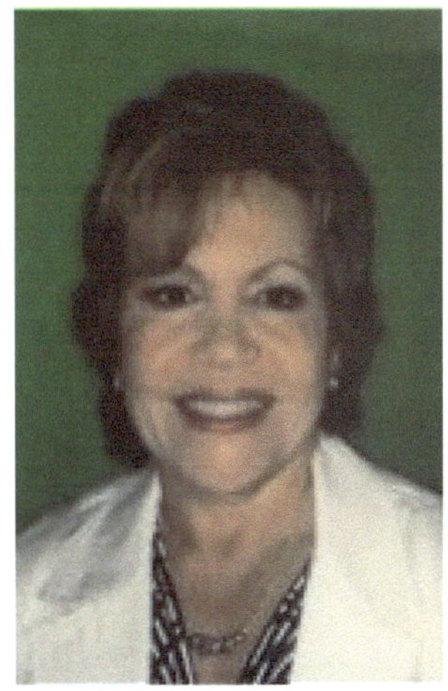

Nina C. Ramirez, MD (2000-2002)

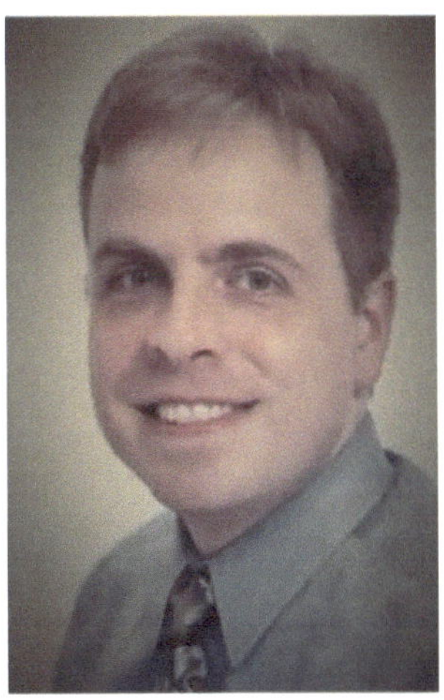

Richard E. Crockett, MD (2000-2003)

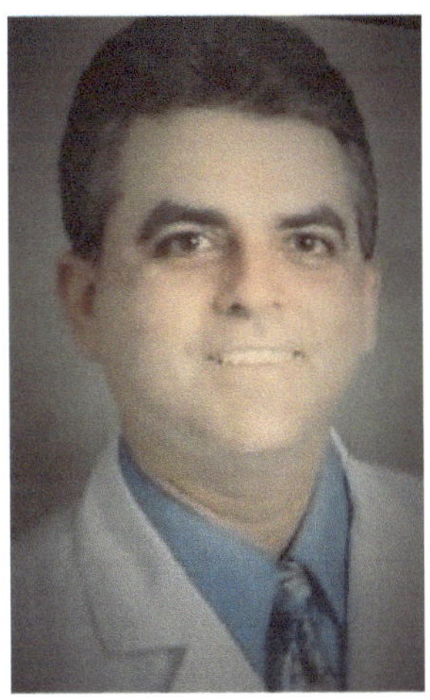

Jose R. Arias, Jr., MD (2001-2003)

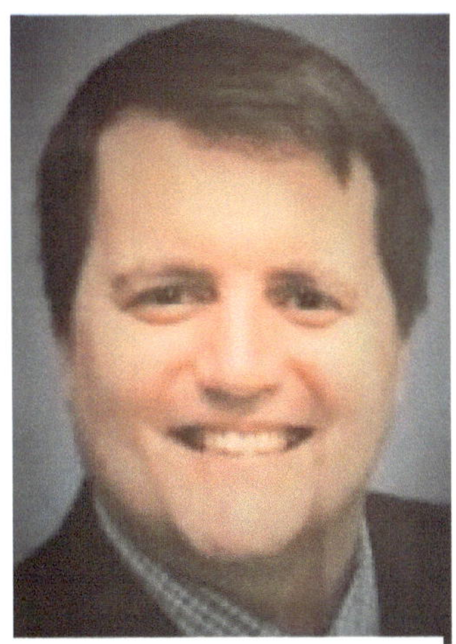

A. Sean McKnight, MD (2002-2004)

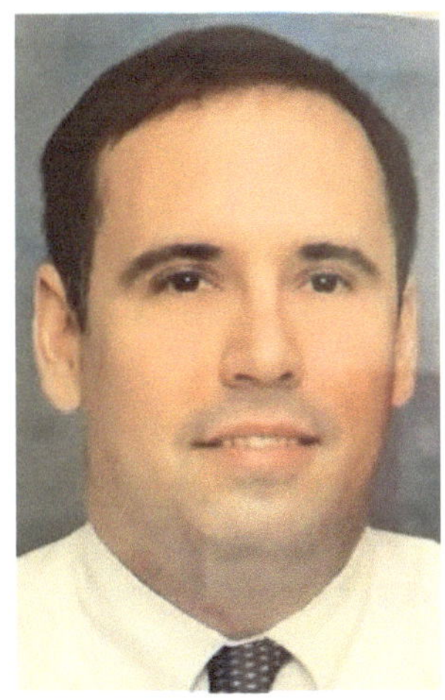

Patrick J. DeMarco, MD (2003-2005)

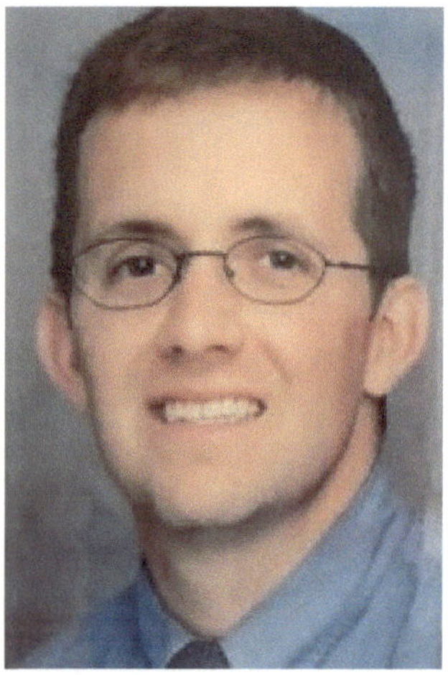

John T. Ramey, MD
(2003-2005)

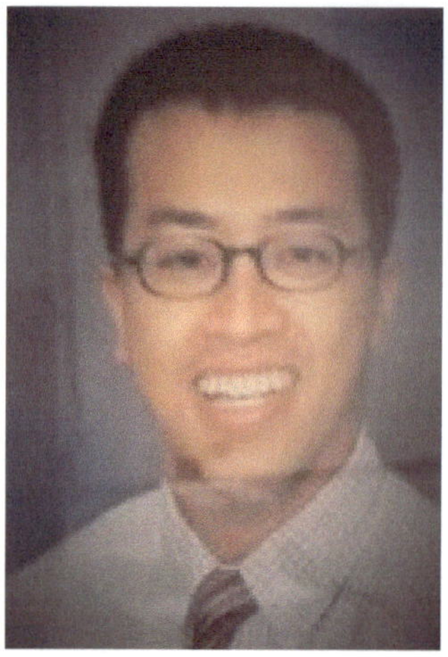

Alex T. Vu, MD
(2004-2006)

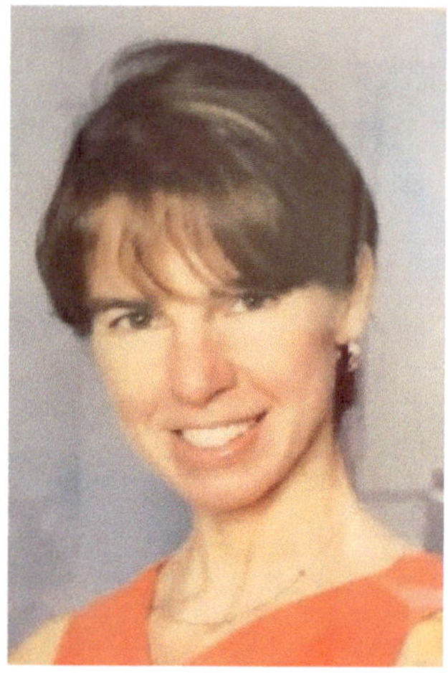

Denise M. Kearney, MD
(2004-2006)

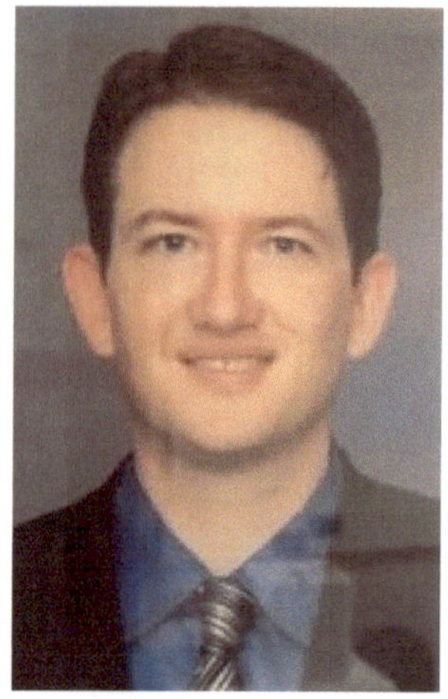

Steven L. Cole, DO
(2005-2007)

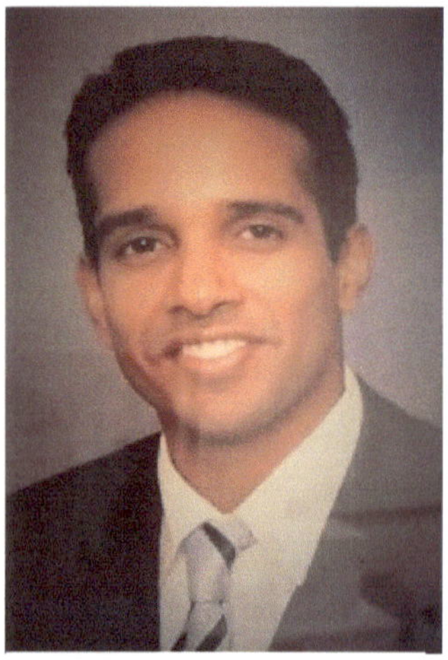

Thomas Chacko, MD
(2005-2007)

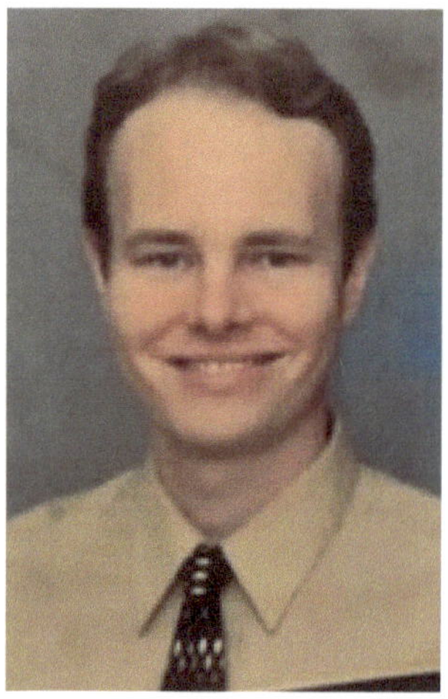

Andrew Bagg, MD
(2006-2008)

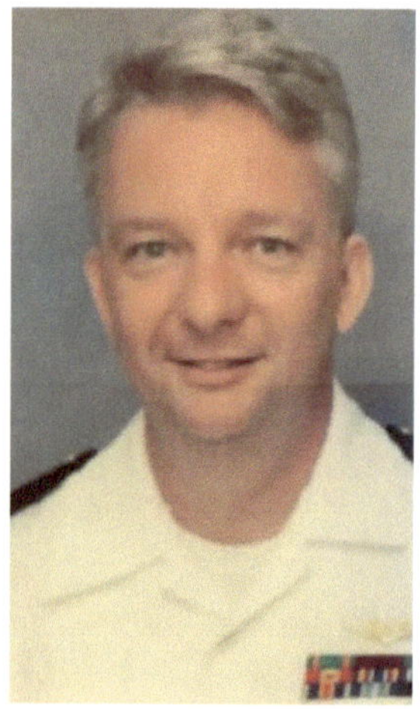

Ronald Purcell, MD
(2006-2008)

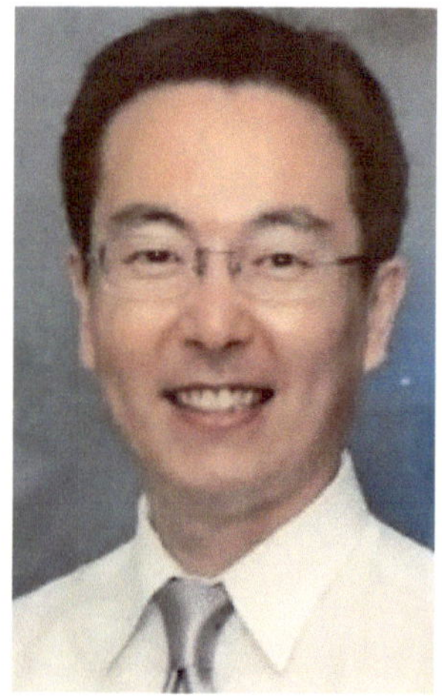

Byol Shin, DO
(2006-2008)

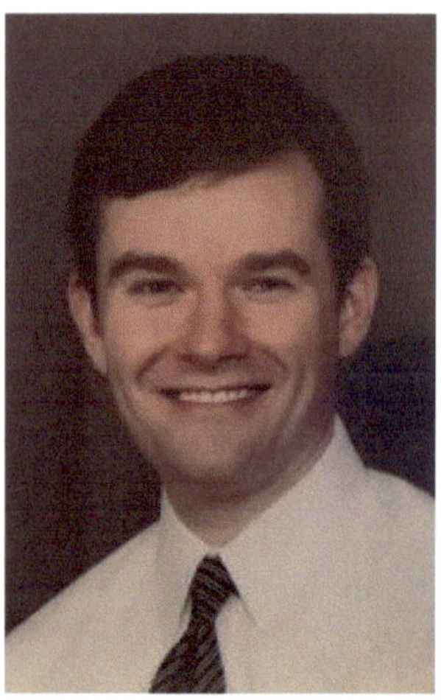

Joshua Phillips, MD
(2007-2009)

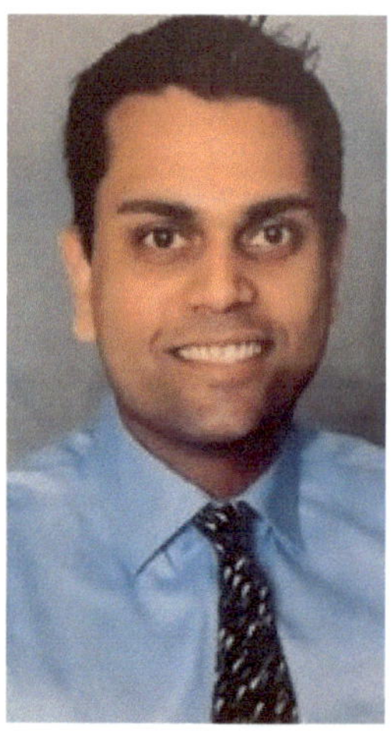

Mathew Varghese, MD
(2007-2009)

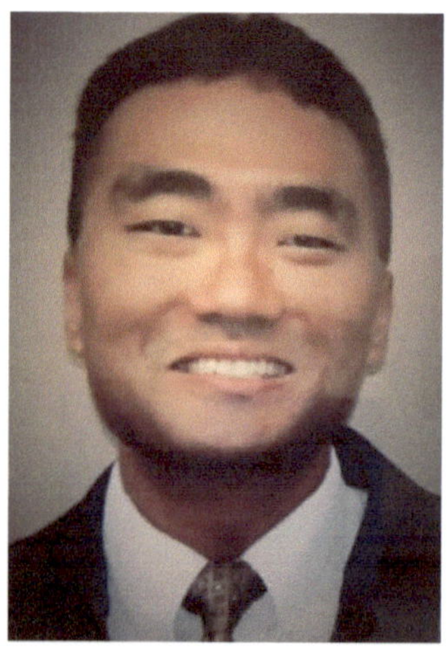

Dennis Kim, MD
(2008-2010)

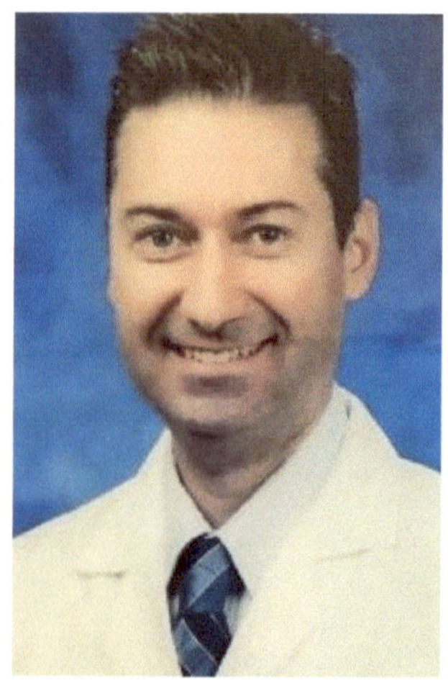

Efren Rael, MD
(2008-2010)

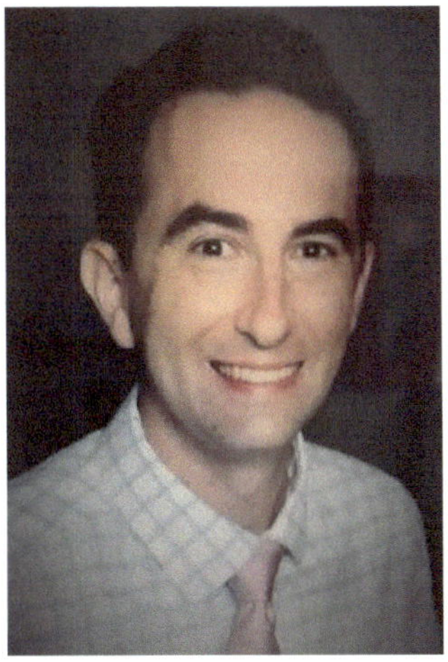

Robert (Robbie) Pesek, MD
(2009-2011)

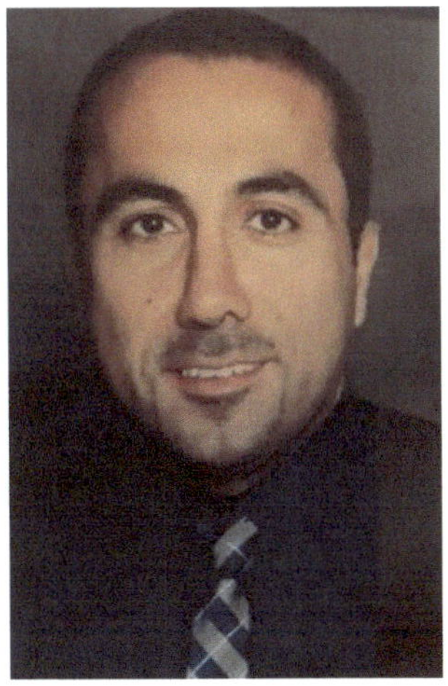

Michel Alkhalil, MD
(2009-2011)

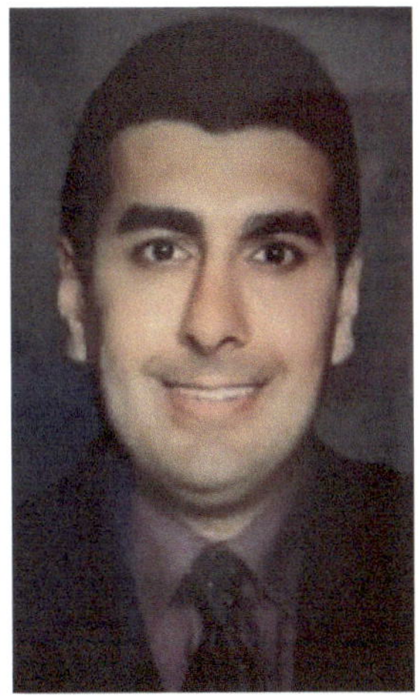

Ahmed Butt, MD
(2010-2012)

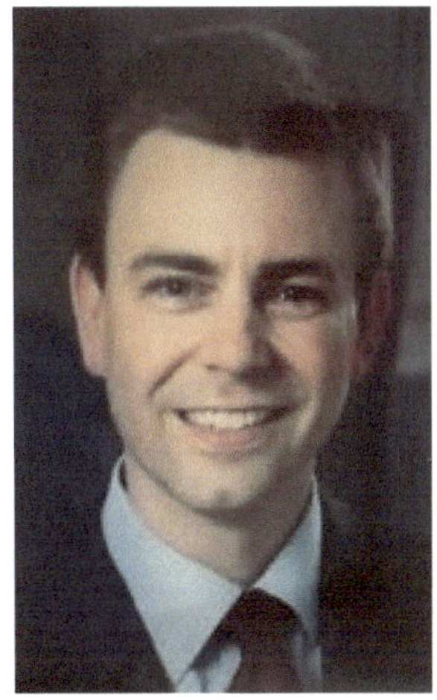

David Fitzhugh, MD
(2010-2012)

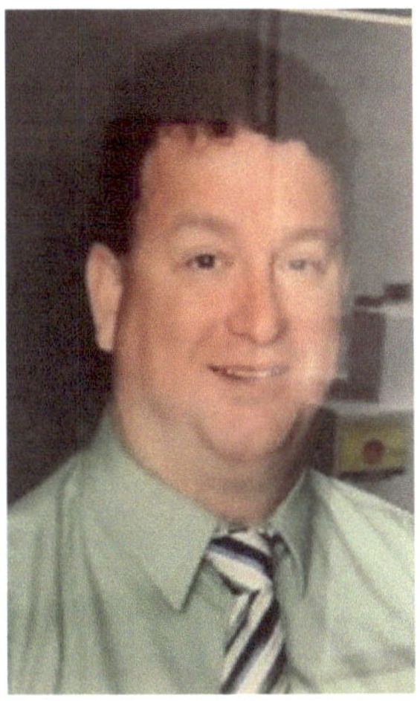

James Parkerson, DO
(2010-2012)

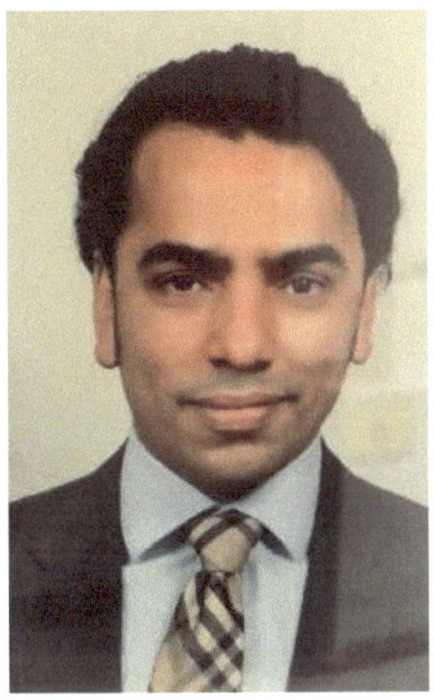

Salman Aljubran, MD
(2010-2013)

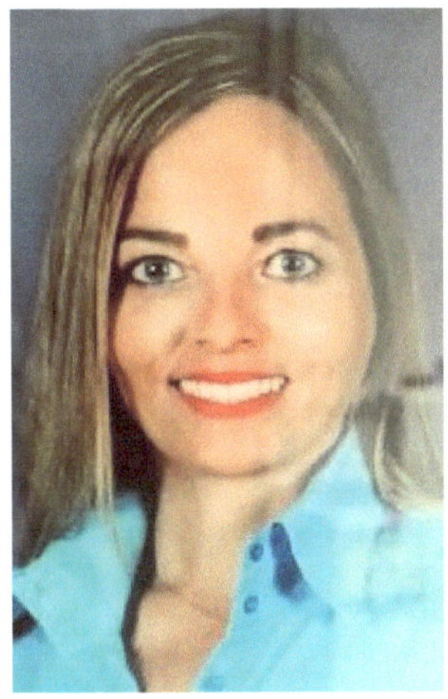

Susan Culverhouse, MD
(2011-2013)

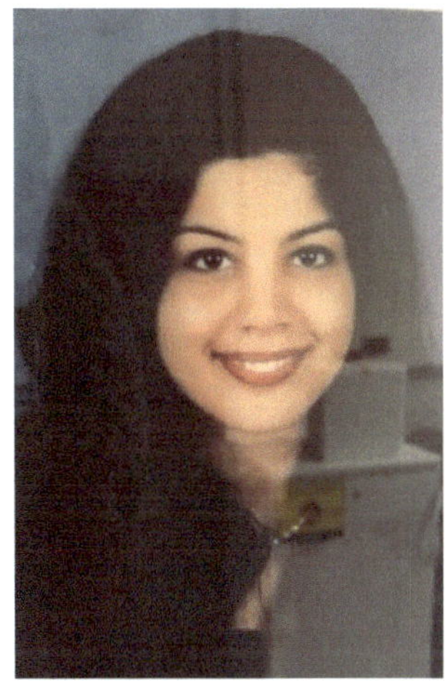

Neetu Talreja, MD
(2011-2013)

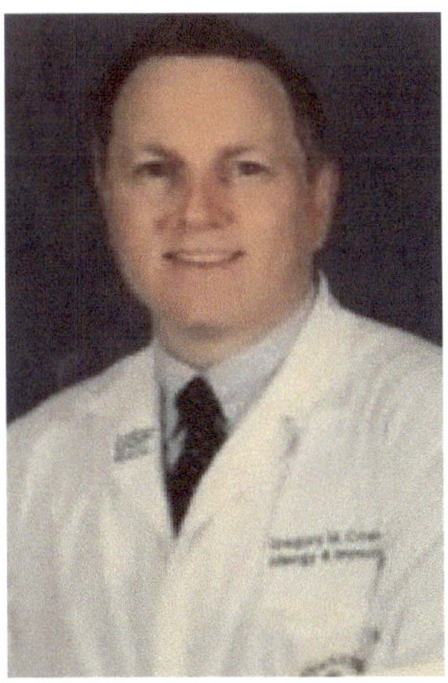

Gregory M. Cowan, MD
(2012-2014)

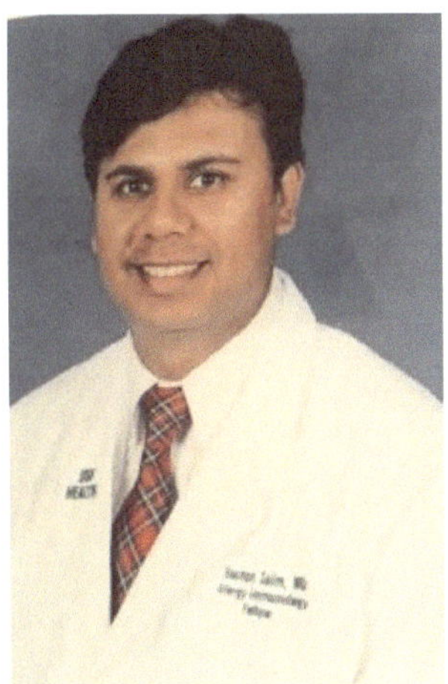

Nauman Salim, MD
(2012-2014)

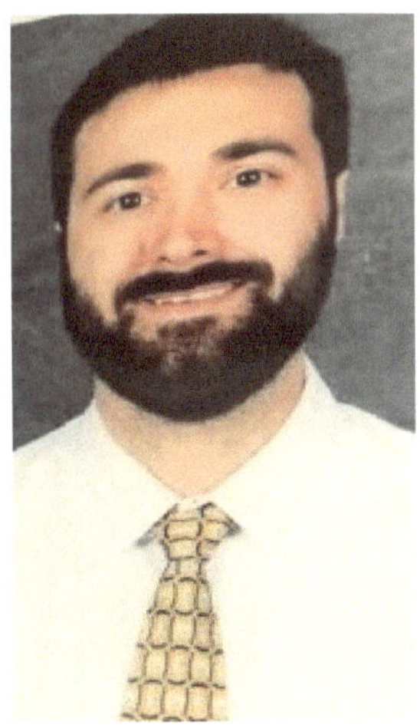

Michael C. Balduzzi, MD
(2013-2015)

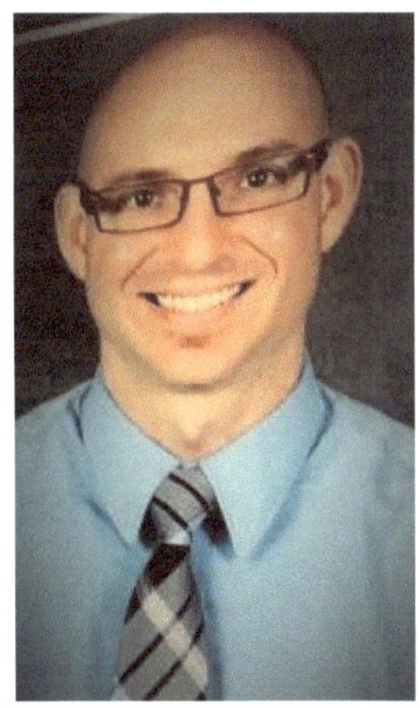

Adam C. Updegraff, DO
(2013-2015)

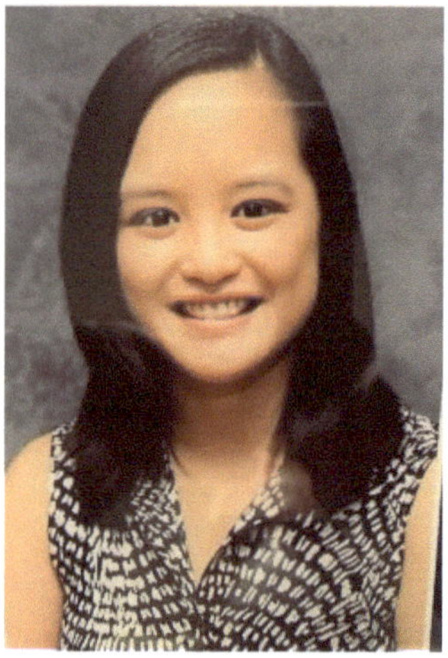

Jennifer E. Fergeson, DO
(2014-2016)

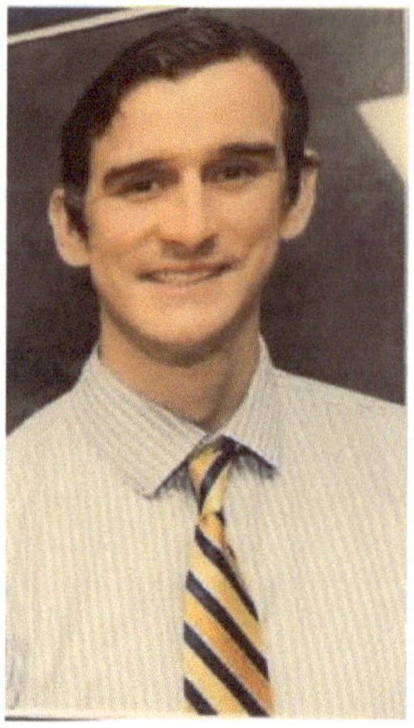

Andrew J. Cooke, MD
(2014-2016)

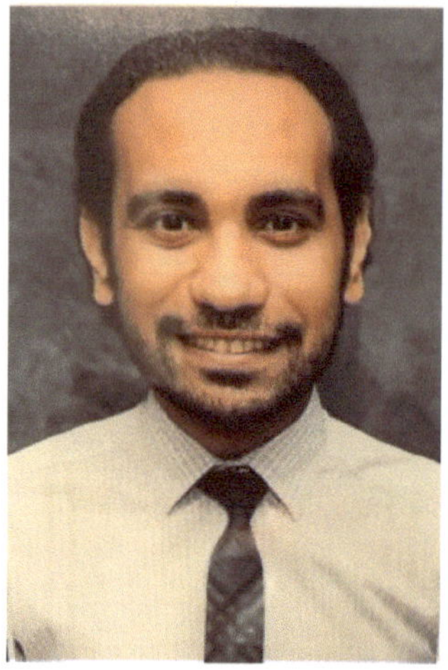

Adeeb A. Bulkhi, MD
(2014-2017)

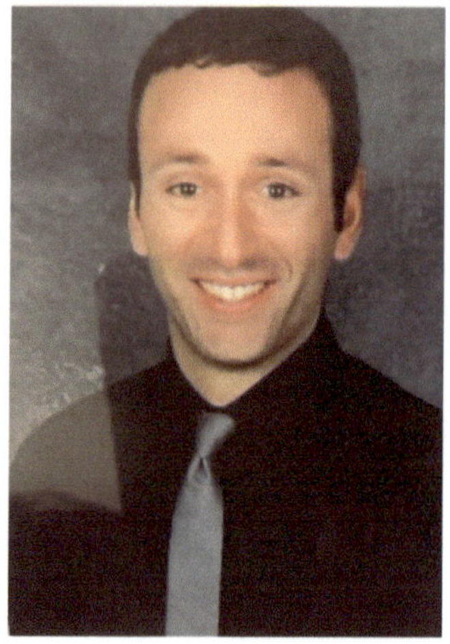

Peter Ricketti, DO
(2015-2017)

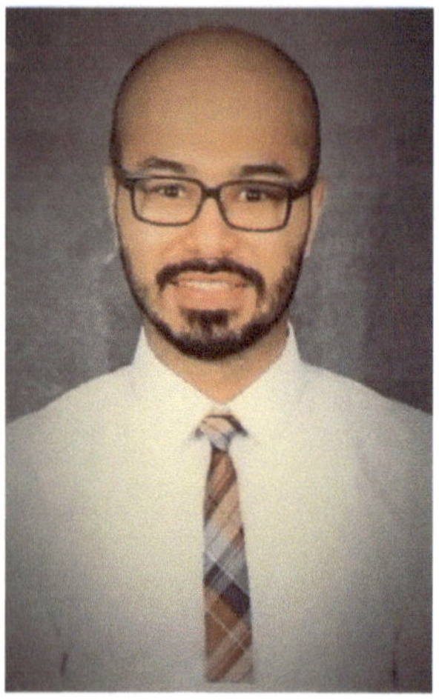

Sultan Alandijani, MD
(2015-2017)

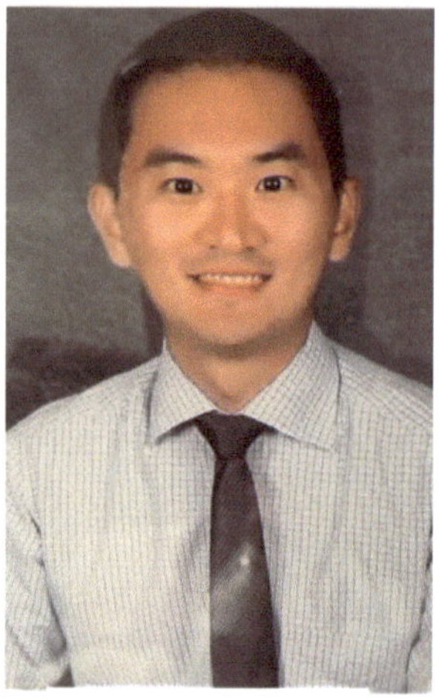

Chen Lin, MD
(2015-2017)

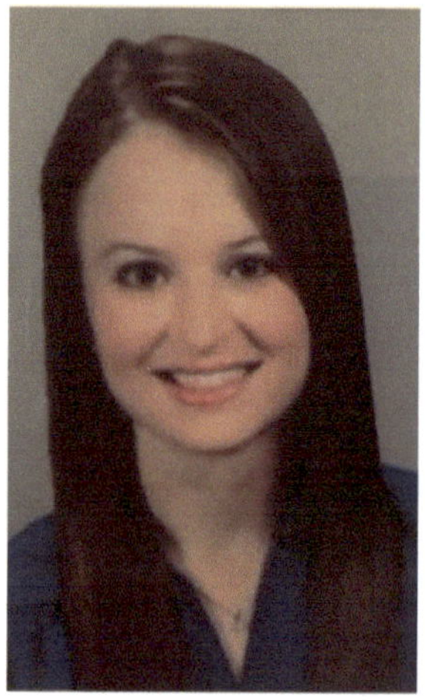

Amber N. Pepper, MD
(2016-2018)

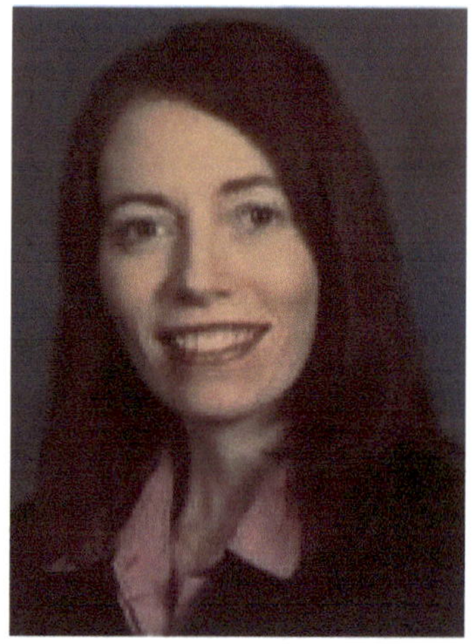

Emma Westermann-Clark, MD
(2016-2018)

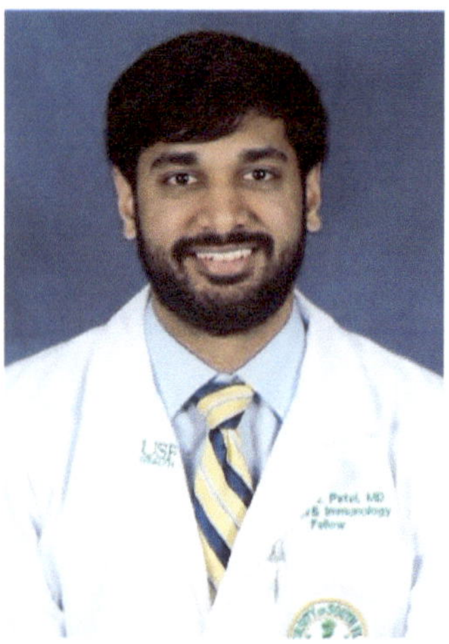

Shiven S. Patel, MD
(2017-2019)

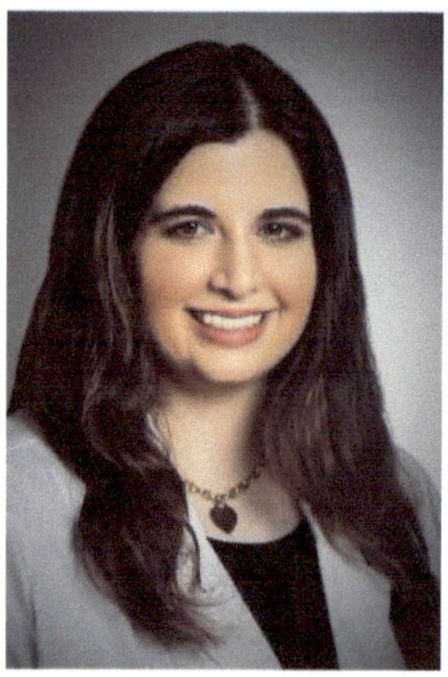

Tara V. Saco, MD
(2017-2019)

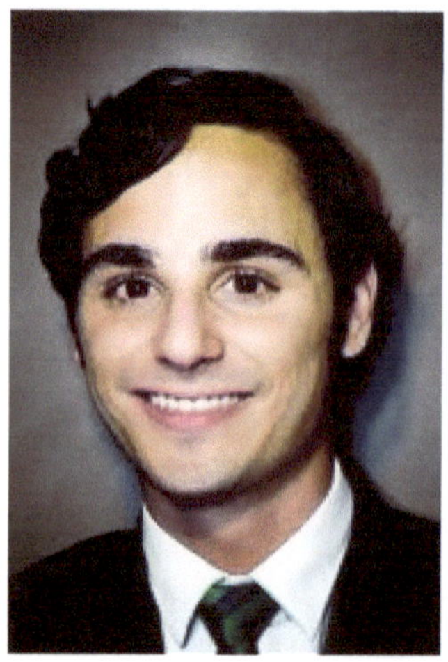

Raul S. Villarreal, MD
(2018-2020)

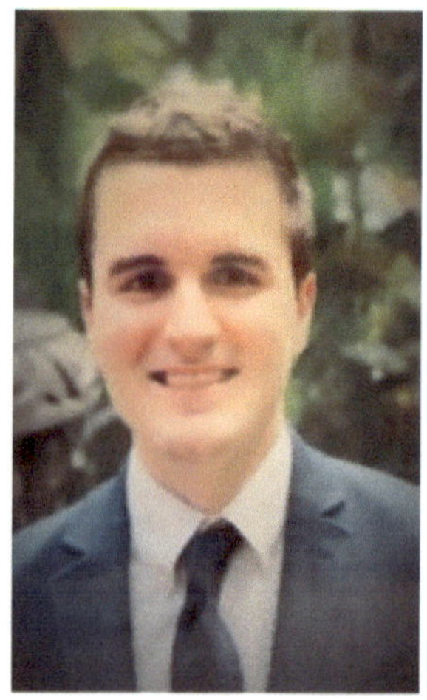

Kirk V. Shepard, II, MD
(2017-2019)

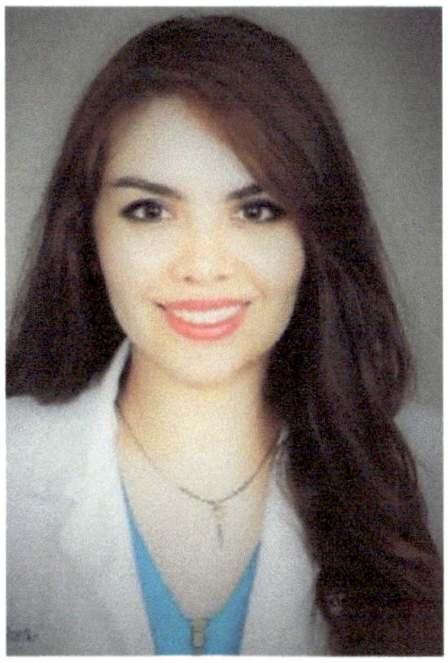

Claudia Gaefke, MD
(2018-2020)

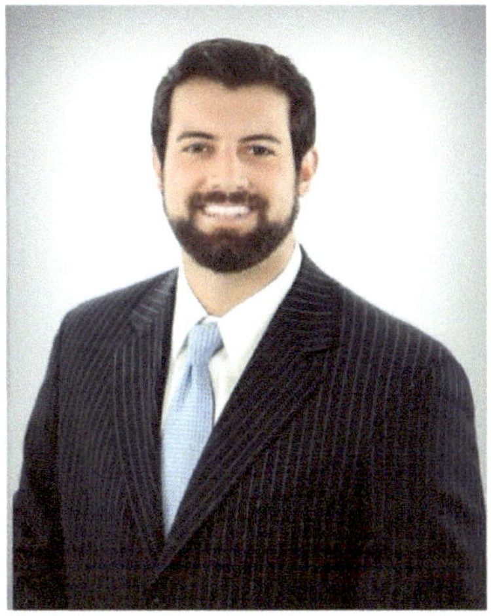

Nicholas Kolinsky, DO
(2019-2021)

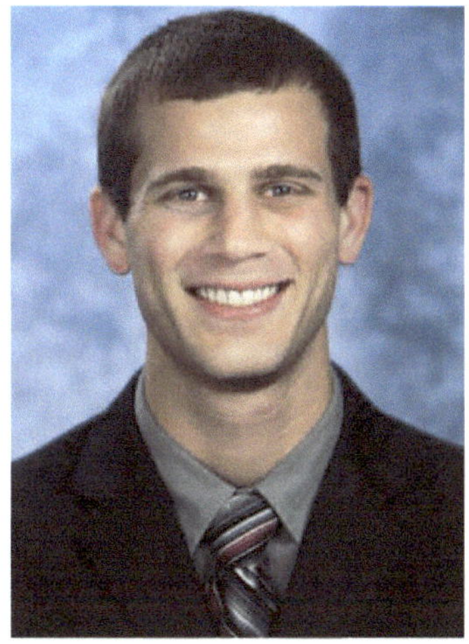

David Gubernick, MD
(2019-2021)

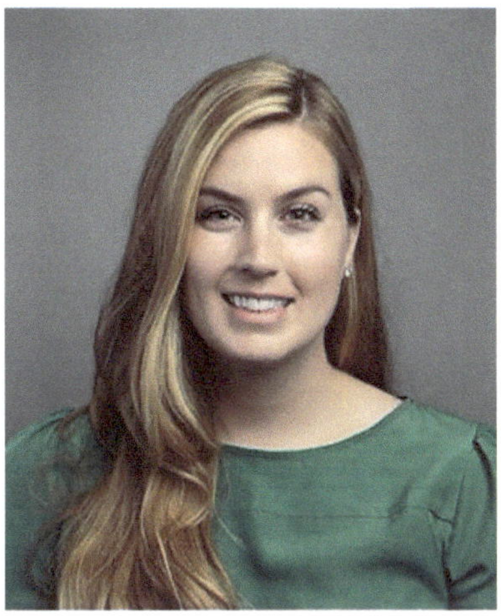

Stephanie Hudey, MD
(2019-2021)

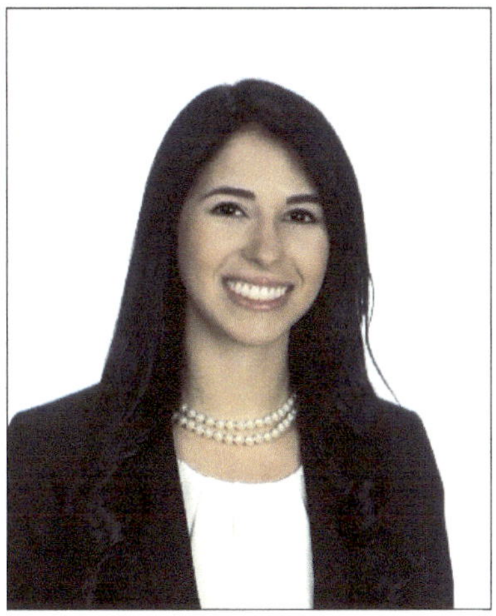

Natalie Diaz-Cabrera, MD
(2020-2022)

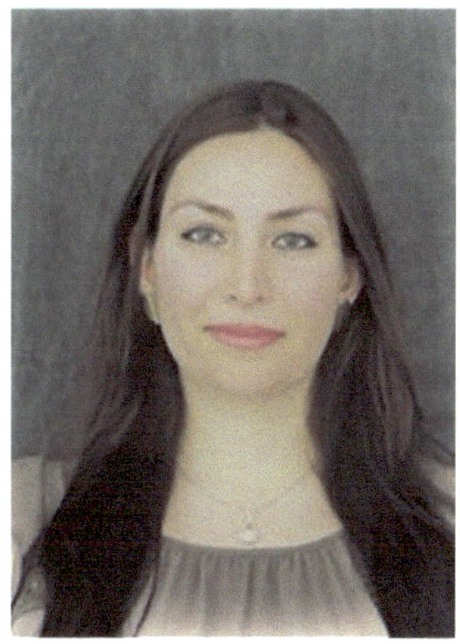

Donya Imanirad, MD
(2020-2022)

Chapter 5: Additional Pictures of Internal Medicine Allergy and Immunology Fellows

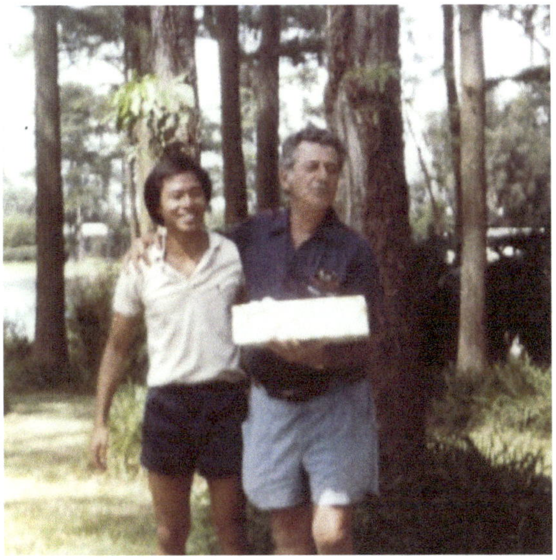

Left to right: Steven J. Louie, MD (1981-1983); Samuel C. Bukantz, MD; graduation party for Dr. Louie; June 1983.

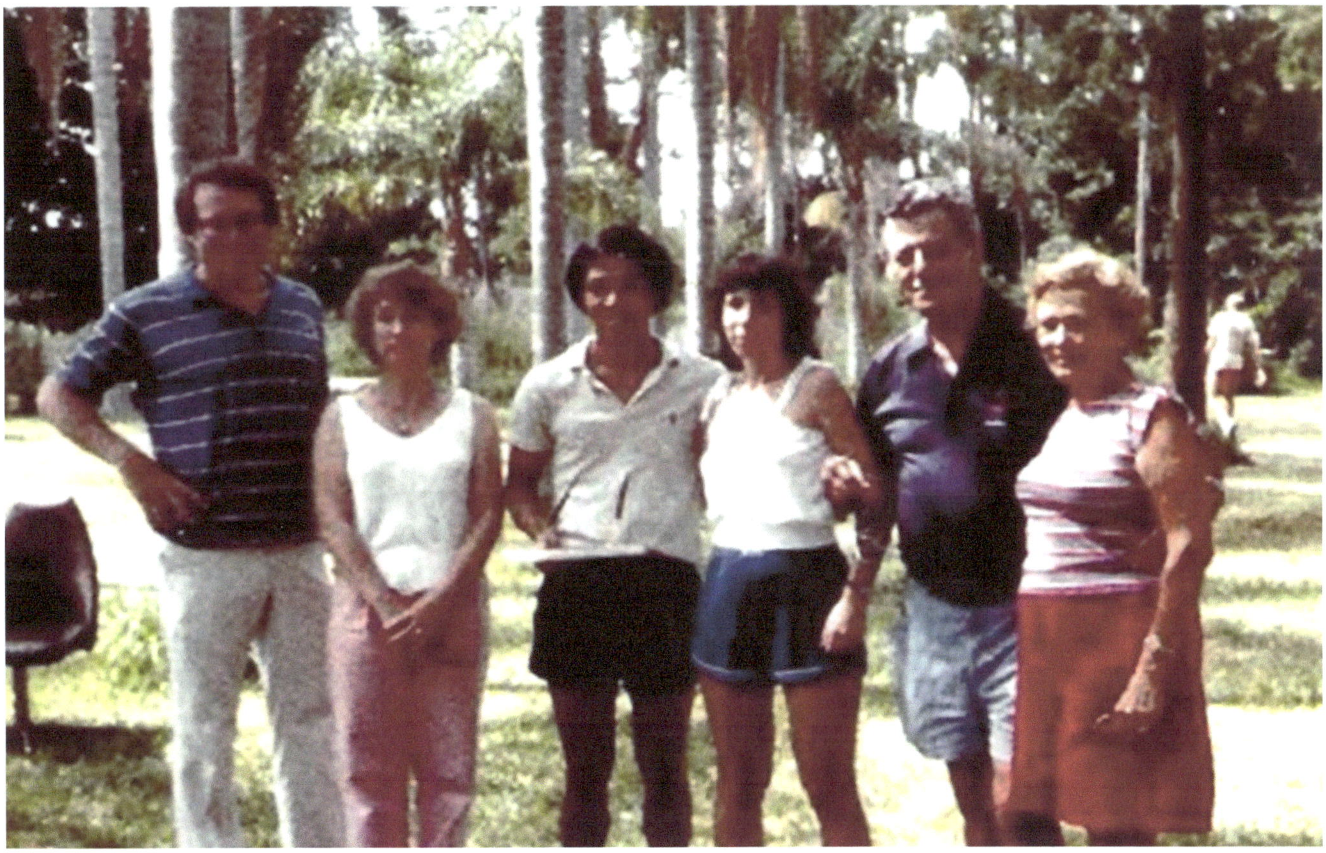

Left to right: Richard F. Lockey, MD, MS; Carol Lee Lockey; Steven J. Louie, MD (1981-1983); Barbara Louie; Samuel C. Bukantz, MD; Jewell Bukantz; graduation party for Dr. Louie; June 1983.

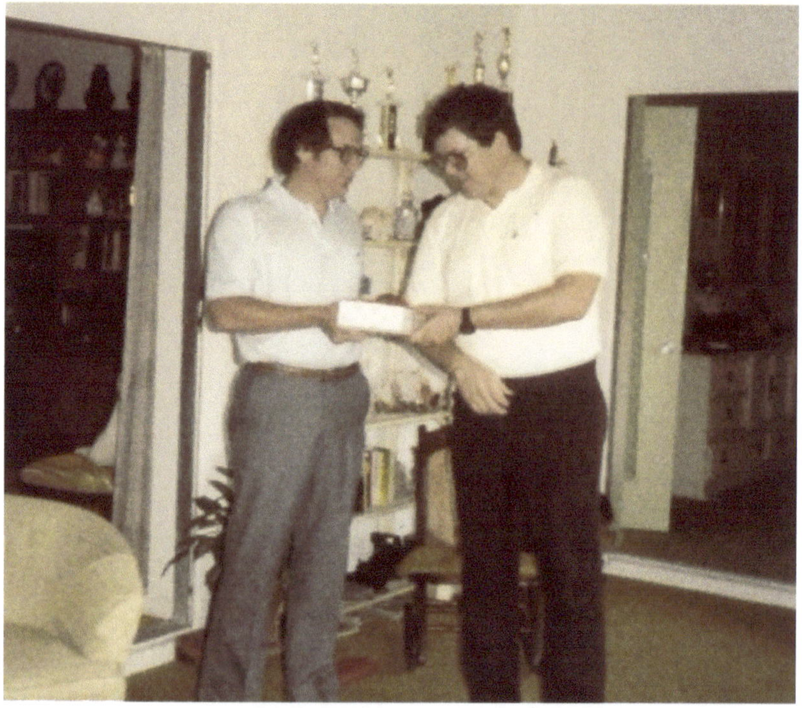

Left to right: Richard F. Lockey, MD, MS; Albert E. Hensel, MD (1982-1984); graduation party; June 1984.

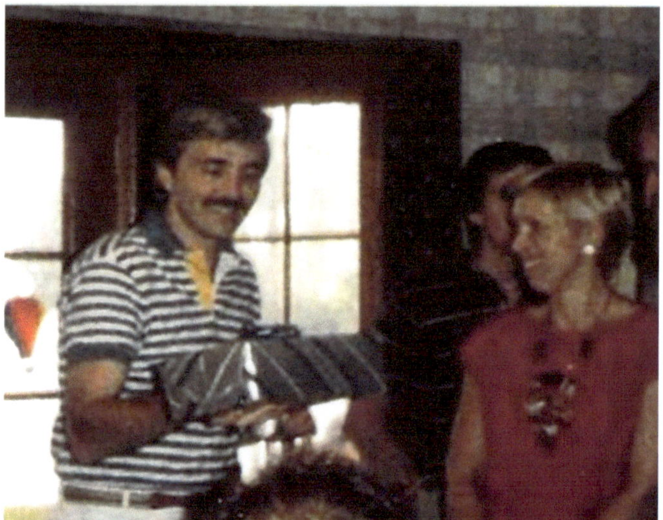

Left to right: Dennis K. Ledford, MD (1983-1985); Ann Rogers (VA Allergy nurse); graduation party for Dr. Ledford; June 1985.

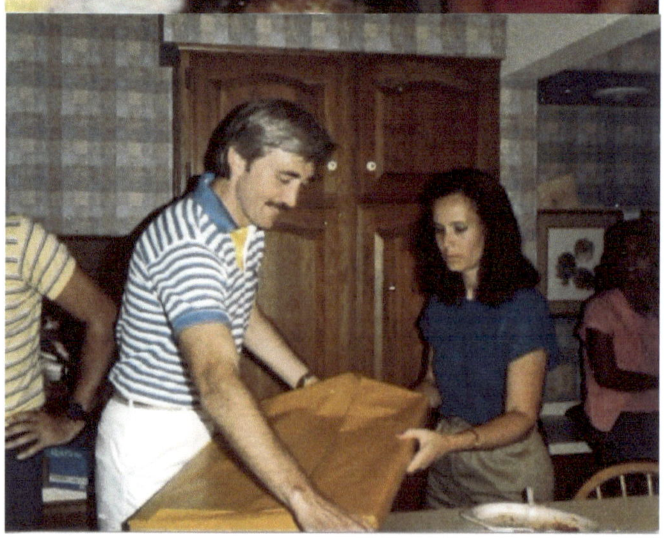

Left to right: Dennis K. Ledford, MD (1983-1985); Jennifer Ledford; graduation party for Dr. Ledford; June 1985.

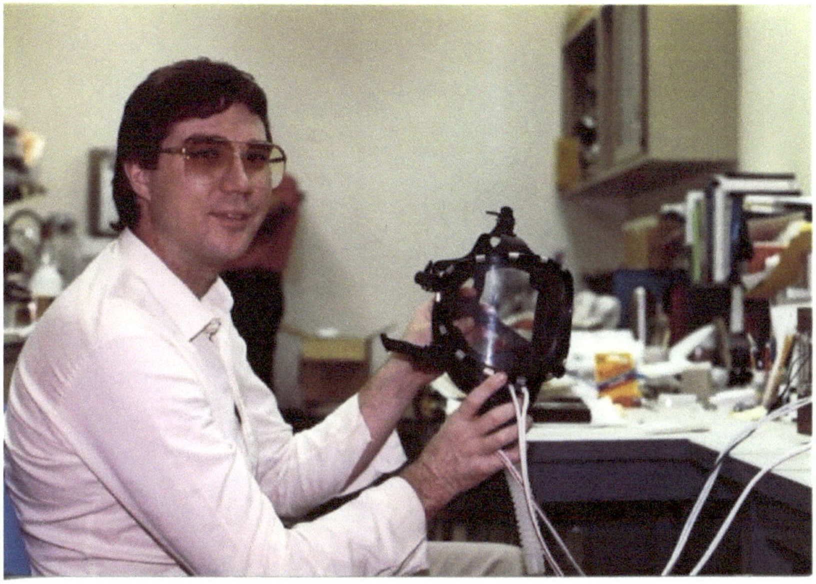

Robert P. Nelson, MD (1985-1987).

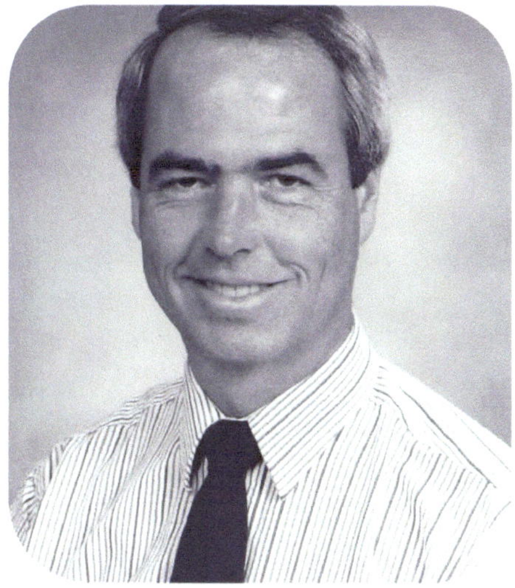

John J. Stablein, MD
(1979–1981)

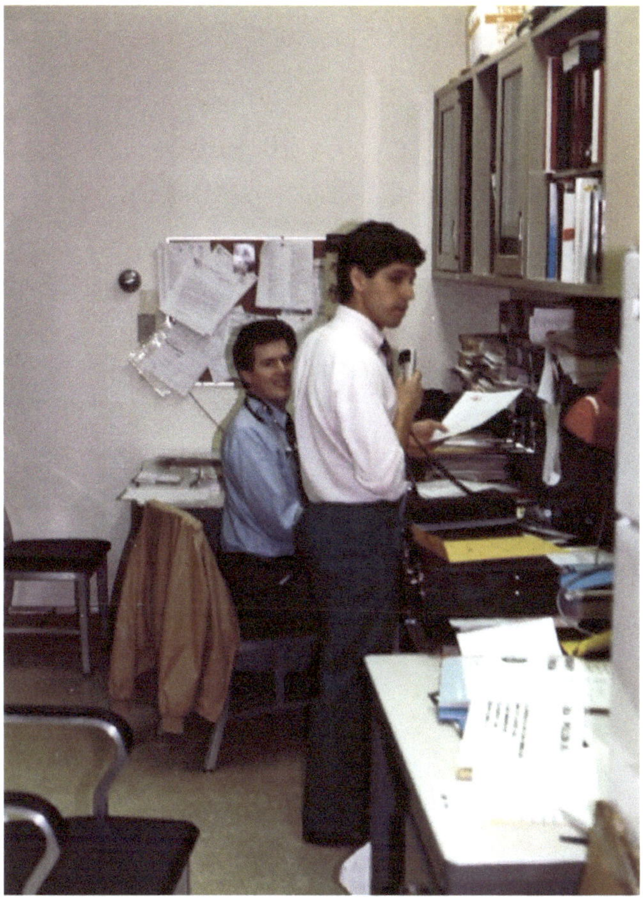

Left to right; Mark W. Minor, MD (1985-1987); Joseph D. Diaz, MD (1986-1988); Fellows' Room in the Research Building; circa 1986.

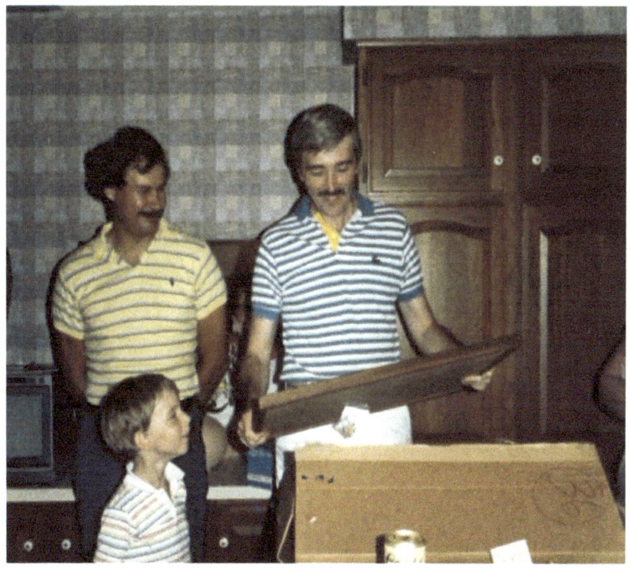

Front: Michael Ledford. Back, left to right: Gerald A. Bucholtz, MD (1980-1982); Dennis K. Ledford, MD (1983-1985); graduation party for Dr. Ledford; June 1985.

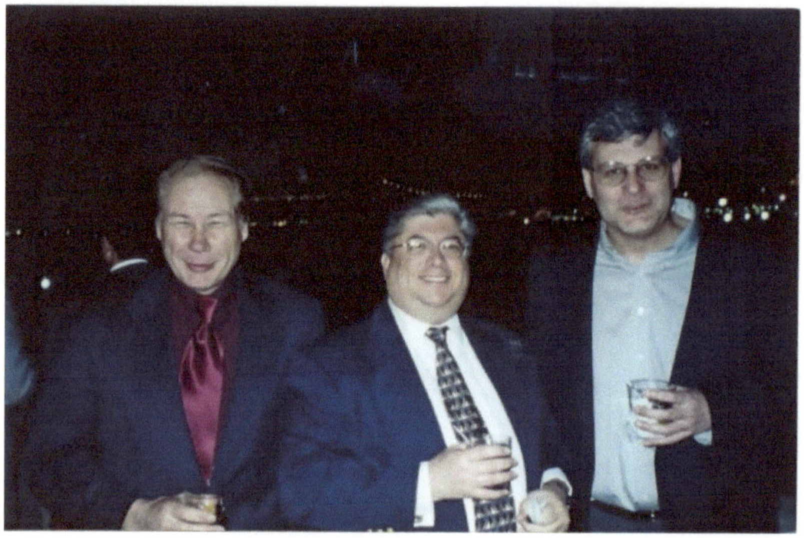

Left to right: Gerald A. Bucholtz, MD (1980-1982); Jack Parrino, MD (1977-1979); David N. Wright, MD (1988-1991); circa 1990.

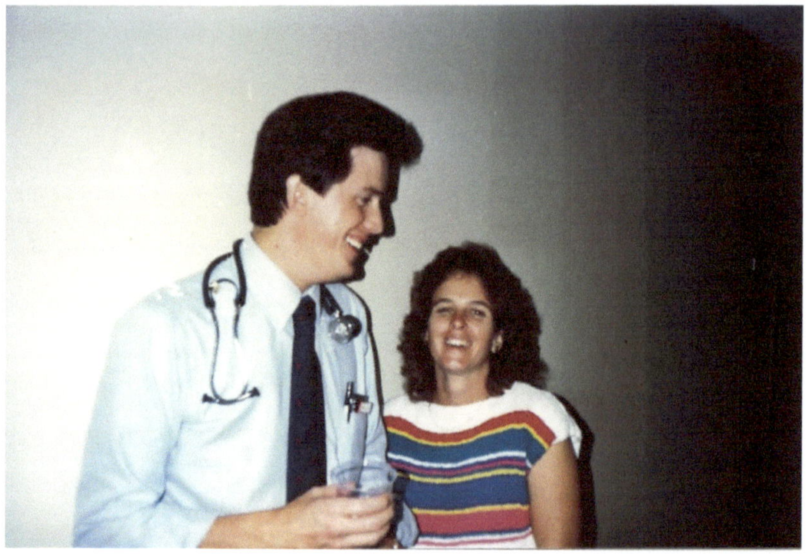

Left to right: Mark W. Minor, MD (1985-1987); Pat Walsh; circa 1986.

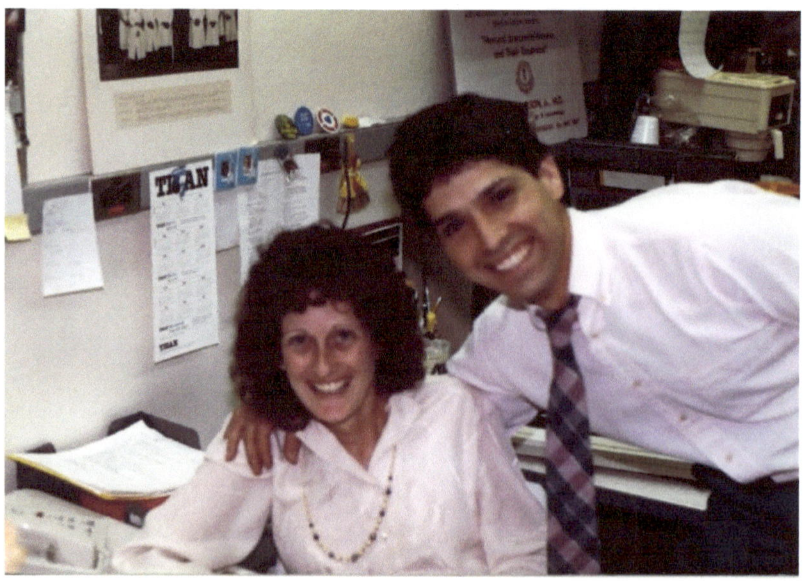

Left to right: Peggy Hales; Joseph D. Diaz, MD (1986-1988); circa 1986.

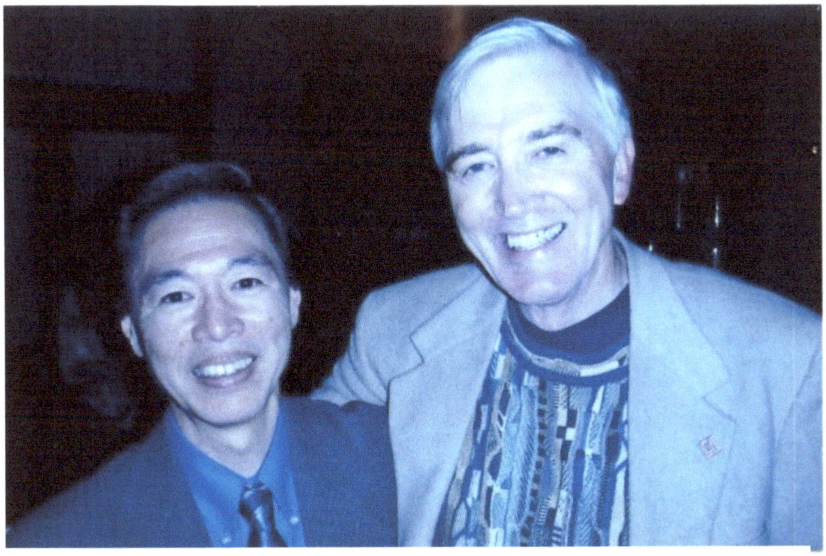

Steven J. Louie, MD (1981-1983); Dennis K. Ledford, MD (1983-1985); circa 1990.

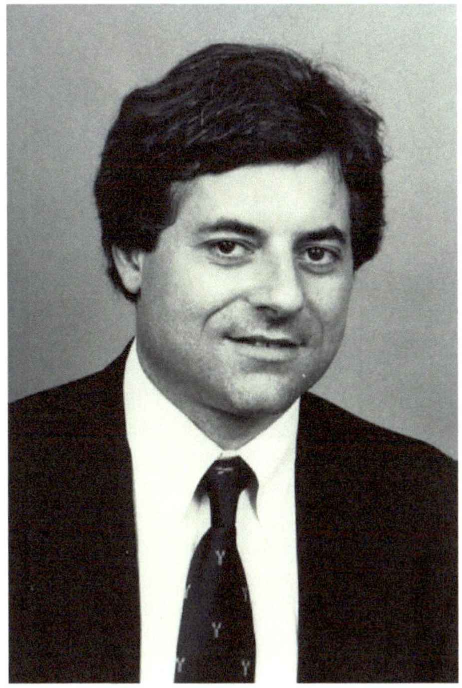

Donald W. Russell, MD (1987-1990).

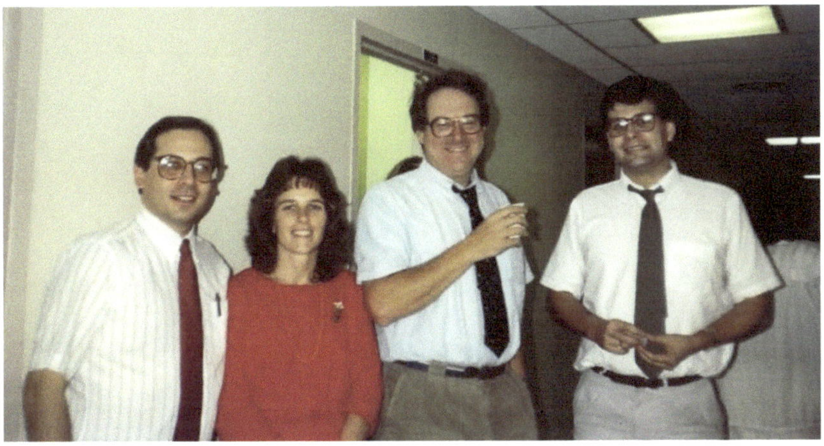

Left to right: Richard P. Silton, MD (1988-1990); Pat Walsh; Richard F. Lockey, MD, MS; David N. Wright, MD (1988-1991); Christmas party 1989.

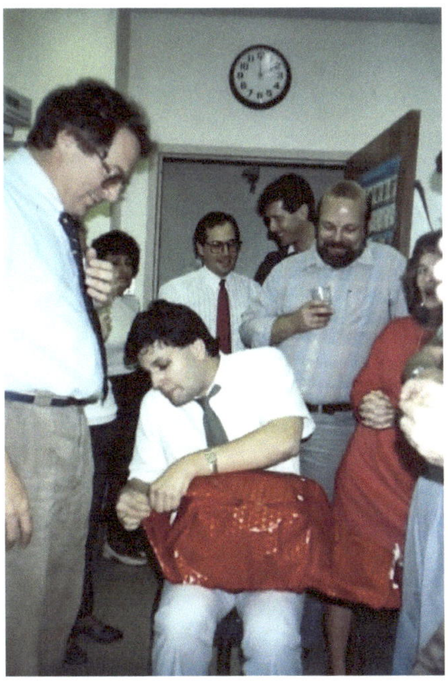

Front (left to right): Richard F. Lockey, MD, MS; David N. Wright, MD (1988-1991). Back (left to right): name unknown; Richard P. Silton, MD (1988-1990) Enrique Fernandez-Caldas, PhD; Walter Trudeau, MS; Pat Walsh; Christmas party 1989.

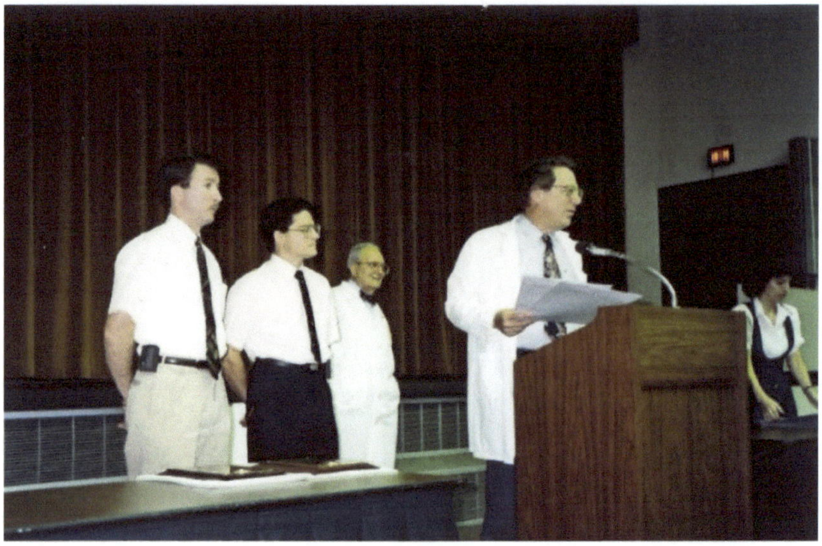

Front: Richard F. Lockey, MD, MS. Back (left to right): Thomas B. Edwards, MD (1990-1992); Carlos M. Jacinto, MD (1990-1992); Roy H. Behnke, MD (Founding Chairman, Department of Internal Medicine); graduation; June 1992.

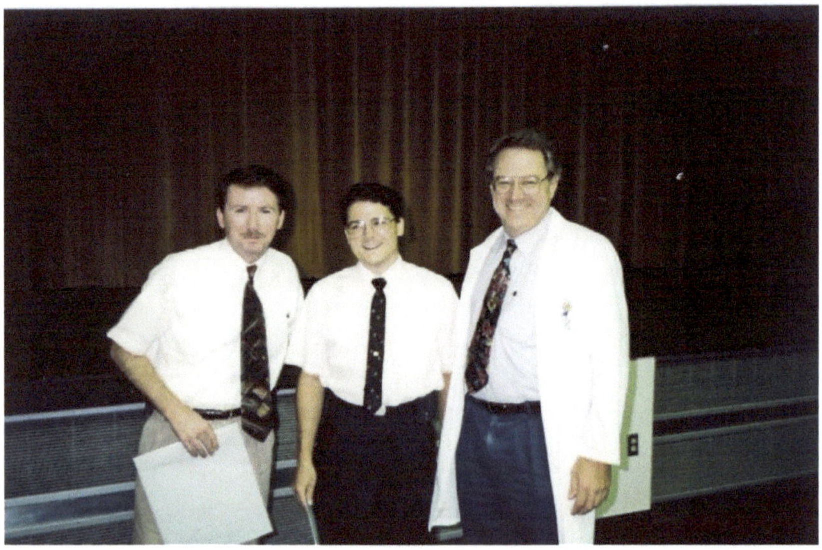

Left to right: Thomas B. Edwards, MD (1990-1992); Carlos M. Jacinto, MD (1990-1992); Richard F. Lockey, MD, MS; graduation; June 1992.

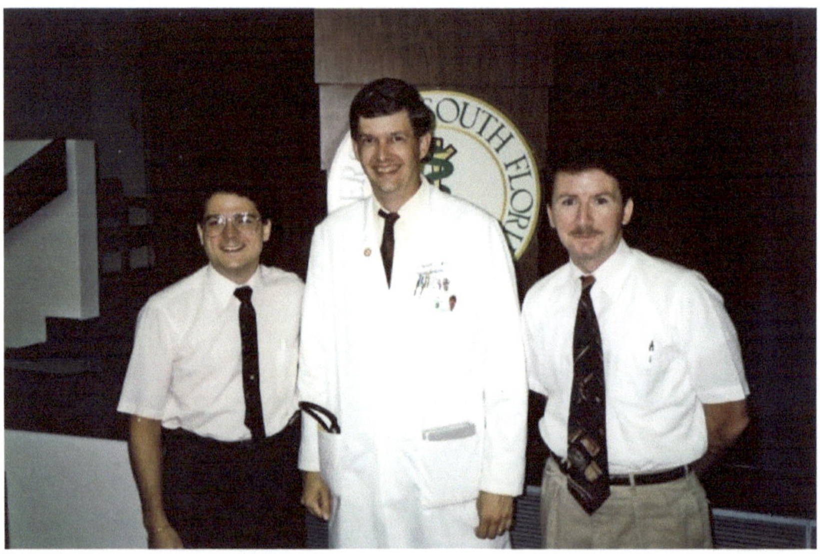

Left to right: Carlos M. Jacinto, MD (1990-1992); G. Edward Stewart, MD (1991-1994); Thomas B. Edwards, MD (1990-1992).

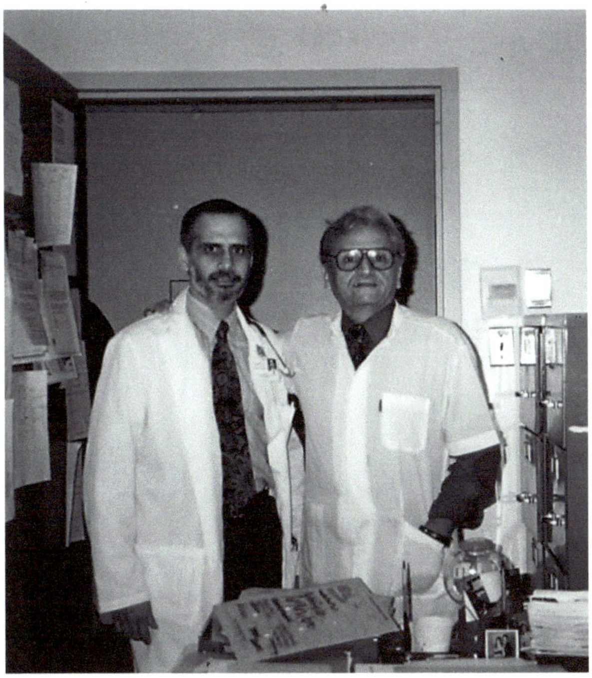

Left to right: Jose Andrade, MD (1992-1995); Sagrado Lamir David, MD (Visiting Research Scholar from Brazil, November 1993).

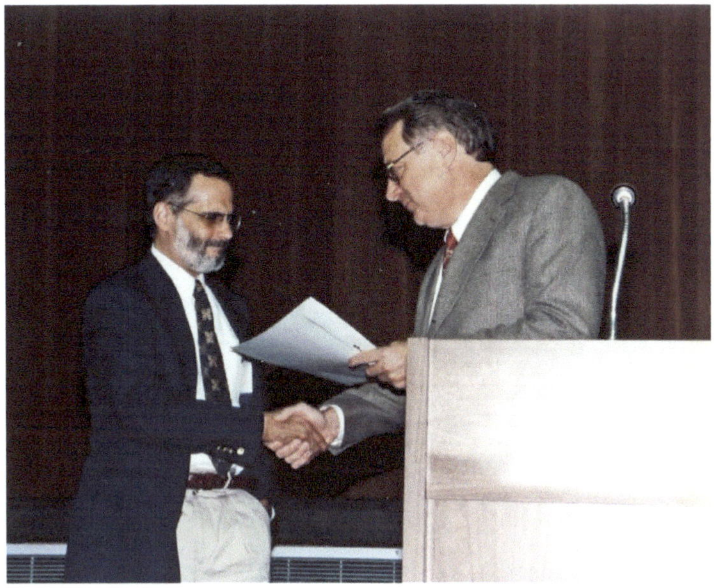

Left to right: Jose Andrade, MD (1992-1995) and Richard F. Lockey, MD, MS; graduation; June 1995.

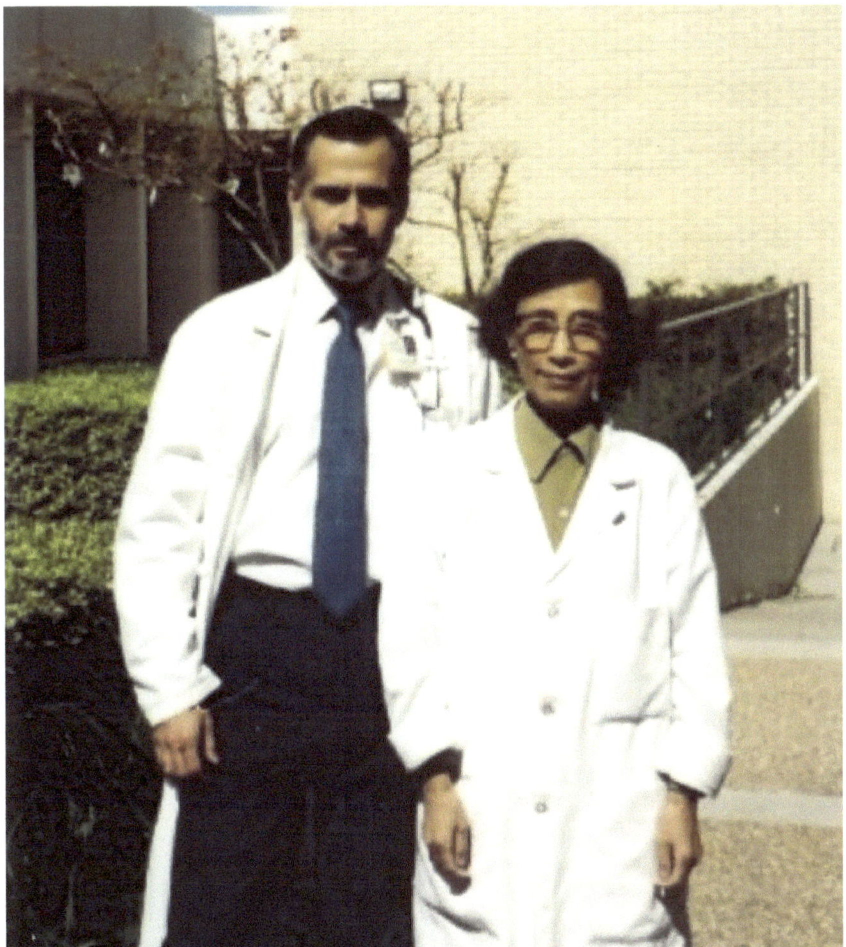

Left to right: Jose Andrade, MD (1992-1995) and Zhaoming Wen, MD (Visiting Research Scholar from China, August 1994 – November 1994).

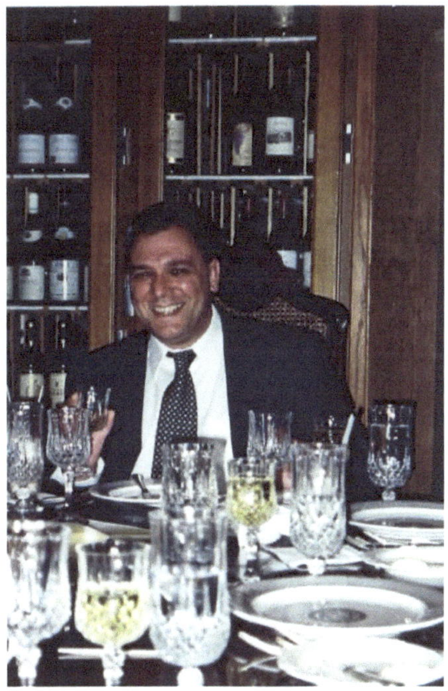

Demetrios S. Theodoropoulos, MD (1997-2000); circa 1998.

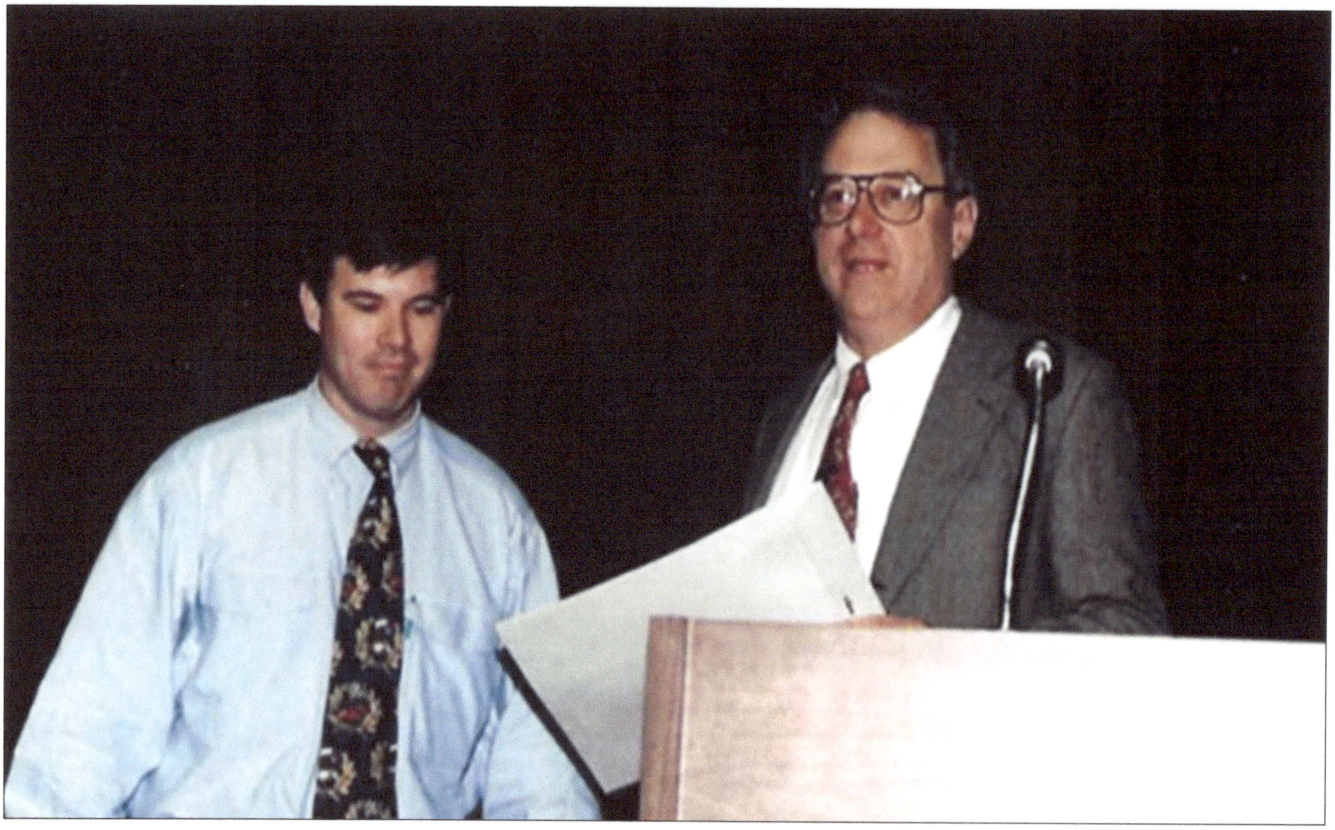

Left to right: Brett E. Stanaland, MD (1992-1995) and Richard F. Lockey, MD, MS; graduation; June 1994 (Allergy and Immunology Fellowship).

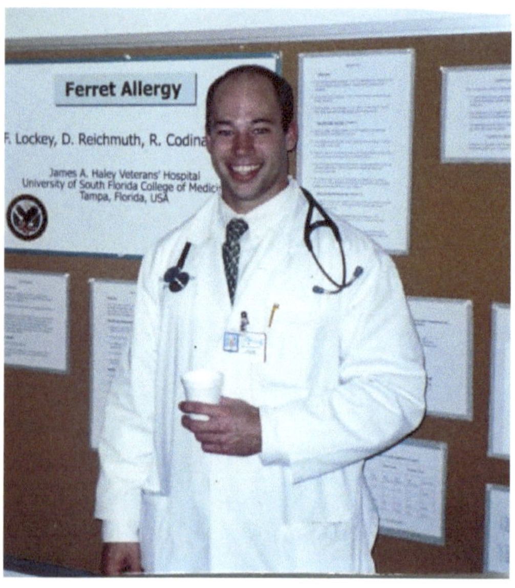

Daniel A. Reichmuth, MD (1999-2002).

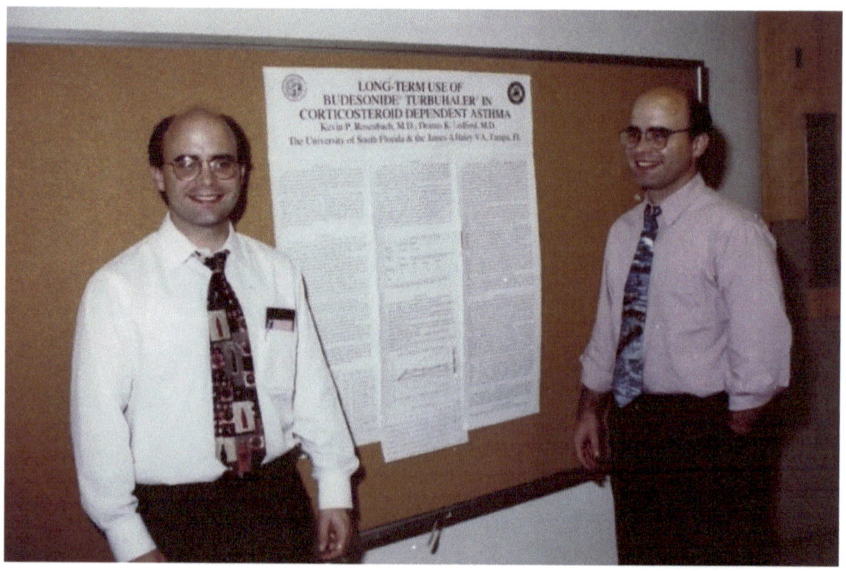

Left to right: Kevin P. Rosenbach, MD (1995-1998) and Keith A. Rosenbach, PhD, MD (twin brother, Infectious Disease fellow); circa 1997.

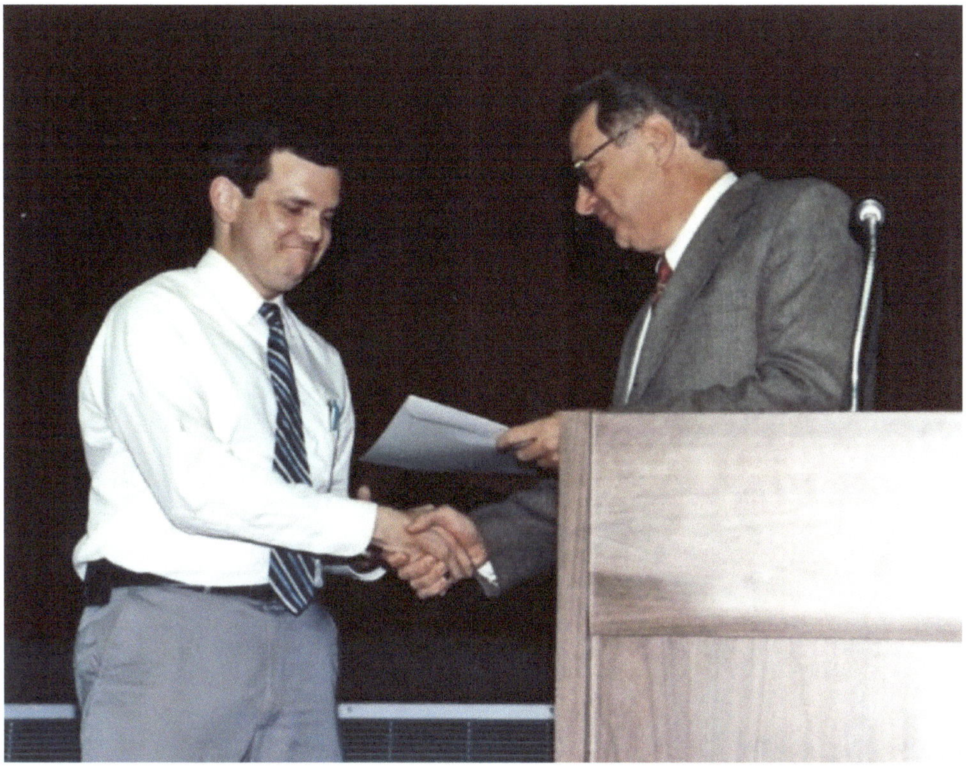

Left to right: Stephen F. Kemp, MD (1993-1996) and Richard F. Lockey, MD, MS; graduation; June 1995 (Allergy and Immunology

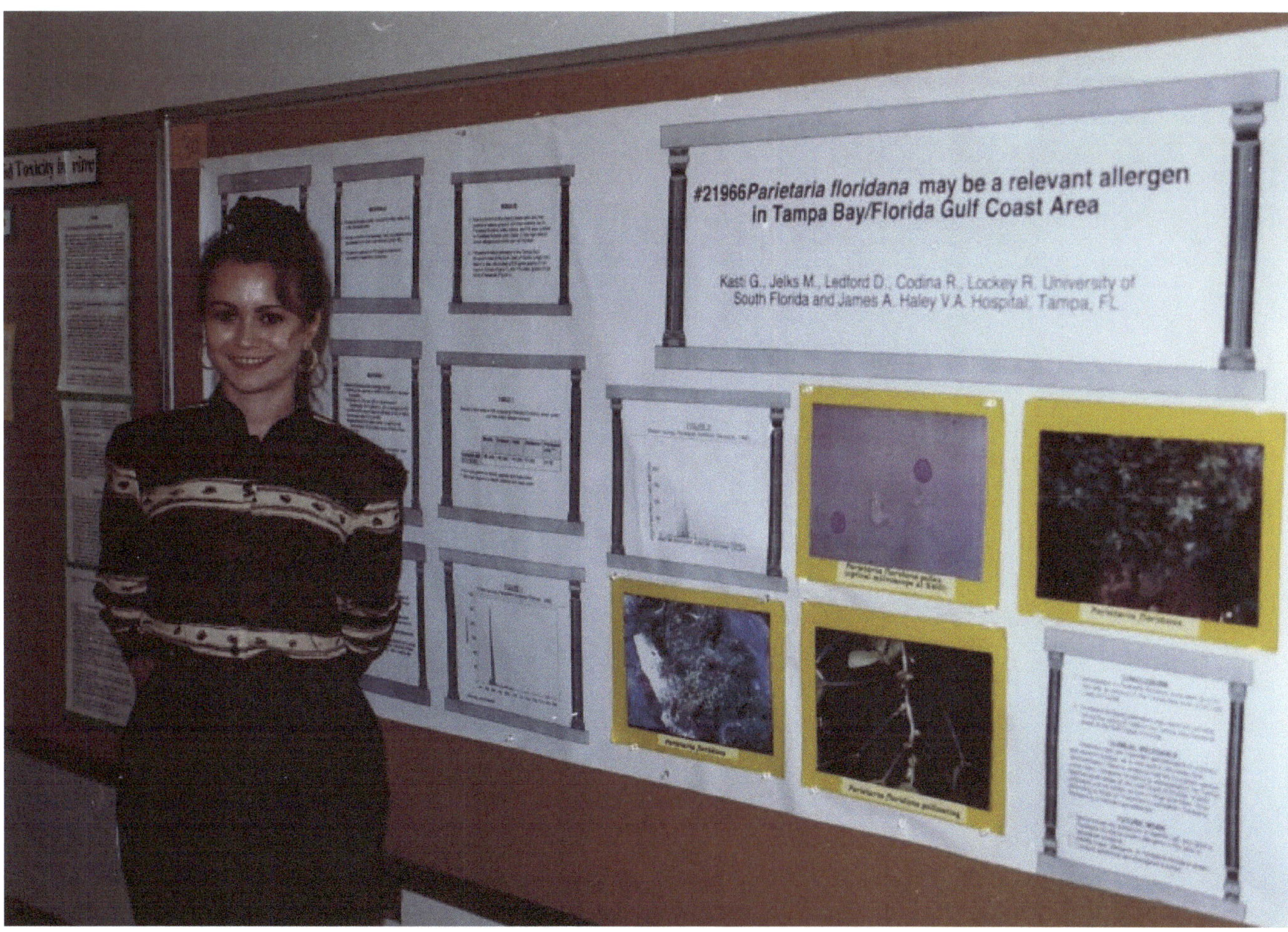
#21966 Parietaria floridana may be a relevant allergen
in Tampa Bay/Florida Gulf Coast Area
Kasti G., Jelks M., Ledford D., Codina R., Lockey R. University of
South Florida and James A. Haley V.A. Hospital, Tampa, FL

Giana L. Nicoara-Kasti, MD (1996-1998); circa 1997.

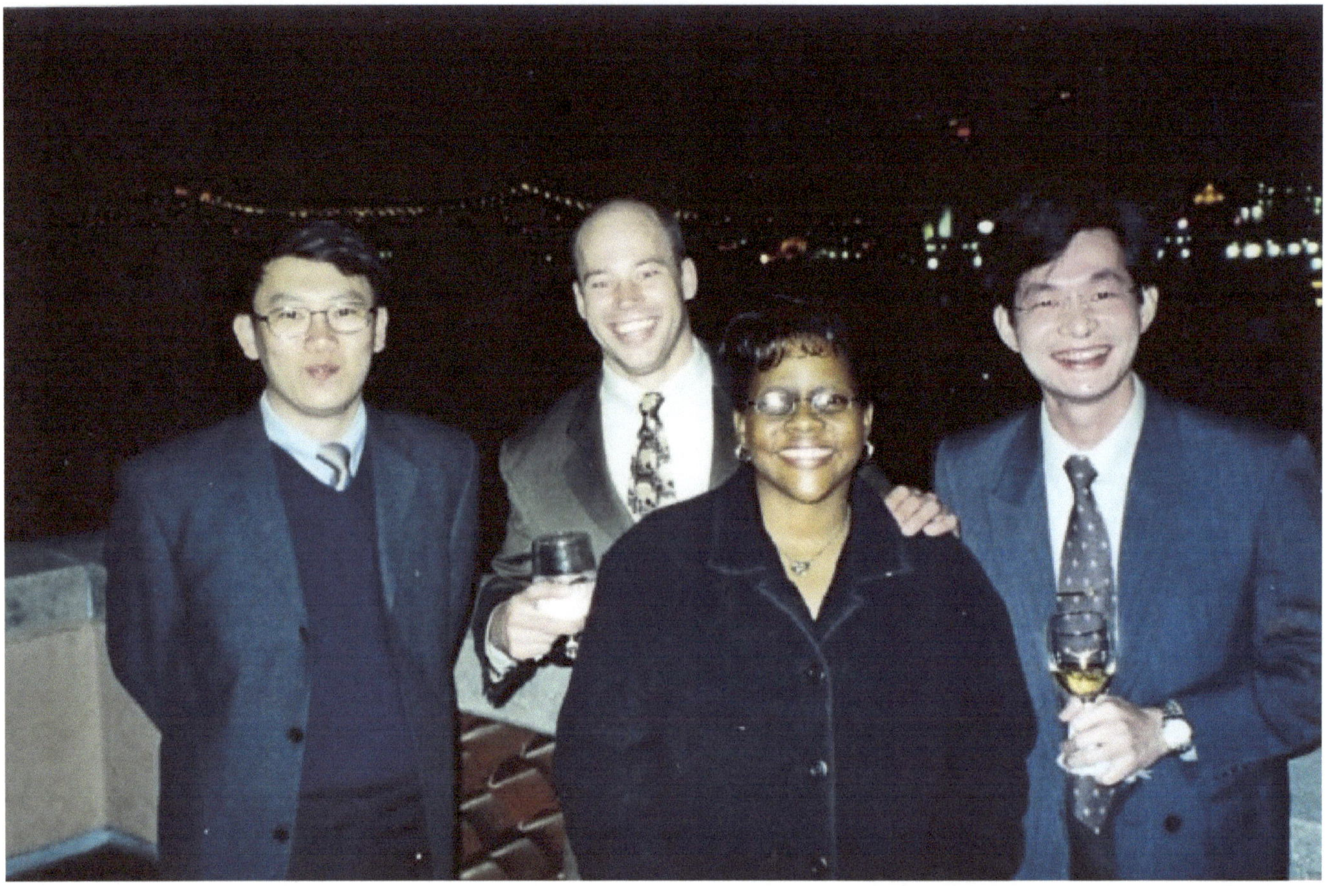

Front: Roselyn M. Hicks, MD (ACH, 2000-2002). Back (left to right): Voravich Luangwedchakarn, MD (ACH, 1998-2001); Daniel A. Reichmuth, MD (1999-2002); Nathan Tang, MD (ACH, 1996-1999). Circa 2000.

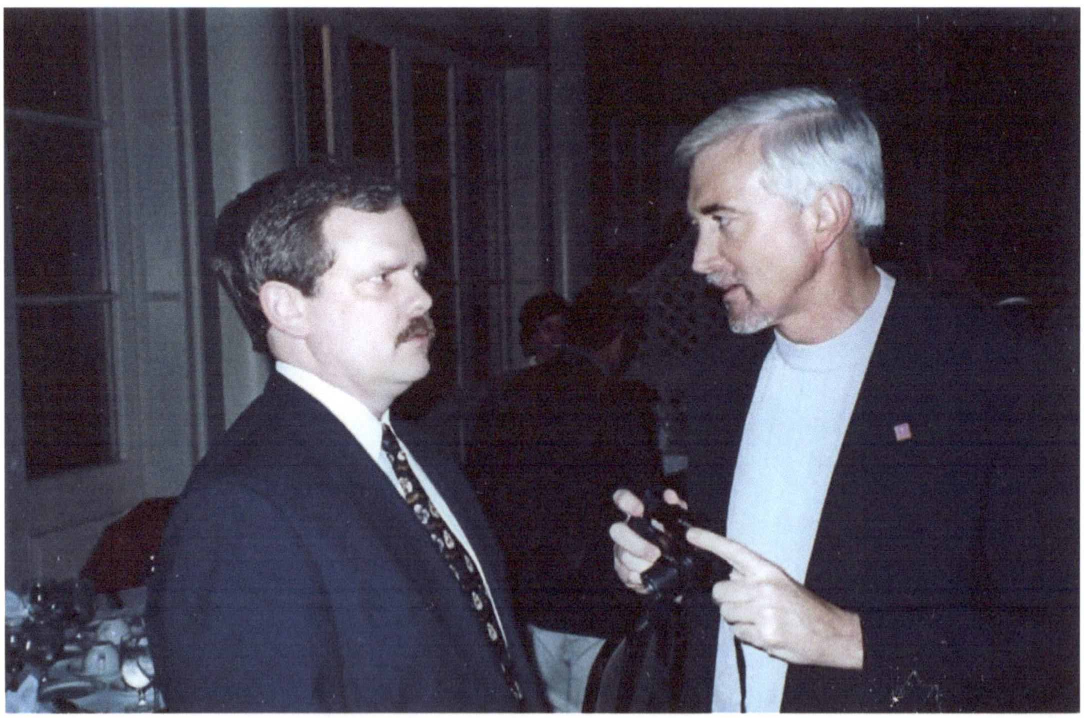

Stephen F. Kemp, MD (1993-1996) and Dennis K. Ledford, MD (1983-1985); circa 2000.

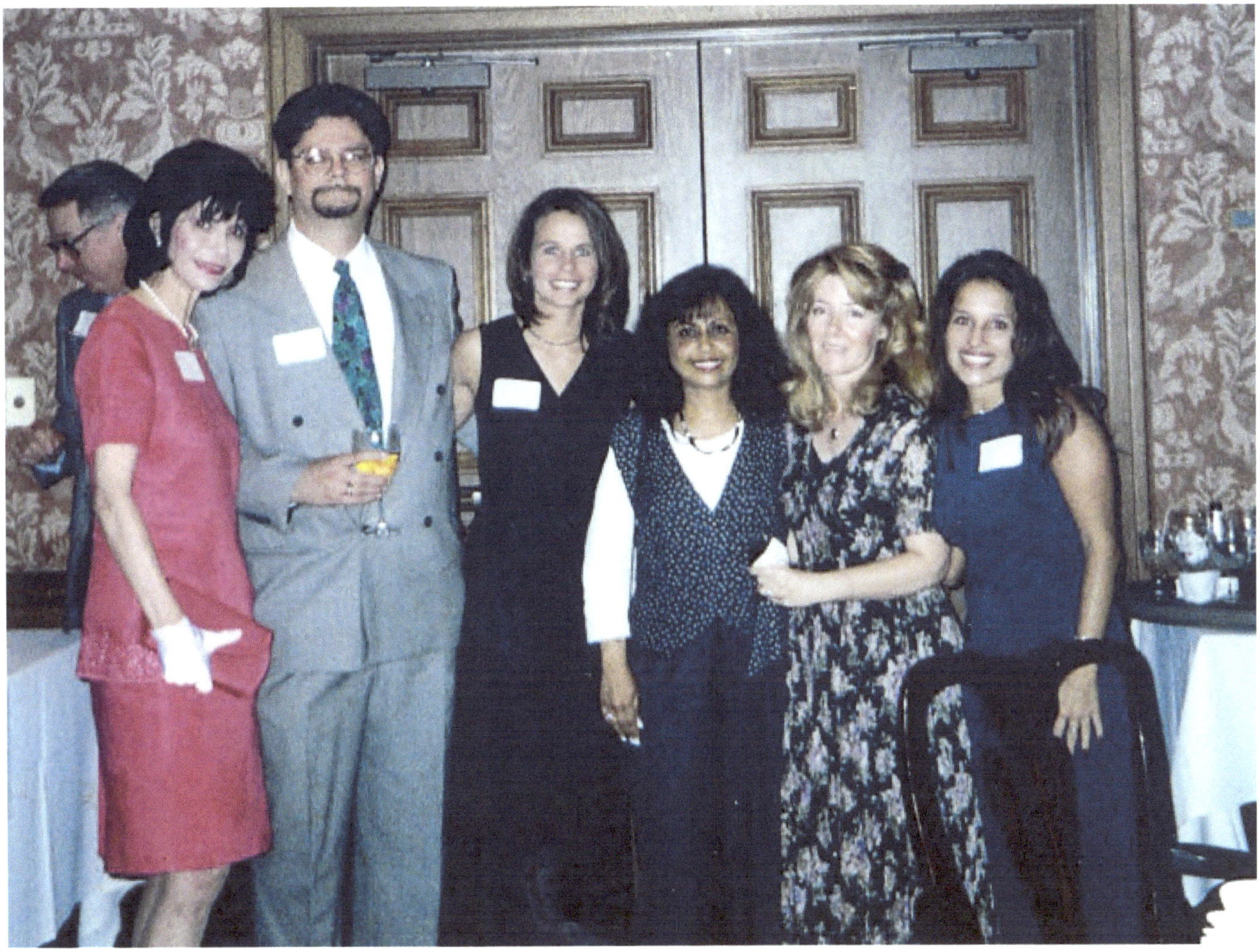

Left to right: Mary Jane Luck; Thomas W. Luck, MD (1999-2001); Diana Miller, Geeta Gehi, Sandra Rocha, Alisa Deicidue; Richard F. Lockey, MD, MS in the background; circa 2000.

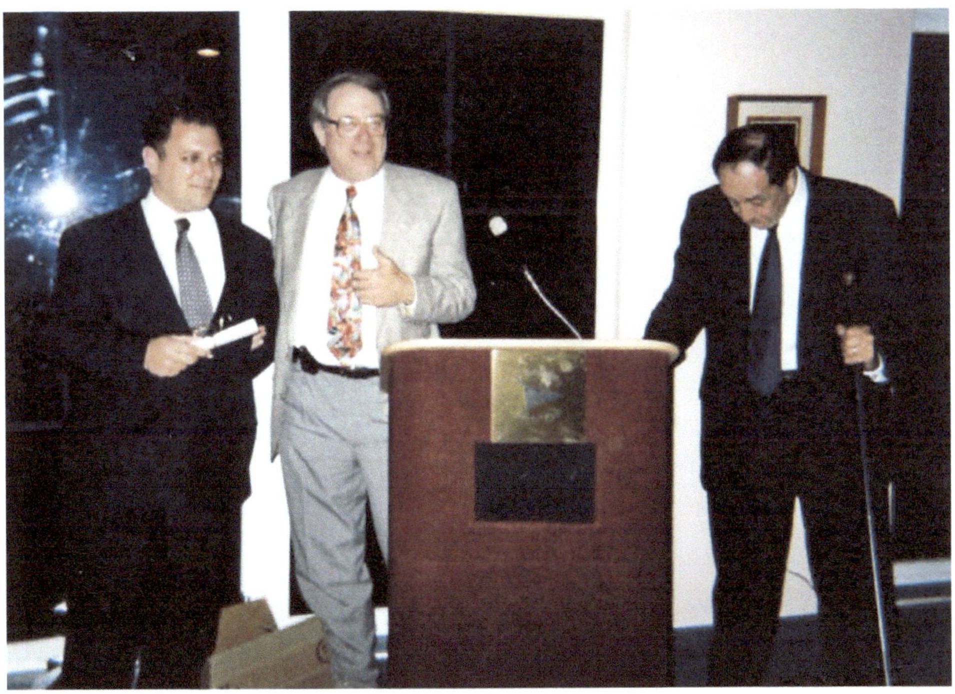

Left to right: Demetrios Theodoropoulos, MD (1997-2000); Richard F. Lockey, MD, MS; Robert A. Good, MD, PhD, DSc; circa 2000.

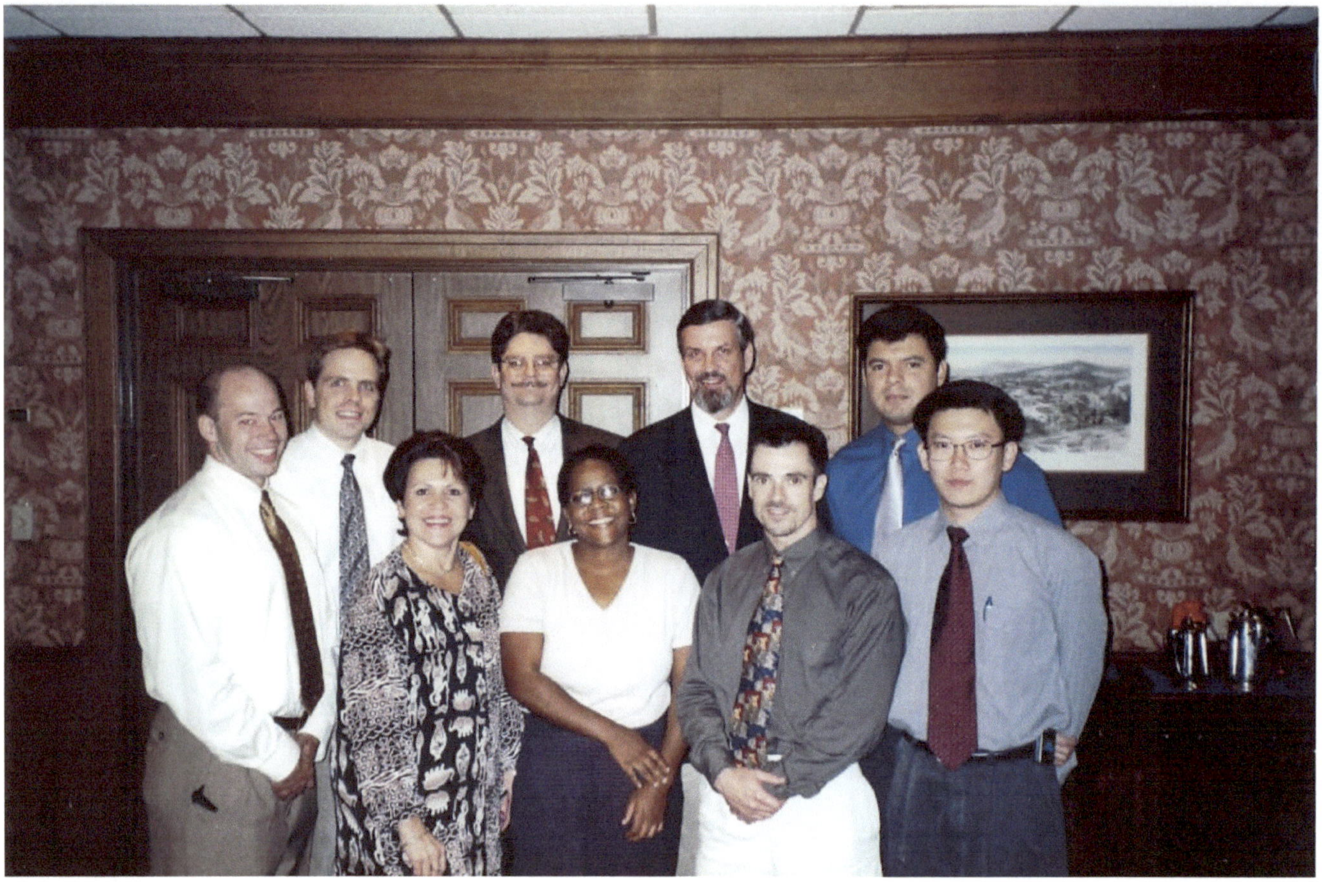

Front row (left to right): Nina Ramirez, MD (2000-2002); Roselyn M. Hicks, MD (ACH, 2000-2002); David Provencher, MD (ACH, 1999-2001); Voravich Luangwedchakarn, MD (ACH, 1998-2001). Back row (left to right): Daniel A. Reichmuth, MD (1999-2002); Richard E. Crockett, MD (2000-2003); Thomas W. Luck, MD (1999-2001); name unknown; Roberto Rivera, MD (ACH, 1999-2001). Circa 2000.

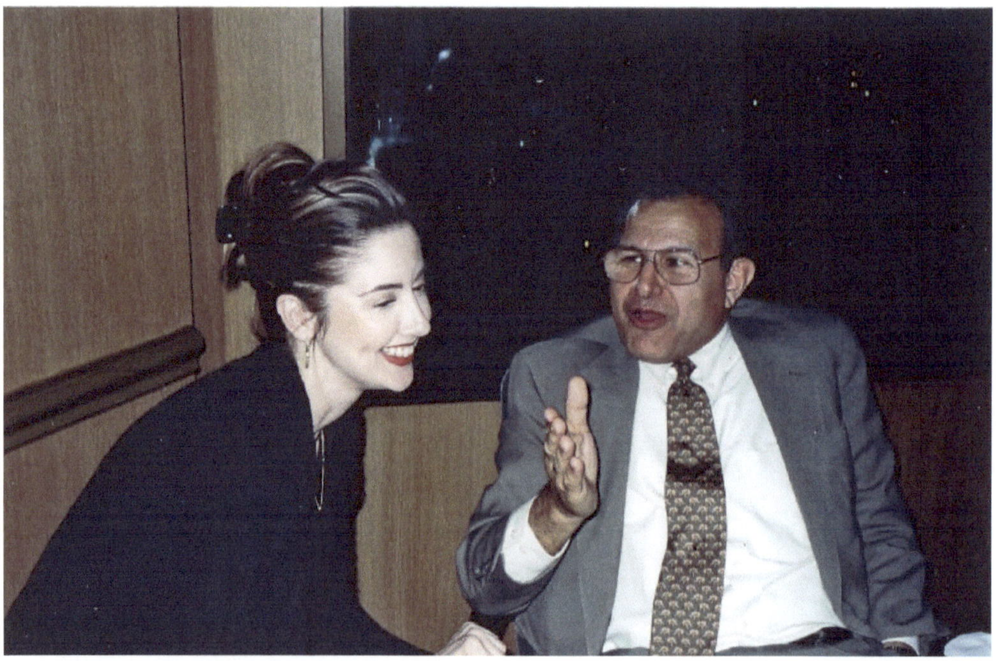

Lizette S. Hernandez, MD (1994-1997 and Sami L. Bahna, MD, DrPH; circa 2000.

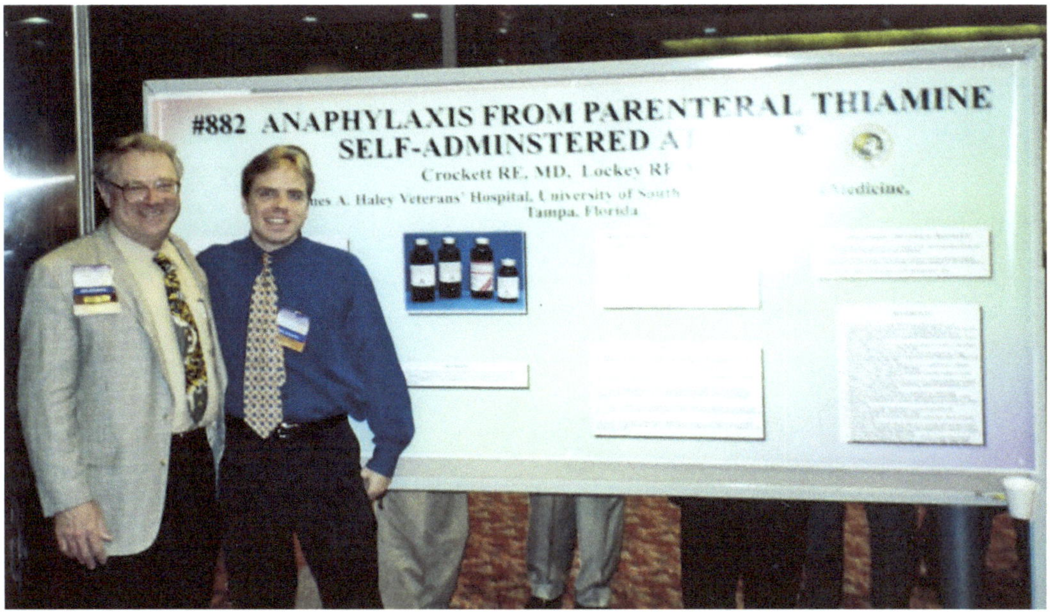

Left to right: Richard F. Lockey, MD, MS and Richard E. Crockett, MD (2000-2003). 2001 American Academy of Allergy Asthma & Immunology Annual Meeting, New Orleans.

Left to right: Shyam S. Mohapatra, PhD and Daniel A. Reichmuth, MD (1999-2002); circa 2000.

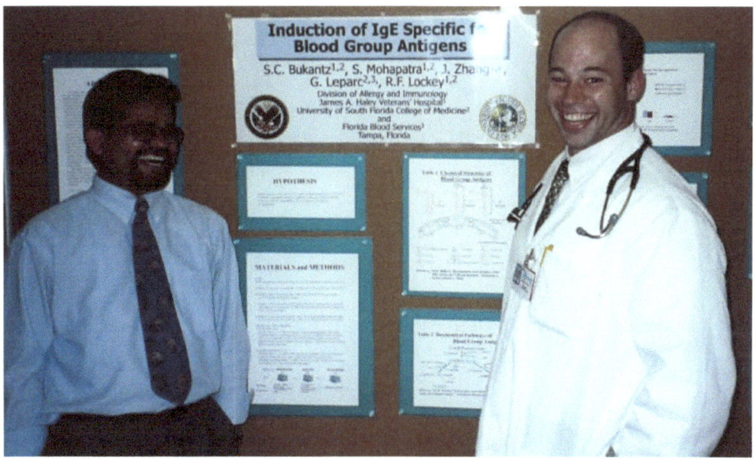

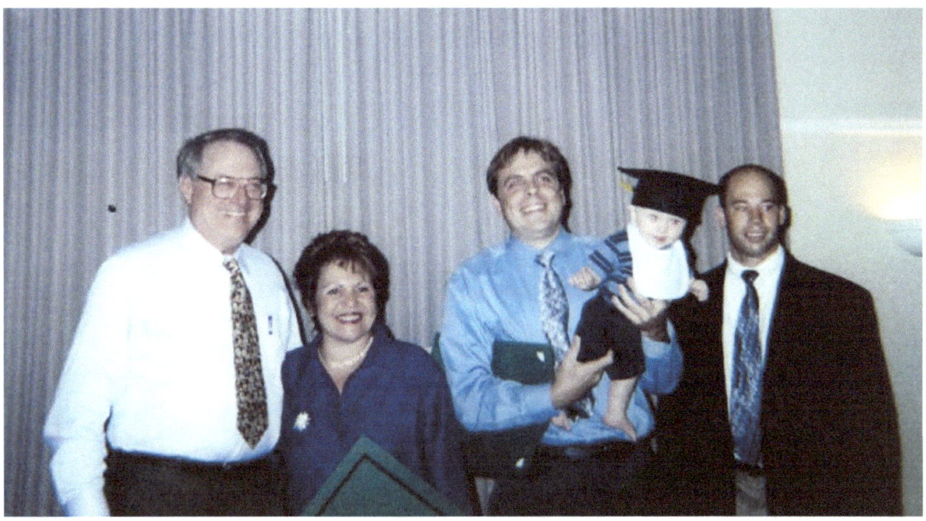

Left to right: Richard F. Lockey, MD, MS; Nina C. Ramirez, MD (2000-2002); Richard E. Crockett, MD (2000-2003) and son; Daniel A. Reichmuth, MD (1999-2002); graduation; June 2002.

Left to right: Geeta Gehi; Sandra Rocha, Nina C. Ramirez, MD (2000-2002); Peggy Hales; graduation; June 2002.

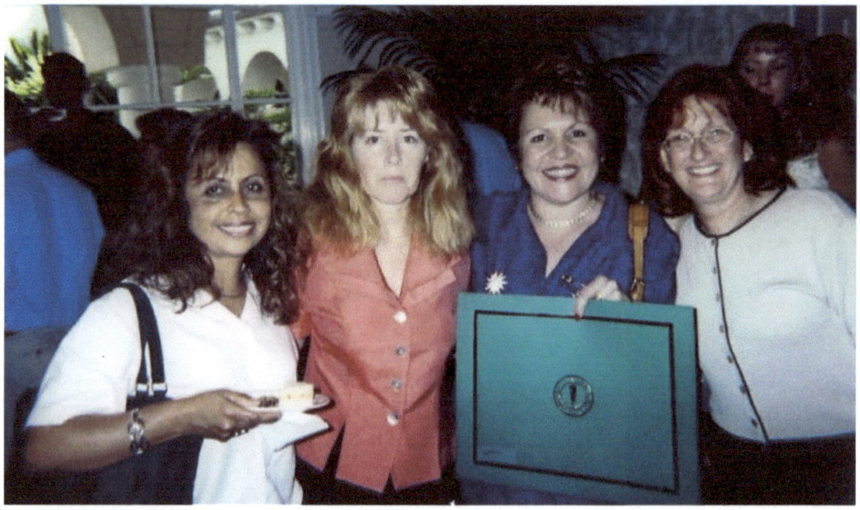

Left to right: Dona Shearer (clinical office, Drs. Lockey, Fox, Ledford); Jose Arias Jr., MD (2001-2003); Nina C. Ramirez, MD (2000-2002); circa 2002.

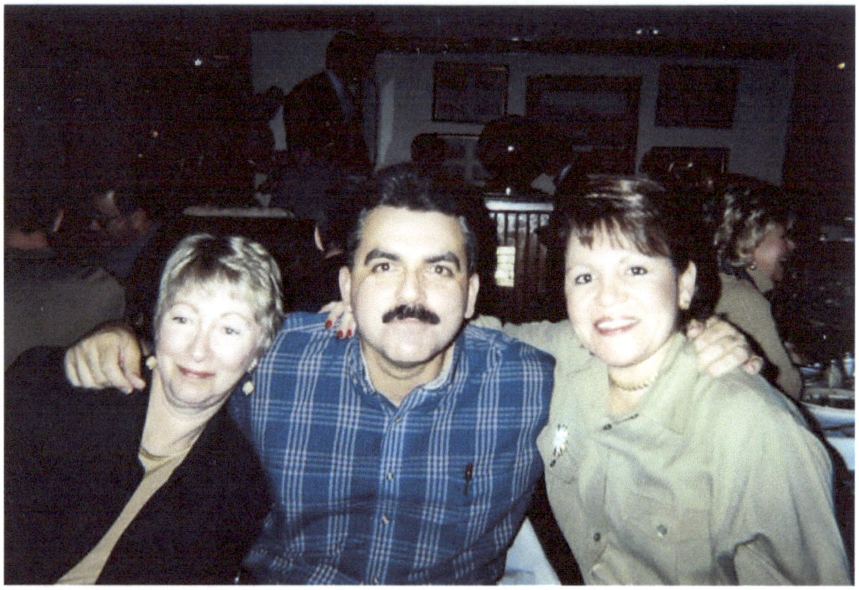

Left to right: Sean McKnight, MD (2002-2004); Dennis K. Ledford, MD (1983-1985); Jennifer Ledford; circa 2004.

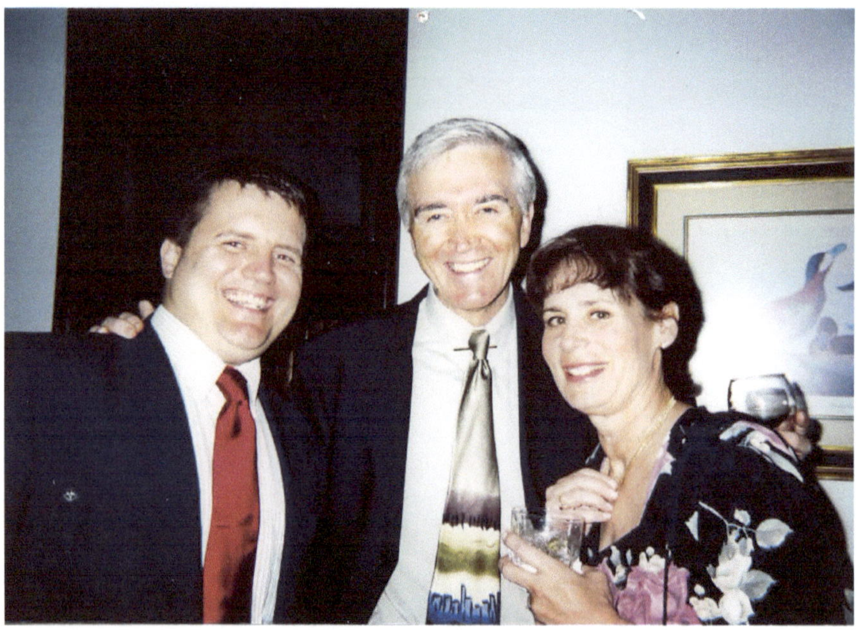

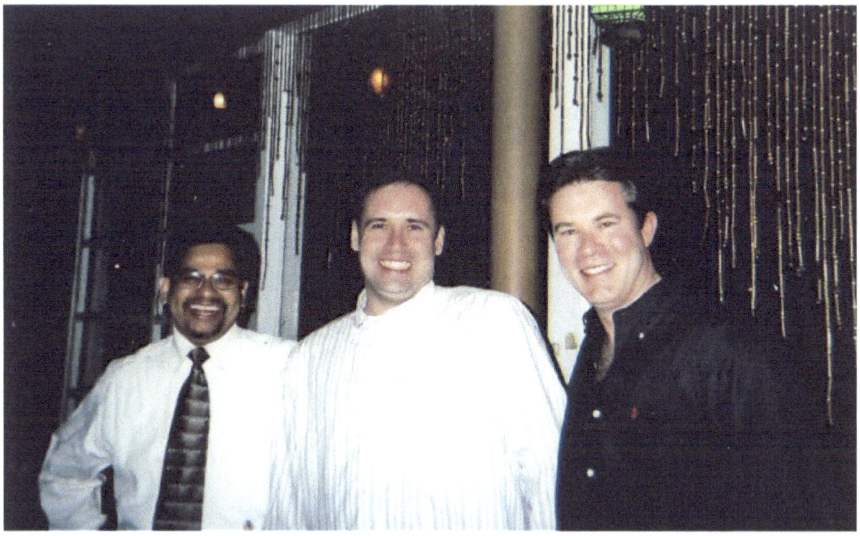

Left to right: Shyam S. Mohapatra, PhD; Patrick J. DeMarco, MD (2003-2005); Brett E. Stanaland, MD (1992-1995); circa 2005.

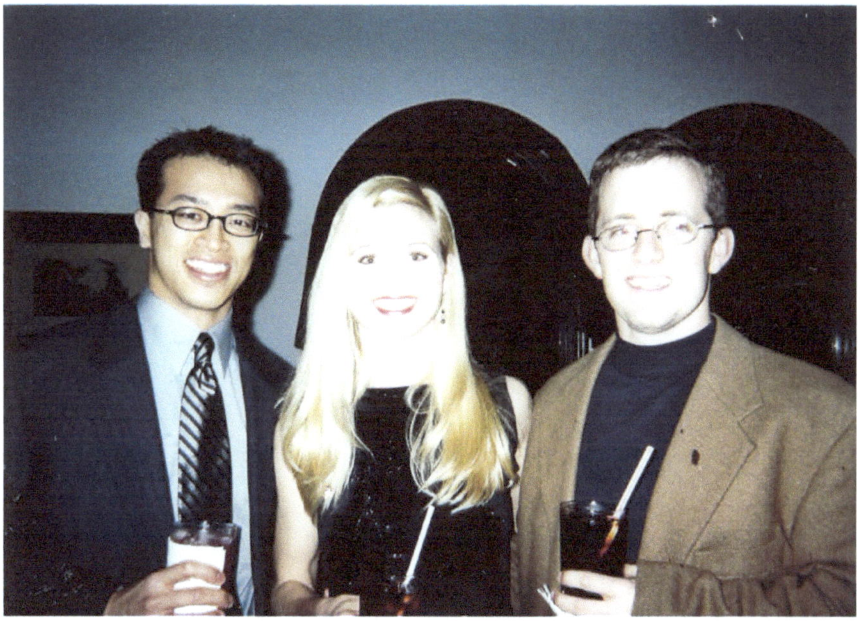

Left to right: Alex T. Vu, MD (2004-2006); Mikki Ramey; John T. Ramey, MD (2003-2005); circa 2005.

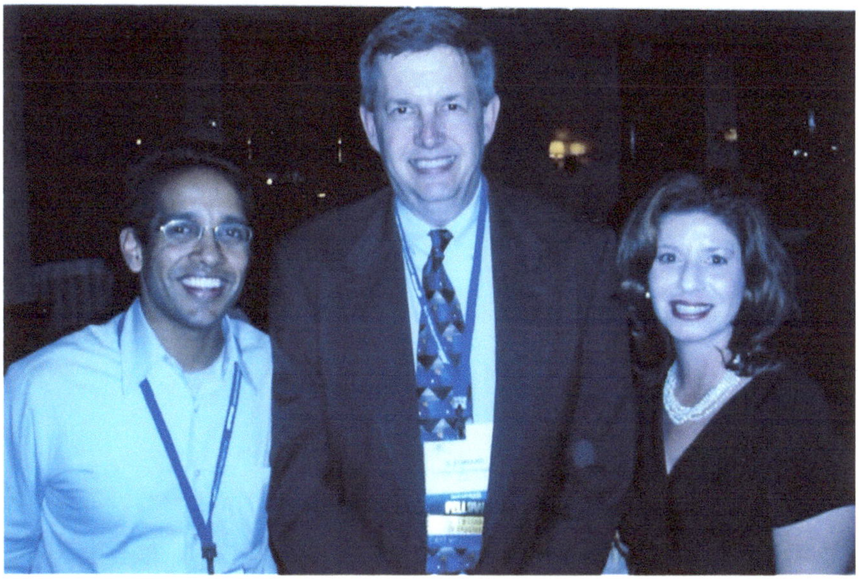

Left to right: Thomas Chacko, MD (2005-2007); G. Edward Stewart, MD (1991-1994); Patti Stewart; circa 2006.

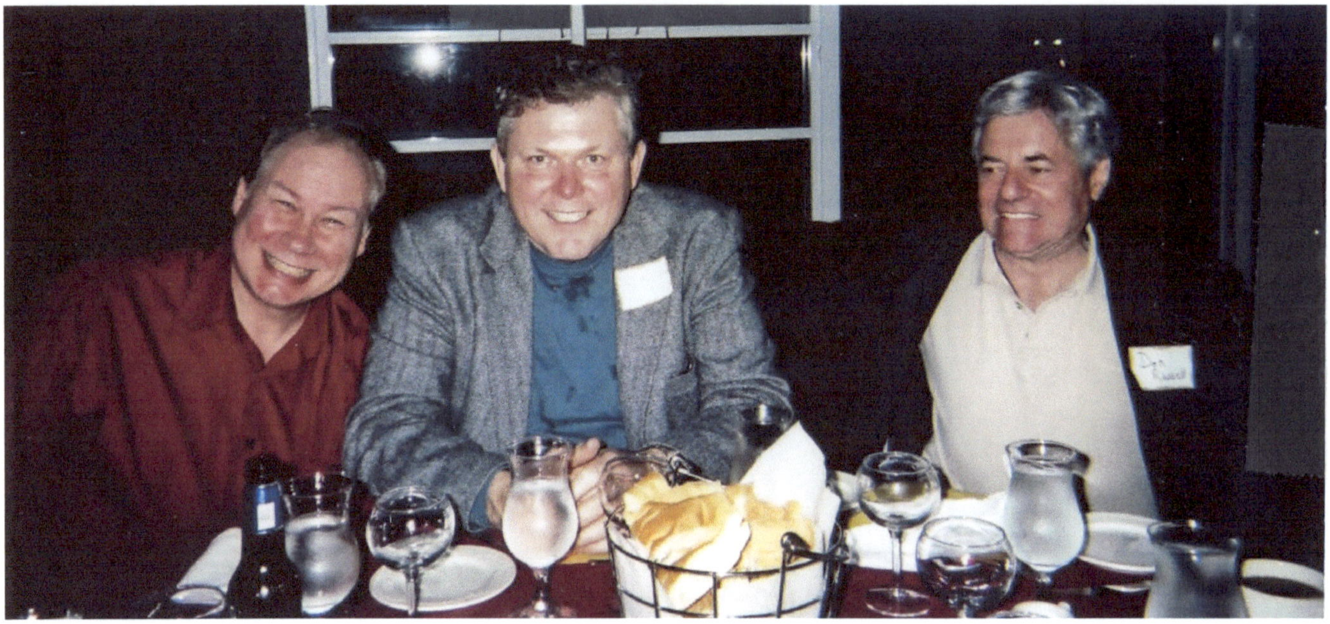

Left to right: Gerald A. Bucholtz, MD (1980-1982); Albert E. Hensel (1982-1984); Donald W. Russell, MD (1987-1990); USF Alumni Dinner, AAAAI Meeting, Miami 2006.

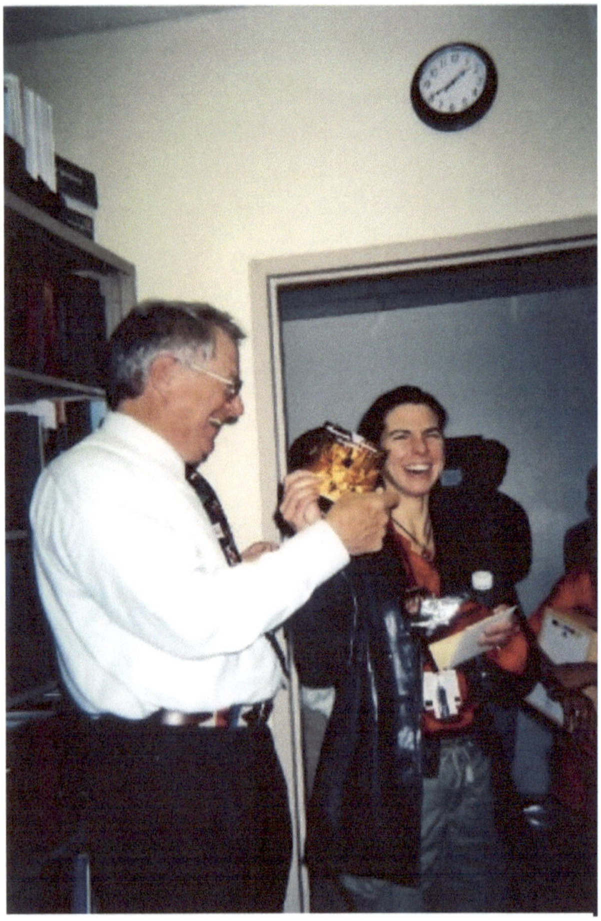

Left to right: Richard F. Lockey, MD, MS and Denise M. Kearney, MD (2004-2006); circa 2005.

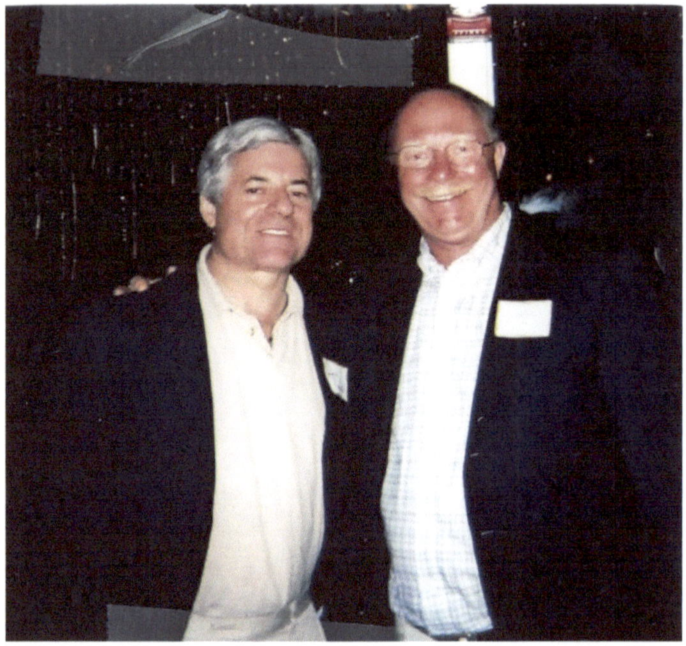

Left to right: Donald W. Russell, MD (1987-1990) and Lionel V. Bonini, MD (ACH 1986-1988); 2006.

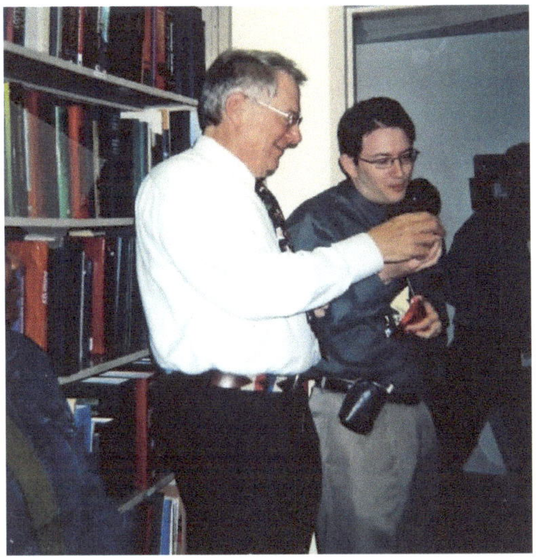

Left to right: Richard F. Lockey, MD, MS and Steven L. Cole, DO (2005-2007).

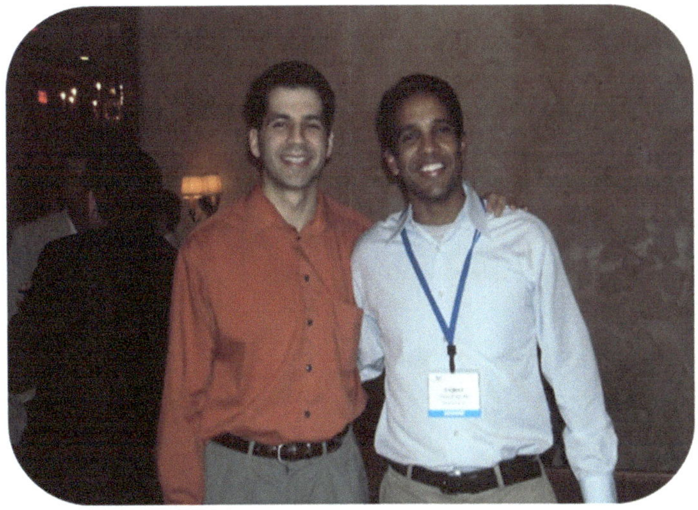

Left to right: Richard Lavi, MD (ACH 2004-2006) and Thomas Chacko, MD (2005-2007); USF Alumni Dinner, 2008 American Academy of Allergy Asthma & Immunology Annual Meeting, Philadelphia.

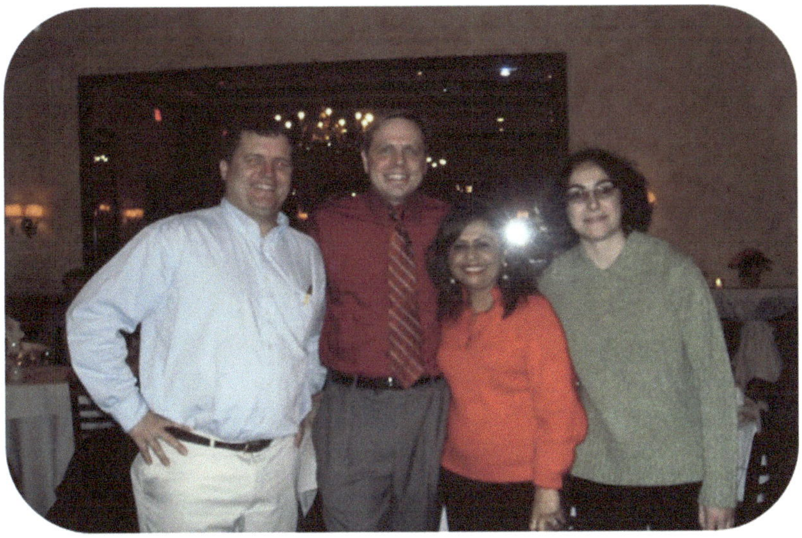

Left to right: Sean McKnight, MD (2002-2004); Richard E. Crockett, MD (2000-2003); Geeta Gehi; Cristina Jaen, PhD; USF Alumni Dinner, 2008 American Academy of Allergy Asthma & Immunology Annual Meeting, Philadelphia.

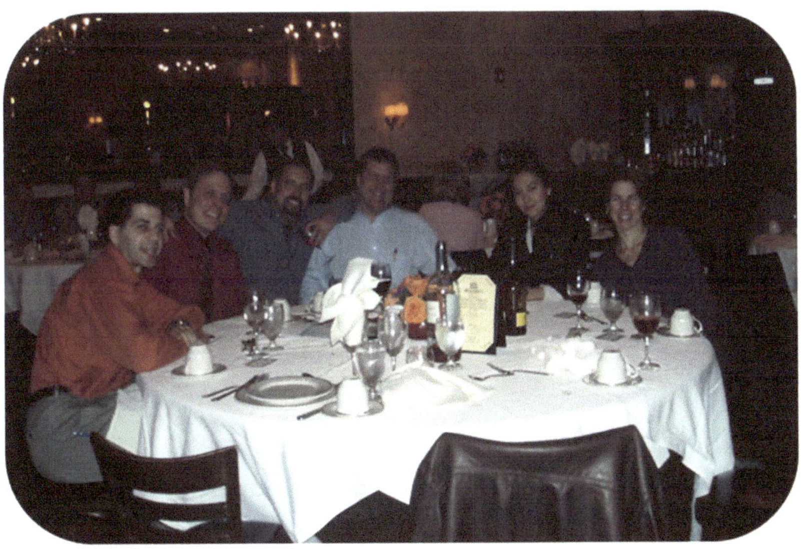

Left to right: Richard Lavi, MD (ACH 2004-2006); Richard E. Crockett, MD (2000-2003); Patrick J. DeMarco, MD (2003-2005); A. Sean McKnight, MD (2002-2004); Morna Dorsey, MD, MMSc (ACH faculty); Denise M. Kearney, MD (2004-2006).

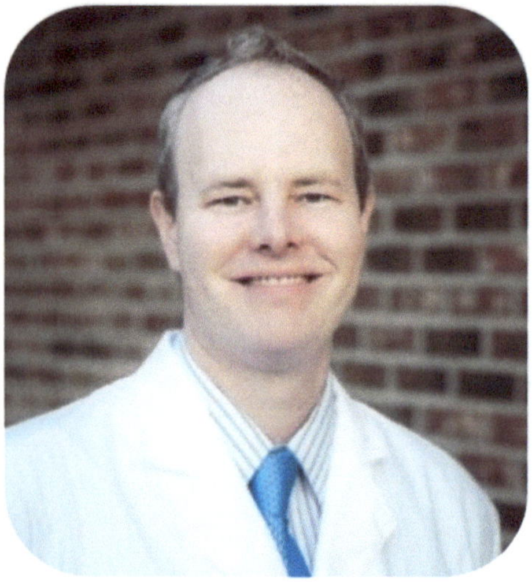

Andrew Bagg, MD (2006-2008).

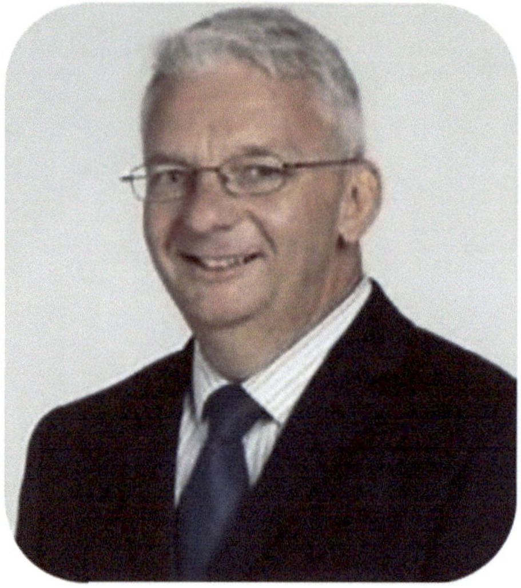

Ronald T. Purcell, MD (2006-2008

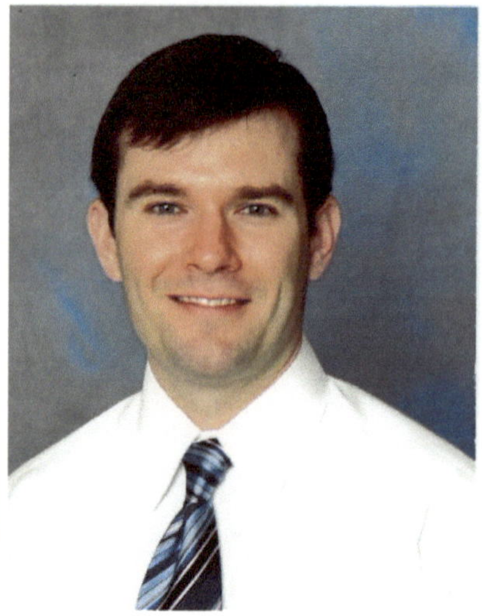

Joshua Phillips, MD (2007-2009).

Byol Shin, DO (2006-2008).

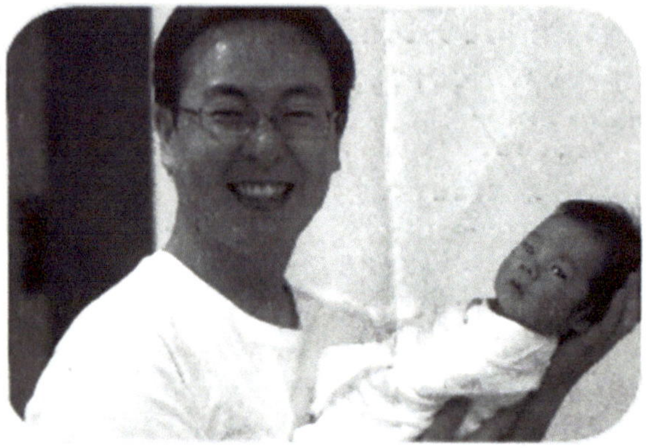

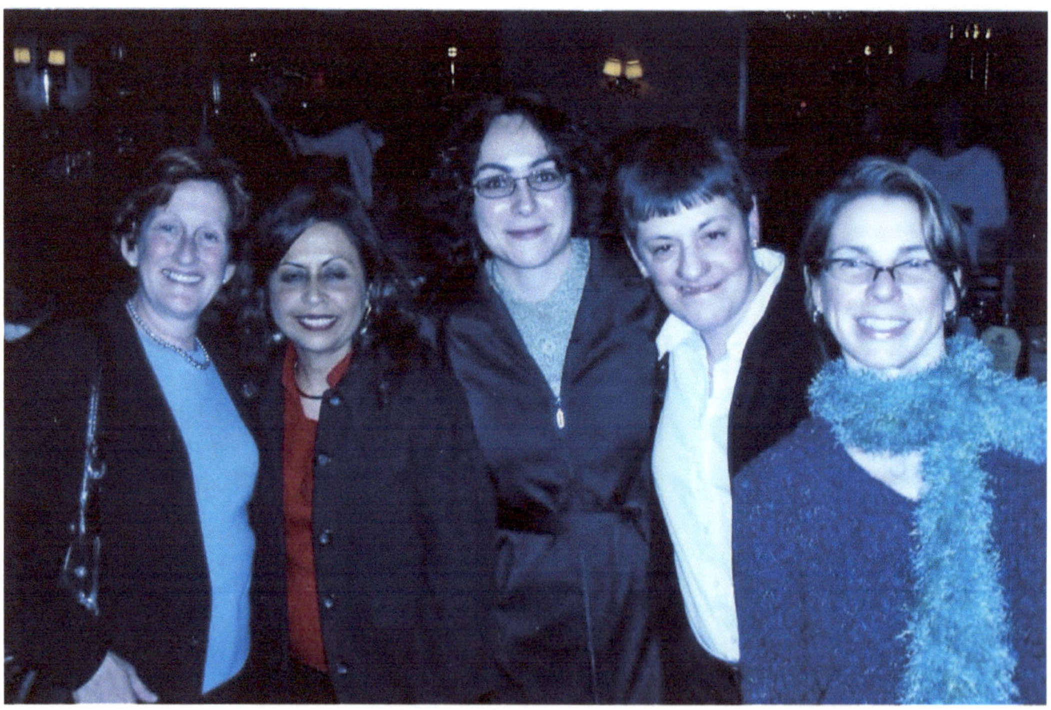

Left to right: Peggy Hales, Geeta Gehi, Cristina Jaen, PhD; Rosa Codina, PhD; Denise M. Kearney, MD (2004-2006); circa 2008.

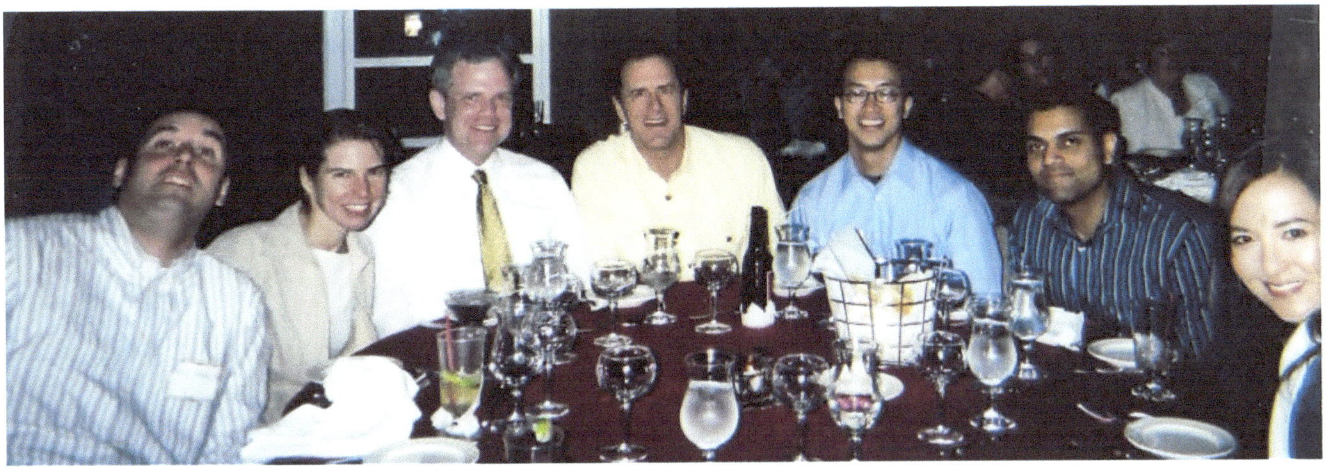

Left to right: Patrick J. Demarco, MD (2003-2005); Denise M. Kearney, MD (2004-2006); Stephen F. Kemp, MD (1993-1996); Hugh H. Windom, MD (Clinical Affiliate Professor); Alex T. Vu, MD (2004-2006); Mathew Varghese, MD (2007-2009); Morna Dorsey, MD, MMSc, circa 2008.

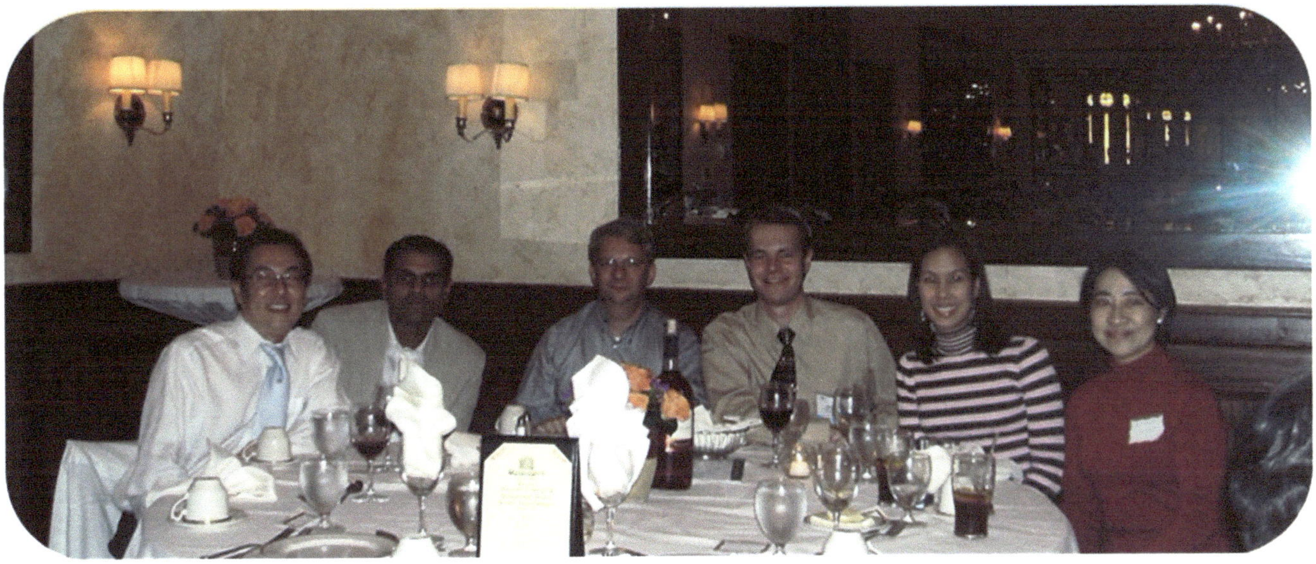

Left to right: Byol Shin, DO (2006-2008); Mathew Varghese, MD (2007-2009); Ronald T. Purcell, MD (2006-2008); Andrew S. Bagg, MD (2006-2008); guests; circa 2008.

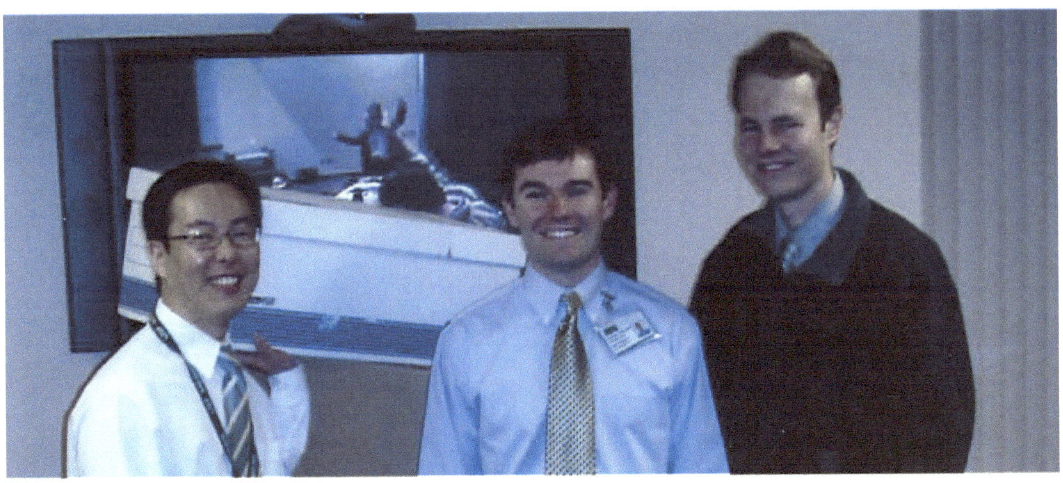

Left to right: Byol Shin, DO (2006-2008); Joshua Phillips, MD (2007-2009); Andrew Bagg, MD (2006-2008); circa 2008.

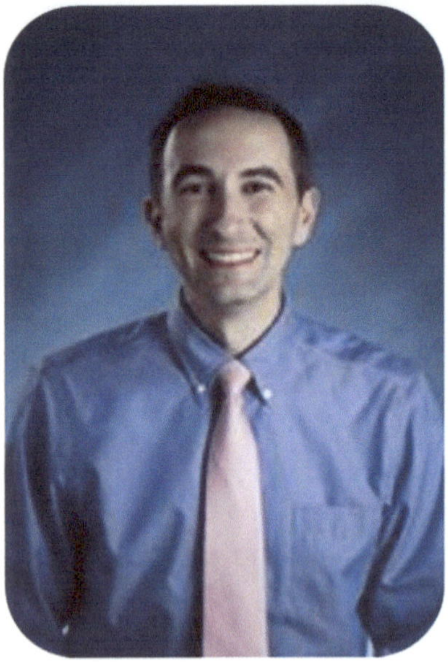

Robert (Robbie) D. Pesek, MD (2009-2011).

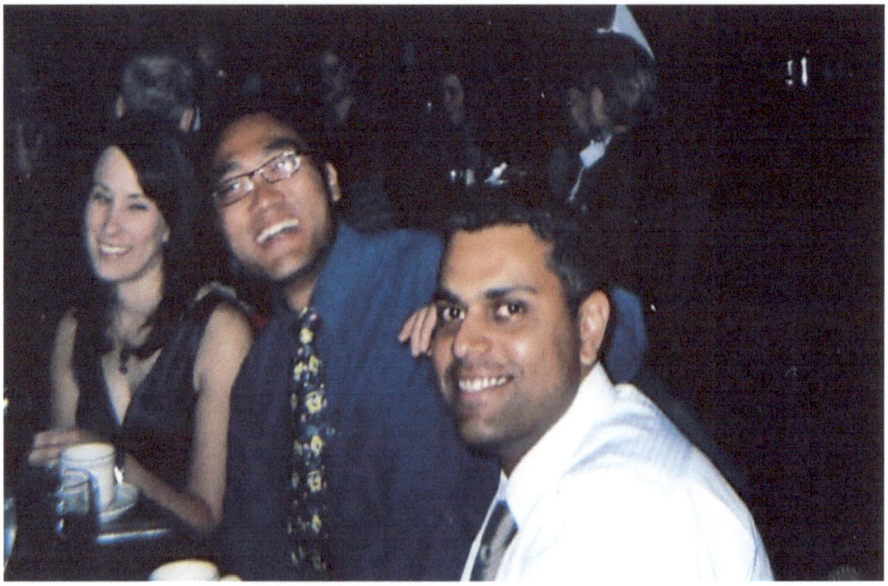

Left to right: Jenny Kim, M.D; Dennis Kim, MD (2008-2010); Mathew Varghese, MD (2007-2009); 2009.

Left to right: Dennis Kim, MD (2008-2010); Jenny Kim, MD; Trace Adkins (featured guest, 2009 Education and Research Trust Fund fund-raising dinner, American Academy of Allergy Asthma & Immunology Annual Meeting, Washington, D.C.); Joshua Phillips, MD (2007-2009).

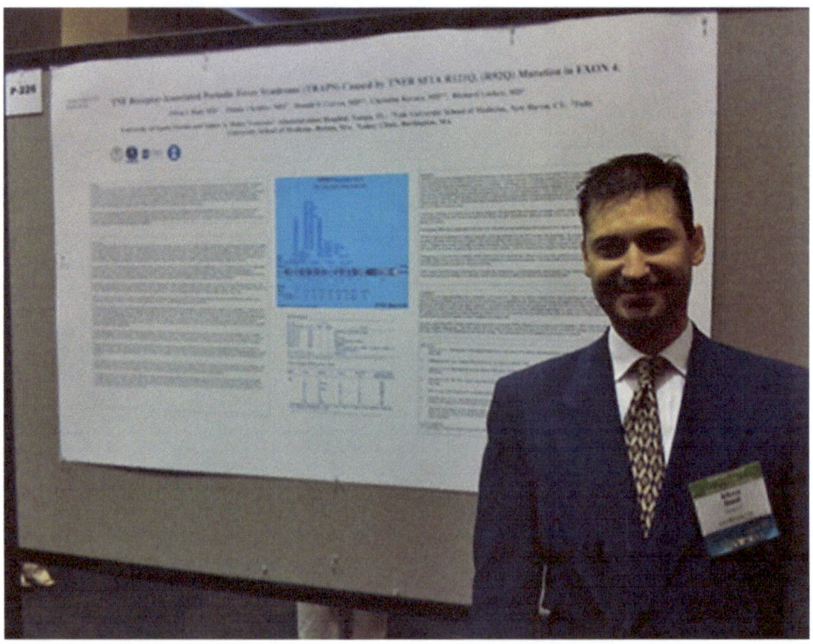

Efren L. Rael, MD (2008-2010); American College of Allergy, Asthma & Immunology Meeting; Seattle, November 2008.

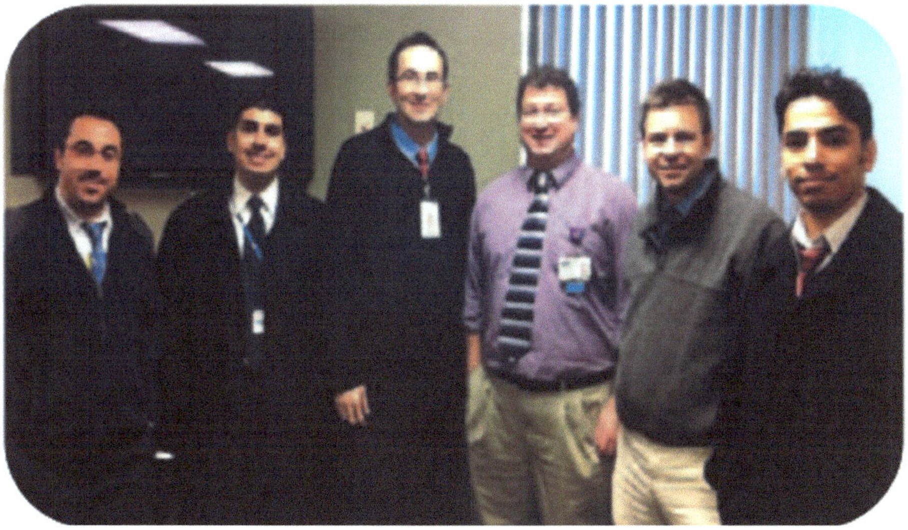

Left to right: Michel Alkhalil, MD (2009-2011); Ahmed Butt, MD (2010-2012); Robert (Robbie) D. Pesek, MD (2009-2011); James Parkerson, DO (2010-2012); David J. Fitzhugh, MD (2010-2012); Salman Aljubran, MD (2010-2013); circa 2010.

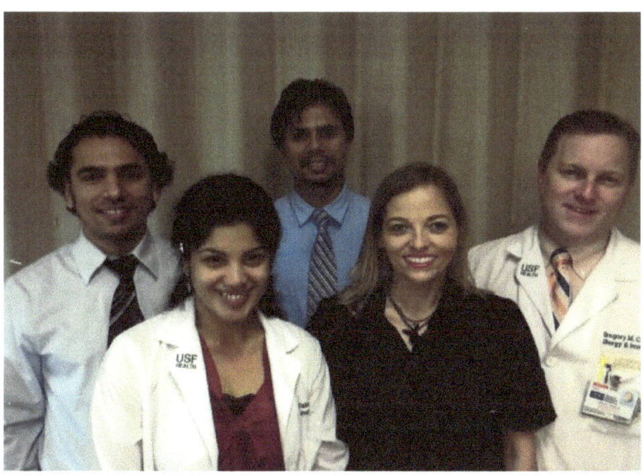

Font row (left to right): Neetu Talreja, MD (2011-2013); Susan Culverhouse, MD (2011-2013). Back row (left to right): Salman Aljubran, MD (2010-2013); Nauman Salim, MD (2012-2014); Gregory Cowan, MD (2012-2014). Circa 2012.

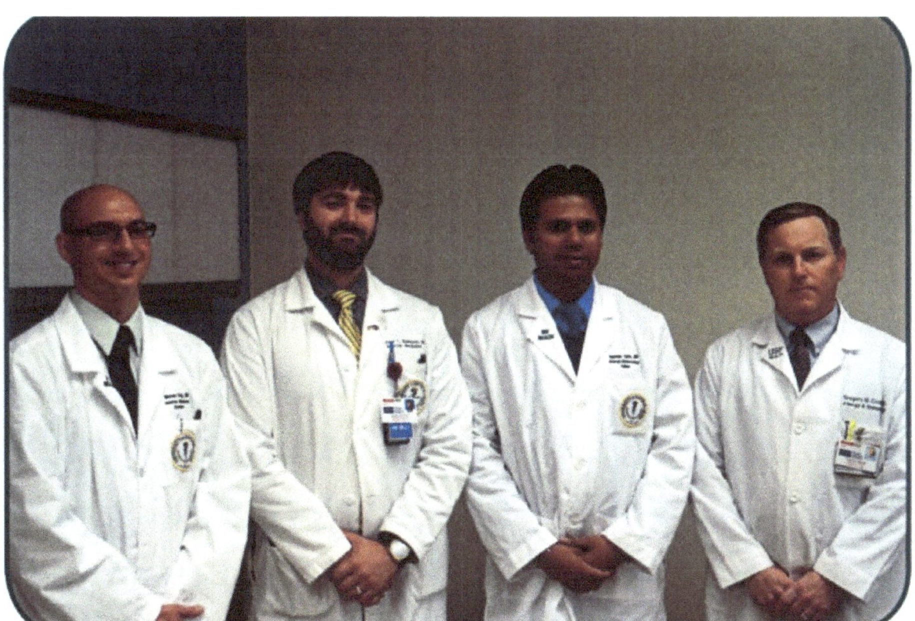

Left to right: Adam C. Updegraff, DO (2013-2015); Michael C. Balduzzi, MD (2013-2015); Nauman Salim, MD (2012-2014); Gregory M. Cowan, MD (2012-2014).

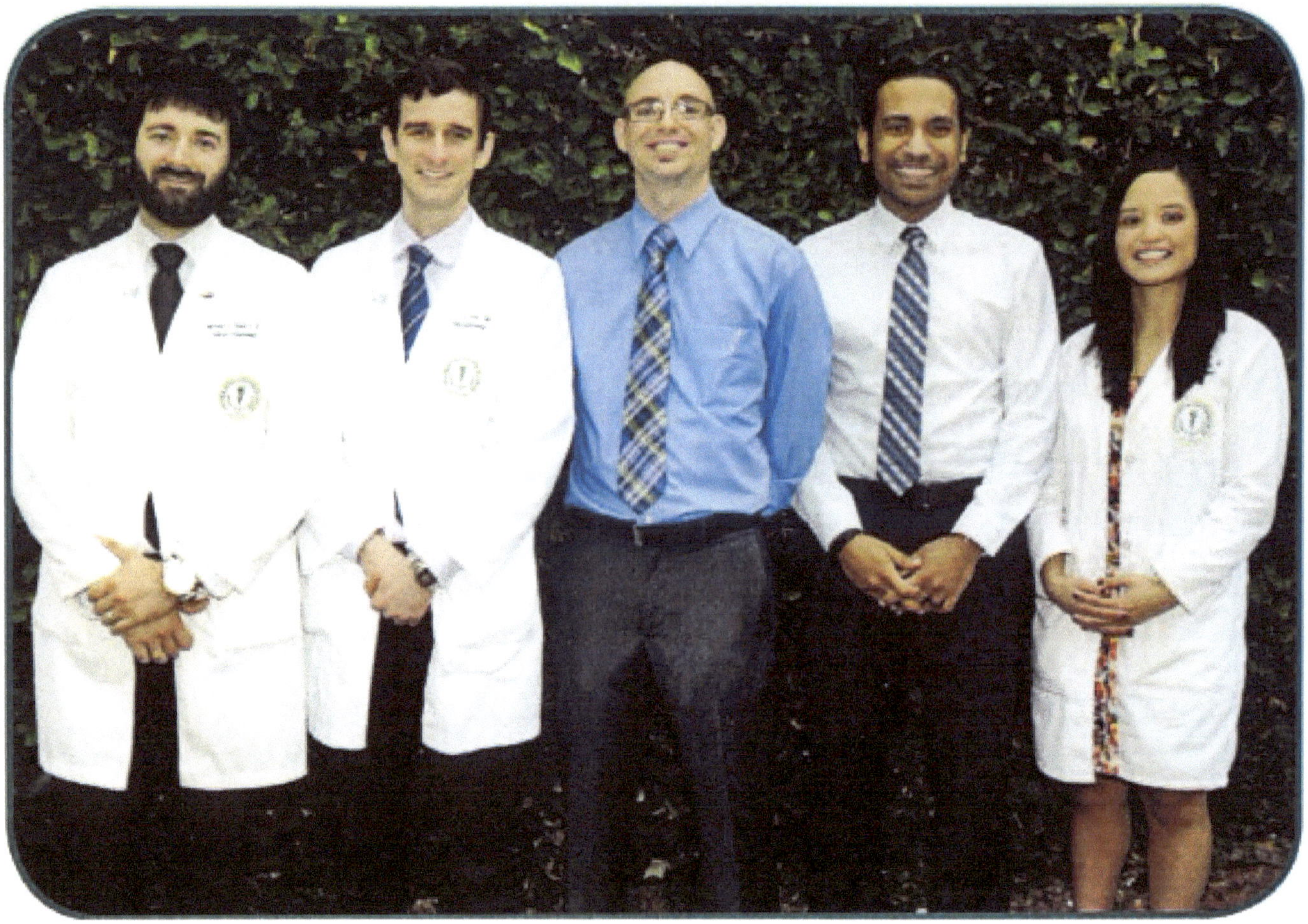

Left to right: Michael Balduzzi, MD (2013-2015); Andrew J. Cooke, MD (2014-2016); Adam C. Updegraff, DO (2013-2015); Adeeb A. Bulkhi, MD (2014-2017); Jennifer E. Fergeson, DO (2014-2016).

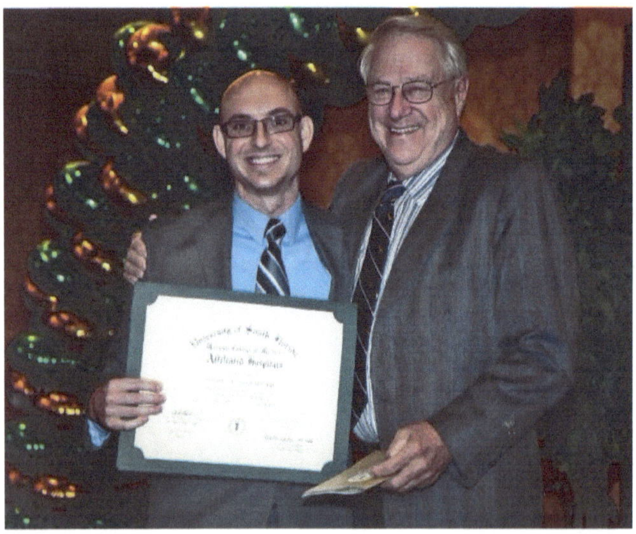

Left to right: Adam C. Updegraff, DO (2013-2015) and Richard F. Lockey, MD, MS; graduation; June 2015.

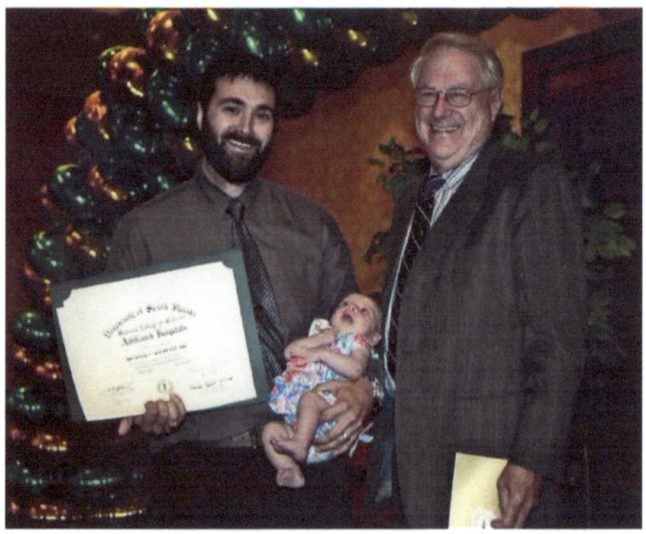

Left to right: Michael C. Balduzzi, MD (2013-2015) and daughter; Richard F. Lockey, MD, MS; graduation; June 2015.

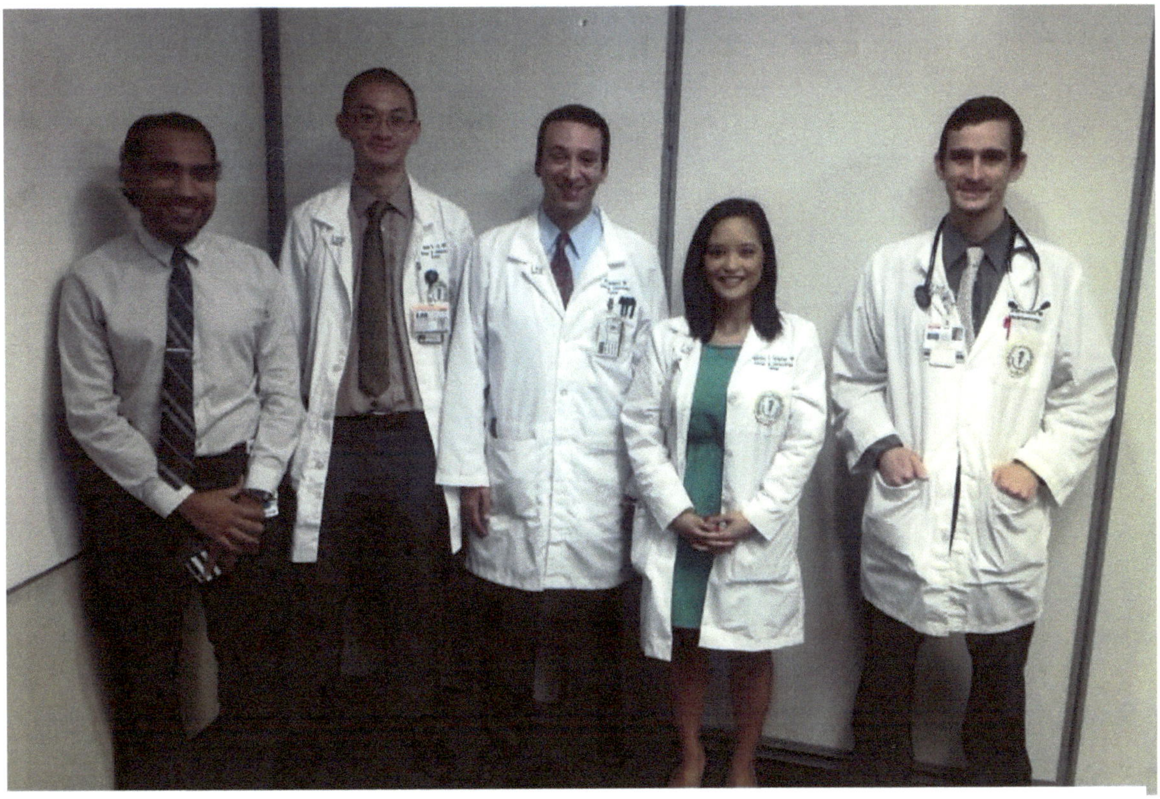

Left to right: Adeeb A. Bulkhi, MD (2014-2017); Chen Lin, MD (2015-2017); Peter Ricketti, DO (2015-2017); Jennifer E. Fergeson, DO (2014-2016); Andrew J. Cooke, MD (2014-2016); 2015.

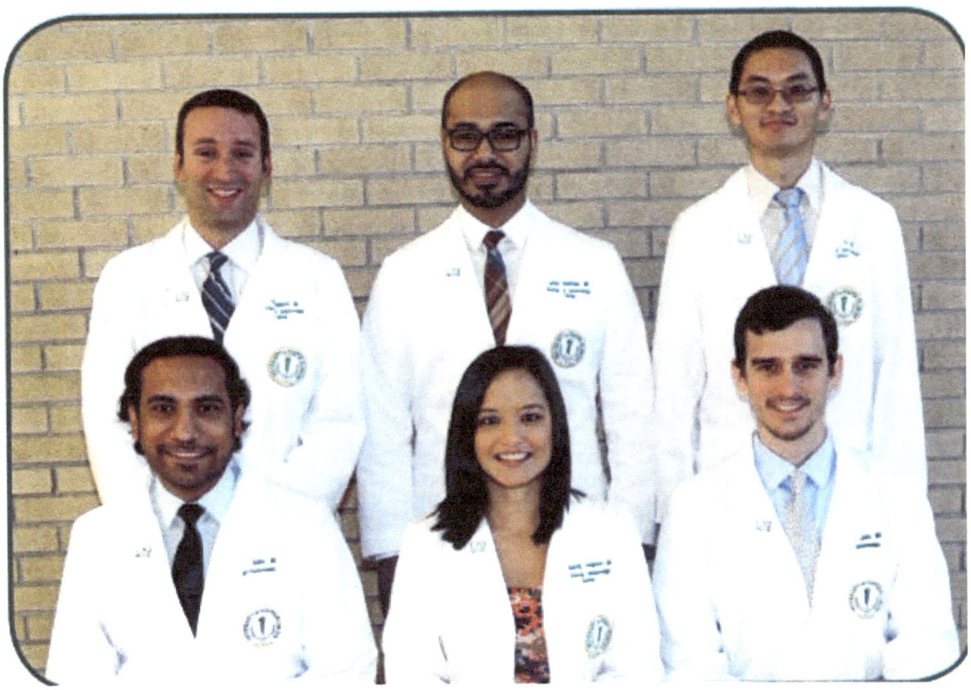

Front row (left to right): Adeeb A. Bulkhi, MD (2014-2017); Jennifer E. Fergeson, DO (2014-2016); Andrew J. Cooke, MD (2014-2016). Back row (left to right): Peter A. Ricketti, DO (2015-2017); Sultan Alandijani, MD (2015-2017); Chen Lin, MD (2015-2017). Circa 2016.

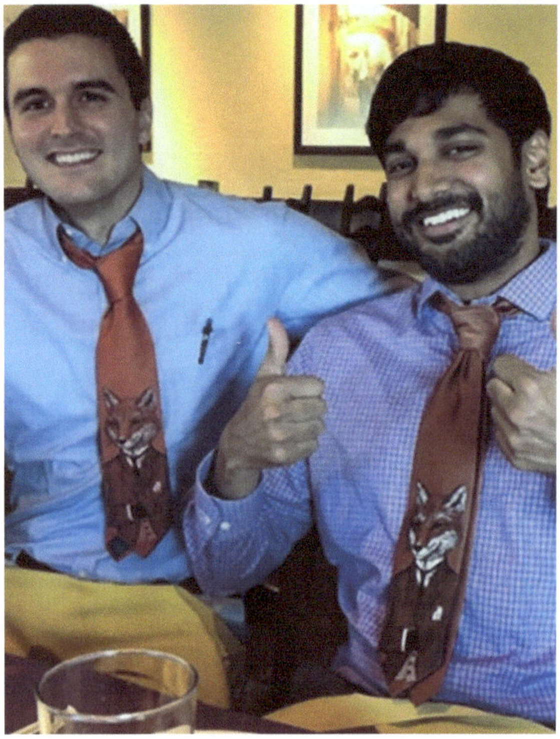

Left to right: Kirk V. Shepard II, MD (2017-2019) and Shiven S. Patel, MD (2017-2019). Graduation dinner; June 2019; graduation gift – famous "Fox" tie.

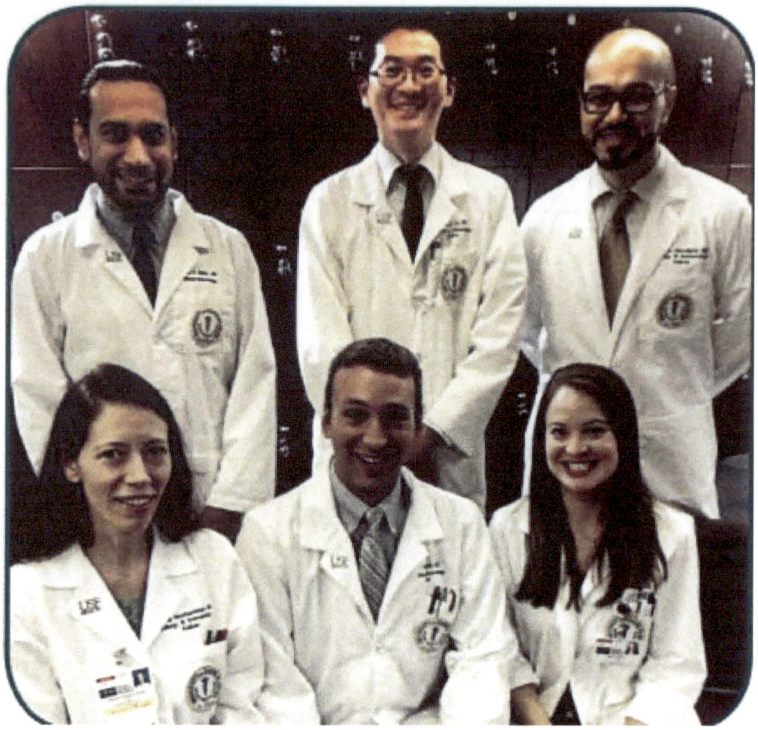

Front row (left to right): Emma Westermann-Clark, MD (2016-2018); Peter A. Ricketti, DO (2015-2017); Amber N. Pepper, MD (2016-2018). Back row (left to right): Adeeb A. Bulkhi, MD (2014-2017); Chen Lin, MD (2015-2017); Sultan Alandijani, MD (2015-2017). Circa 2017.

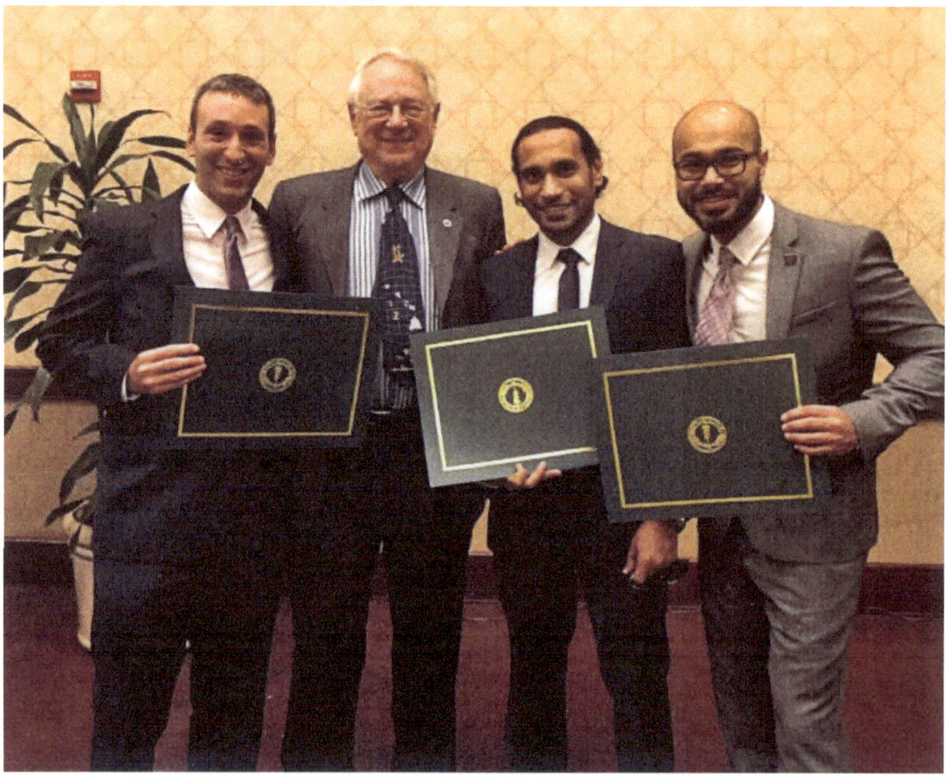

Left to right: Peter Ricketti, DO (2015-2017); Richard F. Lockey, MD, MS; Adeeb Bulkhi, MD (2014-2017); Sultan Alandijani, MD (2015-2017); graduation 2017.

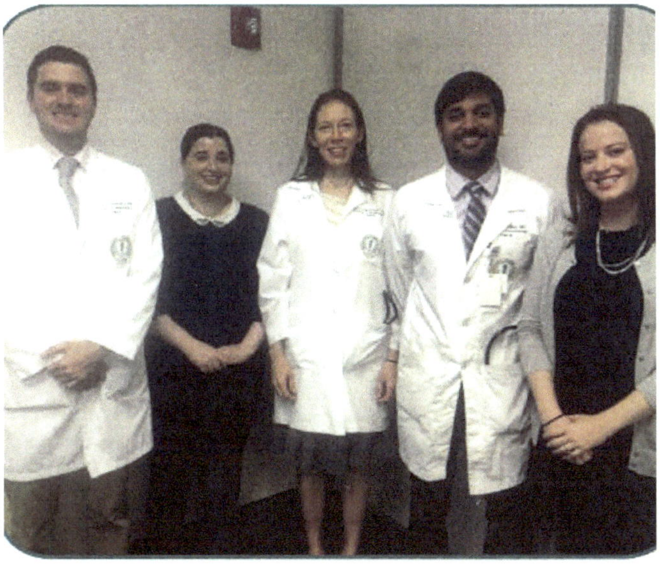

Left to right: Kirk V. Shepard II, MD (2017-2019); Tara V. Saco, MD (2017-2019); Emma Westermann-Clark, MD (2016-2018): Shiven S. Patel, MD; Amber N. Pepper, MD (2016-2018);2017.

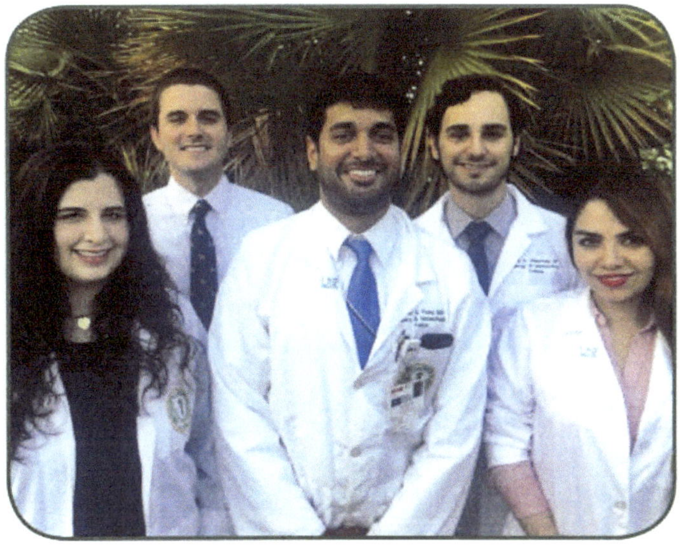

Front row (left to right): Tara V. Saco, MD (2017-2019); Shiven S. Patel, MD (2017-2019); Claudia Gaefke, MD (2018-2020). Back row (left to right): Kirk V. Shepard II, MD (2017-2019); Raul Sergio Villarreal, MD (2018-2020). Circa 2018.

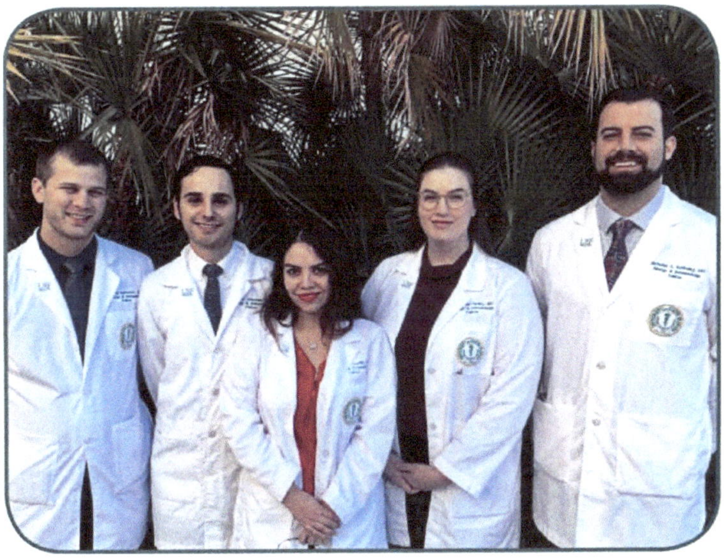

Left to right: David Gubernick, MD (2019-2021); Raul Sergio Villarreal, MD (2018-2020); Claudia Gaefke, MD (2018-2020); Stephanie Hudey, MD (2019-2021); Nicholas Kolinsky, DO (2019-2021); 2019.

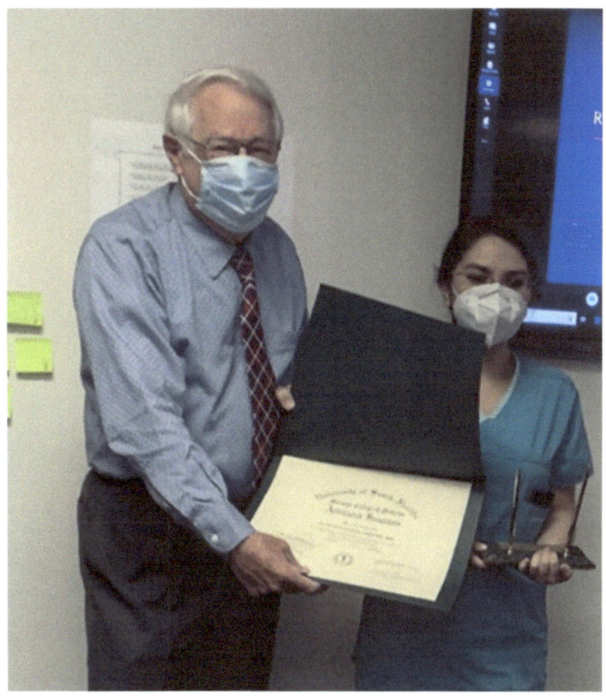

Left to right: Richard F. Lockey, MD, MS; Claudia Gaefke, MD (2018-2020); graduation; June 2020.

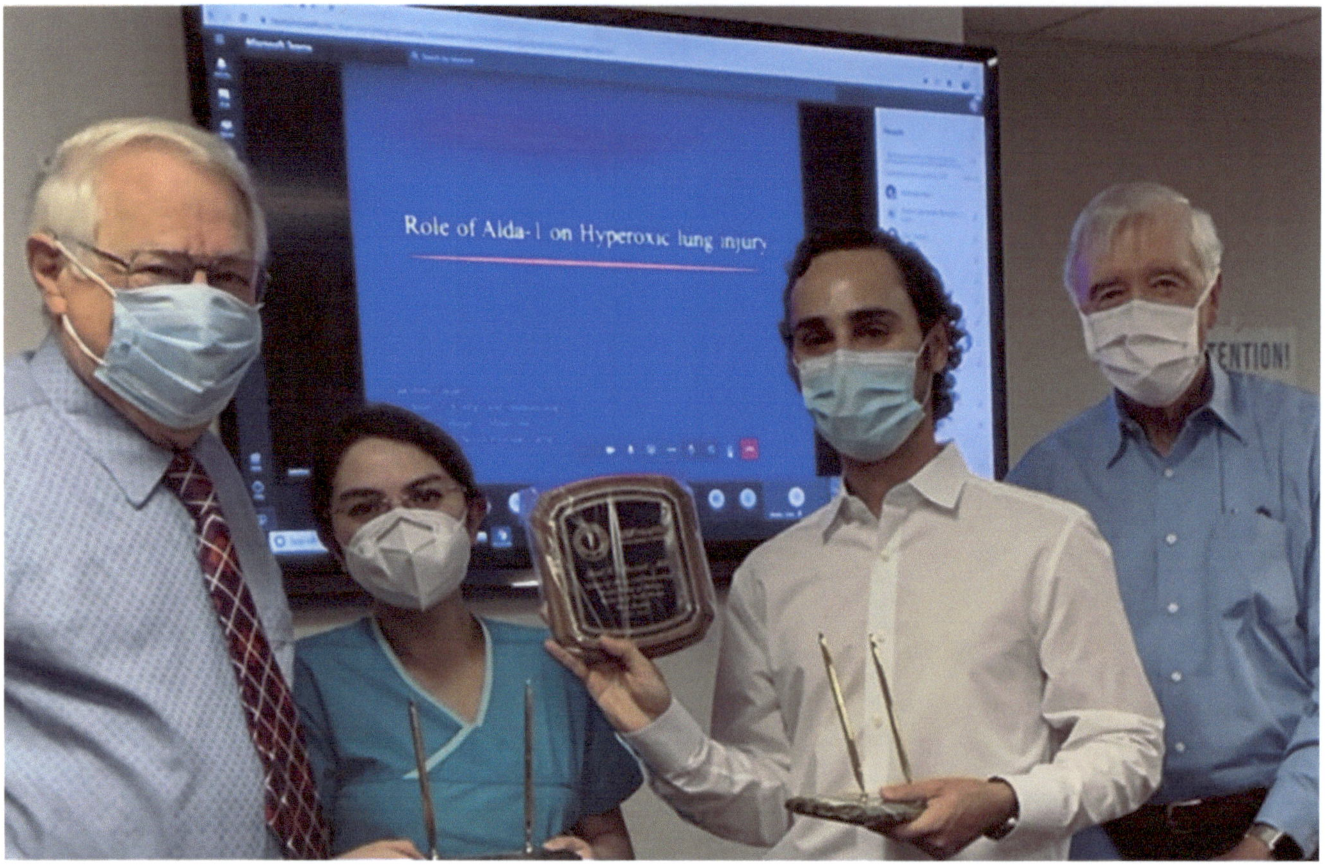

Left to right: Richard F. Lockey, MD, MS; Claudia Gaefke, MD (2018-2020); Raul Sergio Villarreal, MD (2018-2020); Dennis K. Ledford, MD (1983-1985); graduation; June 2020. Drs. Gaefke and Villarreal receiving graduation pen sets; Dr. Villarreal receiving Chief Fellow plaque.

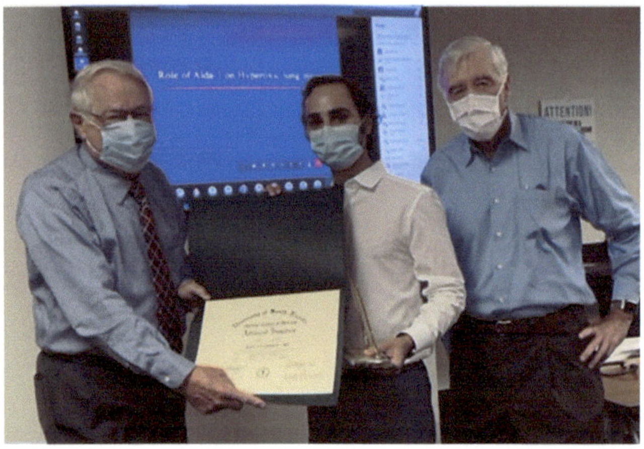

Above, left to right: Richard F. Lockey, MD, MS; Raul Sergio Villarreal, MD (2018-2020); Dennis K. Ledford, MD (1983-1985); graduation; June 2020.

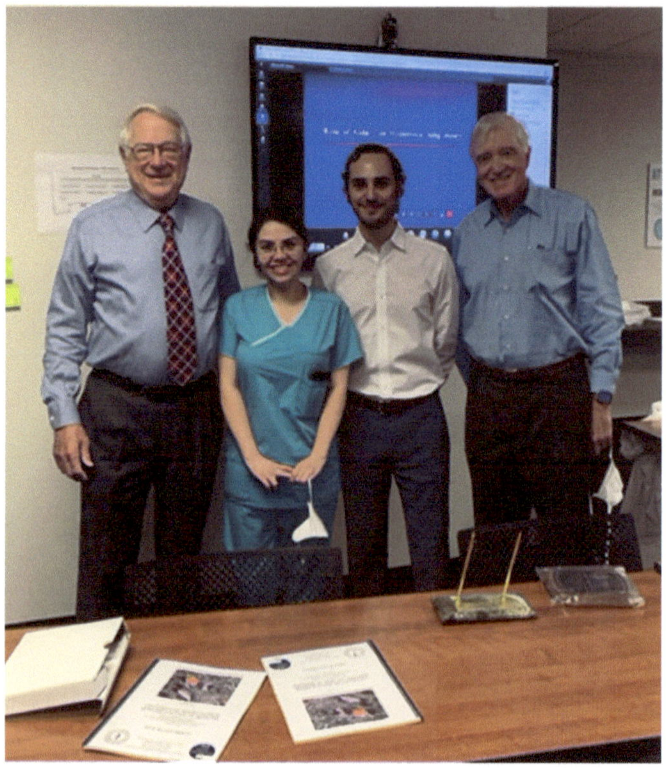

Right, left to right: Richard F. Lockey, MD, MS; Claudia Gaefke, MD (2018-2020); Raul Sergio Villarreal, MD (2018-2020); Dennis K. Ledford, MD (1983-1985); graduation; June 2020.

Chapter 6: Department of Pediatrics, Allergy and Immunology Fellows

Please note that the years listed by the physician's name designate the years fellowship training occurred. Pictures were not necessarily taken during the years indicated.

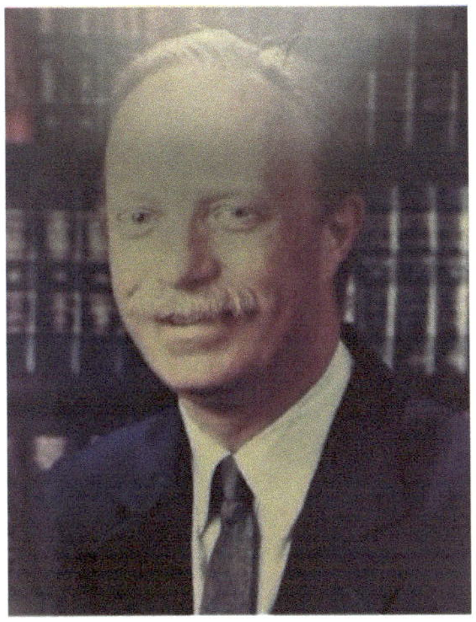

Lionel V. Bonini, MD
(1986-1988)

Ragab Salem Aoun, MD
(1986-1988)

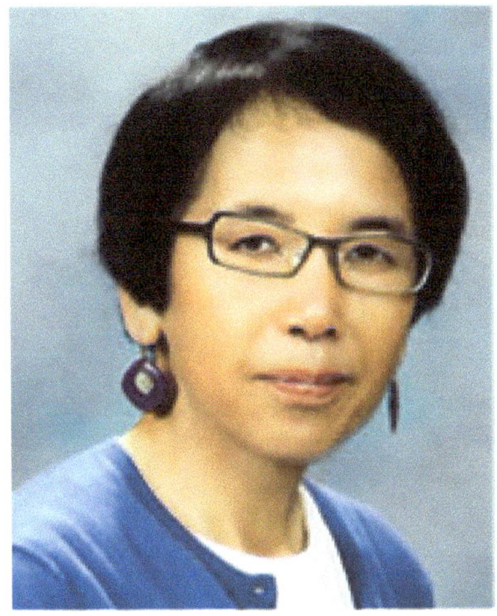

Harumi Jyonouchi, MD
(1987-1989)

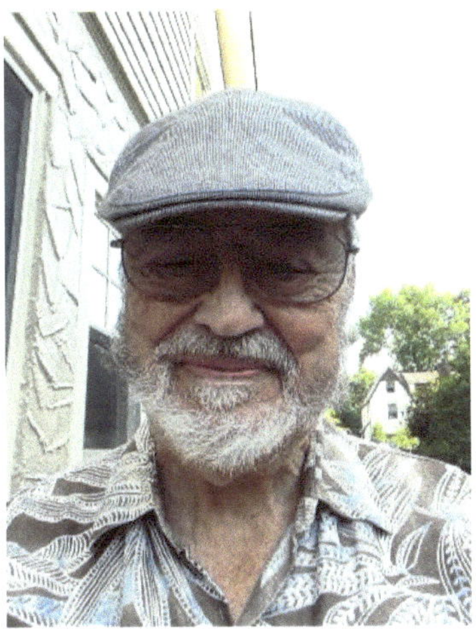

Michael McCann, MD
(1988-1990)

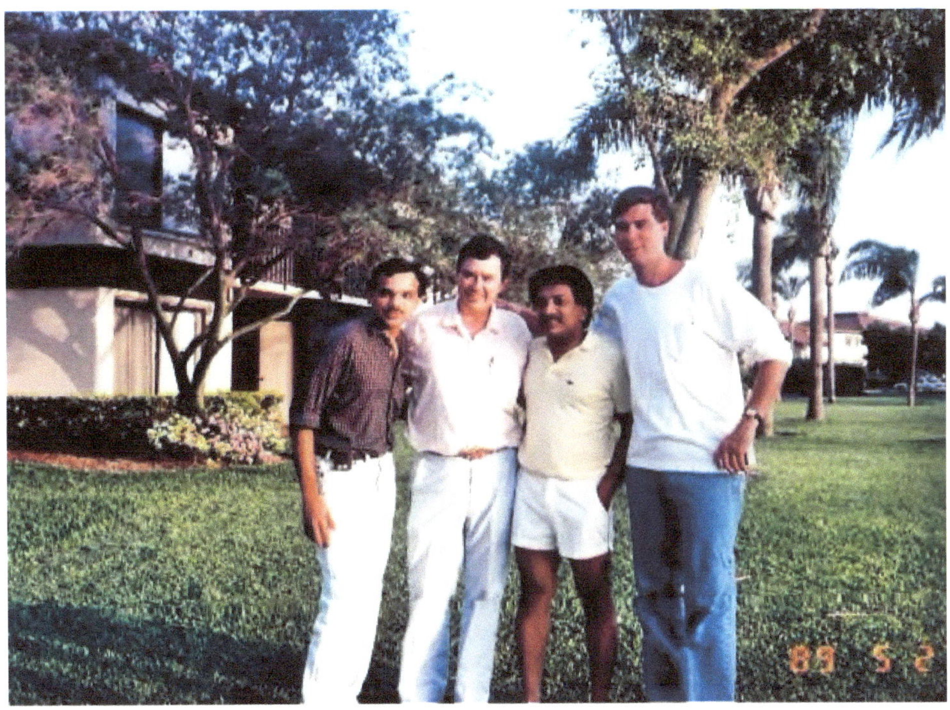

Left to right: Krishna Urval, MD (1988-1990); Michael McCann, MD (1988-1990); Ranjith M. Shetty, MD; (1988-1990); Robert P. Nelson, MD (Tampa, 1985-1987).

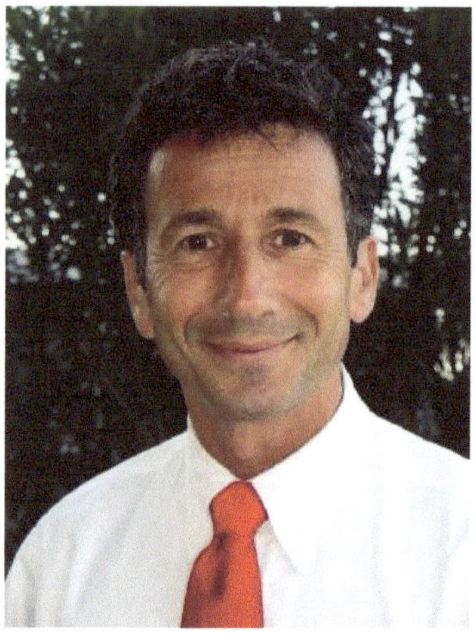

Roberto DiNicolo, MD
(1989-1991)

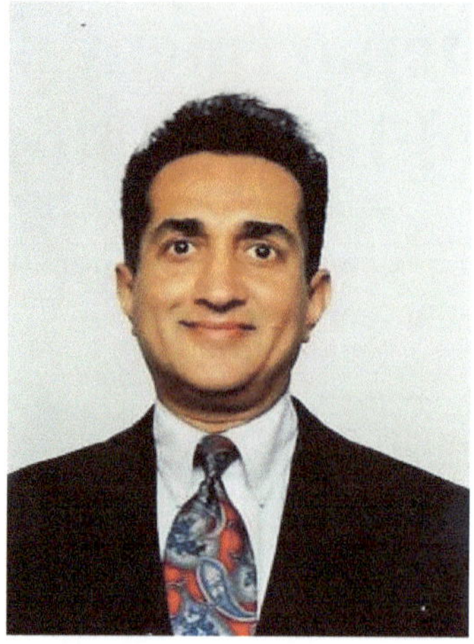

Shivasundara Krishna, MD
(1989-1991)

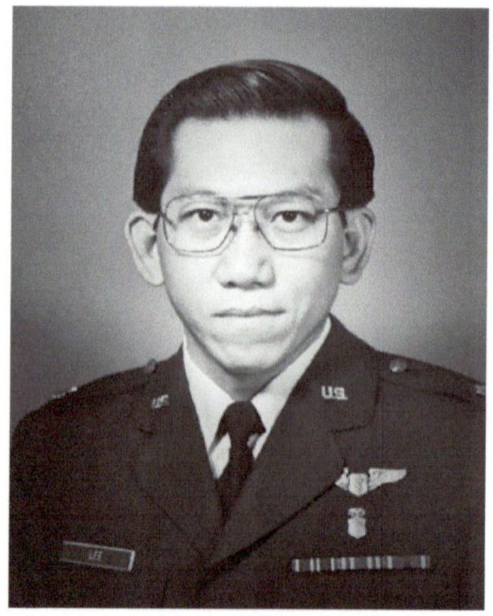

Harry Lee, MD
(1989-1991)

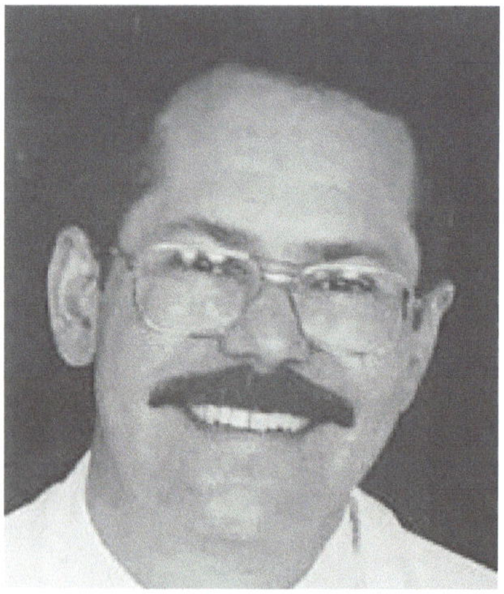

Jose Carro, MD
(1990-1992)

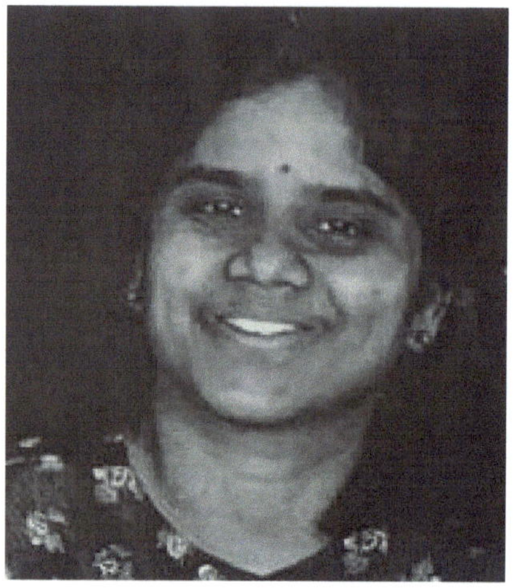

Sai Karlapudi, MD
(1990-1992)

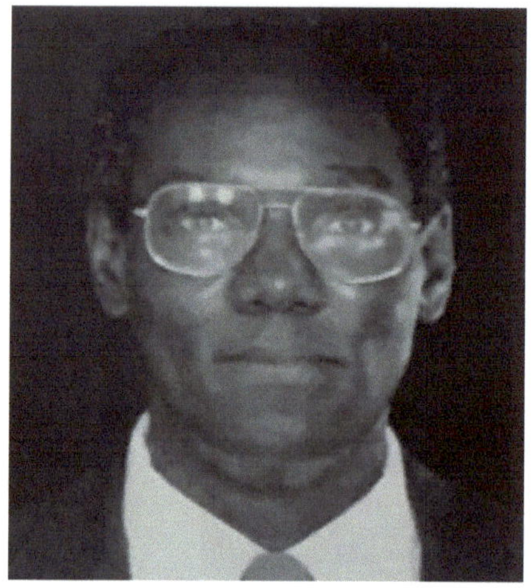

Cleveland Moore, MD
(1990-1992)

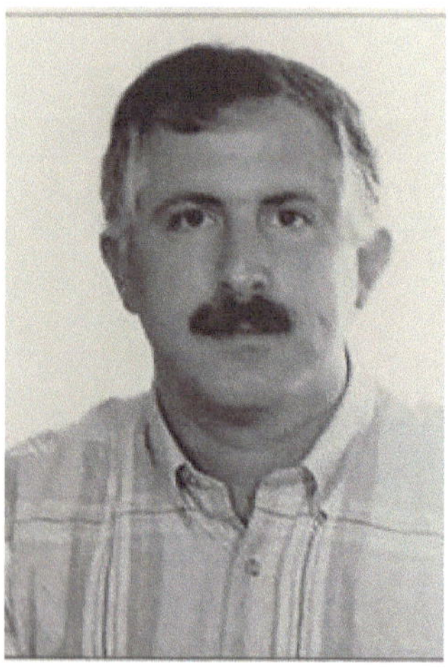

Samuel Gubernick, DO
(1991-1993)

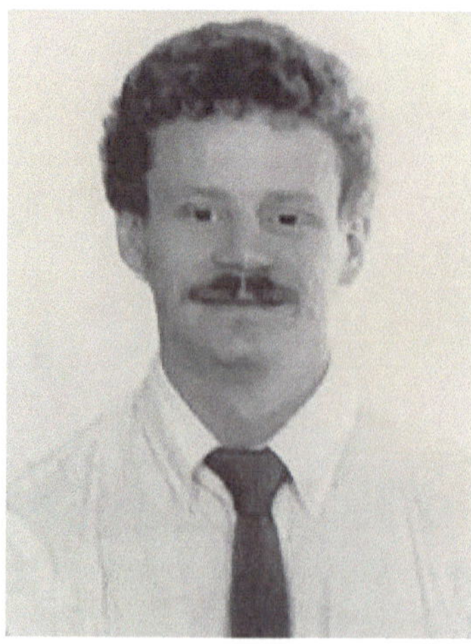

Craig Kalik, MD
(1991-1993)

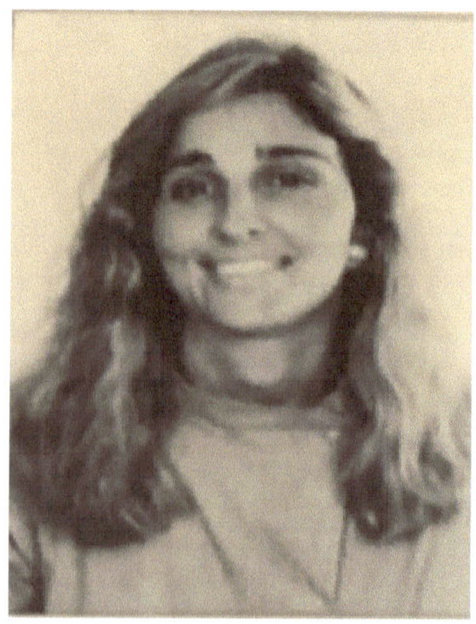

Maria (Maite) Teresa de la Morena, MD
(1991-1995)

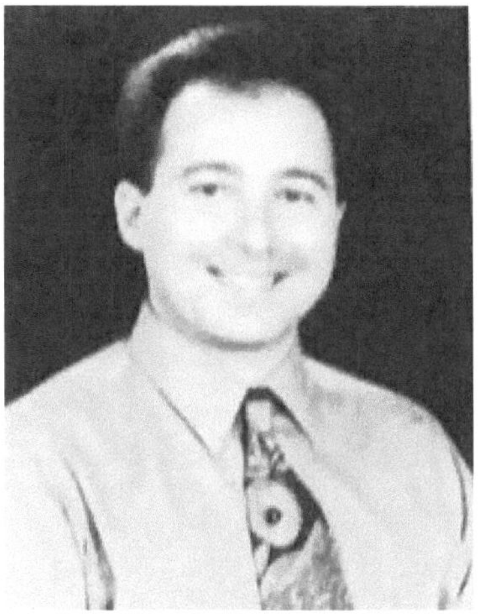

Jamie Kratz, MD
(1992-1994)

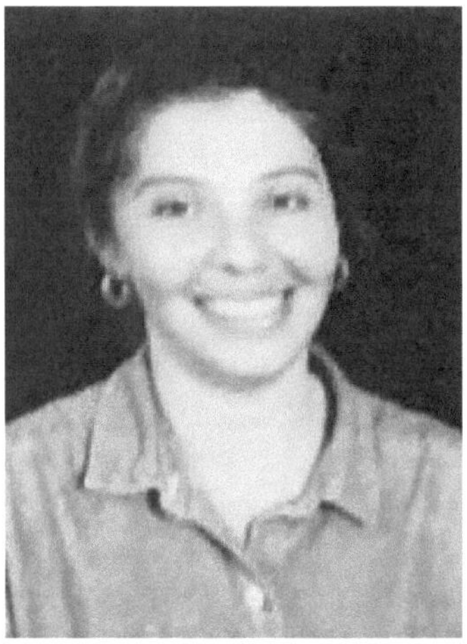

Maria Macias, MD
(1992-1994)

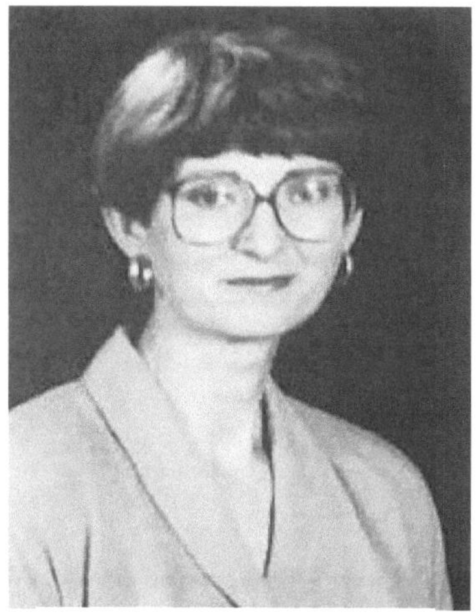

Jeanette Warner, MD
(1992-1994)

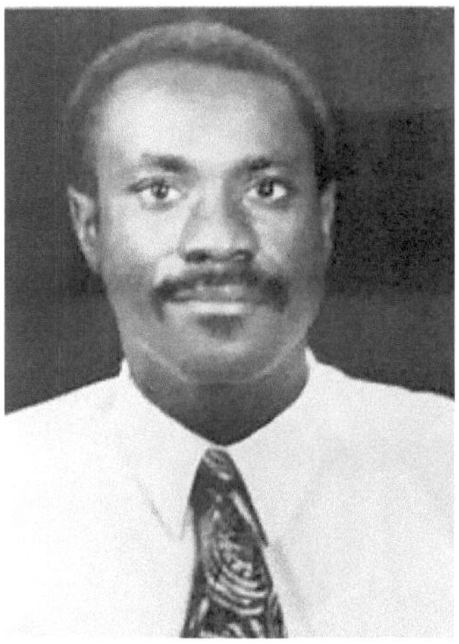

Jocelyn Celestin, MD
(1993-1994)

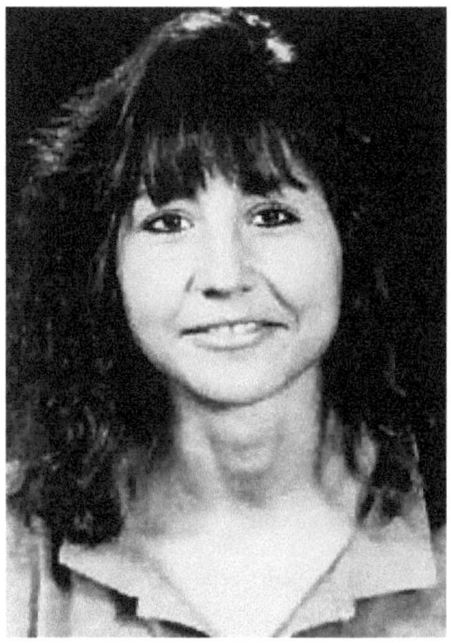

Maria Olivero, MD
(1993-1995)

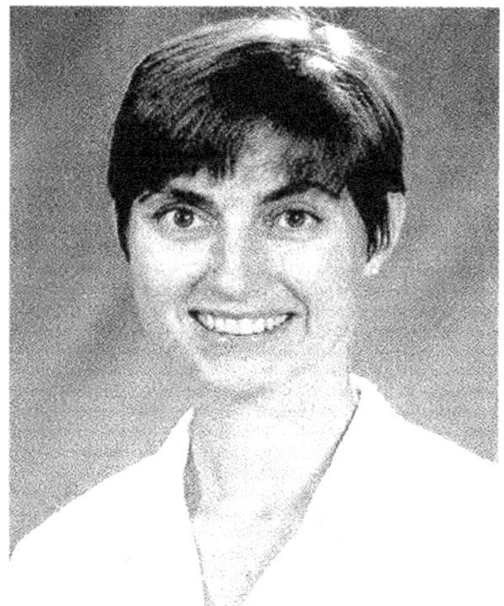

Margaret Kelleher, MD
(1994-1995)

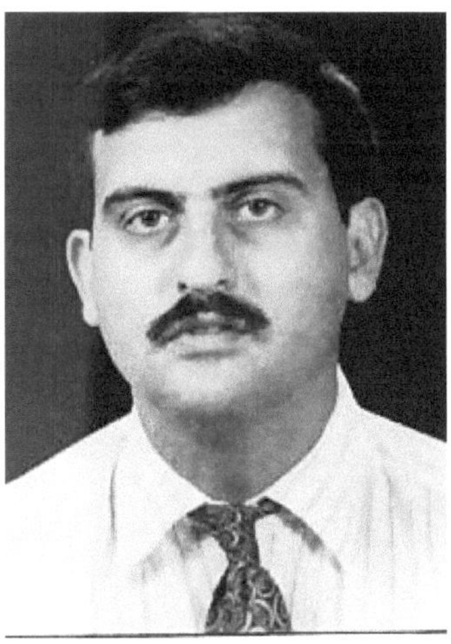

Angelos Koutsonikolis, MD
(1993-1996)

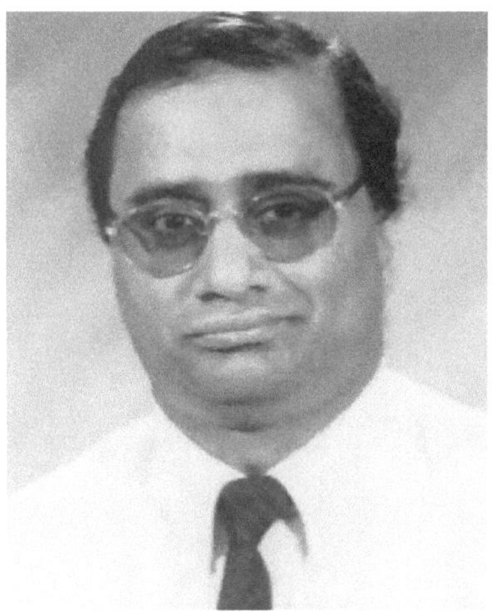

Ramarathinam Nagarajan, MD
(1994-1996)

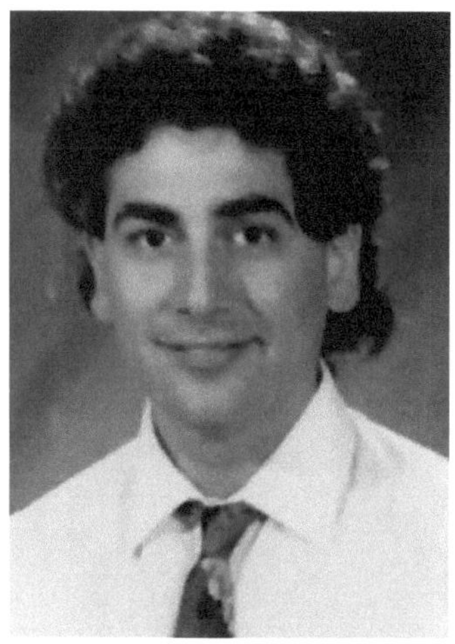

Bernard Zeffren, MD
(1994-1996)

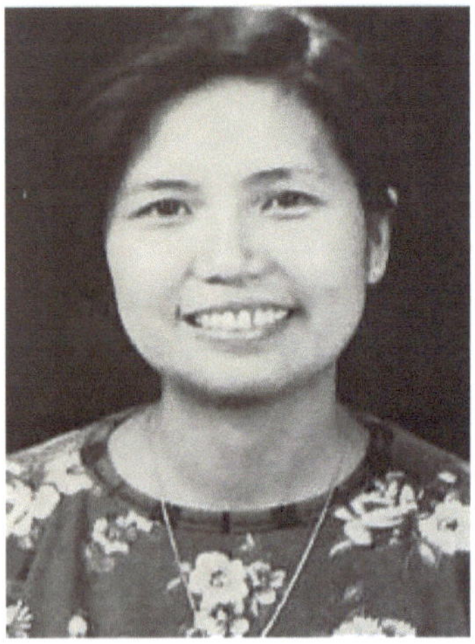

Emerita Brigino-Buenaventura, M.D
(1994-1997)

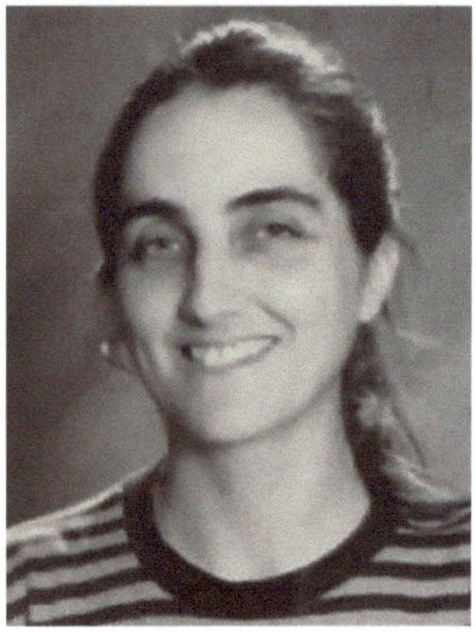

Duygu Uckan, MD
(1994-1997)

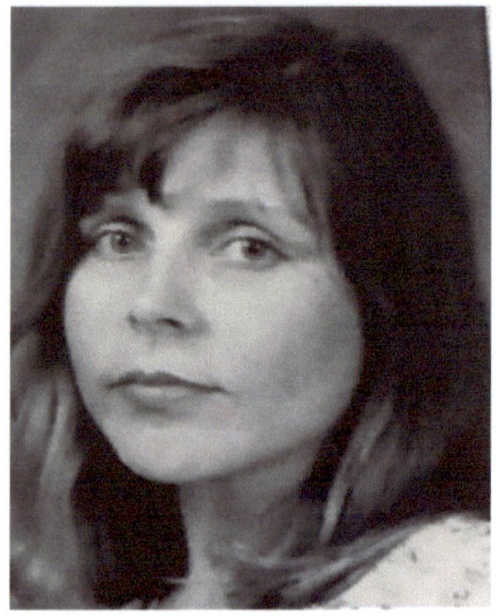

Maria J. Pochcial, MD
(1995-1997)

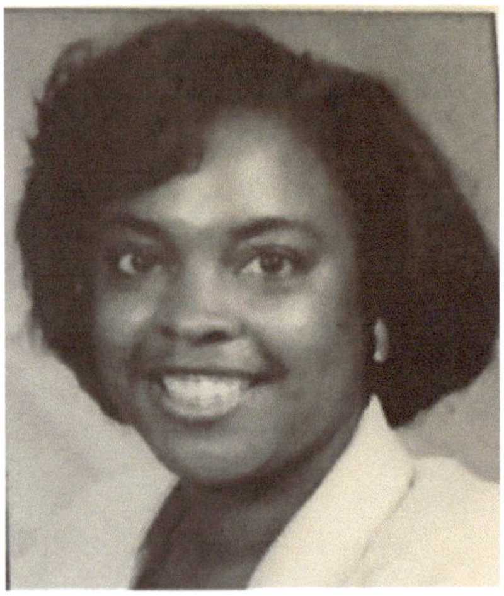

Jada L. Armstrong, MD
(1995-1997)

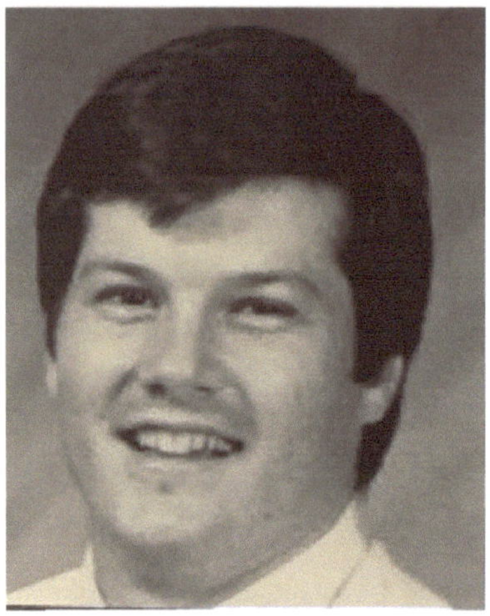

John Duplantier, MD
(1995-1997)

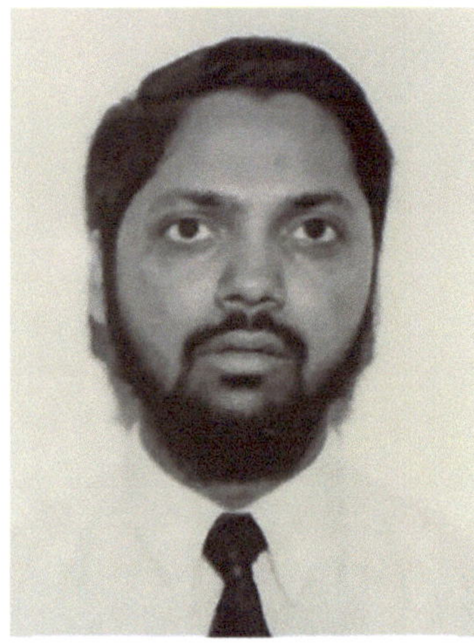

Shafqat Sayeed, MD
(1996-1998)

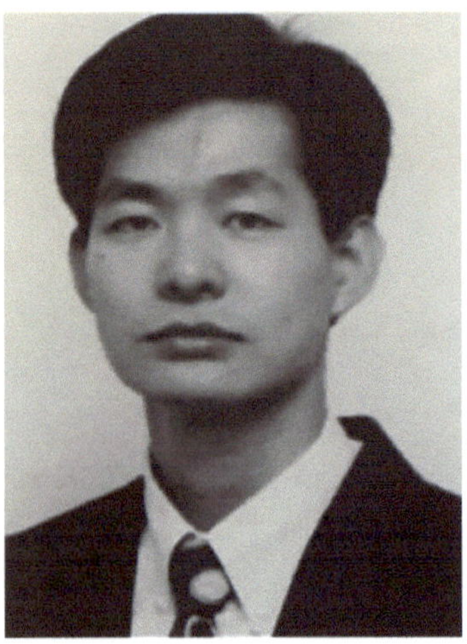

Nathan Tang, MD
(1996-1999)

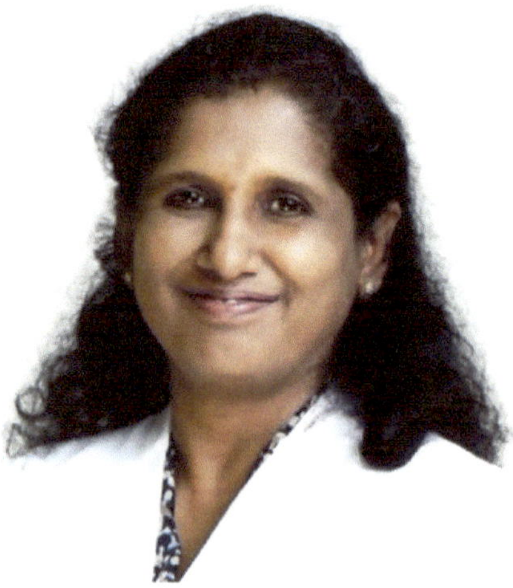

Latha Chamarthy, MD
(1997-1999)

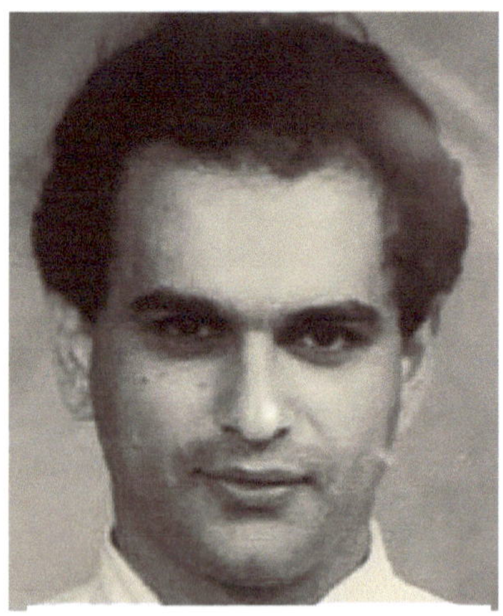

Chris Christodoulou, MD
(1997-1999)

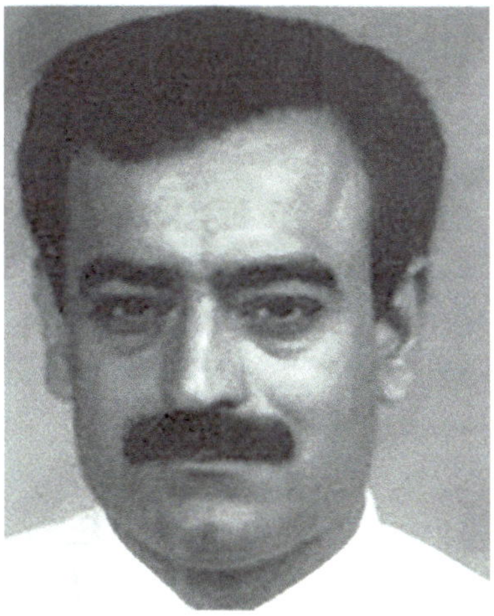

Shahid Iqbal, MD
(1997-2000)

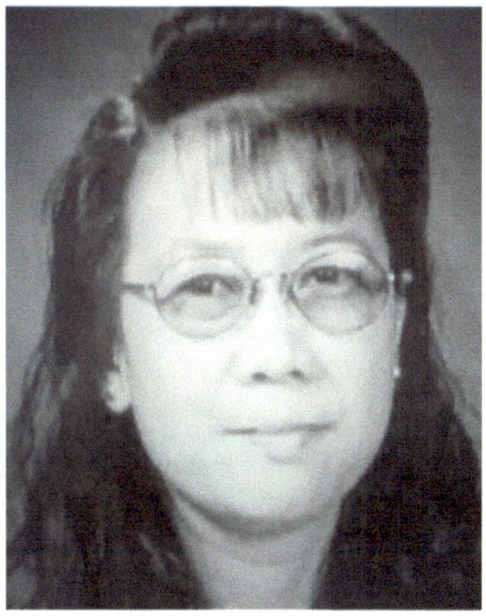

Belen Tan, MD
(1998-2000)

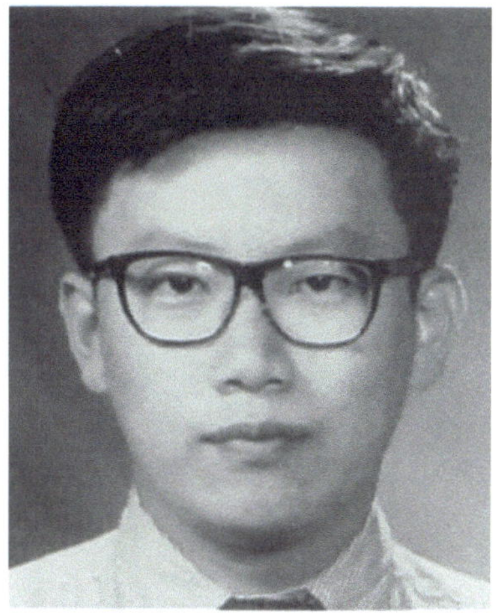

Voravich Luangwedchakarn, MD
(1998-2001)

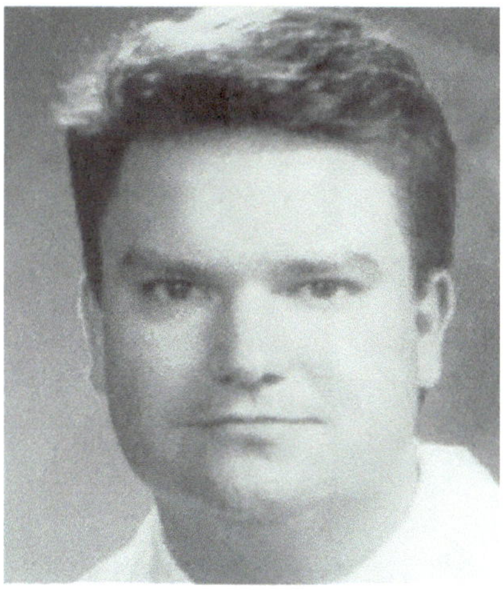

Stuart White, MD
(1998-2001)

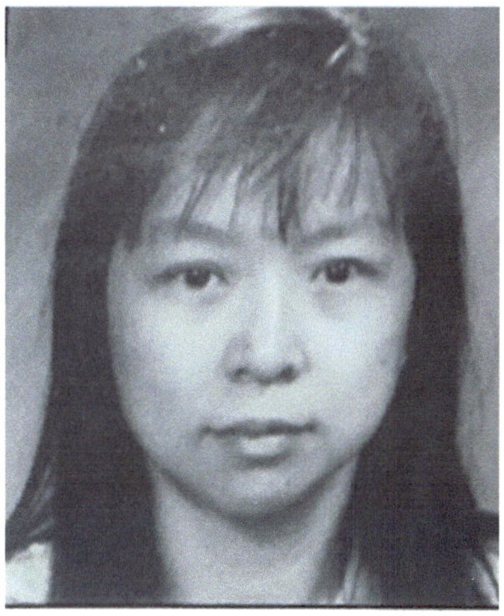

Suwannee Uthaisangsook, MD
(1999-2000)

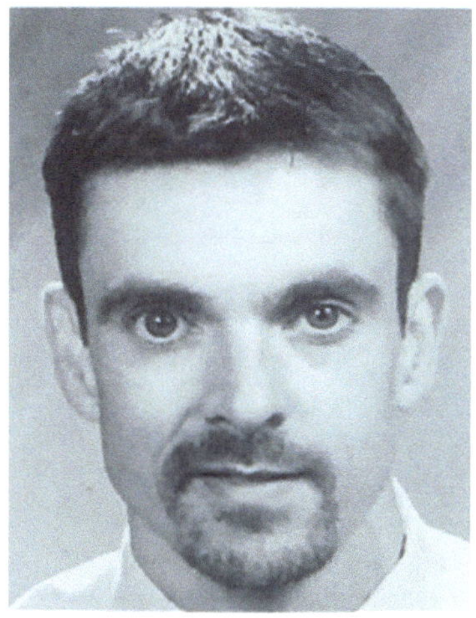

David Provencher, MD
(1999-2001)

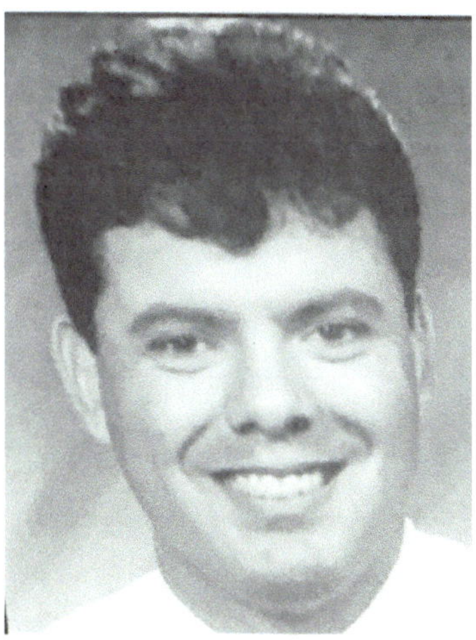

Roberto Rivera, MD
(1999-2001)

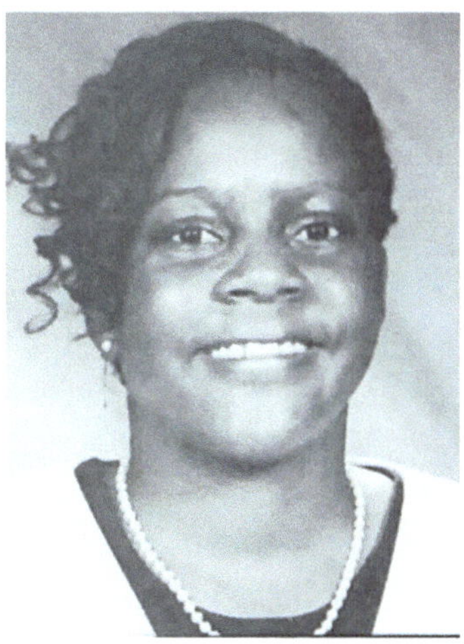

Roselyn M. Hicks, MD
(2000-2002)

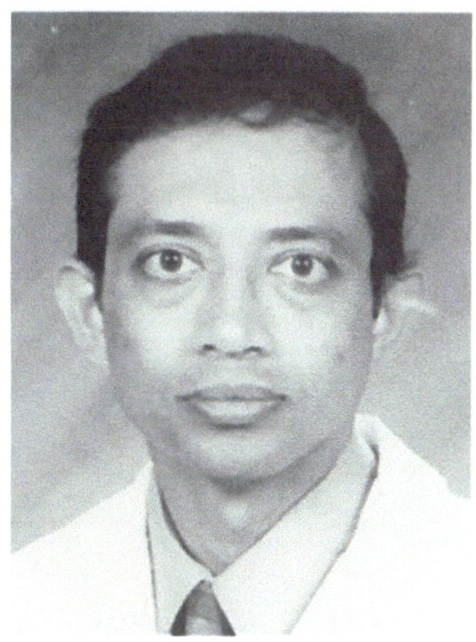

Hyder Ali Khan, MD
(2000-2002)

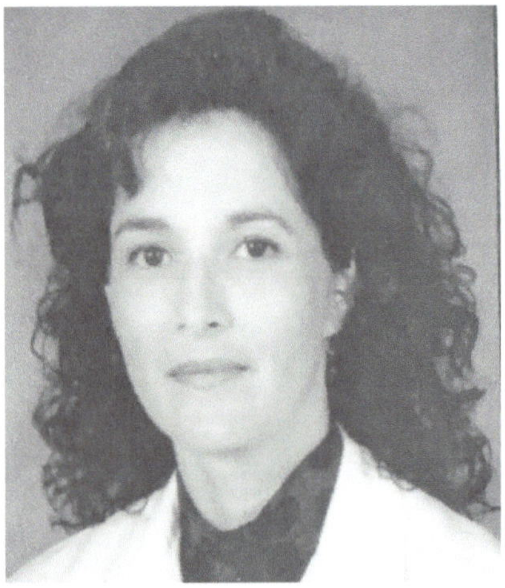

Diana P. Jerez-Martin, MD
(2001-2003)

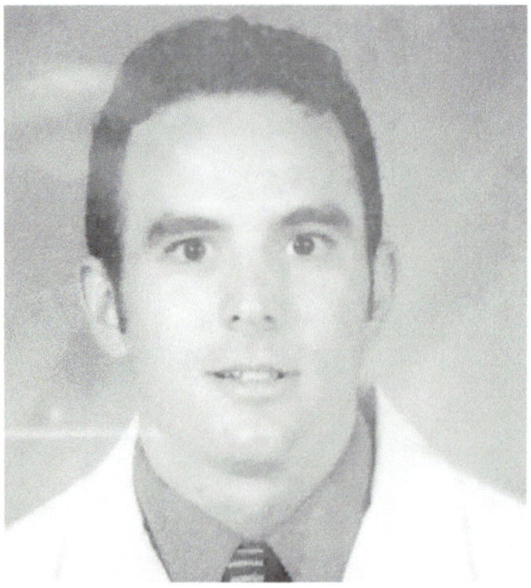

Michael J. Palumbo, MD
(2001-2003)

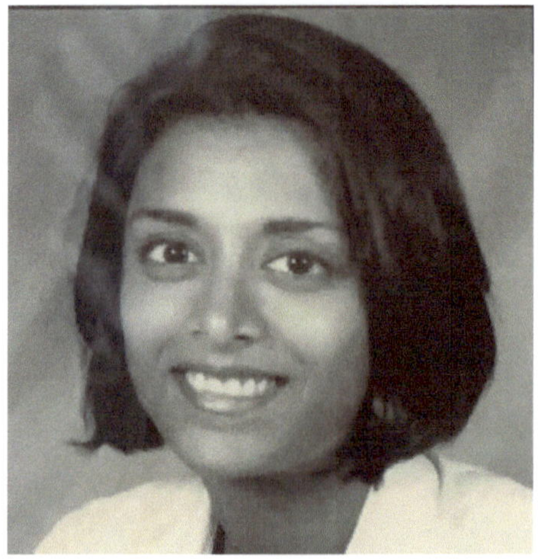

Rajivi Porthiraj Rucker, MD
(2001-2004)

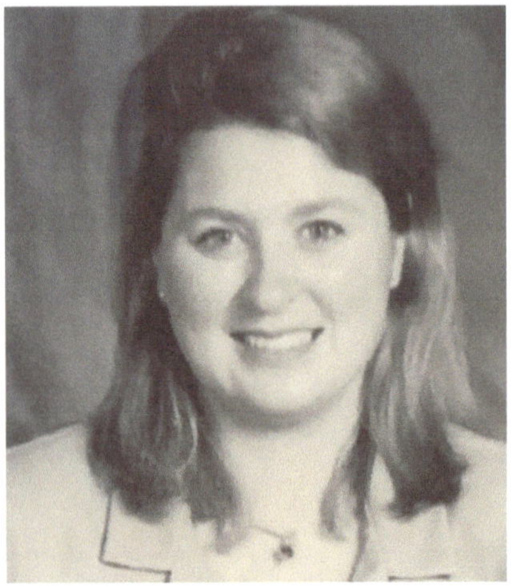

Dawn M. Zacharias, MD
(2002-2004)

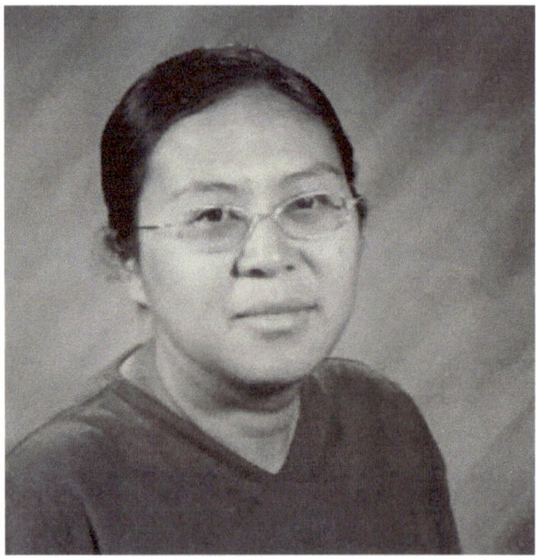

Dareen Siri, MD
(2003-2005)

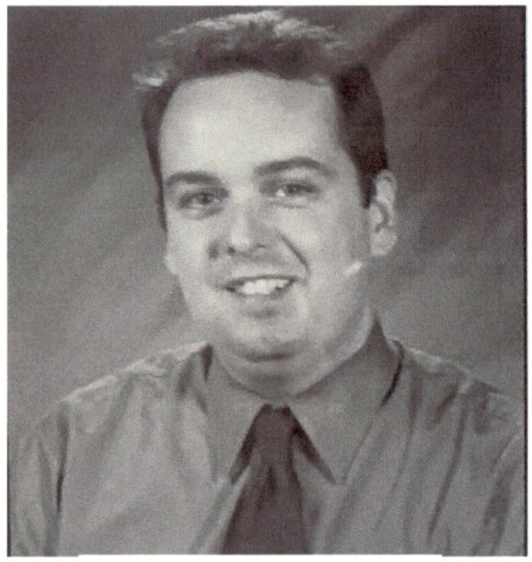

Albert S. Hartel, MD
(2004-2006)

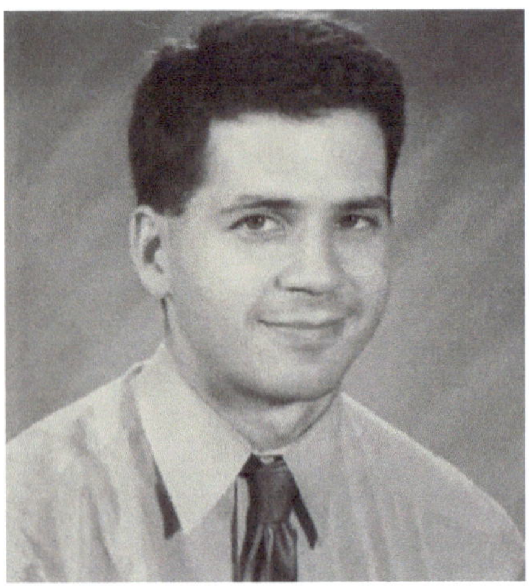

Richard F. Lavi, MD
(2004-2006)

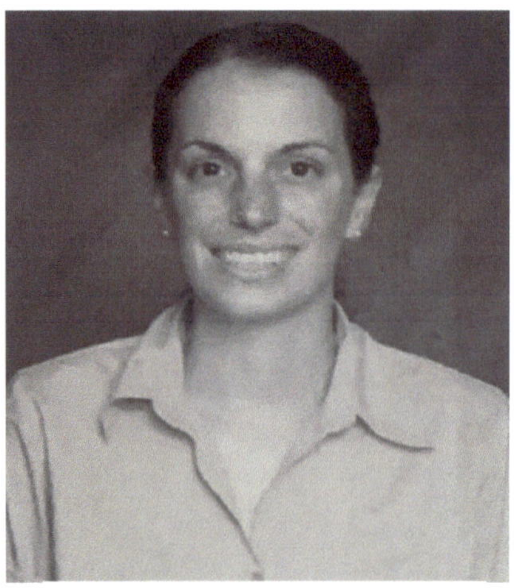

Adriana S. McCubbin, MD
(2005-2007)

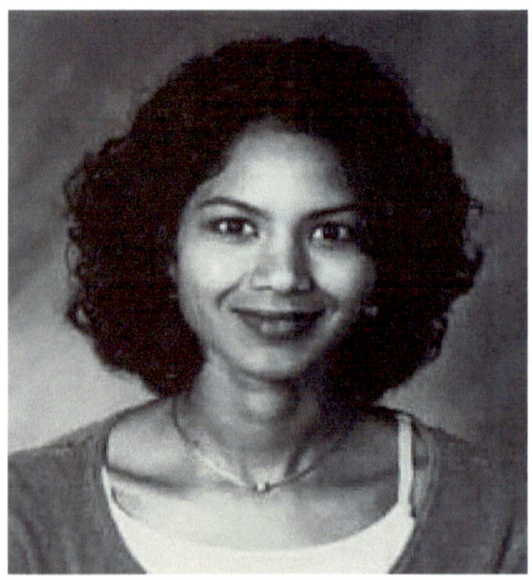

Madhurima Sanka, DO
(2005-2007)

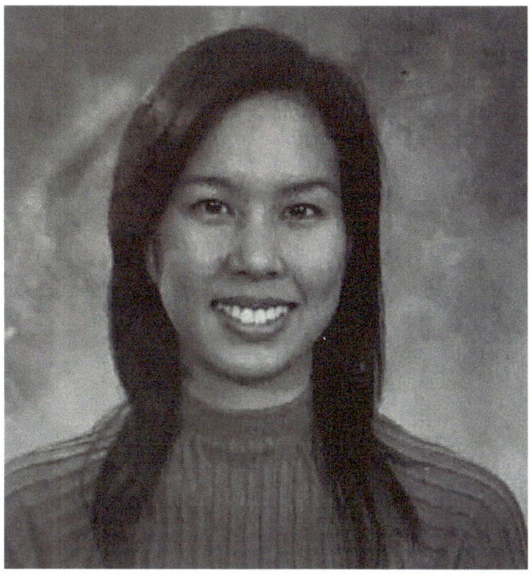

Panida Sriaroon, MD
(2006-2009)

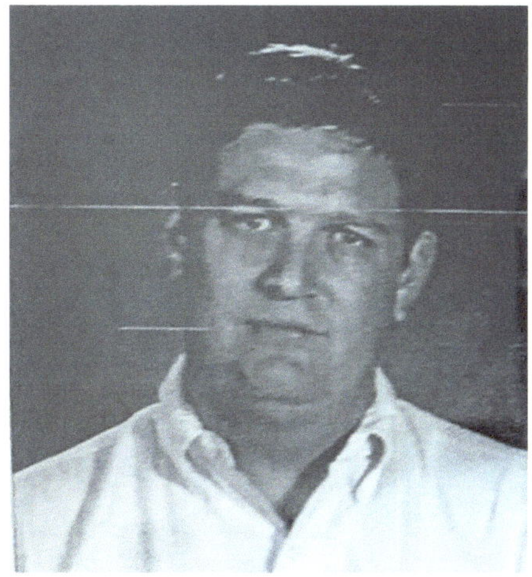

Jason Caldwell, DO
(2007-2009)

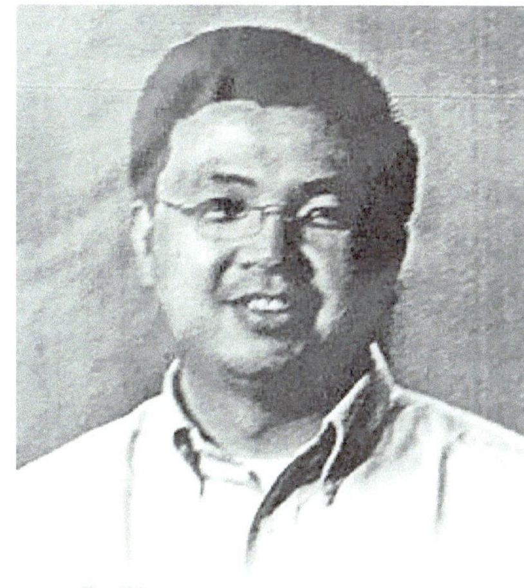

Woei Yeang Gary Eng, MD
(2008-2010)

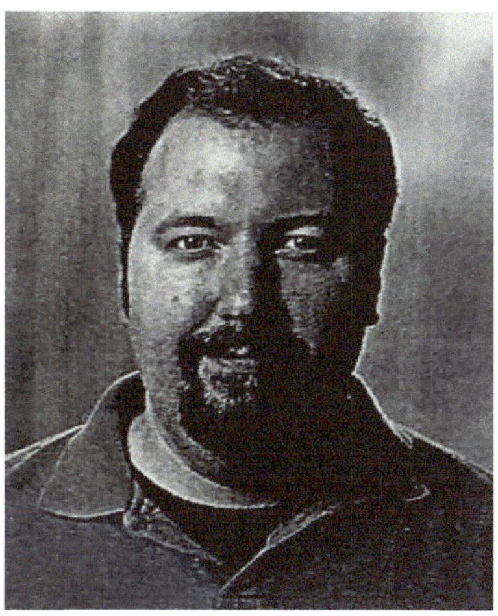

Loren Isakson, MD
(2008-2010)

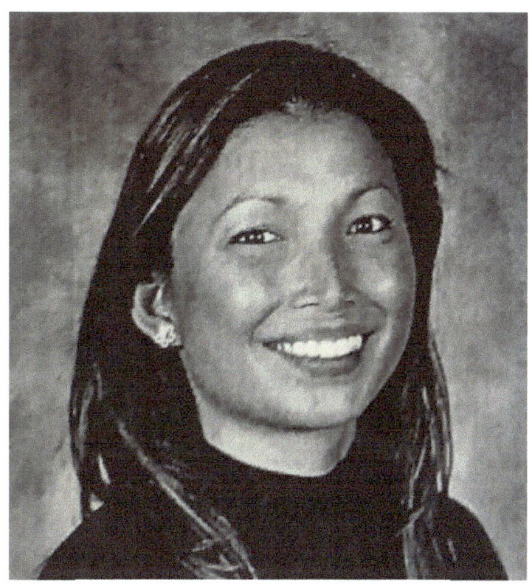

Maliena Longley, MD
(2009-2011)

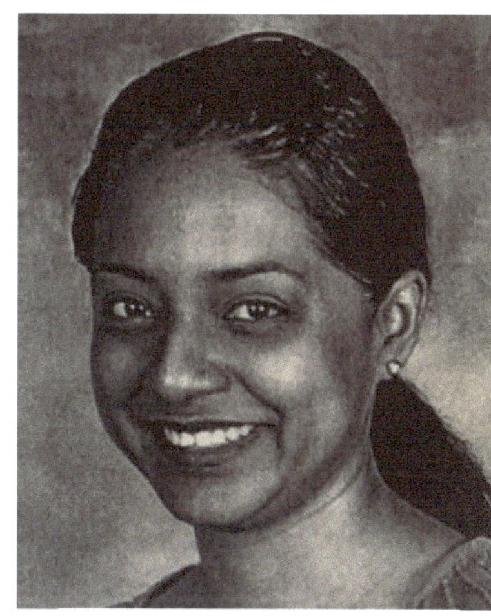

Araceli Elizalde, MD
(2010-2012)

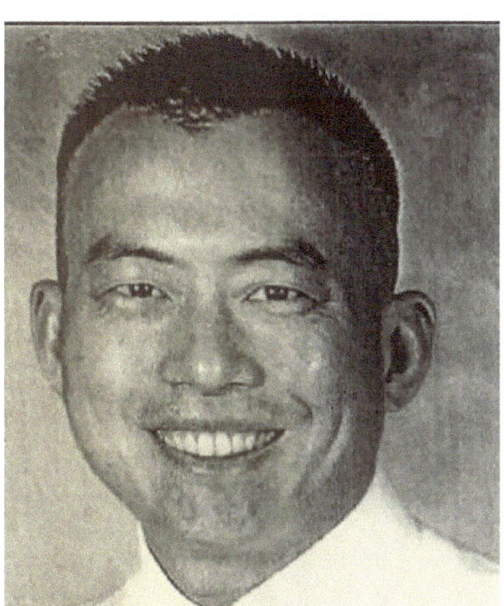

Doanh Nguyen, MD
(2010-2012)

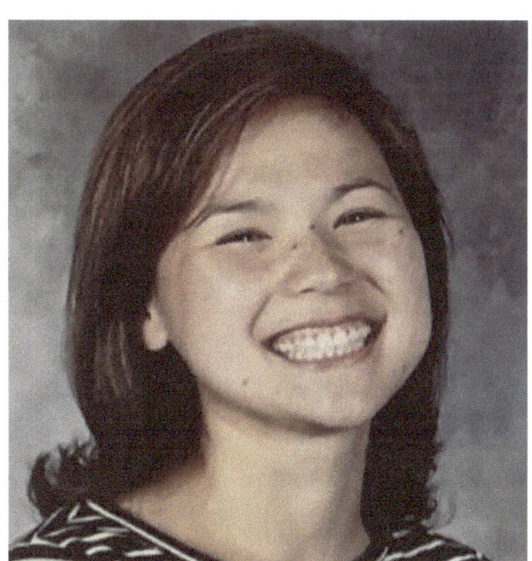

Jean Marie Brown Ly, MD
(2011-2013)

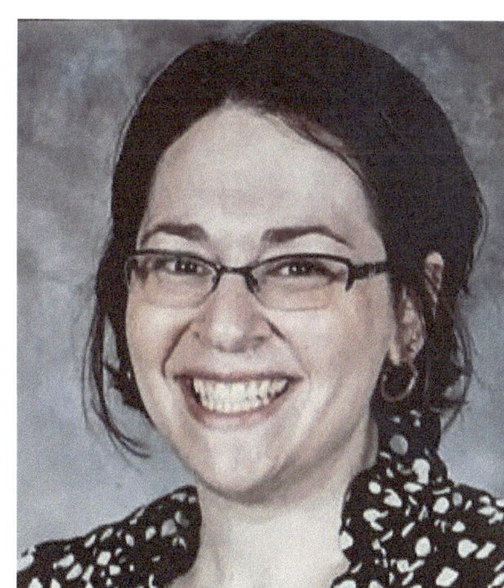

Hava Tillipman Ladinsky, MD
(2011-2013)

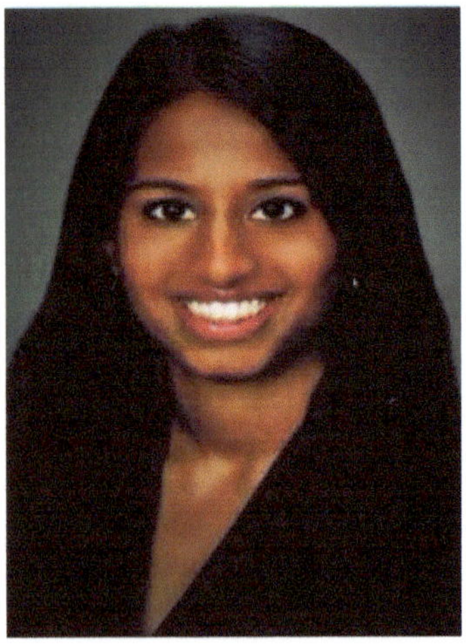

Hana Niebur, MD
(2012-2014)

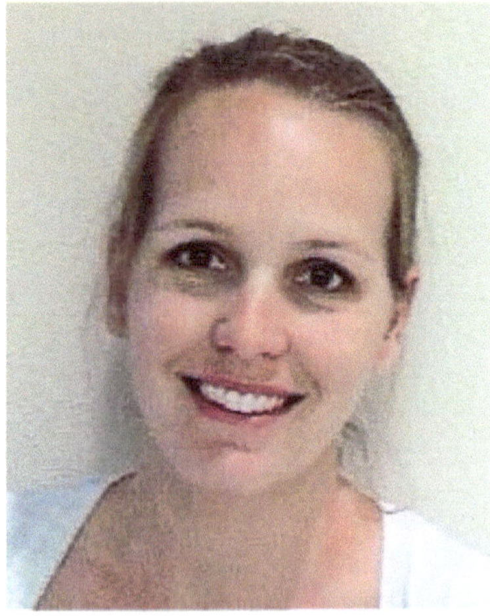

Catherine Kubiak, MD
(2013-2015)

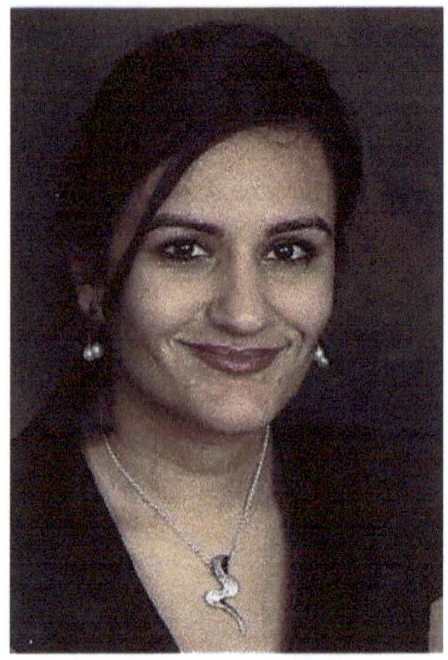

Farnaz Tabatabaian, MD
(2013-2015)

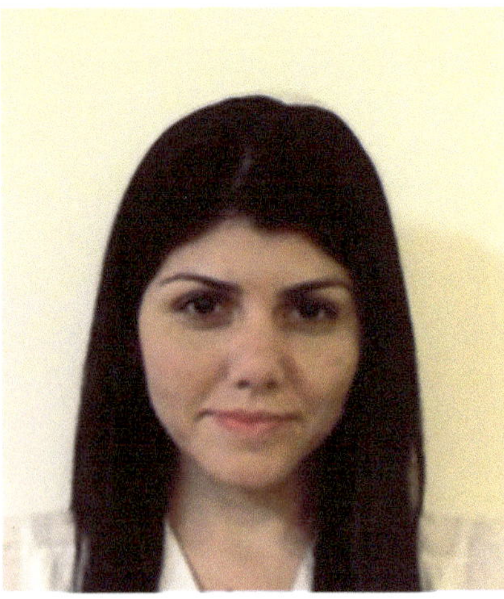

Sheila Bina, MD
(2014-2016)

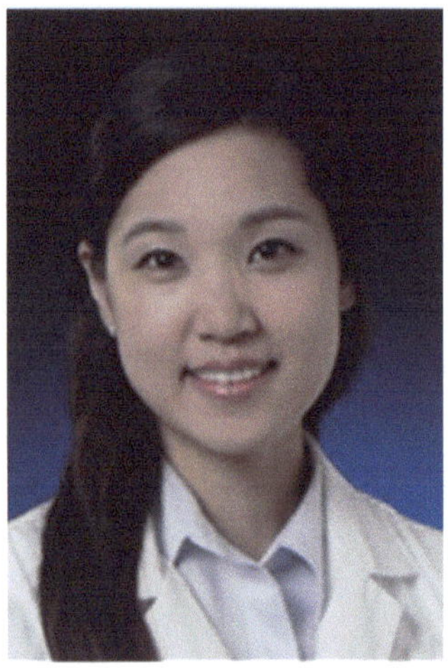

Jenni Yoon, MD
(2014-2016)

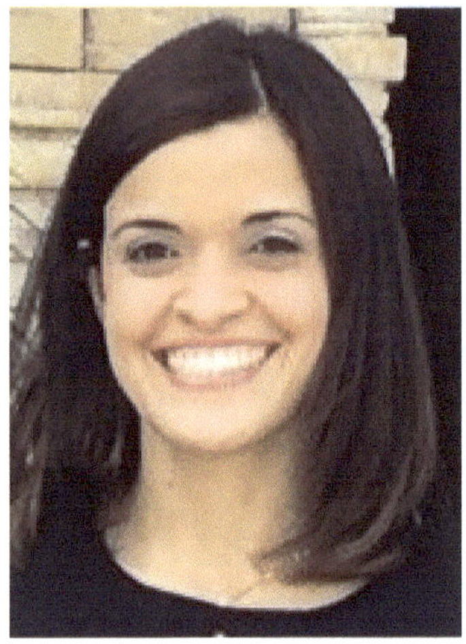

Johana Castro-Wagner, MD
(2015-2017)

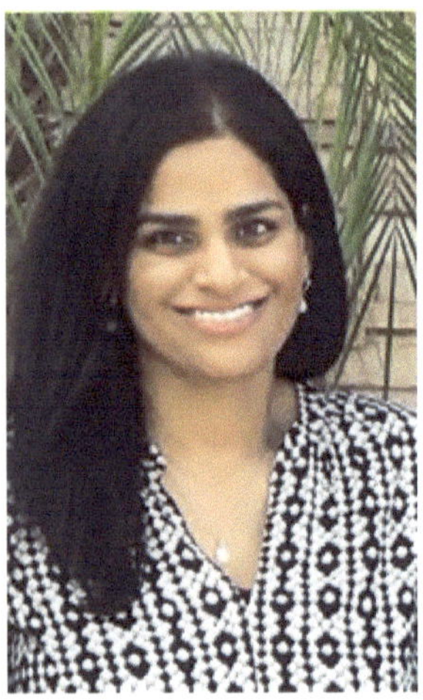

Bhumika Patel, MD
(2015-2017)

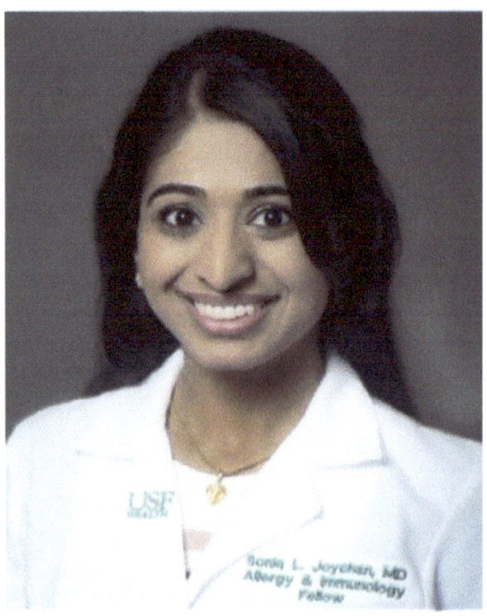

Sonia Joychan, MD
(2016-2018)

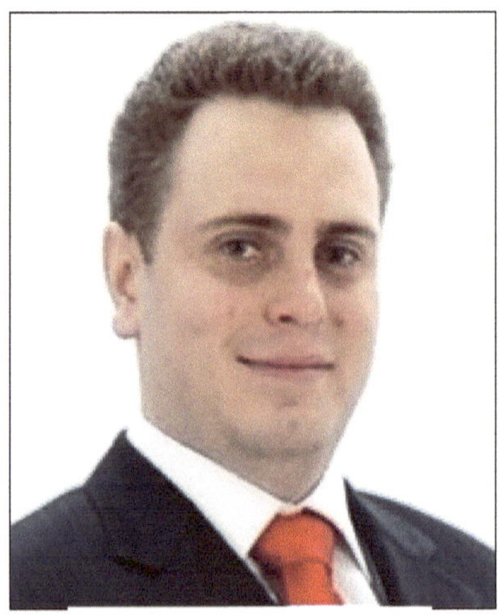

David Lindsay, MD
(2016-2018)

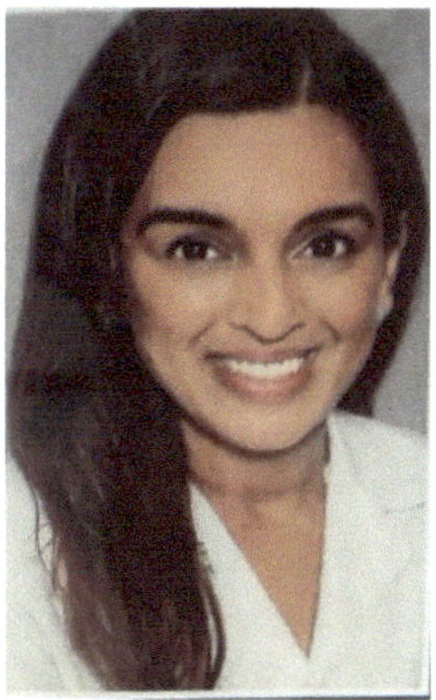

Fatima Khan, MD
(2017-2019)

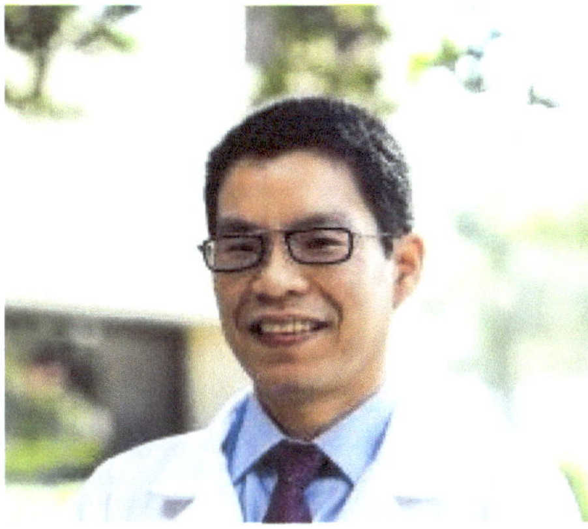

Warit Jithpratuck, MD
(2017-2019)

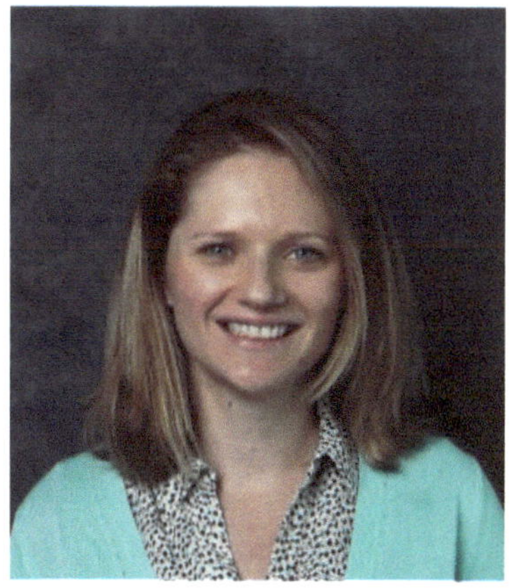

Irina Dawson, MD
(2018-2020)

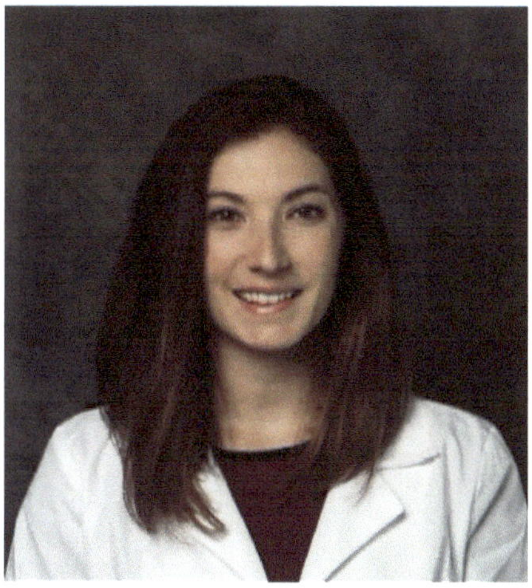

Jacqueline Squire, MD
(2018-2020)

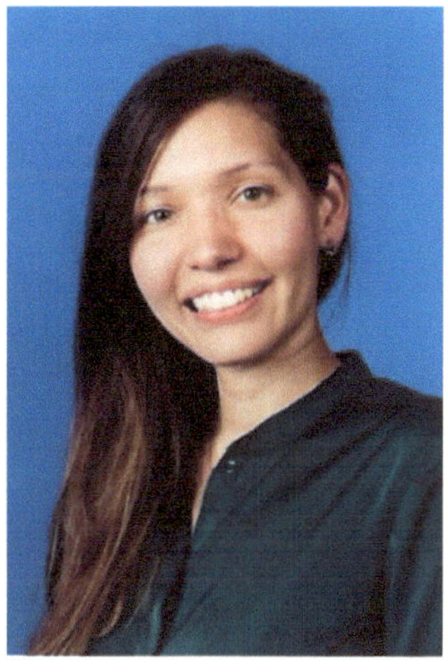

Priyanka Timothy MD
(2020-2022)

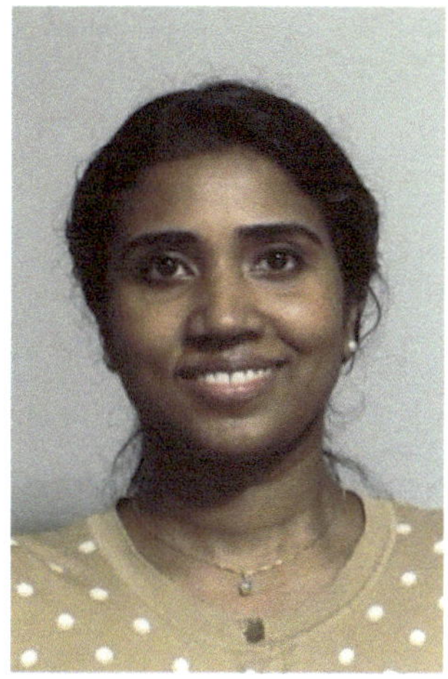

Maria Chitty-Lopez, MD
(2019-2021)

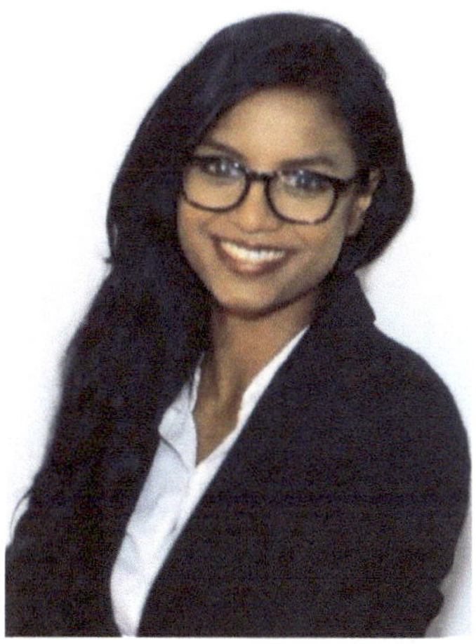

Mary Ann Miranda, MD
(2020-2022)

Chapter 7: All Children's Hospital Allergy and Immunology Pediatric and Internal Medicine Fellows

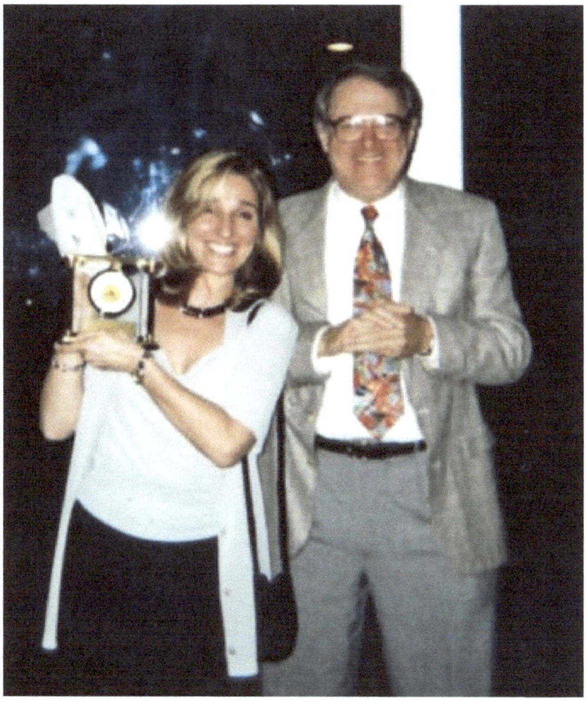

Left to right: Maria Teresa de la Morena, MD (ACH, 1991-1995) and Richard F. Lockey, MD, MS; circa 1999.

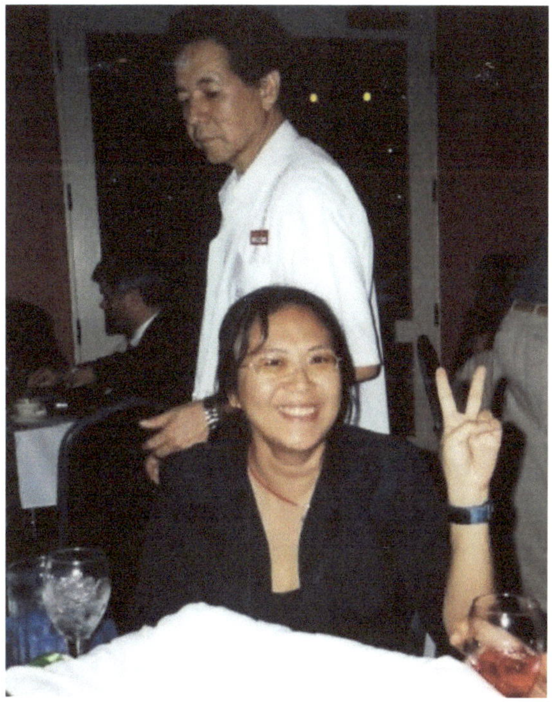

Dareen Siri, MD (ACH, 2003-2005); circa 2010.

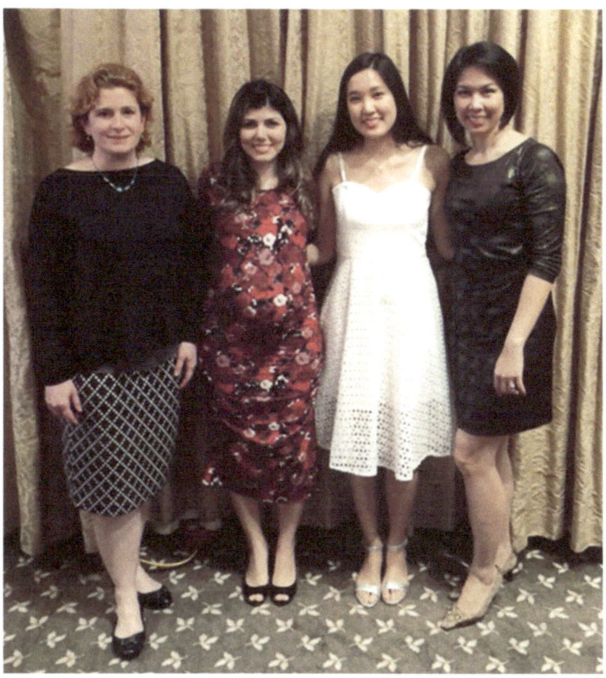

Left to right: Jolan Walter, MD, PhD; Sheila Bina, MD (ACH, 2014-2016); Jenni Yoon, MD (ACH, 2014-2016); Panida Sriaroon, MD (ACH, 2006-2009); 2016.

Left to right: Sheila Bina, MD (ACH, 2014-2016); Bhumika Patel, MD (ACH, 2015-2017); Johana Castro-Wagner, MD (ACH, 2015-2017); Jenni Yoon, MD (ACH, 2014-2016); 2016.

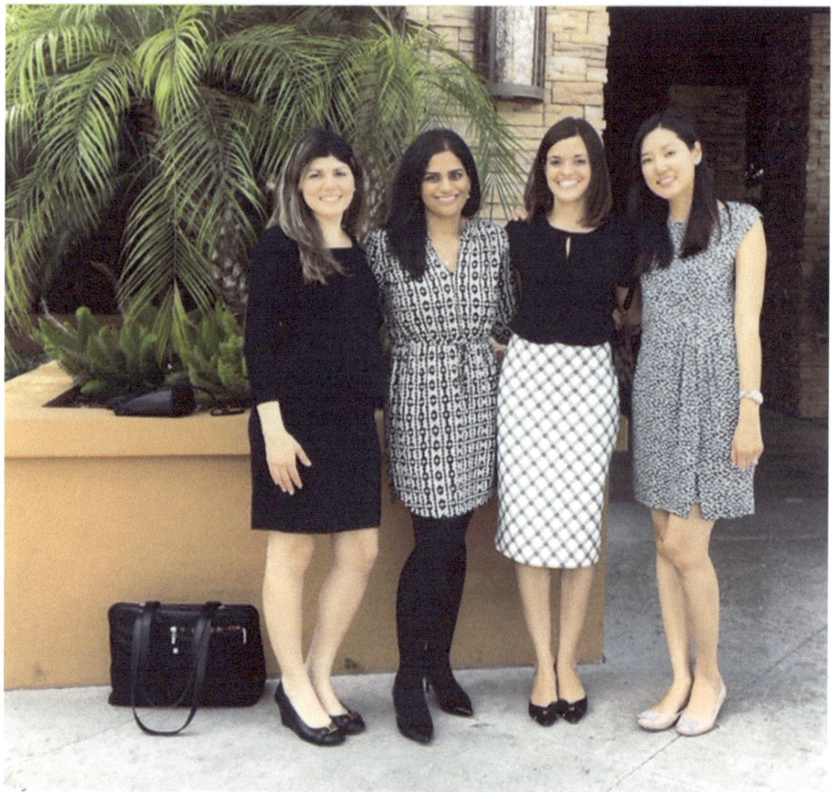

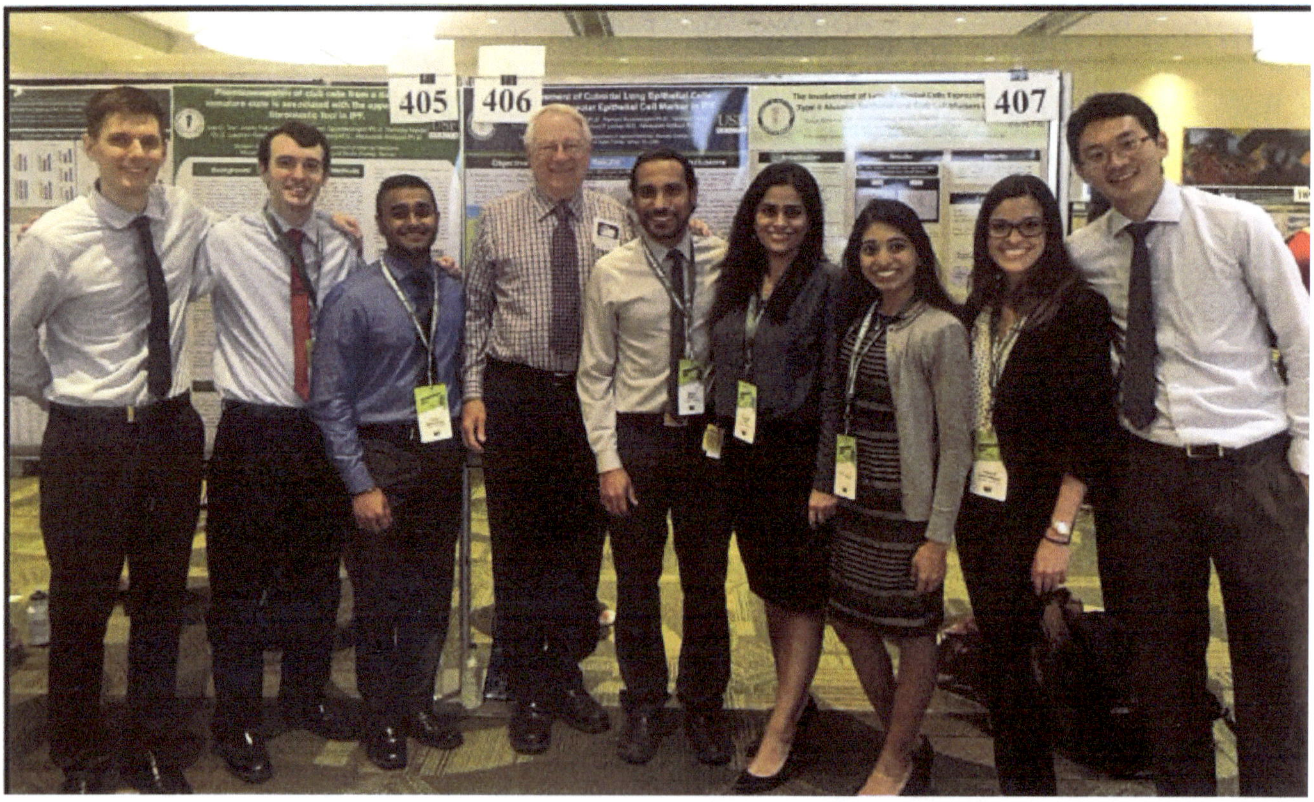

Left to right: Alex Czachor; Travis Herrin; Sanjay Mahendrasah; Richard F. Lockey, MD, MS; Adeeb Bulkhi, MD (2014-2017); Bhumika Patel, MD (ACH, 2015-2017); Sonia Joychan, MD (ACH, 2016-2018); Johana Castro-Wagner, MD (ACH, 2015-2017); Chen Lin, MD (2015-2017); 2017 USF Health Research Day.

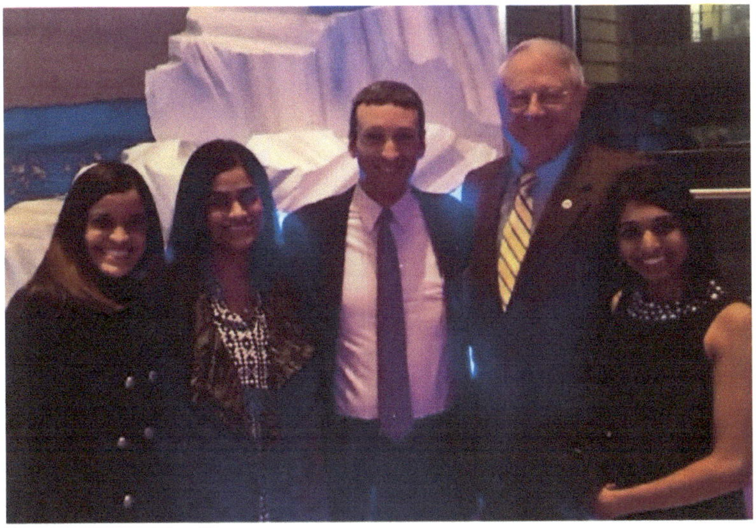

Left to right: Johana Castro-Wagner, MD (ACH, 2015-2017); Bhumika Patel, MD (ACH, 2015-2017); Peter Ricketti, DO (2015-2017); Richard F. Lockey, MD, MS; Sonia

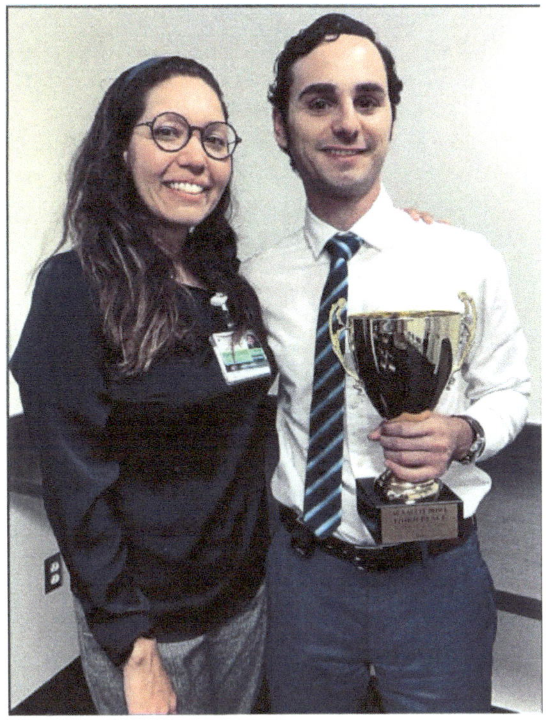

Left to right: Maria Chitty-Lopez, MD (ACH, 2019-2021) and Raul S. Villarreal, MD (2018-2020); 3rd place; American College of Allergy Asthma & Immunology (ACAAI) 2019 Annual Meeting, Fellows-in-Training Bowl, Houston, TX.

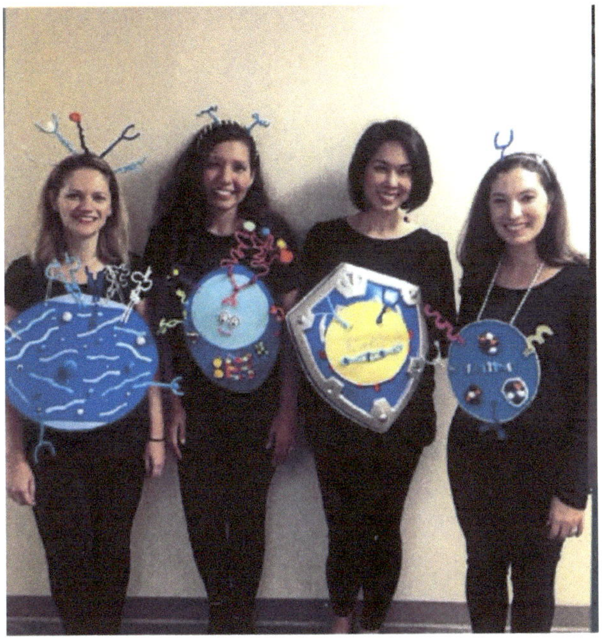

Left to right: Irina Dawson, MD (ACH, 2018-2020); Maria Chitty-Lopez, MD (ACH, 2019-2021); Panida Sriaroon, MD (ACH, 2006-2009); Jacqueline Squire, MD (ACH, 2018-2020); 2019.

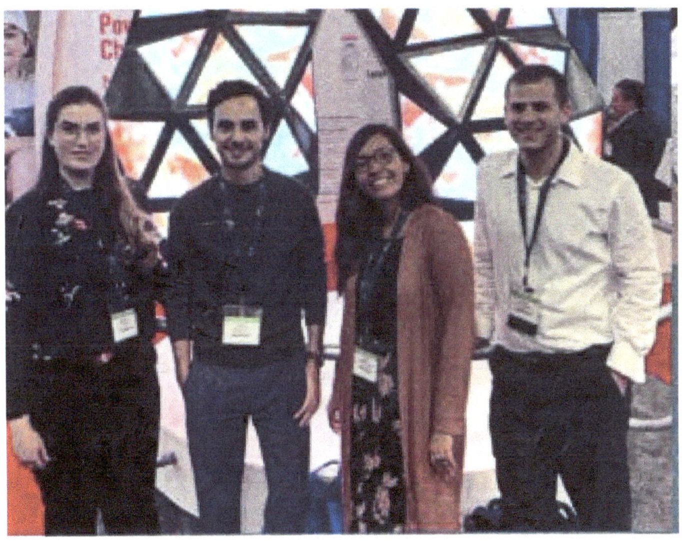

Left to right: Stephanie Hudey (2019-2021); Raul S. Villarreal, MD (2018-2020); Maria Chitty-Lopez, MD (ACH, 2019-2021); David Gubernick, (2019-2021); American College of Allergy Asthma & Immunology (ACAAI) 2019 Annual Meeting, Houston, TX.

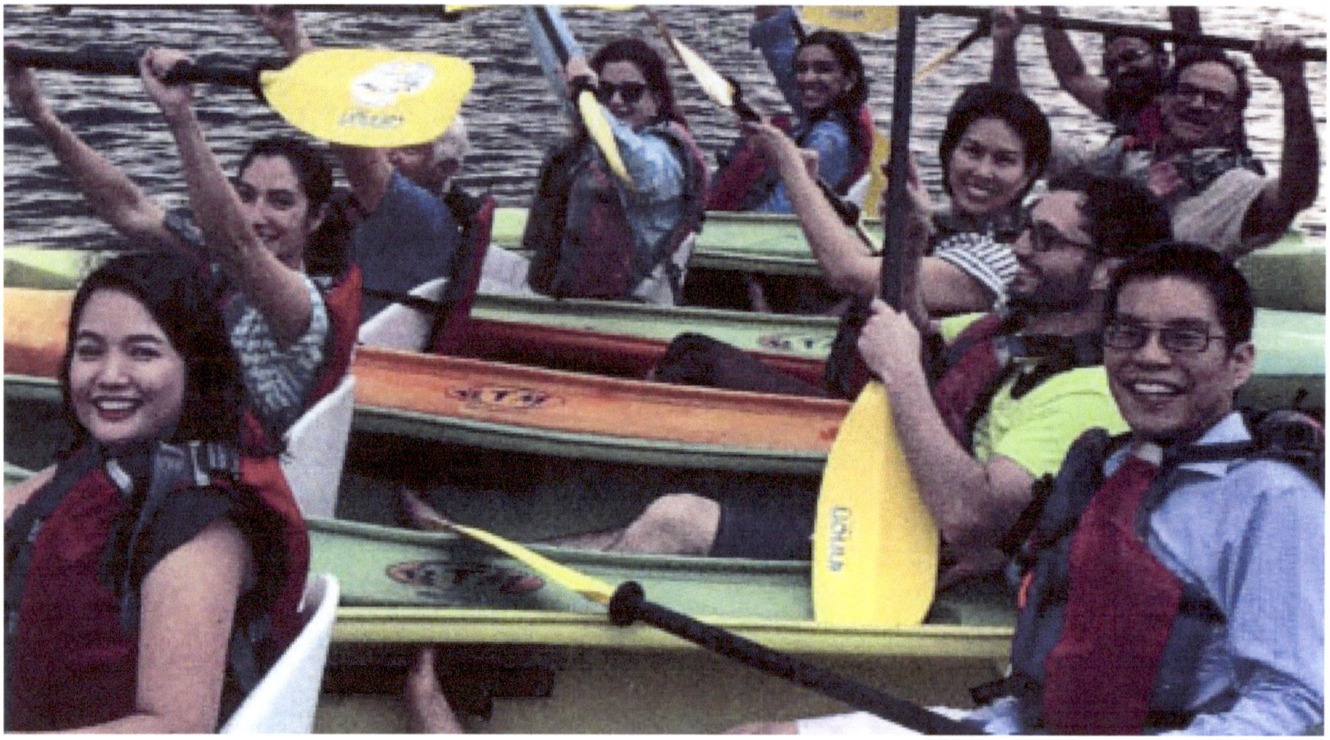

2019 End-of-Year Celebration; Pediatric Fellows and Faculty.

Chapter 8: Division Group Pictures

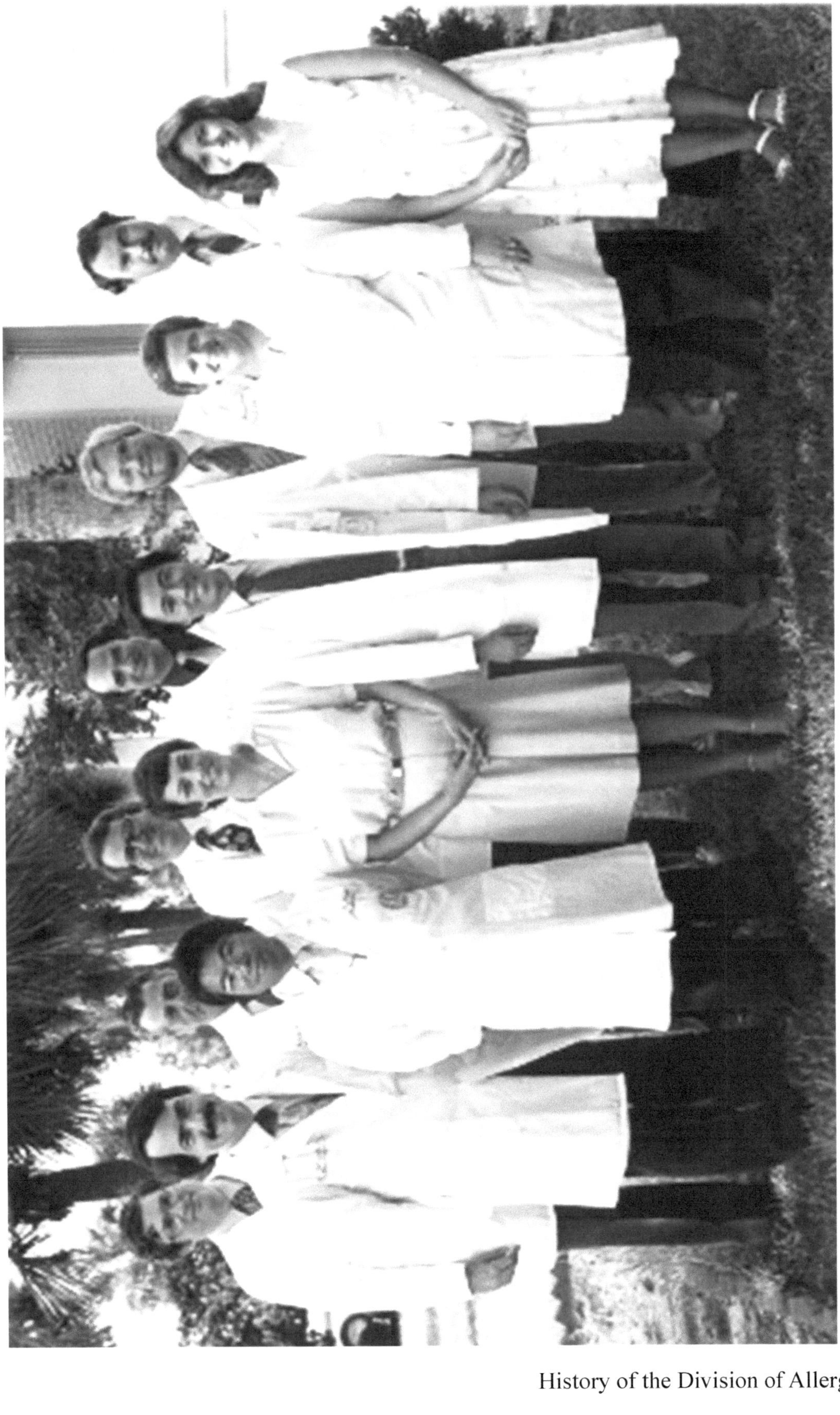

Front row (left to right): John J. Stablein, MD (1979-1981); Sadahiro Asai, MD; Judy Bien; Steven J. Louie, MD (1981-1983); Irene Baird-Warren; Ginger Montuoro. Back row (left to right): R. Lawrence Siegel, MD, PhD; Samuel C. Bukantz, MD; Richard F. Lockey, MD, MS; Saber Samaan, PhD; Roger W Fox, MD (1978-1980); Gerald A. Bucholtz, MD (1980-1982). Circa 1982.

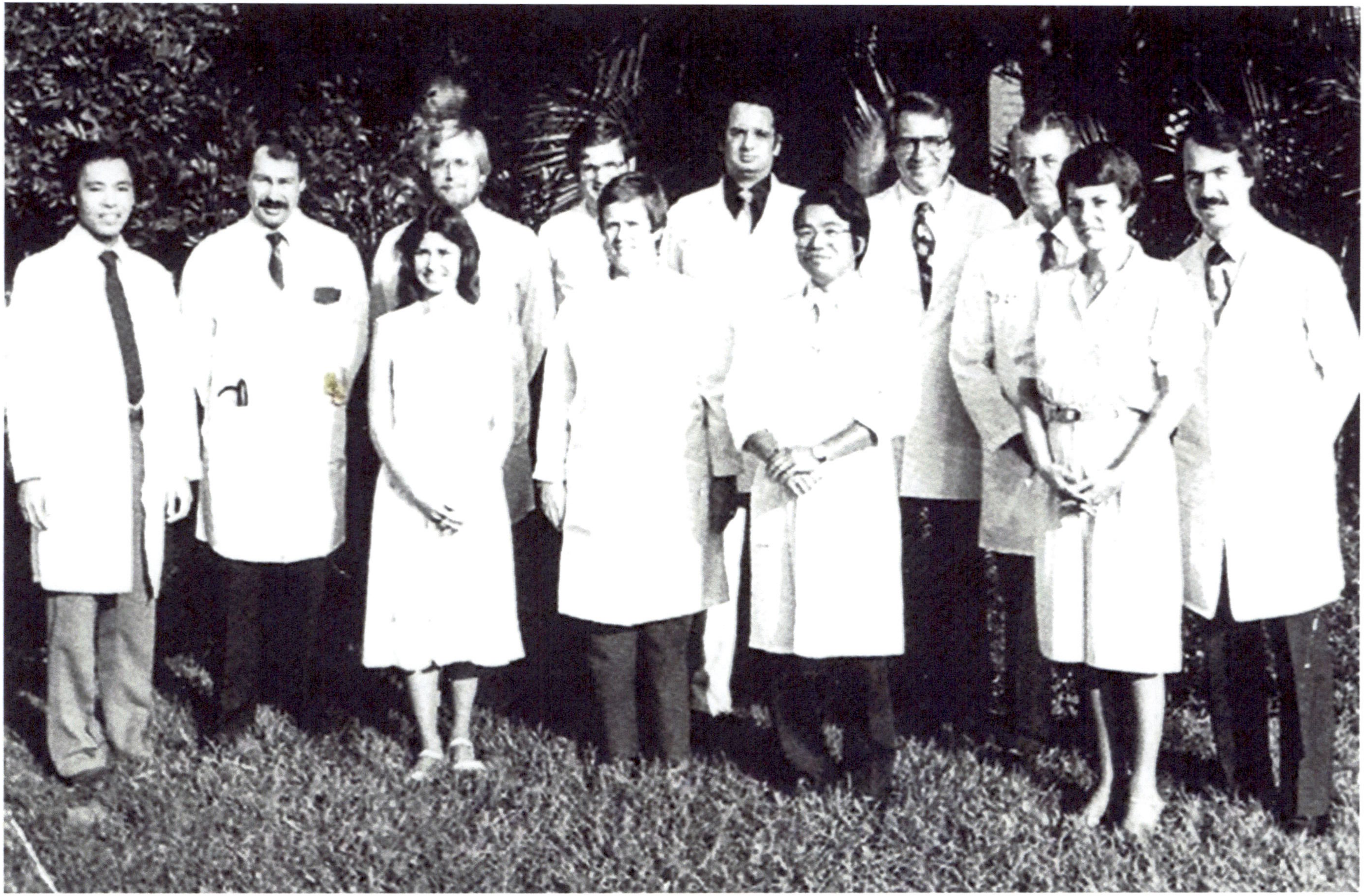

Front row (left to right): Ginger Montuoro; Irene Baird-Warren; Sadahiro Asai, MD; Judy Bien. Back row (left to right): Steve J. Louie, MD (1981-1983); Gerald A. Bucholtz, MD (1980-1982); Roger W. Fox, MD (1978-1980); R. Lawrence Siegel, MD, PhD; Saber Samaan, PhD; Richard F. Lockey, MD, MS; Samuel C. Bukantz, MD; John J. Stablein, MD (1979-1981). Circa 1982.

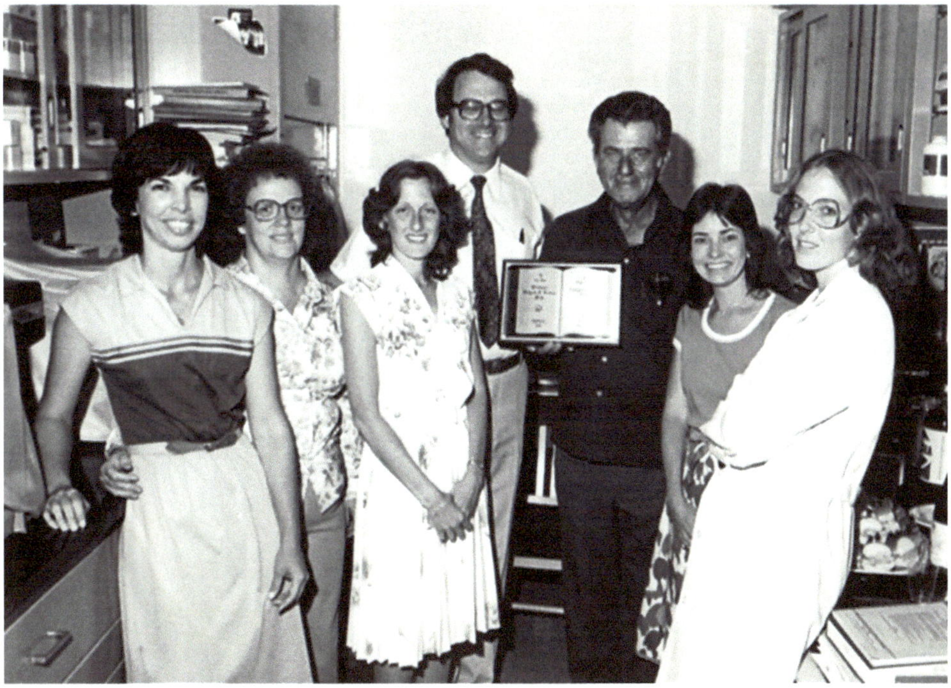

Celebration of Dr. Lockey's promotion to Professor, July 1983. Left to right: Debbie Serbousek; Irene Baird-Warren; Peggy Hales; Richard F. Lockey, MD, MS; Samuel C. Bukantz, MD; Ginger Montuoro; Cindy (surname unknown).

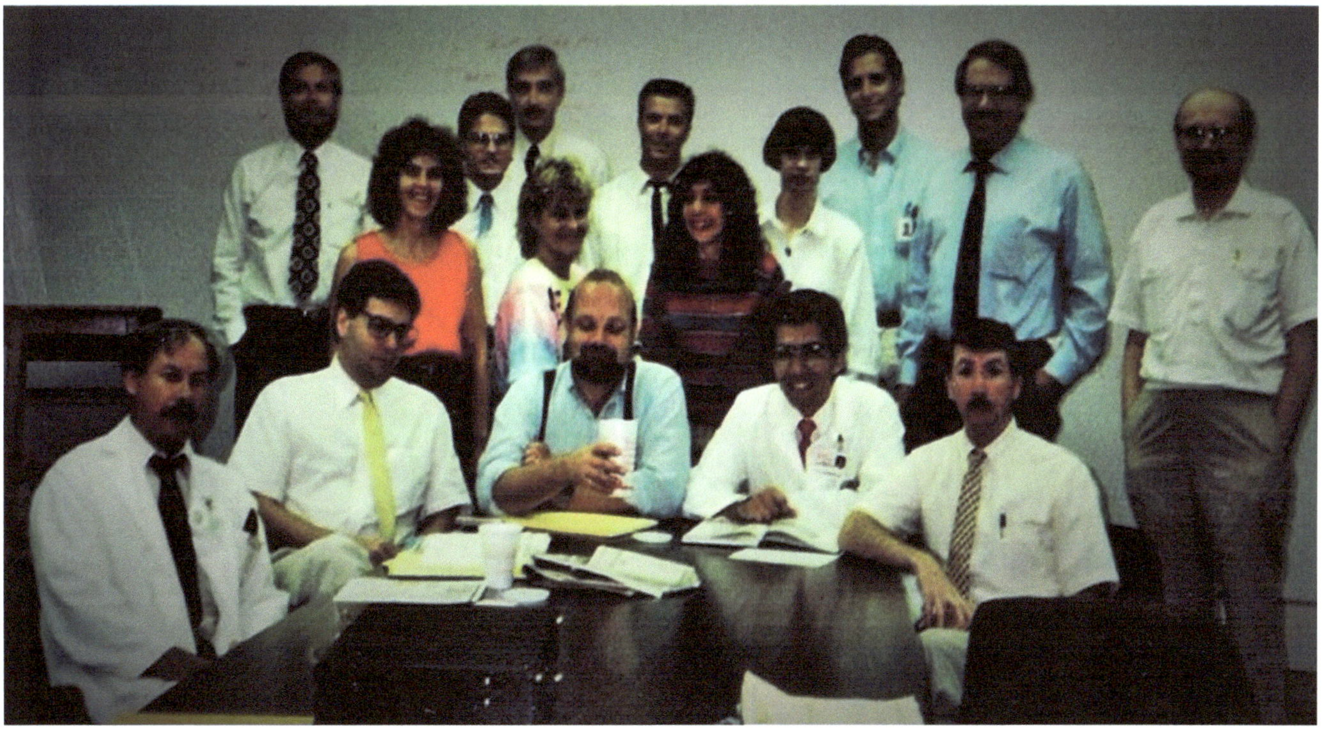

7:30 AM Division Meeting, 1991. Front row (left to right): Gerald A. Bucholtz, MD (1980-1982); David N. Wright, MD (1988-1991); Walter Trudeau, MS; Eduardo Calderon, MD; Thomas B. Edwards, MD (1990-1992). Middle row (left to right): Pat Walsh; Alesha (surname unknown); Sharon Siegel, Rita Johnson. Back row (left to right): Roger W. Fox, MD (1978-1980); Carlos M. Jacinto, MD (1990-1992); Dennis K. Ledford, MD (1983-1985); name unknown; Enrique Fernandez-Caldas, PhD; Richard F. Lockey, MD, MS; Andor Szentivanyi, MD.

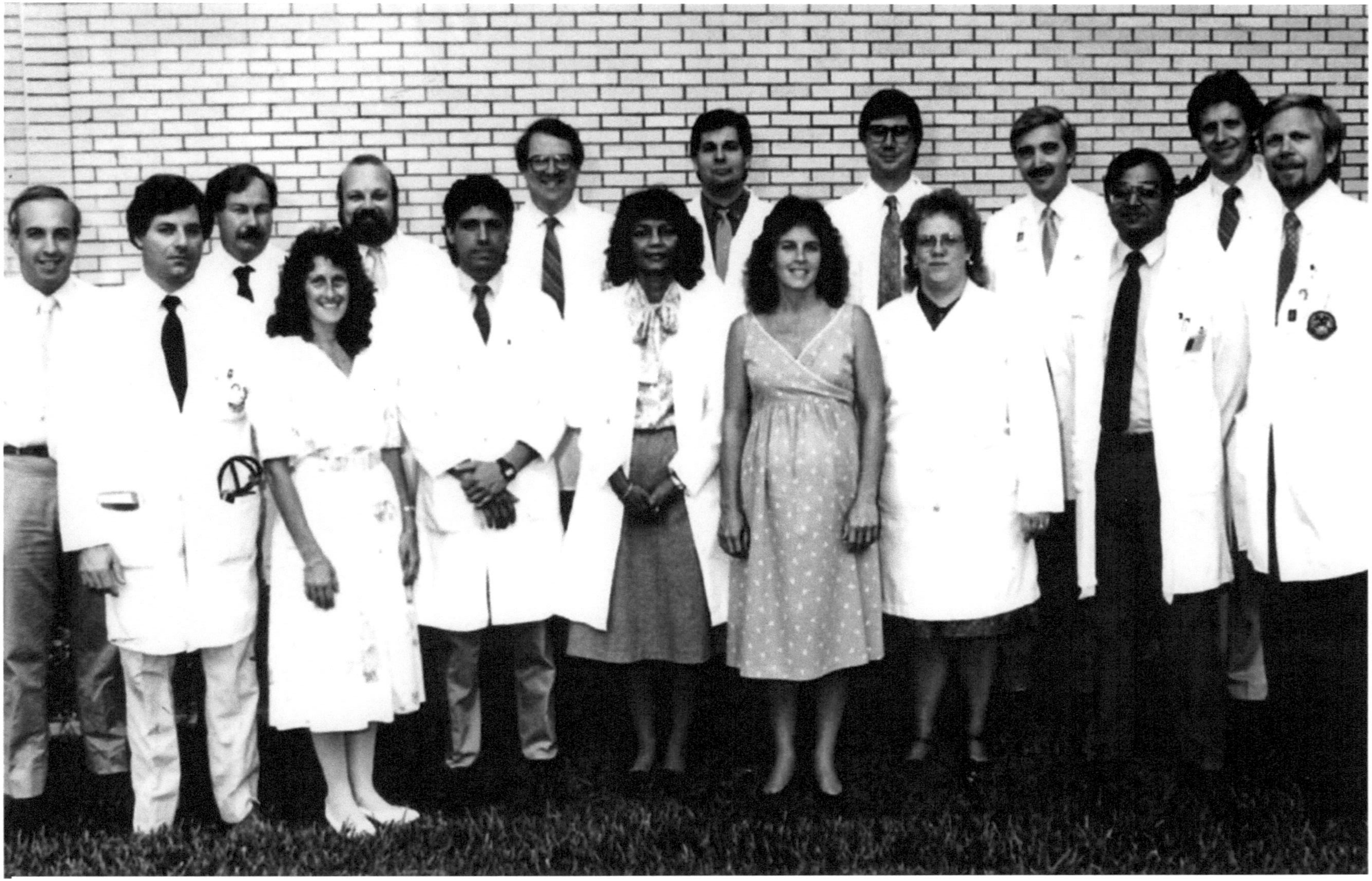

Front row (left to right): Donald W. Russell, MD (1987-1990); Peggy Hales; Joseph D. Diaz, MD (1986-1988); Rama Ganguly, PhD; Pat Walsh; Irene Baird-Warren; Donnie Banerji, MD; Roger W. Fox, MD (1978-1980). Back row (left to right): Mitchel Seleznick, MD; Gerald A. Bucholtz, MD (1980-1982); Walter Trudeau, MS; Richard F. Lockey, MD, MS; David N. Wright, MD (1988-1991); Robert P. Nelson, MD (1985-1987); Dennis K. Ledford, MD (1983-1985); Enrique Fernández-Caldas, PhD. Circa 1987.

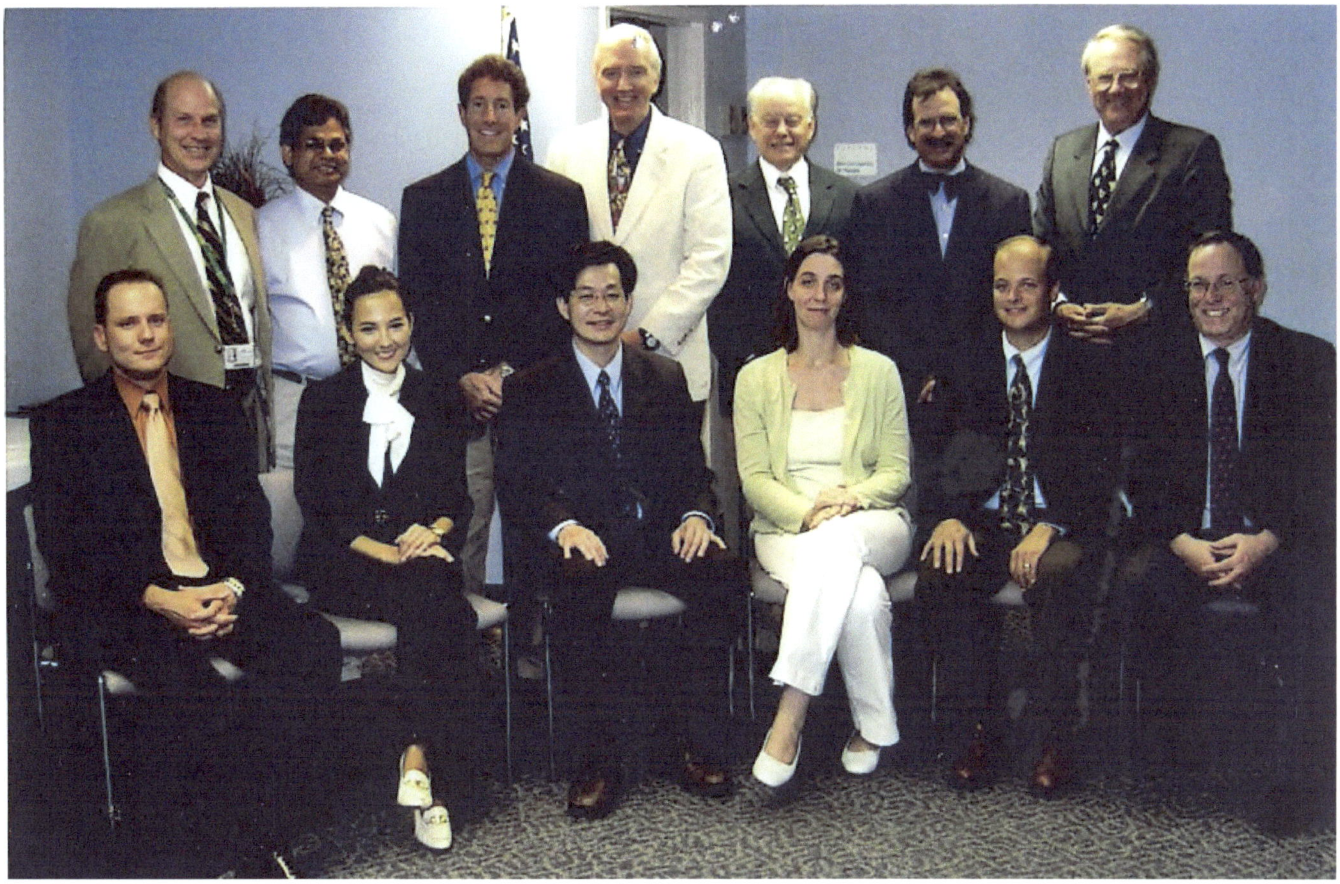

Front row (left to right): Matthew Morrow; Morna Dorsey, MD, MMSc; Nutthapong Tangsinmankong, MD (ACH, 1996-1999); Aleksandra Petrovic, MD; Mark C. Glaum, MD, PhD; Robert Nickeson, MD. Back row (left to right): John W. Sleasman, MD; Shyam S. Mohapatra, PhD; Michael Nieder, MD; Dennis K. Ledford, MD (1983-1985); Monroe J. King, DO; Mandel R. Sher, MD; Richard F. Lockey, MD, MS. Circa 2006.

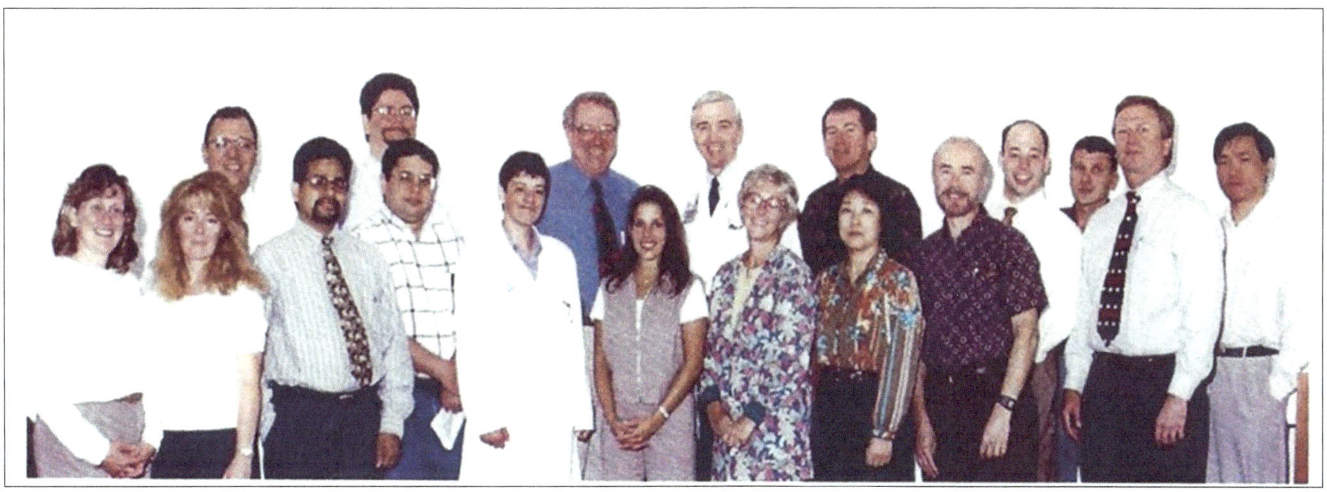

Front row (left to right): Peggy Hales; Sandra Rocha; Shyam Mohapatra, PhD.; Homero San Juan, MD; Rosa Codina, PhD; Alisa Diecidue; Dona Shearer; Xiaoyuan (Sonya) Kong, MD; Gary Hellermann, PhD. Back row (left to right): Demetrios Theodoropoulos, MD (1997-2000); Thomas Luck, MD (1999-2001); Richard F. Lockey, MD, MS; Dennis K. Ledford, MD (1983-1985); Geoffrey Patton, PhD; Daniel Reichmuth, MD (1999-2002); Uknown; Roger W. Fox, MD (1978-1980); Jian Zhang, MD. 1999

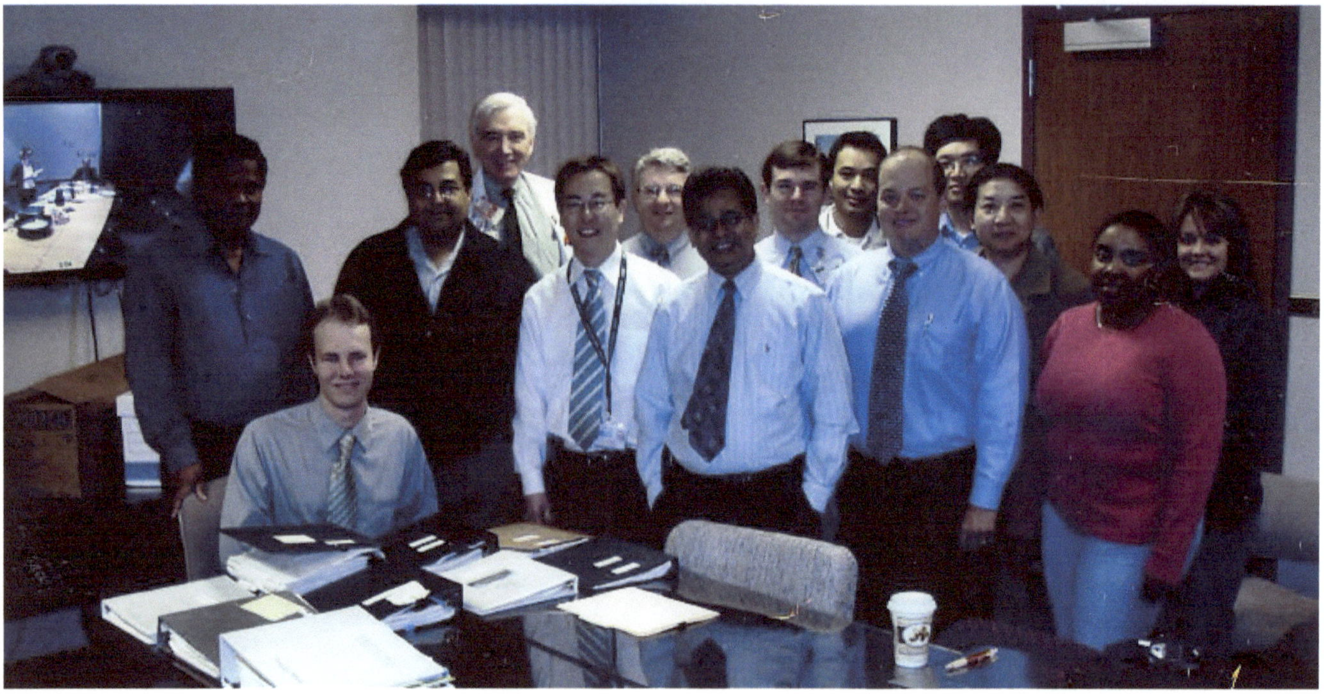

Front row (left to right): Andrew Bagg, MD (sitting) (2006-2008); Byol Shin, DO (2006-2008); Shyam S. Mohapatra, PhD; Mark C. Glaum, MD, PhD, Shawna Shirley; Alison Jones. Back row (left to right): Prasanna Jena, PhD; Arun Kumar, PhD; Dennis K. Ledford, MD (1983-1985); Ronald Purcell, MD (2006-2008); Joshua Phillips, MD (2007-2009); Jia-Wang Wang, PhD; Weidong Zhang, MD, PhD; Guoqing Liu, PhD. Division Research Meeting, circa 2007.

2007 Faculty Retreat; Chinsegut Hill, USF's Conference and Retreat Center; Brooksville, Florida. Front row (left to right): Monroe J. King, DO; Peggy Hales; Stephanie Medley; Dona Shearer; Thomas Chacko, MD (2005-2007). Back row (left to right): Michelle Grandstaff-Singleton; Shyam Mohapatra, PhD; Richard F. Lockey, MD, MS; Roger W. Fox, MD (1978-1980); Hugh Windom, MD; Prasanna Jena, PhD; Arun Kumar, PhD; Steven Cole, DO (2005-2007); Dennis K. Ledford, MD (1983-1985).

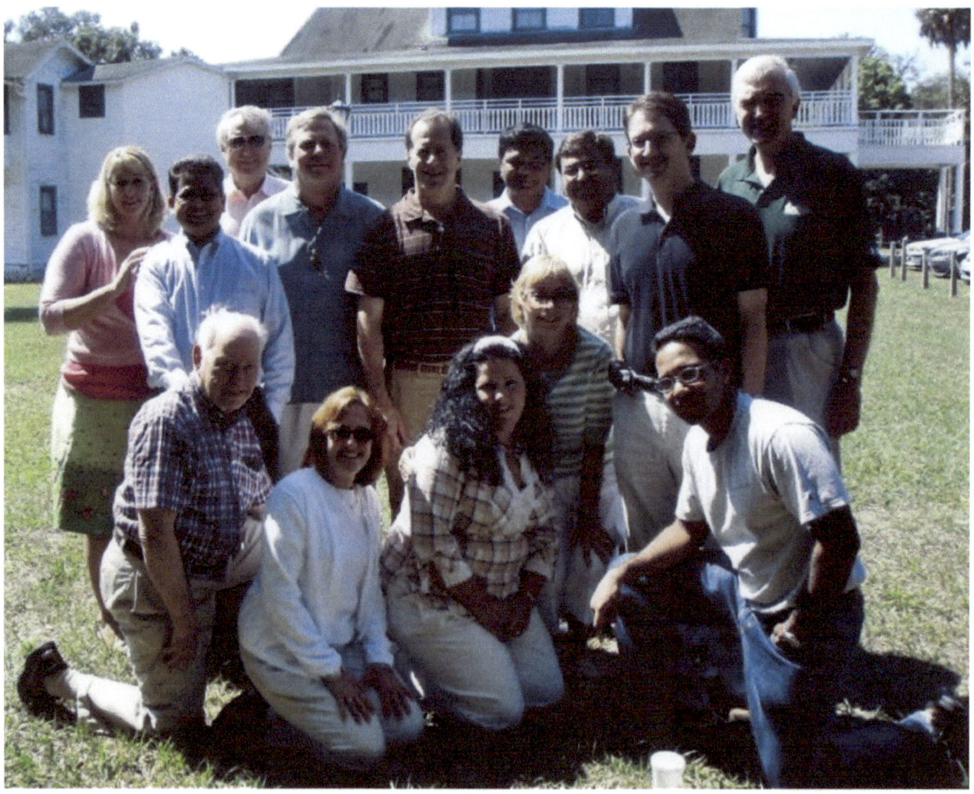

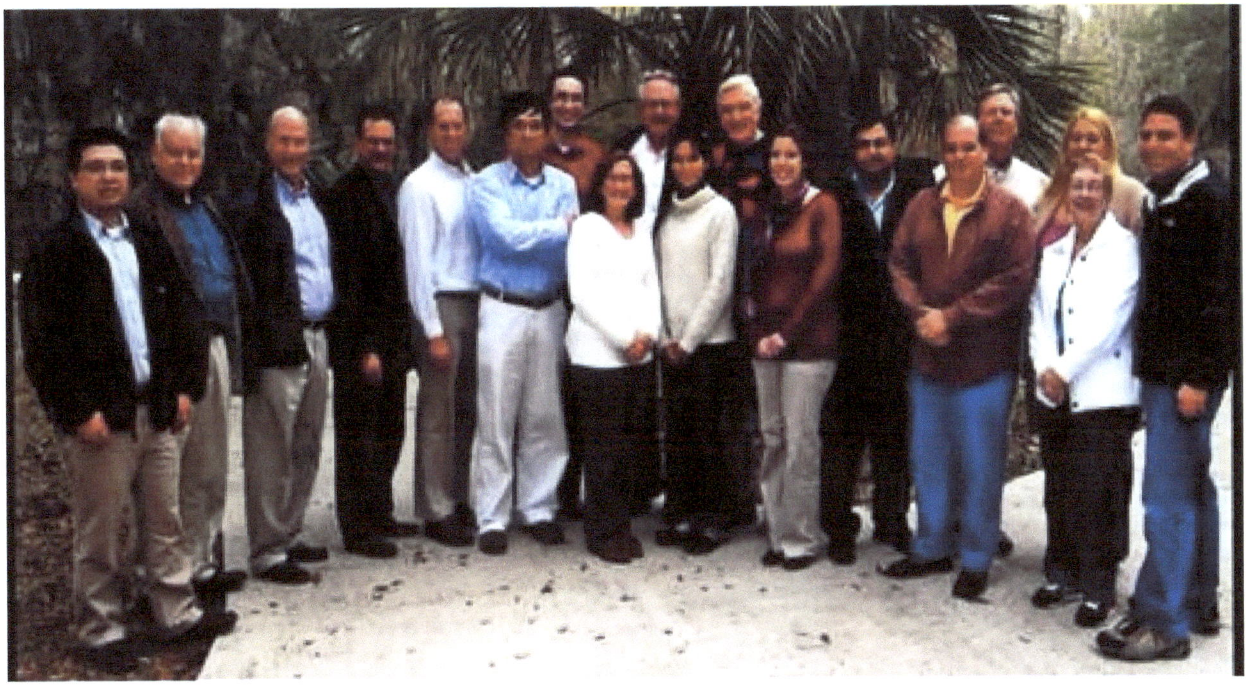

January 2010 Division Retreat; Hillsborough River State Park, Thonotosassa, Florida. Front row (left to right): Weidong Zhang, MD, PhD; Peggy Hales; Morna Dorsey, MD, MMSc; Elena Perez, MD; Arun Kumar, PhD; Mark C. Glaum, MD, PhD; Dona Shearer; Glenn Whelan, PharmD. Back row (left to right): Woei Eng, MD (ACH, 2008-2010); Monroe J. King, DO; John Sleasman, MD; Mandel Sher, MD; Hugh Windom, MD; Robert Pesek, MD (2009-2011); Richard F. Lockey, MD, MS; Dennis K. Ledford, MD (1983-1985); Roger W. Fox, MD (1978-1980); Michelle Grandstaff-Singleton.

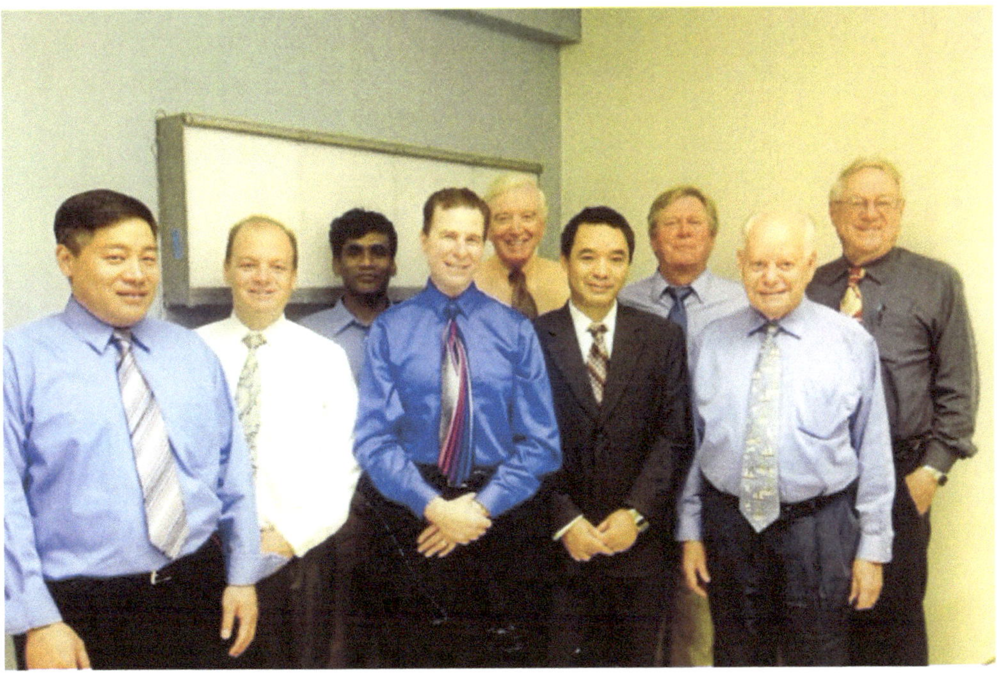

Front row, left to right: Michael Teng, PhD; Mark C. Glaum, MD, PhD; Thomas B. Casale, MD; Jia-Wang Wang, PhD; Monroe J. King, DO. Back row, left to right: Narasaiah Kolliputi, PhD; Dennis K. Ledford, MD (1983-1985); Roger W. Fox, MD (1978-1980); Richard F. Lockey, MD, MS. Circa 2015.

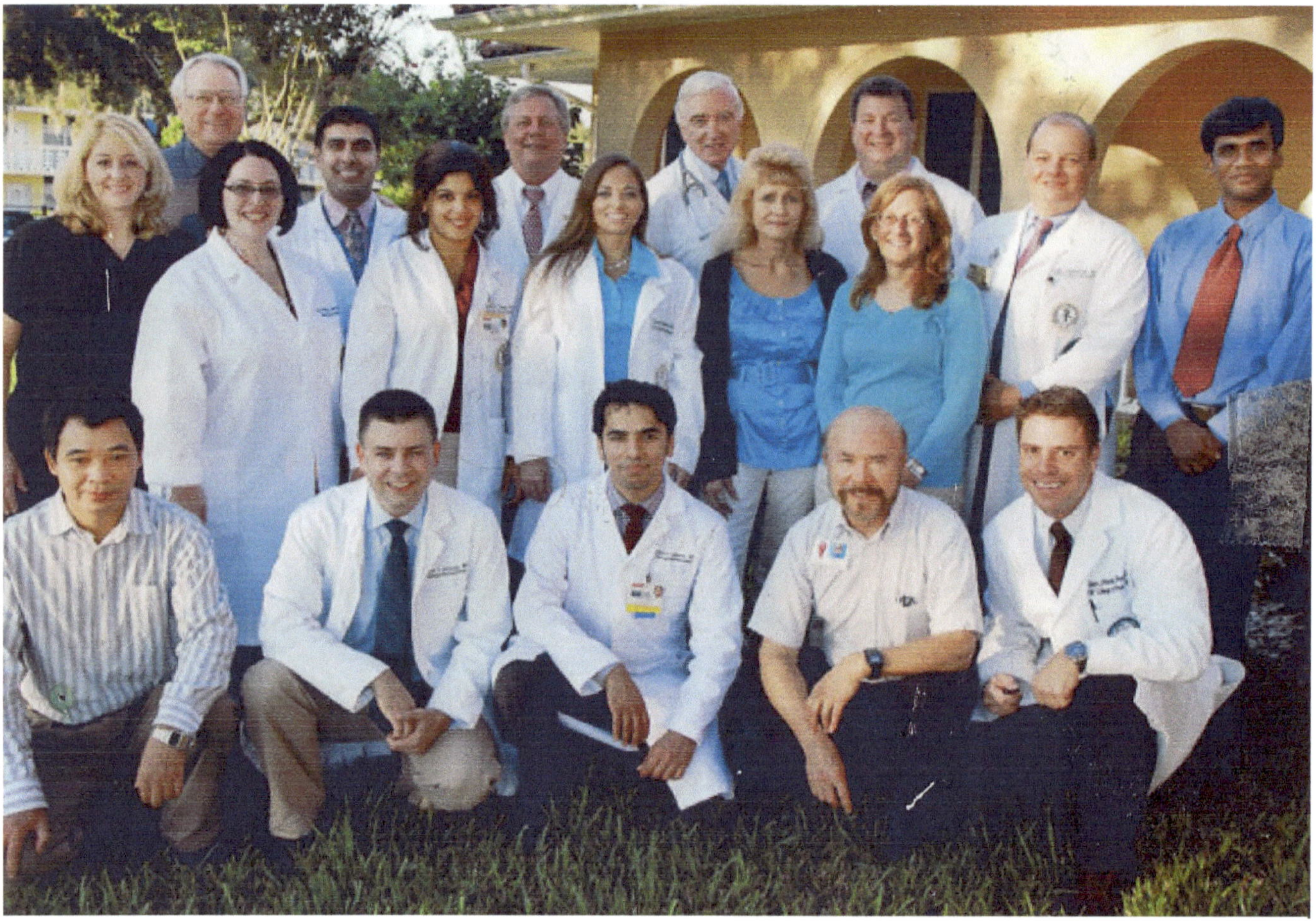

Front row (left to right): Jia-Wang Wang, PhD; David Fitzhugh, MD (2010-2012); Salman Aljubran, MD (2010-2013); Gary Hellermann, PhD; Glenn Whelan, PharmD. Middle row (left to right): Michelle Grandstaff-Singleton; Hava Tillipman Ladinsky, MD (ACH, 2011-2013); Neetu Talreja, MD (2011-2013); Susan Culverhouse, MD (2011-2013); Rebecca Carter-Muncey; Peggy Hales; Mark C. Glaum, MD, PhD; Narasaiah Kolliputi, PhD. Back row (left to right): Richard F. Lockey, MD, MS; Ahmed Butt, MD (2010-2012); Roger W. Fox, MD(1978-1980); Dennis K. Ledford, MD (1983-1985); James Parkerson, DO (2010-2012). Circa 2011.

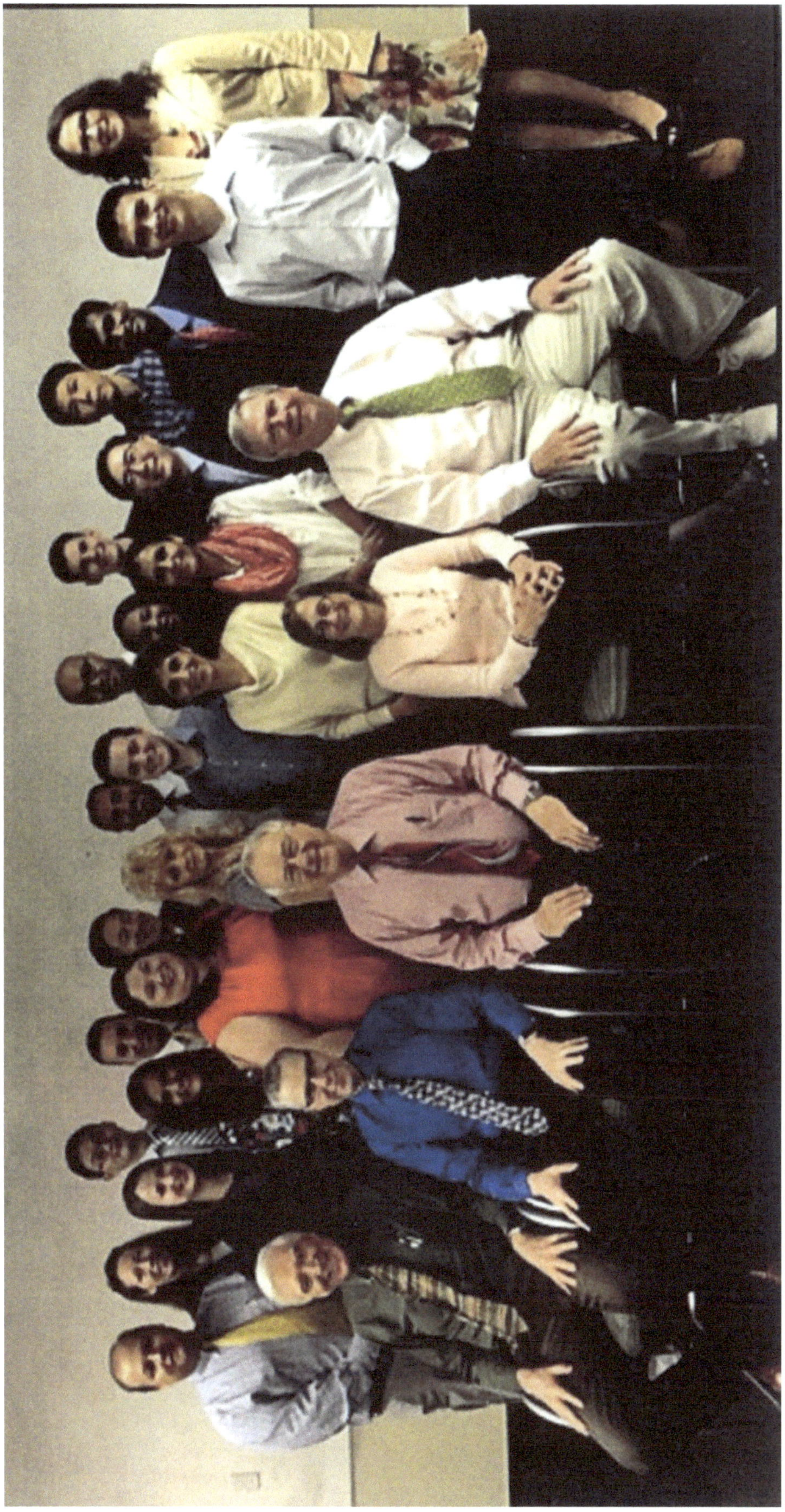

Front row (left to right): Dennis K. Ledford, MD (1983-1985); Thomas B. Casale, MD; Richard F. Lockey, MD, MS; Peggy Hales; Roger W. Fox, MD (1978-1980). Middle row (left to right): Mark C. Glaum, MD, PhD; Emma Westermann-Clark, MD (2016-2018); Amber N. Pepper, MD (2016-2018); Farnaz Tabatabaian, MD (ACH, 2013-2015); Renee Smith; Rebecca Carter; Mason Breitzig; Blanca Camoretti-Mercado, PhD; Andrea N. McCray, PhD; Ramani Soundararajan, PhD; Seong H. Cho, MD; Narasaiah Kolliputi, PhD; Lee Tan, Michelle Twitmyer. Back row (left to right): Chen Lin, MD (2015-2017); Peter Ricketti, DO (2015-2017); Michael Teng, PhD; Adeeb Bulkhi, MD (2014-2017); Sultan Alandijani, MD (2015-2017); Alex Czachor; Jutaro Fukumoto, MD, PhD. January 2017.

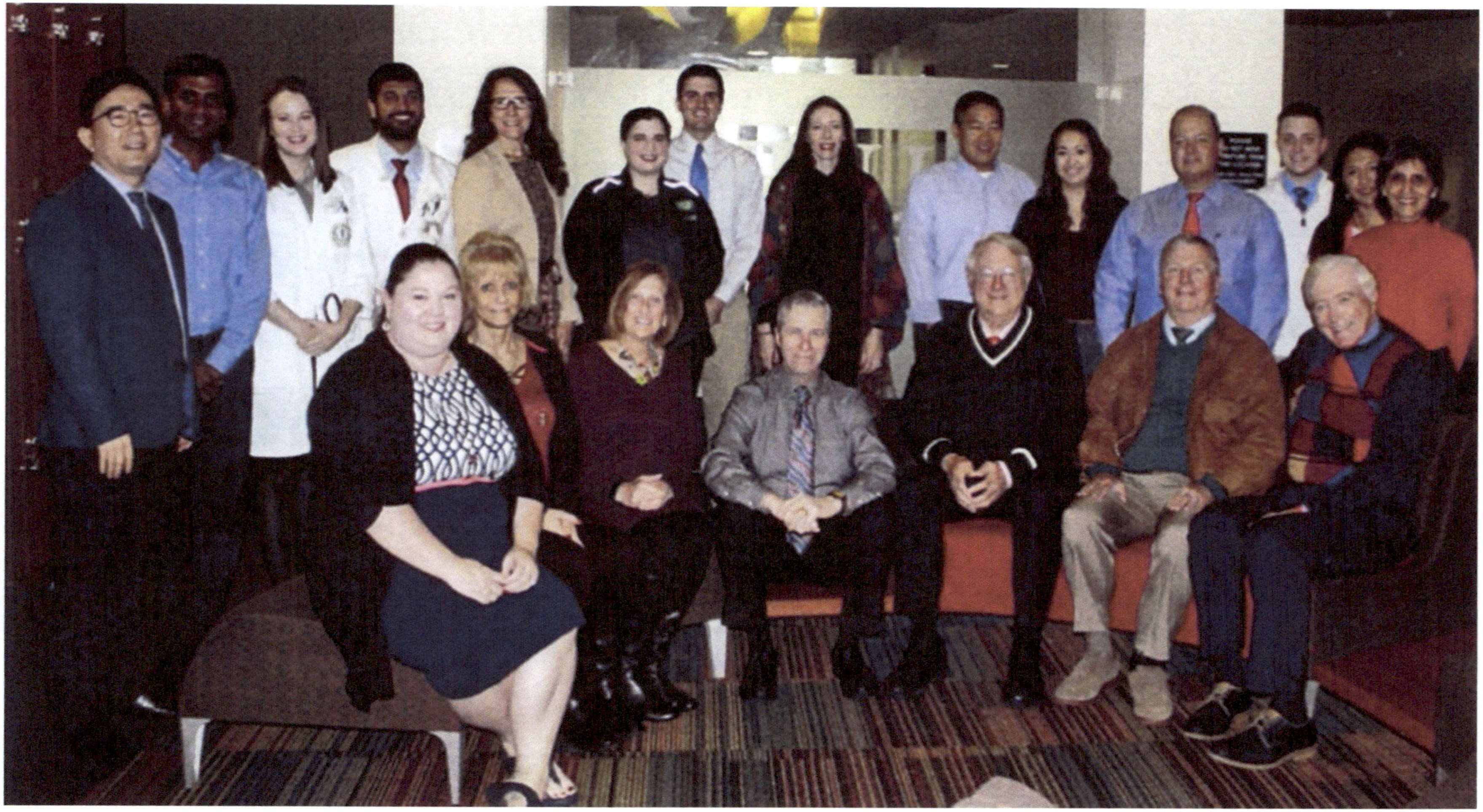

Front row (left to right): Catherine Renee Smith; Rebecca Carter Muncey; Peggy Hales; Thomas B. Casale, MD; Richard F. Lockey, MD, MS; Roger W. Fox, MD (1978-1980); Dennis K. Ledford, MD (1983-1985). Back row (left to right): Seong H. Cho, MD; Narasaiah Kolliputi, PhD; Amber Pepper, MD (2016-2018); Shiven Patel, MD (2017-2019); Michelle Twitmyer; Tara Saco, MD (2017-2019); Kirk Shepard, MD (2017-2019); Emma Westermann-Clark, MD (2016-2018); Michael N. Teng, PhD; Tiffani Kaage; Mark C. Glaum, MD, PhD; Mason Breitzig; Helena Hernández-Cuervo; Blanca Camoretti-Mercado, PhD. December 2017.

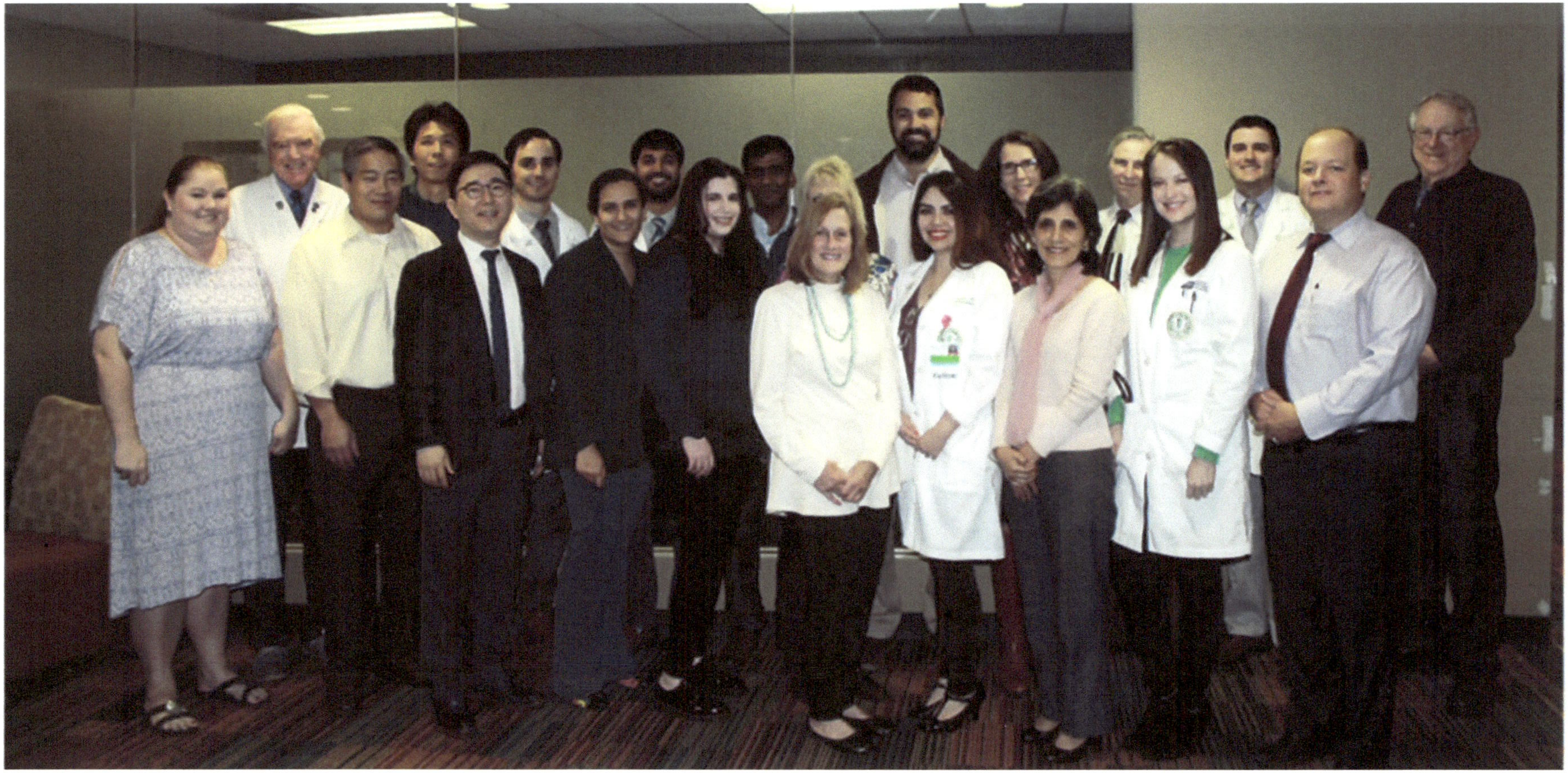

Front row (left to right): Catherine Renee Smith; Michael Teng, PhD; Seong Cho, MD; Farnaz Tabatabaian, MD (ACH, 2013-2015); Tara Saco, MD (2017-2019); Peggy Hales; Claudia Gaefke, MD (2018-2020); Blanca Camoretti-Mercado, PhD; Amber Pepper, MD (2016-2018); Mark C. Glaum, MD, PhD. Back row (left to right): Dennis K. Ledford, MD (1983-1985); Jutaro Fukumoto, MD, PhD; Raul Villarreal, MD (2018-2020); Shiven Patel, MD (2017-2019); Narasaiah Kolliputi, PhD; Juan Carlos Cardet, MD, MPH; Michelle Twitmyer; Thomas B. Casale, MD; Kirk V. Shepard, MD (2017-2019); Richard F. Lockey, MD, MS. Circa 2019.

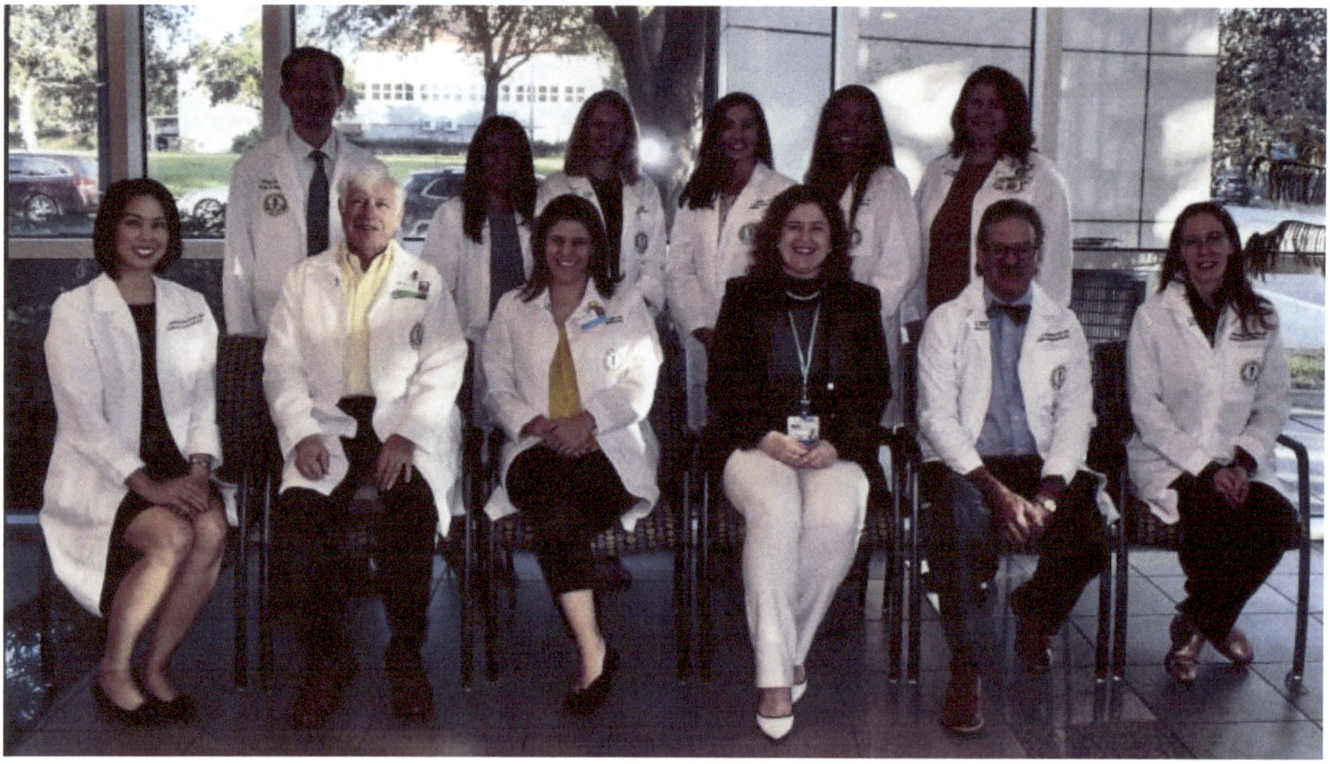

USF Division of Allergy and Immunology, Department of Pediatrics, All Children's Hospital/Johns Hopkins Medicine. Front row (left to right): Panida Sriaroon, MD (ACH, 2006-2009); Mark Ballow, MD; Jennifer Leiding, MD; Jolan Walter, MD, PhD; Mandel Sher, MD; Emma Westermann-Clark, MD (2016-2018). Back row (left to right): Nathan Tang, MD (ACH, 1996-1999); Daime Nieves, APRN; Irina Dawson, MD (ACH, 2018-2020); Jacqueline Squire, MD (ACH, 2018-2020); Maria Chitty-Lopez, MD (ACH, 2019-2021); Carla Duff, ARNP. Circa 2020.

Chapter 9: The Clinical Research Unit (CRU)
A Collection of Memories, Pictures and Brochures

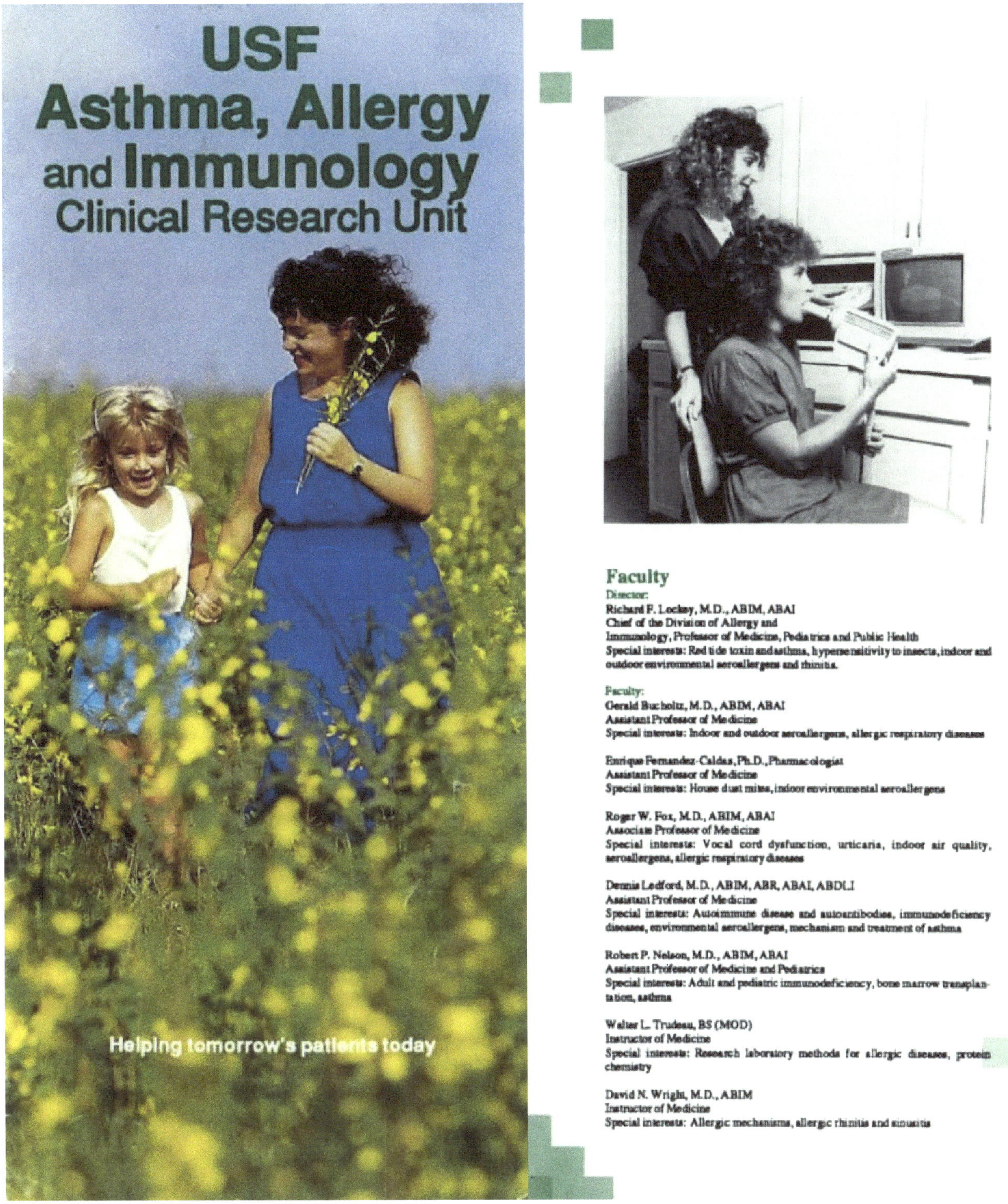

USF
Asthma, Allergy
and Immunology
Clinical Research Unit

Helping tomorrow's patients today

Faculty

Director:

Richard F. Lockey, M.D., ABIM, ABAI
Chief of the Division of Allergy and
Immunology, Professor of Medicine, Pediatrics and Public Health
Special interests: Red tide toxin and asthma, hypersensitivity to insects, indoor and outdoor environmental aeroallergens and rhinitis.

Faculty:

Gerald Bucholtz, M.D., ABIM, ABAI
Assistant Professor of Medicine
Special interests: Indoor and outdoor aeroallergens, allergic respiratory diseases

Enrique Fernandez-Caldas, Ph.D., Pharmacologist
Assistant Professor of Medicine
Special interests: House dust mites, indoor environmental aeroallergens

Roger W. Fox, M.D., ABIM, ABAI
Associate Professor of Medicine
Special interests: Vocal cord dysfunction, urticaria, indoor air quality, aeroallergens, allergic respiratory diseases

Dennis Ledford, M.D., ABIM, ABR, ABAI, ABDLI
Assistant Professor of Medicine
Special interests: Autoimmune disease and autoantibodies, immunodeficiency diseases, environmental aeroallergens, mechanism and treatment of asthma

Robert P. Nelson, M.D., ABIM, ABAI
Assistant Professor of Medicine and Pediatrics
Special interests: Adult and pediatric immunodeficiency, bone marrow transplantation, asthma

Walter L. Trudeau, BS (MOD)
Instructor of Medicine
Special interests: Research laboratory methods for allergic diseases, protein chemistry

David N. Wright, M.D., ABIM
Instructor of Medicine
Special interests: Allergic mechanisms, allergic rhinitis and sinusitis

Clinical Research Unit Brochure, circa 1992.

Research

A drug trial involves several people, including the doctor and patient, the drug manufacturer, representatives from the Food and Drug Administration (FDA) and other organizations responsible for overseeing clinical research at the University.

The drug company submits a proposal to the FDA that is reviewed for its safety and effectiveness. The proposal is examined by the University's Institutional Review Board for similar safety checks and protection of individual rights. That board includes local people who are not health professionals.

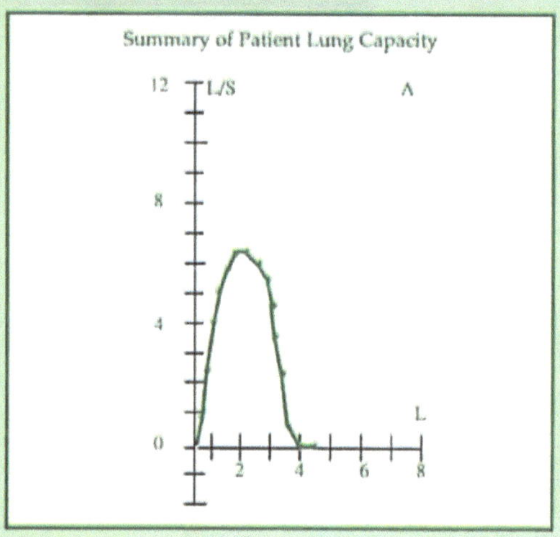

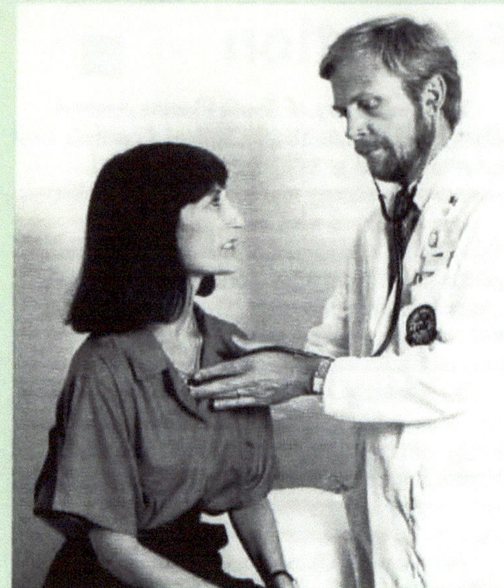

Photos by James Phillips

Patient Care

Once a drug trial proposal is approved and the clinical trial is about to begin, the patient and doctor review detailed information about the drug being tested so that everyone is fully informed about possible benefits from the medication as well as any known risks involved in its use.

Participation in research is vital to improved health care and the advancement of medical science in this country. Physicians around the world study the work done by researchers in the United States, just as our health professionals keep up with breakthroughs in other countries.

With your help, we can continue to make contributions to improve your health and that of your family.

Education

The University of South Florida Asthma, Allergy and Immunology Clinical Research Unit was established in 1977 for the benefit of patients with allergy and immunology problems.

It is affiliated with the College of Medicine's Department of Internal Medicine and the physicians who work at the center are faculty in that department. They examine and treat patients, educate medical students, residents and fellows, and conduct research.

By the early 1980s, the center's researchers were able to begin testing new medications for allergy and immunology problems such as asthma, hay fever, hives and AIDS. Some of the medications are so new that they are not yet available to the general public.

People with allergy and immunology problems can make an important contribution to their own health care and to the advancement of medical science by participating in these clinical drug trials.

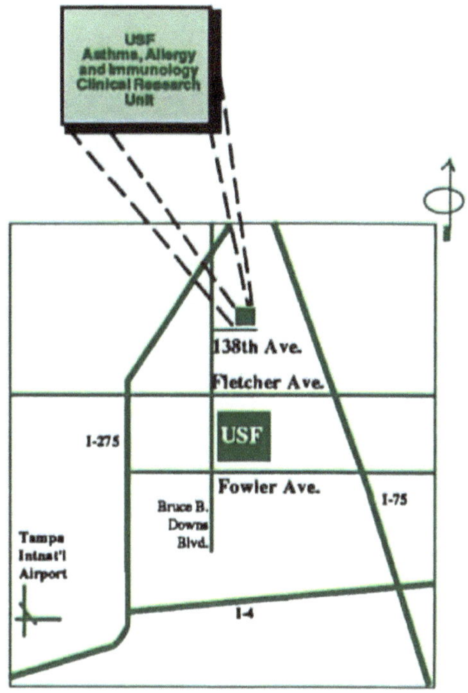

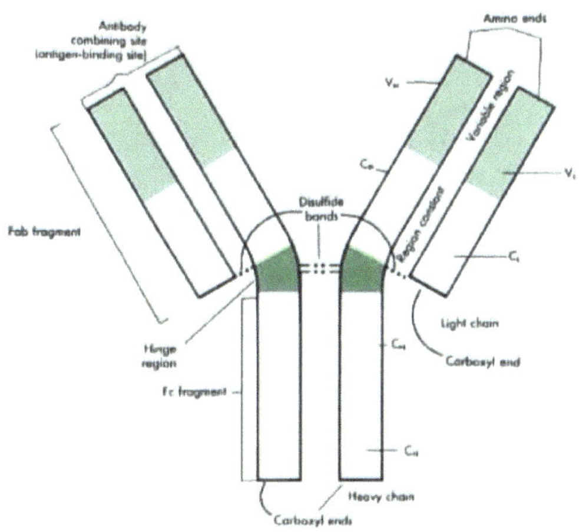

Antibody

USF

Asthma, Allergy and Immunology
Clinical Research Unit
3010 E. 138th Ave., Suite 12
Tampa, FL 33613
(813) 972-8857

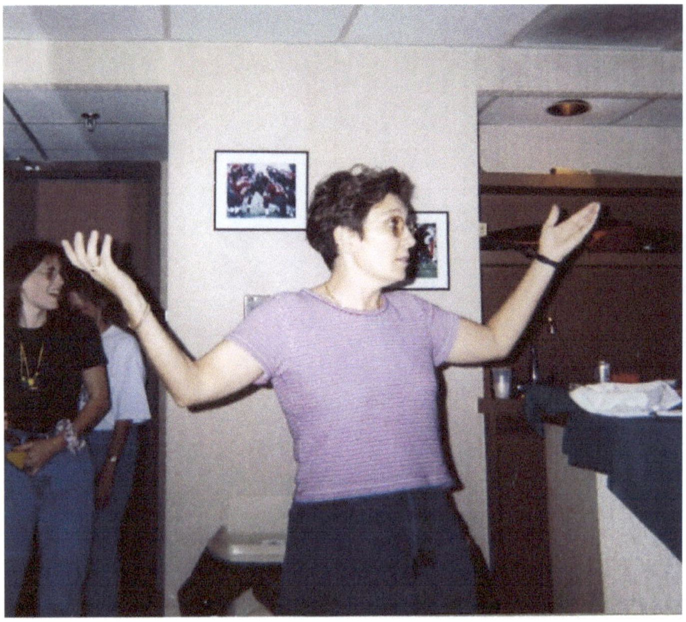

Cindy Reichart, Clinical Research Administrator, circa 2000.

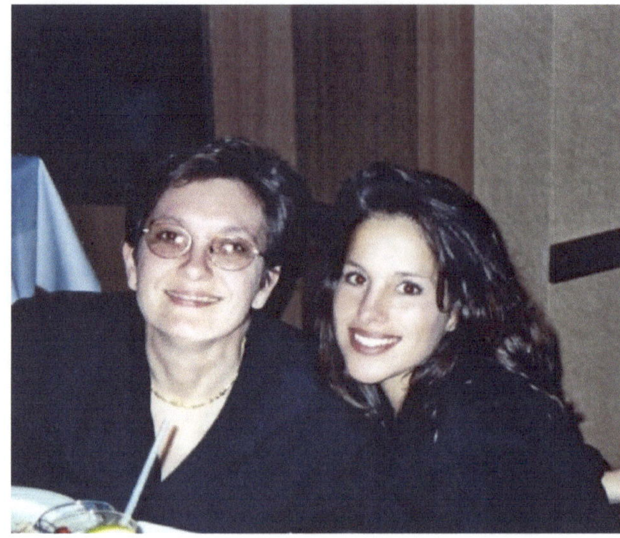

Left to right: Cindy Reichart, Clinical Research Administrator and Alisa Diecidue, Clinical Research Coordinator, circa 1998.

Left to right: Tracy (surname unknown), Clinical Research Coordinator; Yvette Meunier, Regulatory Coordinator; Cindy Reichart, Clinical Research Administrator; Alisa Diecidue, Clinical Research Coordinator, circa 2000.

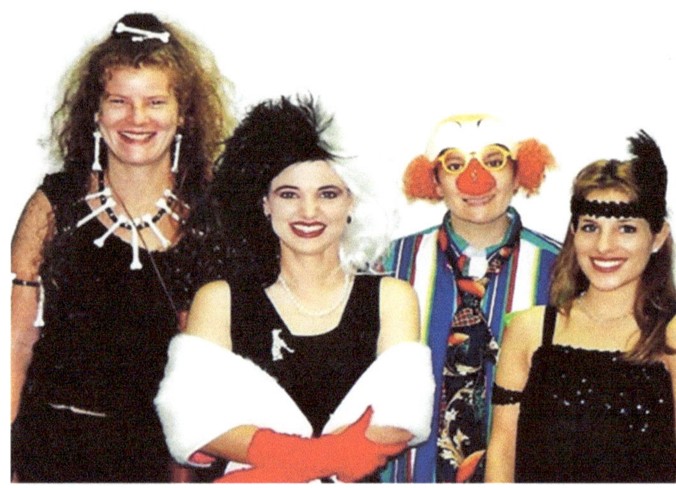

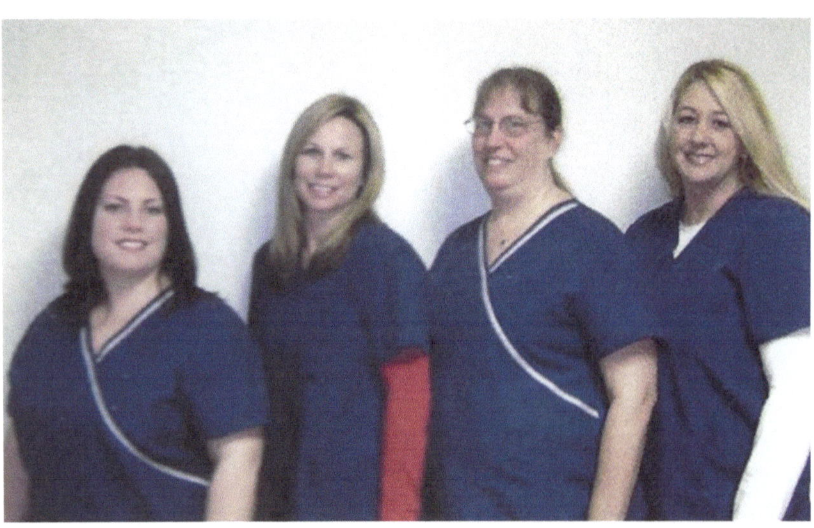

Left to right: Sarah Lewis, Regulatory Coordinator; Diana Miller; Clinical Research Coordinator; Shirley McCullough, Clinical Research Coordinator; Michelle Grandstaff-Singleton, Clinical Research Administrator, circa 2008.

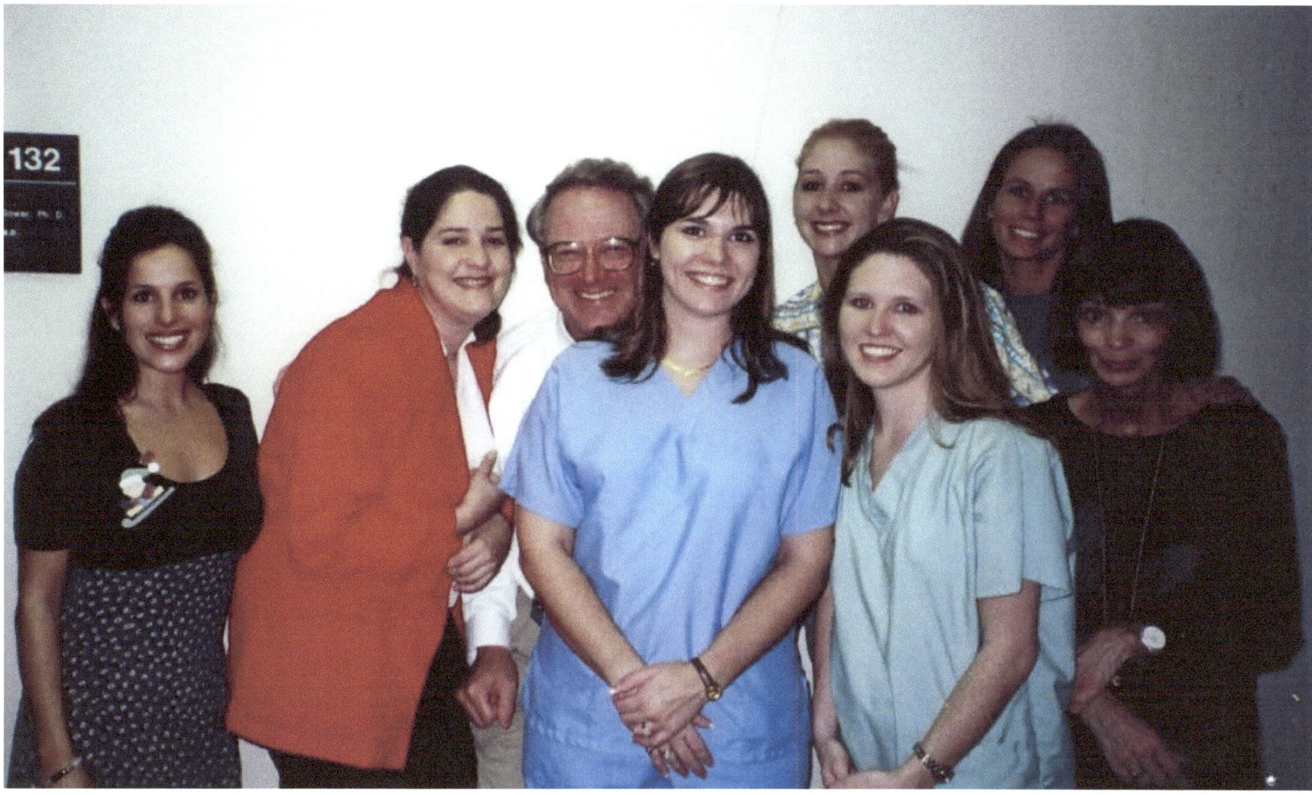

Front row (left to right): Brooke Fimbel, Clinical Research Coordinator; Michelle Hernandez, Clinical Research Coordinator; Pam Nu, Clinical Research Coordinator. Second row (left to right): Alisa Diecidue, Clinical Research Administrator; Menayra Caro, Regulatory Coordinator; Richard F. Lockey, MD, MS; Michelle Grandstaff-Singleton, Clinical Research Coordinator; Diana Miller, Clinical Research Coordinator. Circa 2002.

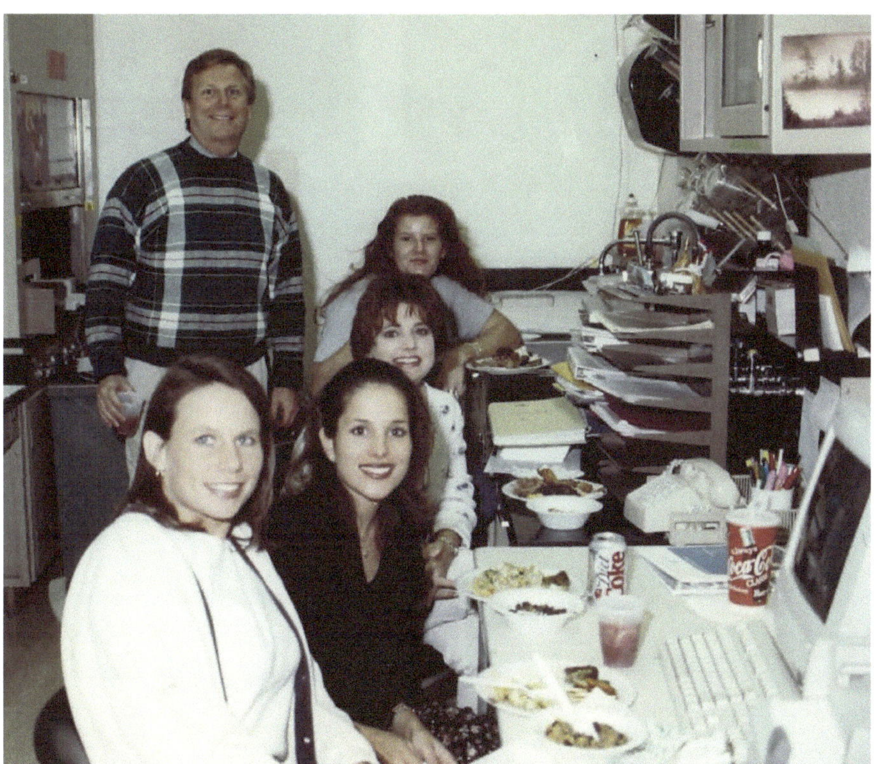

Front to back: Diana Miller, Clinical Research Coordinator; Alisa Diecidue, Clinical Research Administrator; Yvette Meunier, Regulatory Coordinator; Tracy (surname unknown), Clinical Research Coordinator; Roger W. Fox, MD, circa 2002.

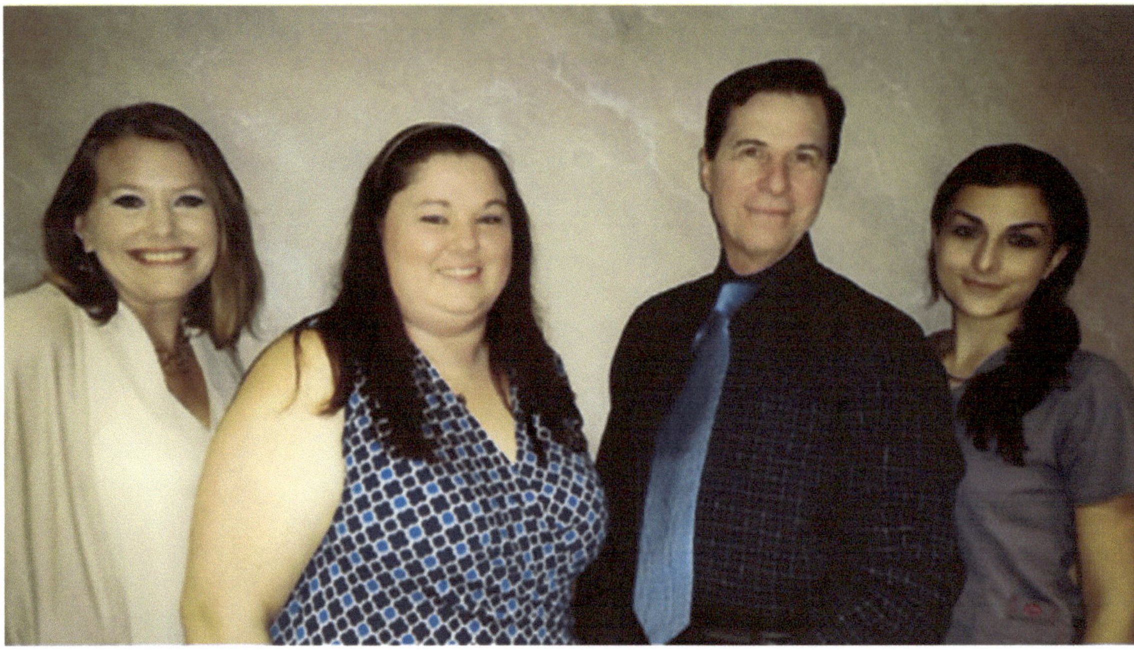

Left to right: Shawna Atha, Clinical Research Administrator; Catherine Renee Smith, Clinical Research Coordinator; Thomas B. Casale, MD, Director, Clinical Research Unit; Jeaneen Ahmad, Clinical Research Coordinator, circa 2014.

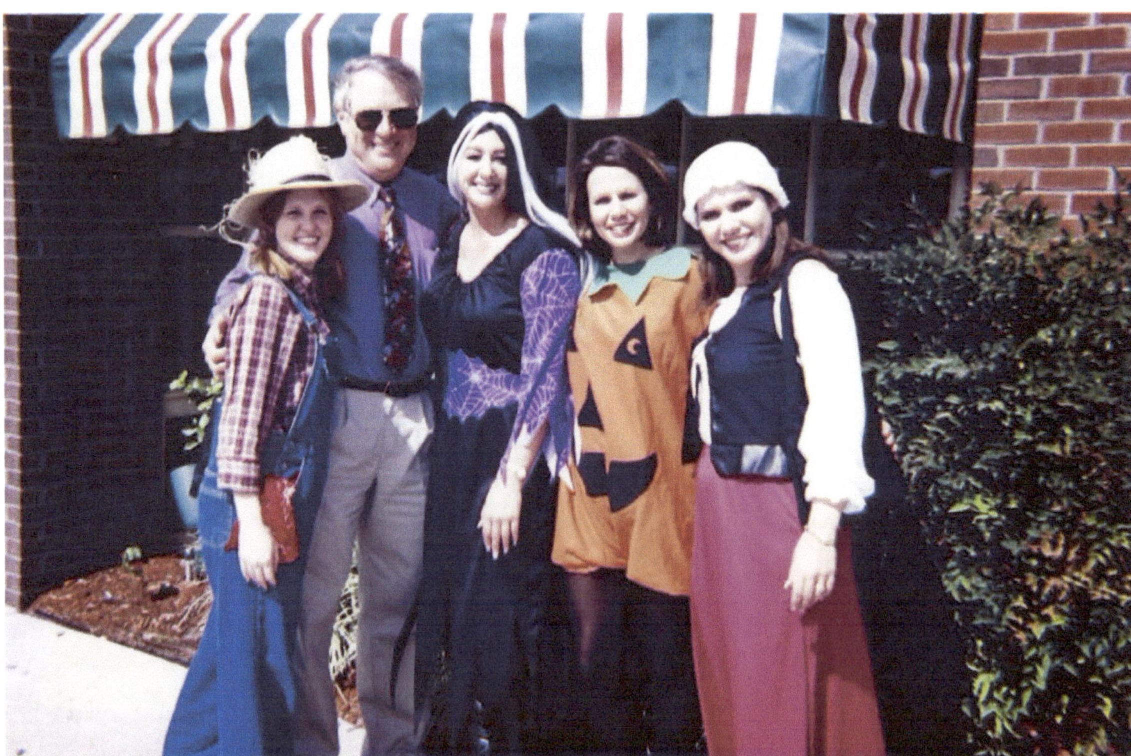

Left to right: Michelle Hernandez, Clinical Research Coordinator; Richard F. Lockey, MD, MS; Michelle Grandstaff-Singleton, Clinical Research Administrator; Diana Miller, Clinical Research Coordinator; Brooke Fimbel, Clinical Research Coordinator, circa 2006.

Clinical Research Unit Brochure, circa 2014.

University of South Florida

Division of Allergy and Immunology

Clinical and Translational Research Unit

The Joy McCann Culverhouse
Airway Disease Research Center

Department of Internal Medicine

USF® HEALTH

Clinical Research Faculty

Thomas B. Casale, M.D.
tbcasale@health.usf.edu

- Director, Clinical Research
- Professor of Medicine
- Board certified in Internal Medicine and Allergy and Immunology

Richard F. Lockey, M.D.
rlockey@health.usf.edu

- Associate Director, Clinical Research
- Director, Division of Allergy and Clinical Immunology
- Distinguished University Health Professor
- Professor of Medicine, Pediatrics, and Public health
- Joy McCann Culverhouse Chair of Allergy and Immunology
- Board Certified in Internal Medicine and Allergy and Immunology

Dennis K. Ledford, M.D.
dledford@health.usf.edu

- Professor of Medicine and Pediatrics
- Mabel and Ellsworth Simmons Professor Allergy and Immunology
- Board certified in Internal Medicine, Allergy and Immunology, and Rheumatology

Roger W. Fox, M.D.
rfox@health.usf.edu

- Professor of Medicine, Pediatrics, and Public Health
- Board certified in Internal Medicine and Allergy and Immunology

Mark C. Glaum, M.D., Ph.D.
mglaum@health.usf.edu

- Associate Professor of Medicine and Pediatrics
- Board certified in Internal Medicine and Allergy and Immunology

Basic Research Faculty

Michael Teng, Ph.D.

- Associate Professor of Medicine and Pediatrics

Narasaiah Kolliputi, Ph.D.

- Associate Professor of Medicine and Pediatrics

Jia Wang, Ph.D.

- Associate Professor of Medicine and Pediatrics

CLINICAL EXPERTISE	CLINICAL PROCEDURES		LABORATORY CAPABILITIES	
• Allergic rhinitis • Allergen immunotherapy • Angioedema, acute and chronic • Asthma • Atopic eczema • Bronchitis, acute and chronic • Contact dermatitis • COPD • Exercise-induced asthma • Hereditary angioedema • Headaches (migraine and tension) • Immunodeficiency • Insect allergy • Nasal polyps • Non-allergic rhinitis • Osteoporosis • Sinusitis, acute and chronic • Temporomandibular joint syndrome • Urticaria, acute and chronic	• Acoustic rhinometry • Allergen challenge (lung) • Allergen challenge (nasal, using acoustic rhinometry) • Allergy skin test • Asthma control test • Blood draw • ECG • End-point skin titration • Exercise challenge • Exhaled nitric oxide • Hypertonic saline challenge • Impedance oscillometry • Mannitol challenge • Methacholine challenge • Microscopy • Nasal scraping • Nasal secretion collection	• Pollen counts • Rhinoscopy • Rhinomanometry • Spirometry with pre- and post- bronchodilation • Sputum induction • Study drug infusion • Urine drug screen • Urine hCG	• Flow cytometry ➤ Cell surface phenotyping of peripheral blood mononuclear cells (PBMC), up to 14 parameters (BD FACS Canto II) ➤ Intracellular cytokine staining of PBMC ➤ Apoptosis/cell cycle assays ➤ Functional analysis of lymphocyte populations ➤ Magnetic (Miltenyi Automacs Pro) or flow cytometric (BD FACS Aria II) sorting of lymphocyte subsets • Antigen-specific and nonspecific lymphocyte proliferation/differentiation • Chemokine/cytokine assays • Cytometric bead arrays for cytokines/ chemokines	• Real-time quantitative PCR ➤ Analysis of PBMC cytokine/ chemokine mRNA expression (individual cytokines genes or PCR arrays) ➤ Identification and quantification of plasma miRNA (proprietary TaqMan assay) • ELISA ➤ Detection of serum / body fluid cytokine and chemokine levels ➤ Detection of serum antibody subtypes • Biomarker assessment

We do clinical research; we do it well!

CENTER HISTORY

The Division of Allergy and Immunology was established in the Department of Internal Medicine at the University of South Florida College of Medicine, Tampa, Florida in 1972, one year after the College of Medicine was founded. Professor Samuel C. Bukantz, M.D., founder of the Division, recruited Richard F. Lockey, M.D. in 1973 as a second faculty member, and these two internationally acclaimed physician scientists established the Clinical Research unit in 1977 and a training program for physicians to become allergists/immunologists in 1977. The Department of Internal Medicine program has five current trainees, and with the Pediatric section at All Children's Hospital in St Petersburg, have trained over 90 allergists/immunologists and numerous American and foreign post-graduate and graduate research scholars. Many of these trainees are now faculty members in academic centers throughout the world. Both the medicine and pediatric sections are supported by funds donated for teaching, research, and patient care and by secured grants for research from the National Institutes of Health (NIH), by the American Lung Association (ALA), various foundations, and industry. The research program expanded in the late 1990s when endowments were donated by grateful friends, Joy McCann Culverhouse and George and Sandy Simmons. In June, 2000, the Clinical Research Unit was selected as one of 19 American Lung Association's Asthma Clinical Research centers, a network of academic asthma research centers dedicated to conduct multicenter clinical research trials in asthma and other airway diseases that are relevant to practical questions about treatment.

RESEARCH EMPHASIS

Basic and clinical research interests include the pathogenesis and treatment of asthma and allergic diseases, aerobiology, primary and secondary immunodeficiency diseases, HIV, bone marrow transplantation, insect hypersensitivity, allergen immunotherapy, co-morbid conditions affecting asthma and upper airway disease, chronic obstructive lung disease, viral respiratory tract infection and asthma, asthma and allergy in the elderly, hereditary angioedema, chronic urticaria and angioedema, atopic eczema, sleep apnea, nasal polyposis, pulmonary artery hypertension and drug allergy.

CLINICAL RESEARCH UNIT

The Division of Allergy and Immunology Clinical Research Unit is a 1600 square foot facility, located just off the main campus, in which pharmaceutical sponsored, divisional clinical research projects and federal and non-federal grant funded clinical research projects are conducted. The main goal of the Center is to bring together basic and clinical scientists who translate bench and clinical research into improved treatment of patients who suffer from asthma and allergic and immunologic diseases. All studies performed are done under the supervision of the physicians and the staff and approved by the University's Human Research Committee. All trainees in allergy and immunology are required to participate in clinical research throughout their training to foster their careers as clinician scientists. Over the past several decades, the Clinical Research faculty have conducted over 500 Phase I, II, III and IV clinical trials and established a working relationship with more than 40 pharmaceutical sponsors, NIH, ALA, VA and many other funding sources.

Staffed by five USF clinician scientists, the Division and the Clinical Research Unit are affiliated with various institutions in the Tampa Bay Area including the H. Lee Moffitt Cancer Center, James A. Haley Veterans' Hospital, Tampa General Hospital, Florida Hospital, the University of South Florida Morsani Center for Advanced Healthcare, and All Children's Hospital.

RESEARCH CAPABILITIES

- Exceeding enrollment requirements is our commitment to quality research.
- Research is conducted in accordance with Good Clinical Practice Guidelines and the highest ethical standards are followed.
- 40 years of experience in over 500 phase I-IV trials.
- Experienced clinical research coordinators.
- Full-time regulatory coordinator which facilitates timely start-up of new studies.
- On-site IRB meets weekly for new protocols; expedited review for amendments and informed consent changes.
- Contracted with Western IRB for multi-center trials.
- Contracted with central IRBs: Quintiles, Quorum & Schulman

Meeting enrollment requirements is standard practice.

POPULATION:

Tampa Bay metropolitan area:
2.5 million population,
Varied ethnic composition,
Easily reached with appropriate media exposure.

MEDICAL PRACTICE

70 new patient and 400 follow-up visits per week

Computerized patient database

LOCATION

The USF campus is 20 minutes from Tampa International Airport and is easily accessible from Interstate 275. We are three blocks north of Fletcher Ave. on the east side of Bruce B. Downs Blvd.

For more information, please contact:

Thomas B. Casale, M.D., Director; any other faculty member or **Shawna Atha**, Clinical Research Unit Administrator at the Division of Allergy and Immunology, Department of Internal Medicine, University of South Florida Clinical Research Unit.

PHONE: (813) 631-4024
FAX: (813) 631-4030
13801 Bruce B. Downs Blvd., Suite 505
Tampa, Florida 33613

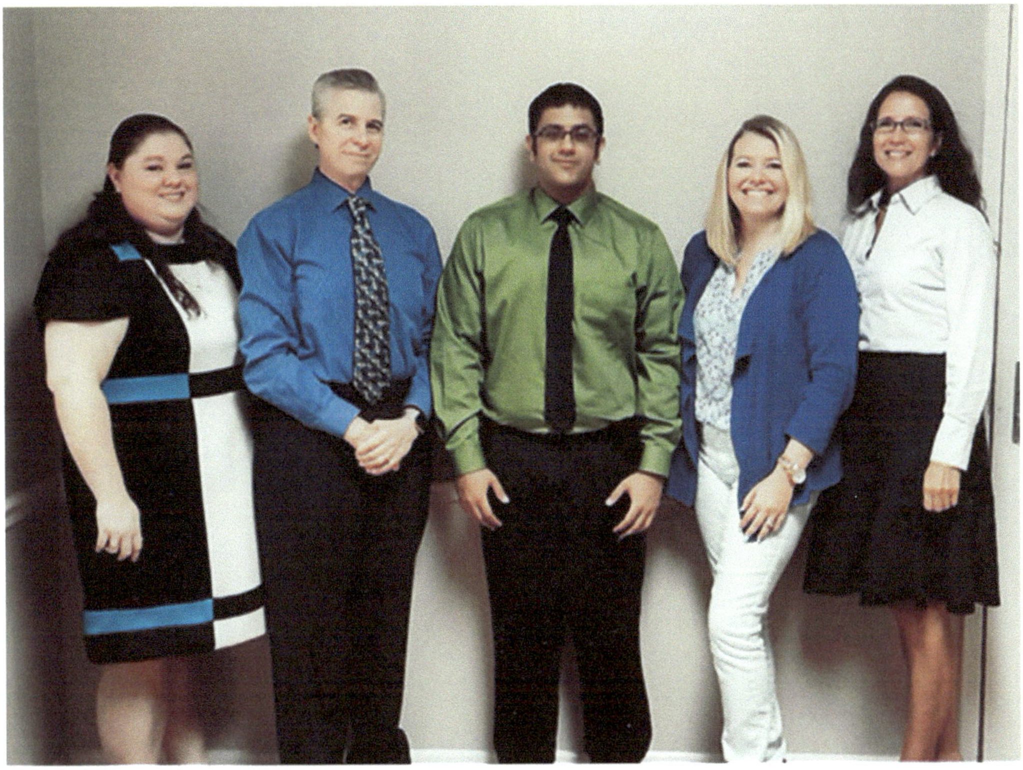

Left to right: Catherine Renee Smith, Clinical Research Coordinator; Thomas B. Casale, MD, Director, Clinical Research Unit; Rikesh Patel, Clinical Research Coordinator; Shawna Atha, Clinical Research Administrator; Michelle Twitmyer, Clinical Research Coordinator, circa 2015.

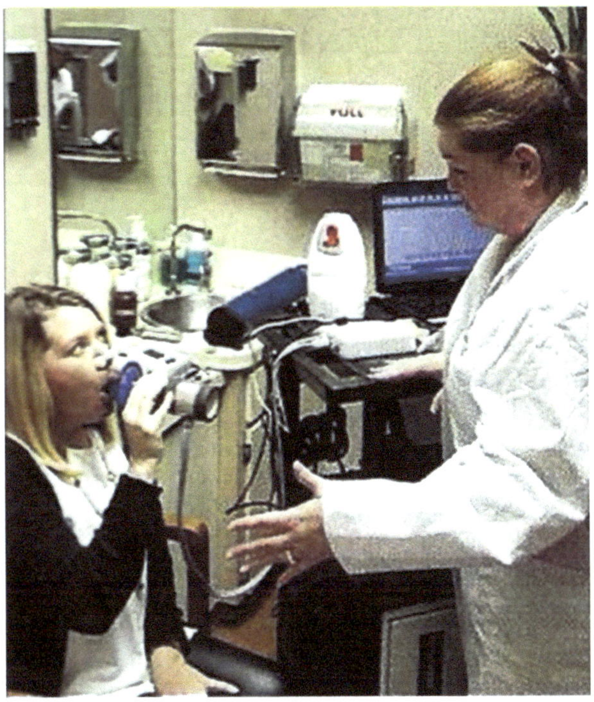

Spirometry in 2015.

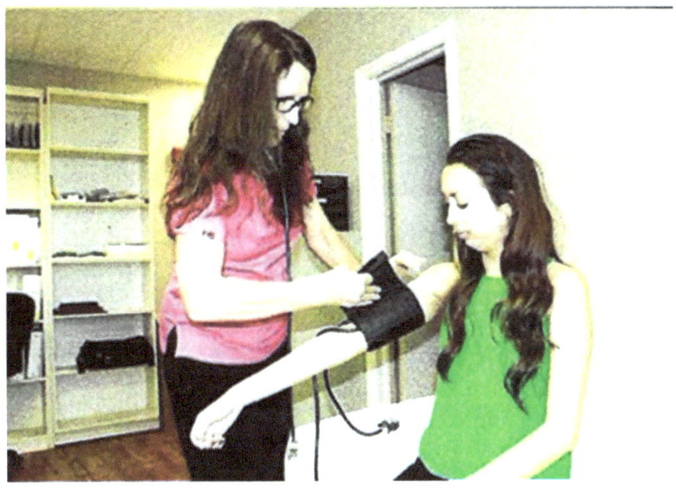

Blood pressure check at Clinical Research office.

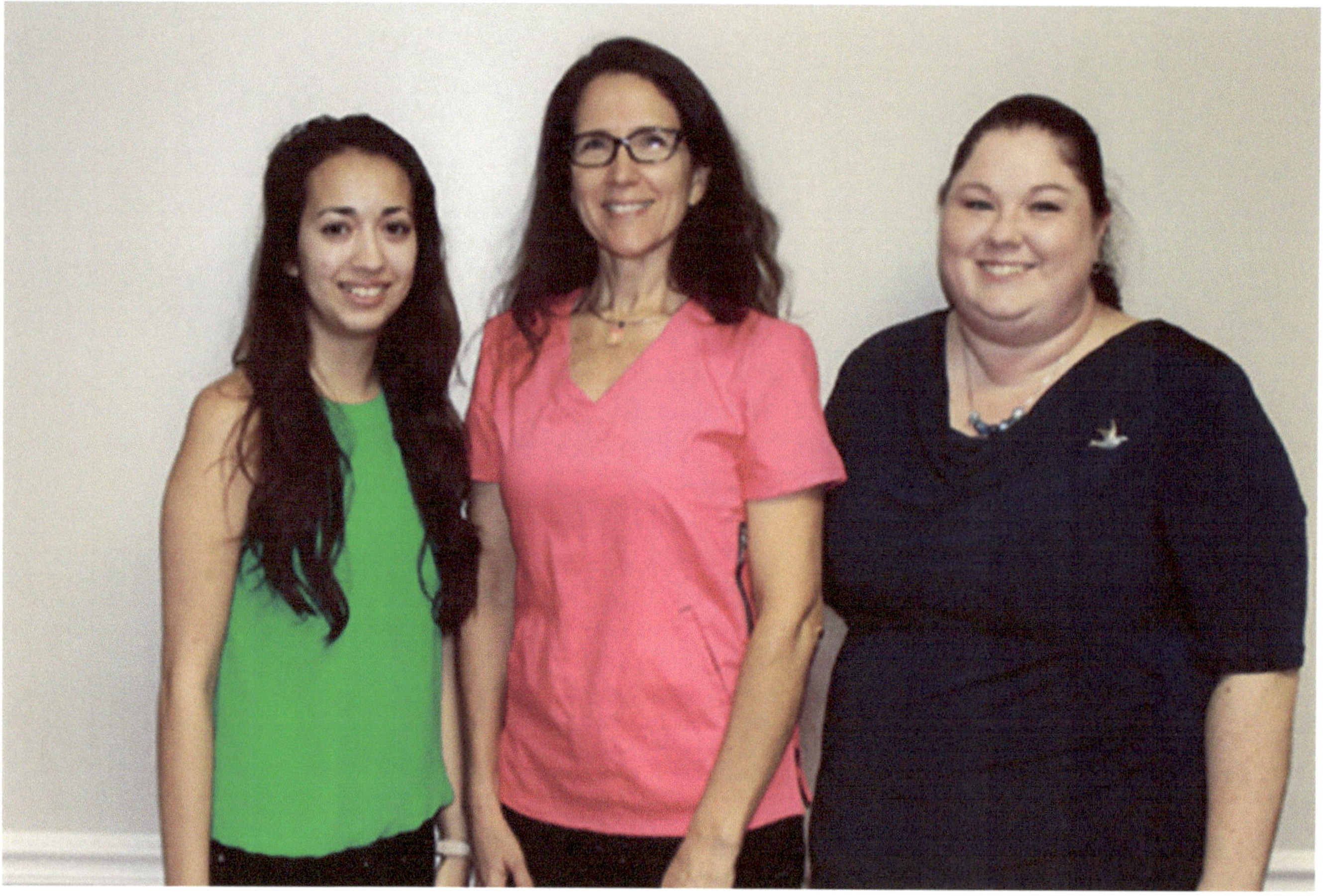

Left to right: Tiffani Kaage, Clinical Research Coordinator; Michelle Twitmyer, Clinical Research Coordinator; Catherine Renee Smith, Clinical Research Administrator, 2016.

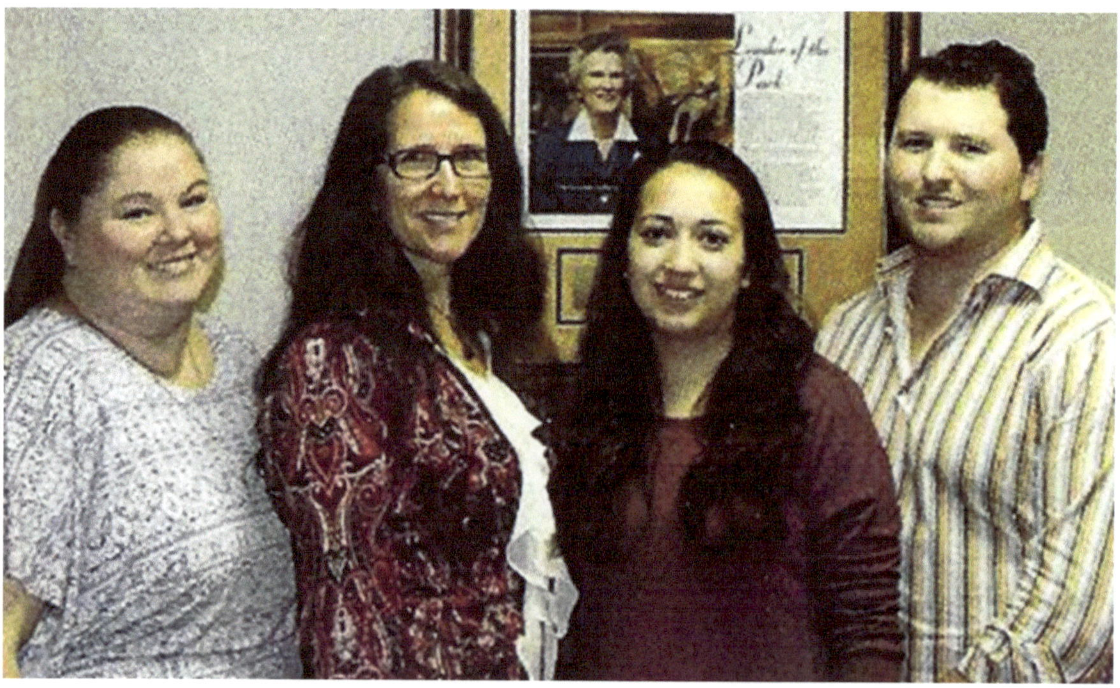

Left to right: Catherine Renee Smith, Clinical Research Administrator; Michelle Twitmyer, Clinical Research Coordinator; Tiffani Kaage, Clinical Research Coordinator; Matt Baker, Clinical Research Coordinator, 2018.

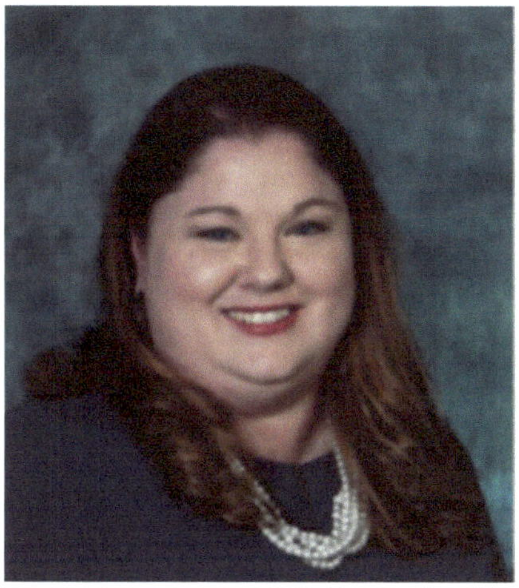

Catherine Renee Smith, CMA, CCRC Clinical Research Administrator, 2019.

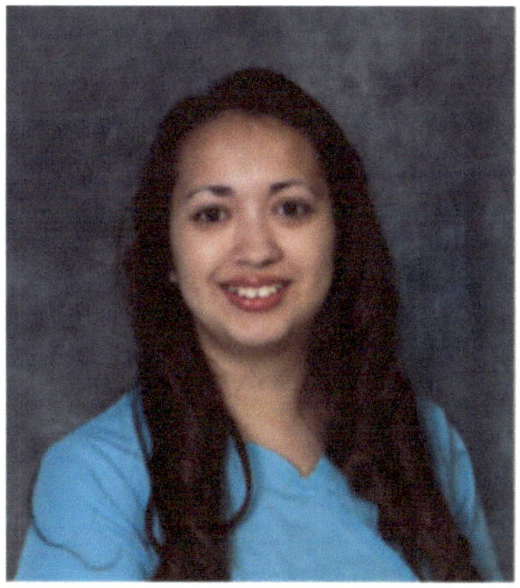

Tiffani Kaage, BS, CCRC, Clinical Research Coordinator, 2019.

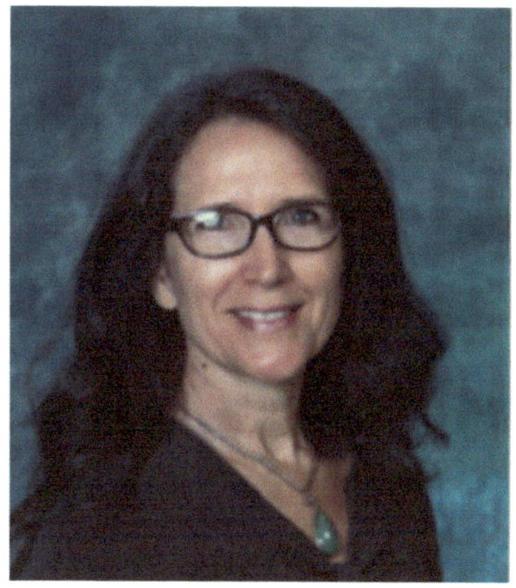

Michelle Twitmyer, BS, CCRC, Clinical Research Coordinator, 2019.

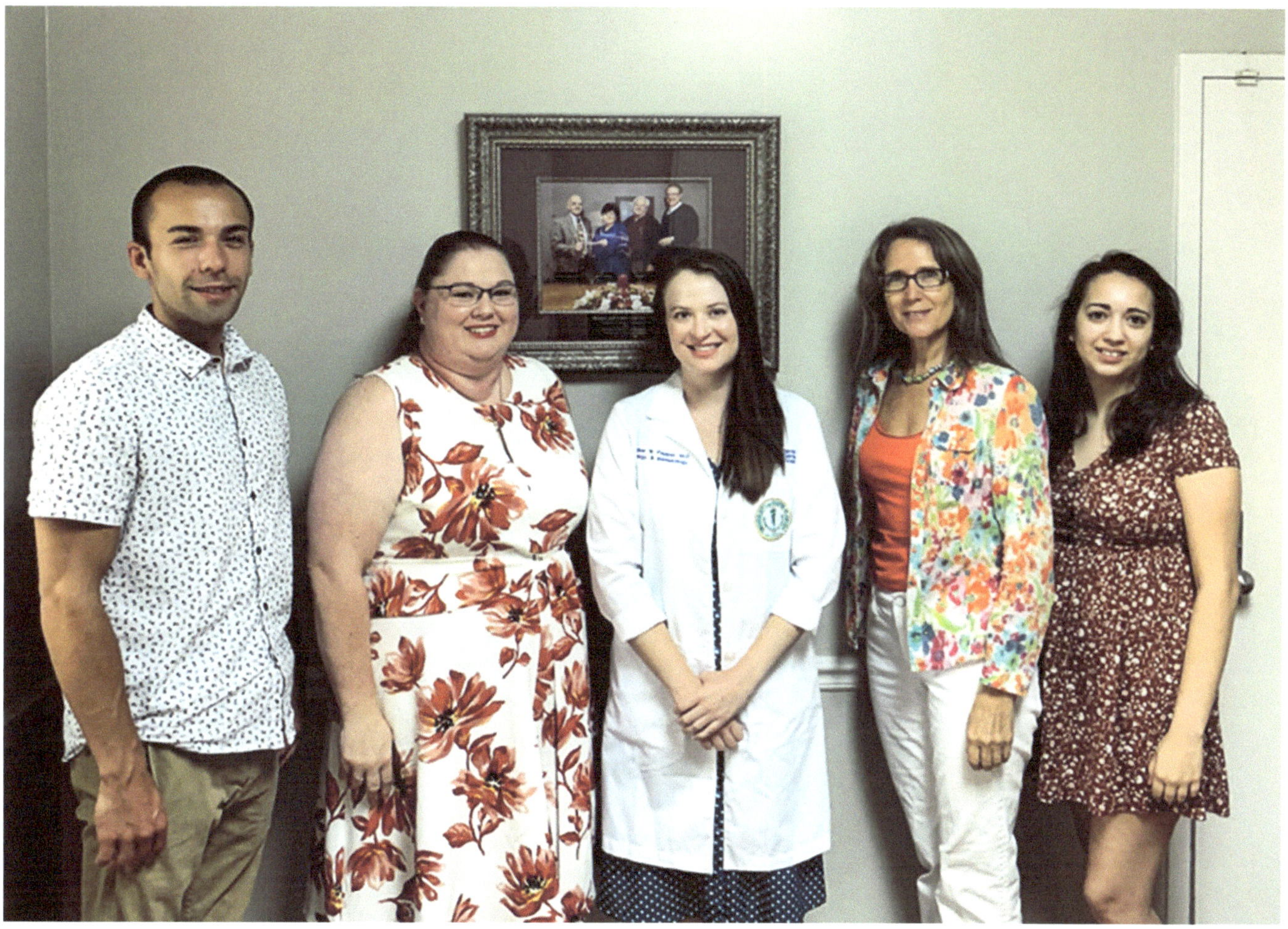

Left to right: Ray Heromin, Lab Technician; Catherine (Renee) Smith, Clinical Research Administrator; Amber Pepper, MD, Assistant Director, Clinical Research Unit; Michelle Twitmyer, Clinical Research Coordinator; Tiffani Kaage, Clinical Research Coordinator, 2020.

Chapter 10: International Visitors

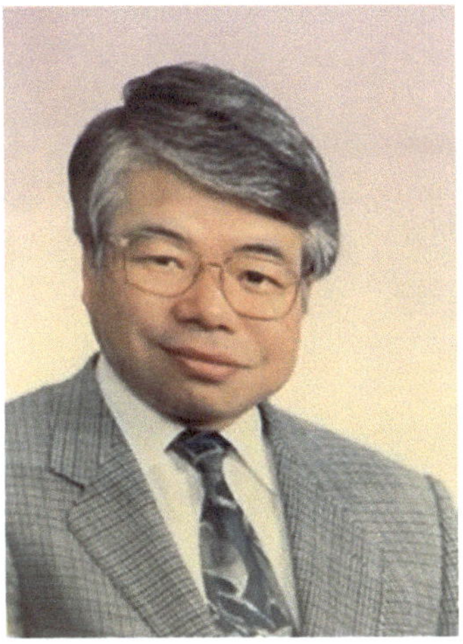

Sadahiro Asai, MD (Exchange Visitor, 1979-1981)

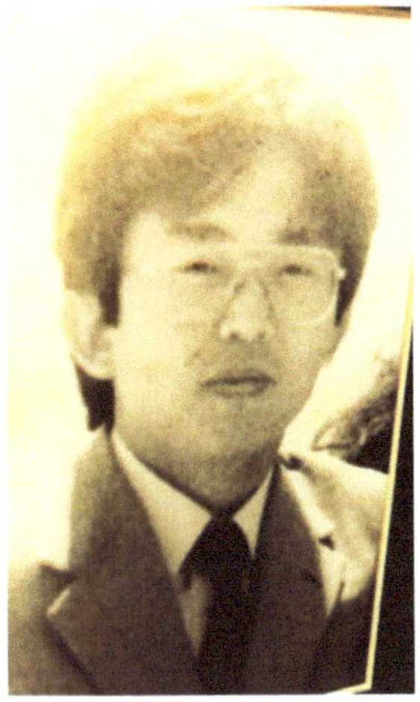

Yuji Sakamoto, MD (Exchange Visitor, 1982-1984)

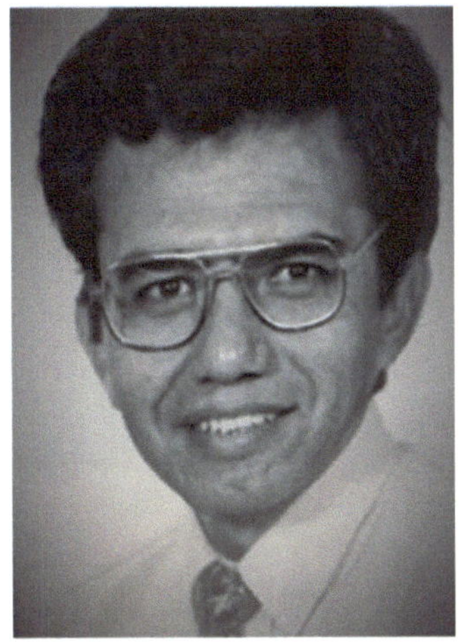

Eduardo G. Calderon, MD (Exchange Visitor, 1988-1993)

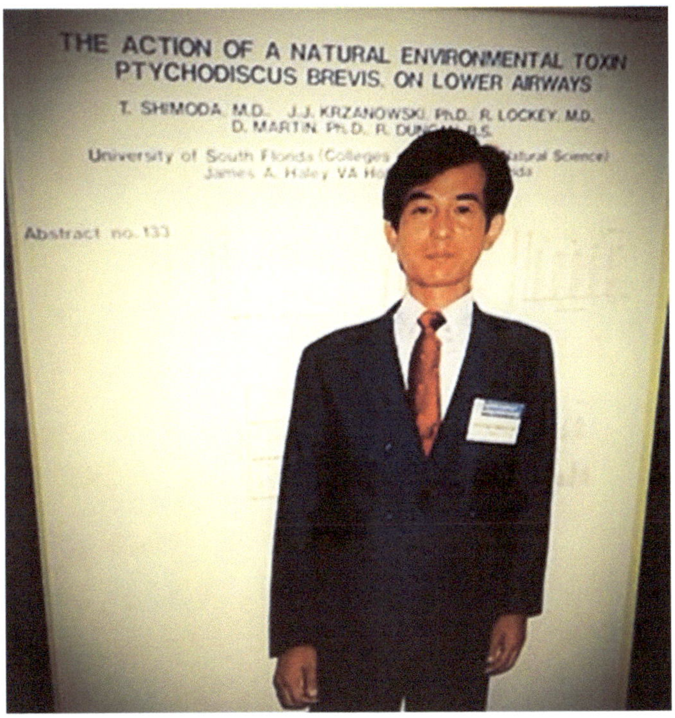

Terufumi Shimoda, MD (Visiting Research Scholar, 1986-1987). Poster: "The Action of a Natural Environmental Toxin, Ptychodiscus brevis on Lower Airways". 1986 American Academy of Allergy & Immunology Annual Meeting.

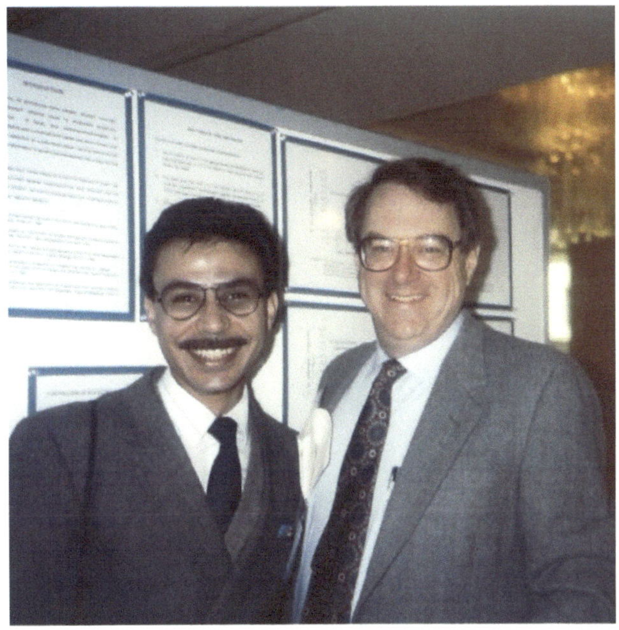

Left to right: Mohammed Askar, MD (Visiting Research Scholar, February 1990 – February 1992) and Richard F. Lockey, MD, MS.

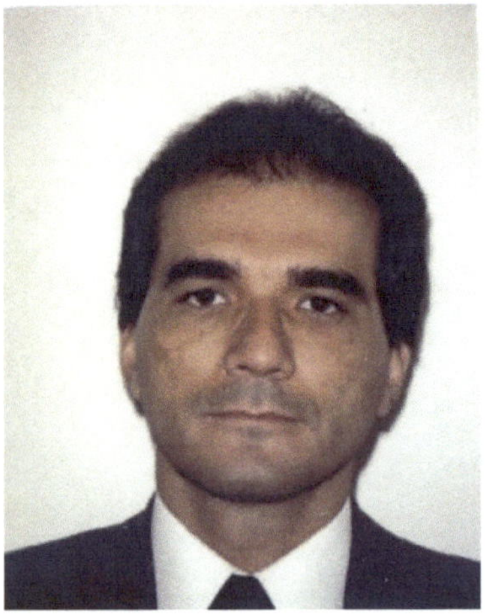

Gustavo Cuadros-Trillos, MB (Exchange Visitor, September 1988 – December 1988 and November 1990 – December 1990).

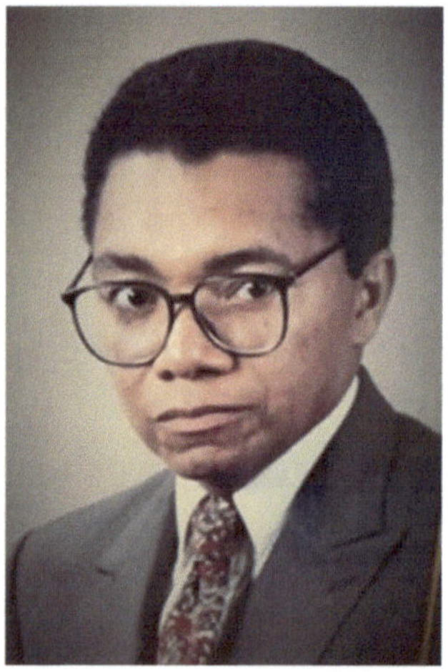

Leonardo Puerta, PhD (Exchange Visitor, 1991; 1993-1995 PhD candidate, University of Cartagena).

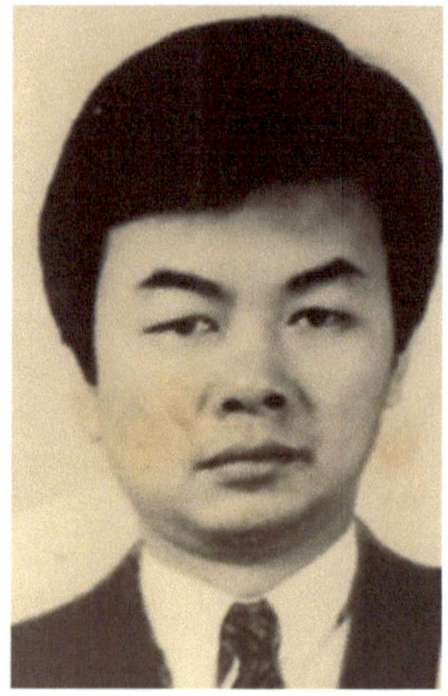

Dong-Keun Lee, MD (Exchange Visitor, 1991-1992).

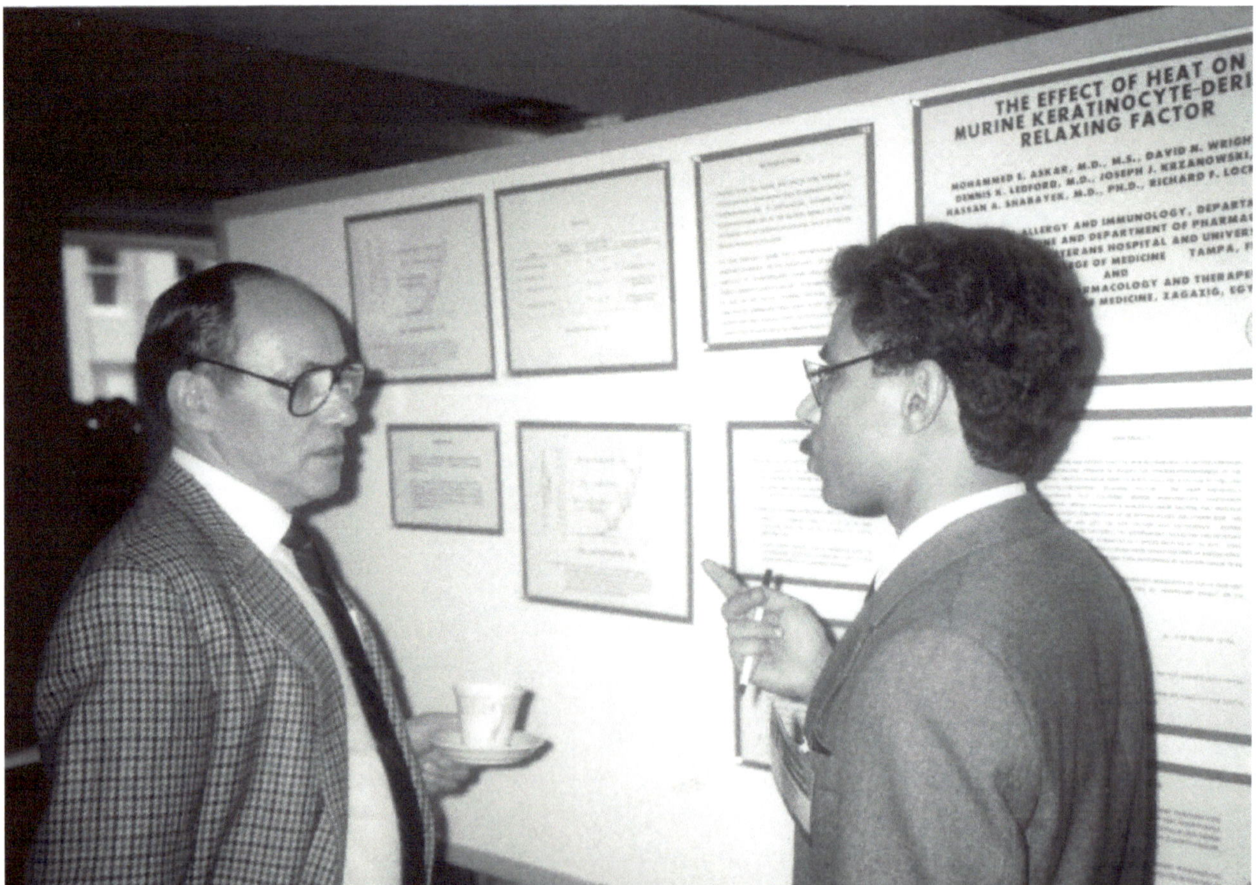

Left to right: Burt Zweiman, MD and Mohammed Askar, MD (Visiting Research Scholar, February 1990 – February 1992). Poster: "The Effect of Heat on Murine Keratinocyte-Derived Relaxing Factor"; 1991 American Academy of Allergy & Immunology Annual Meeting.

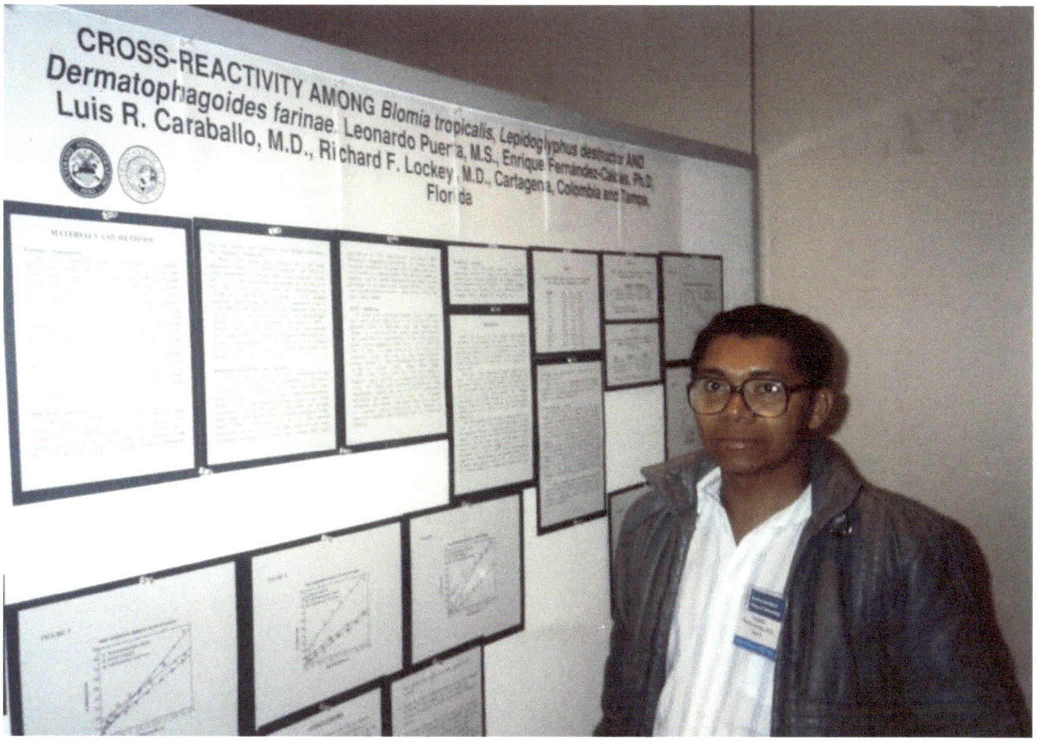

Leonardo Puerta, MS (Exchange Visitor, 1991; 1993 – 1995 PhD candidate, University of Cartagena). Poster: "Cross-Reactivity Among Blomia tropicalis, Lepidoglyphus destructor and Dermatophagoides farina", 1991. American Academy of Allergy & Immunology Annual Meeting.

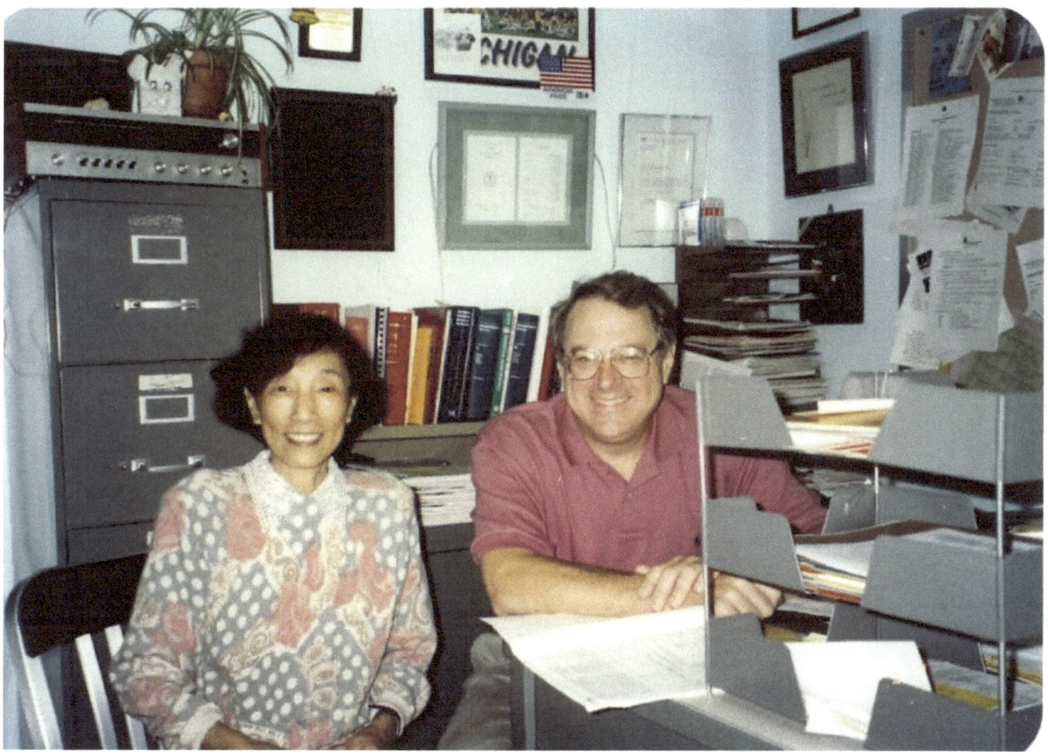

Left to right: Zhaoming Wen, MD (Visiting Research Scholar, August 1994 – November 1994) and Richard F. Lockey MD.

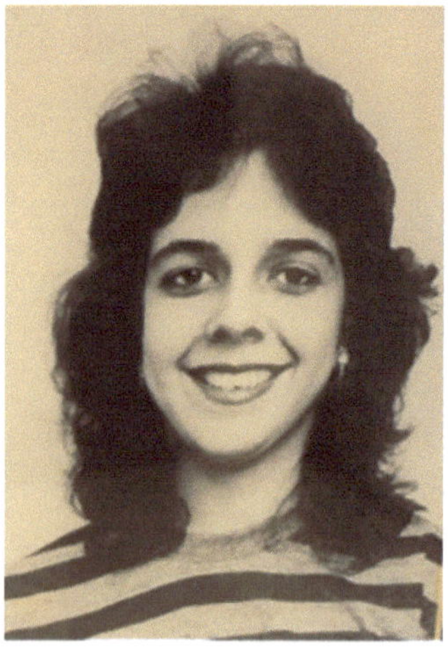

Ingrid P. Cunha M. De Souza Lima, MD (Exchange Visitor, January 1993 – March 1993).

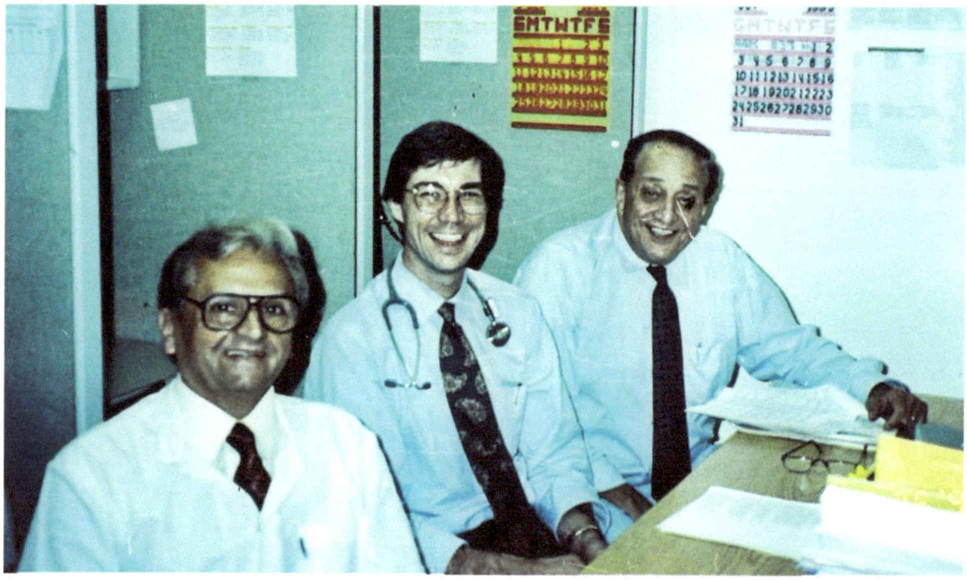

Left to right: Sagrado Lamir David, MD (Visiting Research Scholar, 1993); Robert P. Nelson, MD (1985-1987); Robert A. Good, MD, PhD, DSc.

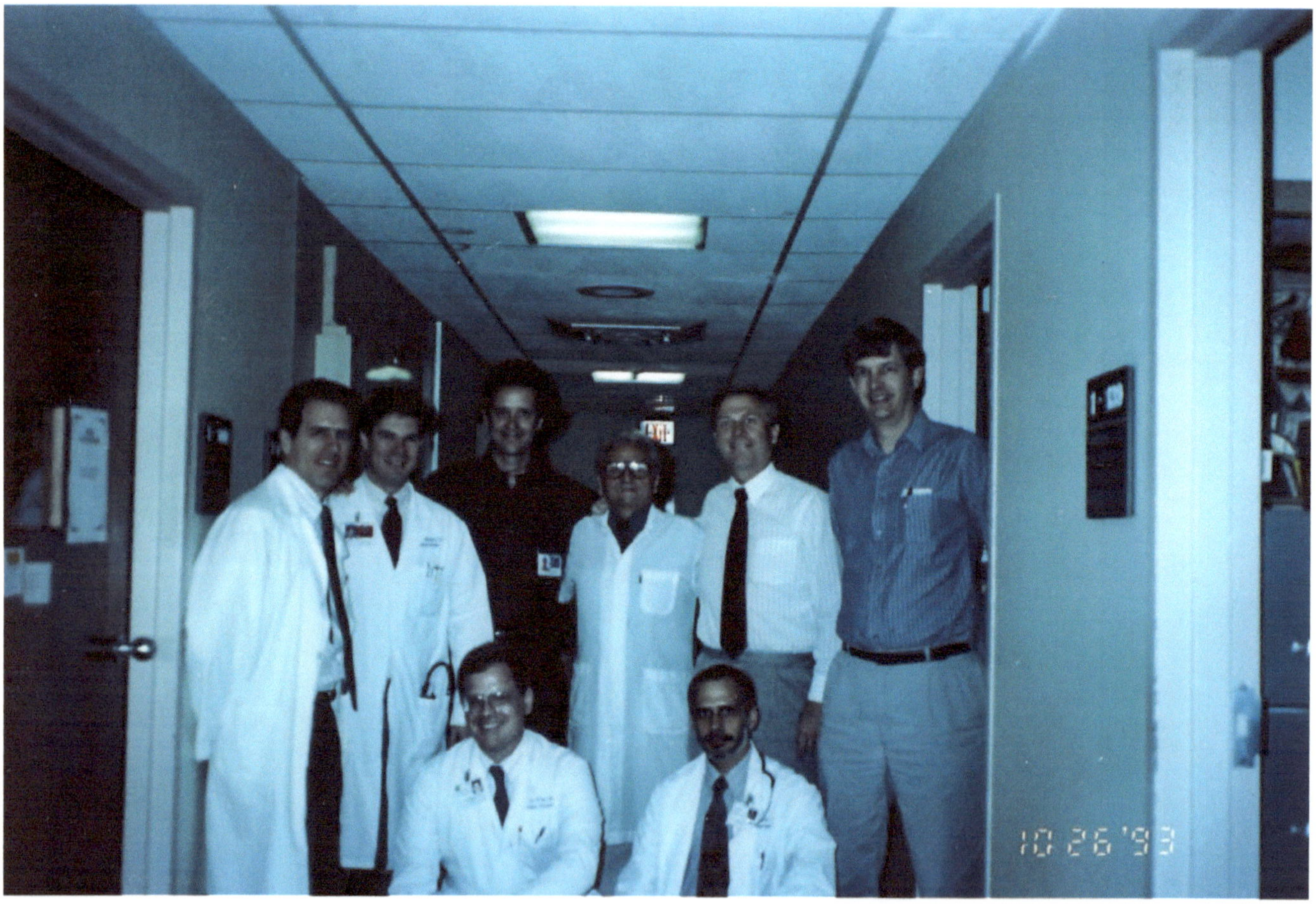

Front row (left to right): Stephen F. Kemp, MD (1993-1996); Jose Andrade, MD (1992-1995). Back row (left to right): Hugh H. Windom, MD; Brett E. Stanaland, MD (1992-1995); Enrique Fernandez-Caldas, PhD; Sagrado Lamir David, MD (Visiting Research Scholar, 1993); Roger W. Fox, MD; G. Edward Stewart, MD (1991-1994).

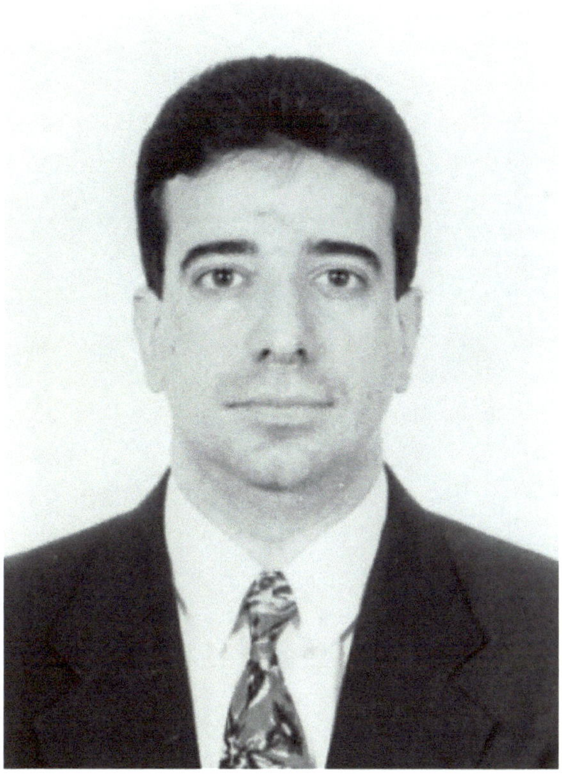

Eduardo Malgalhaes De Souza Lima, MD (Exchange Visitor, January 1993 – March 1993).

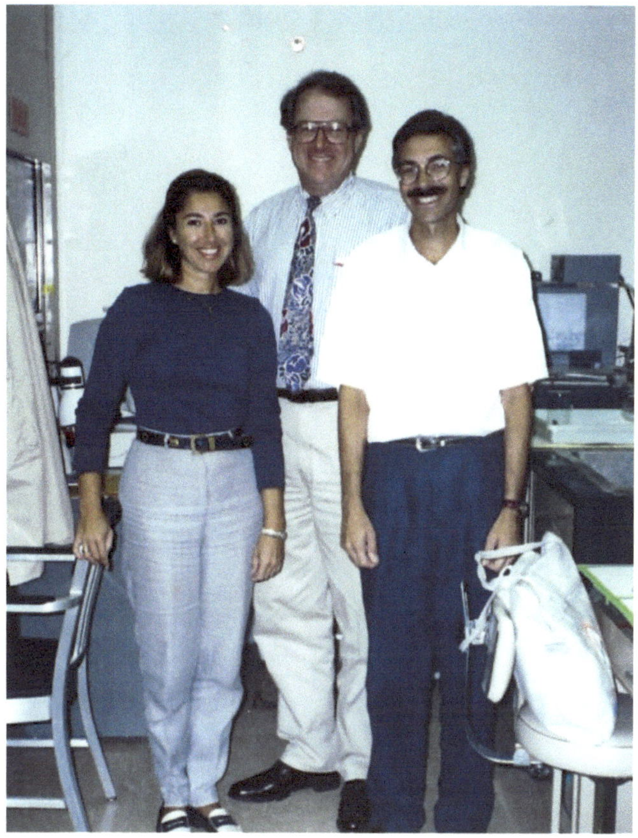

Left to right: Mrs. Albert G. Oehling; Richard F. Lockey, MD, MS; Dr. Albert G. Oehling Jr. (Visiting Research Scholar, 1996).

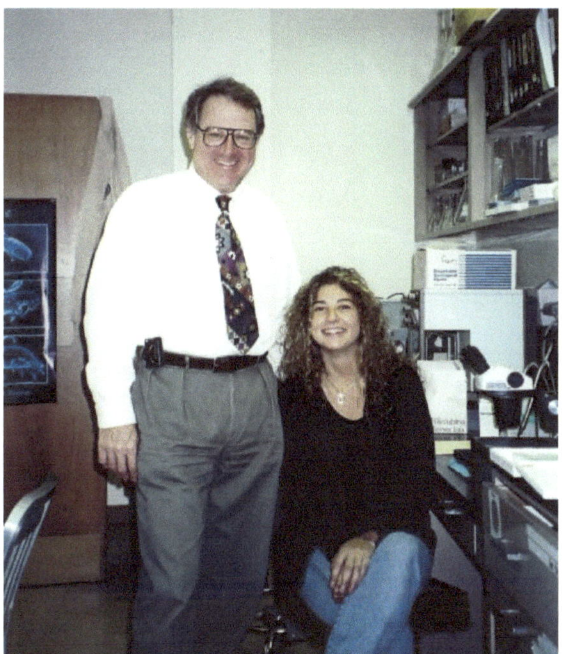

Left to right: Richard F. Lockey, MD, MS and Carina Gabriela Uasuf, MD (Visiting Research Scholar, February 1995 – April 1995).

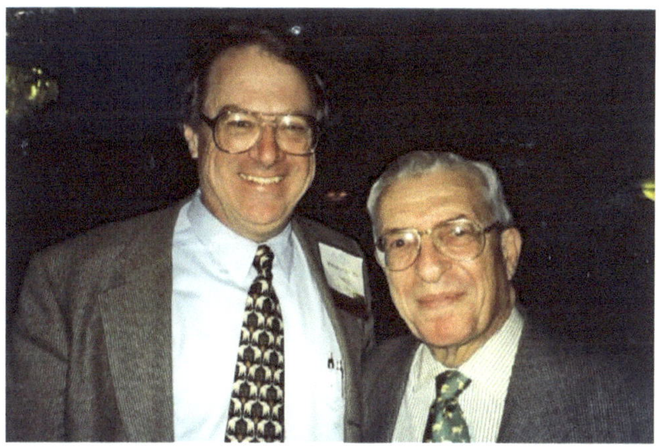

Left to right: Richard F. Lockey and MD; Albert K. Oehling, MD; 1997.

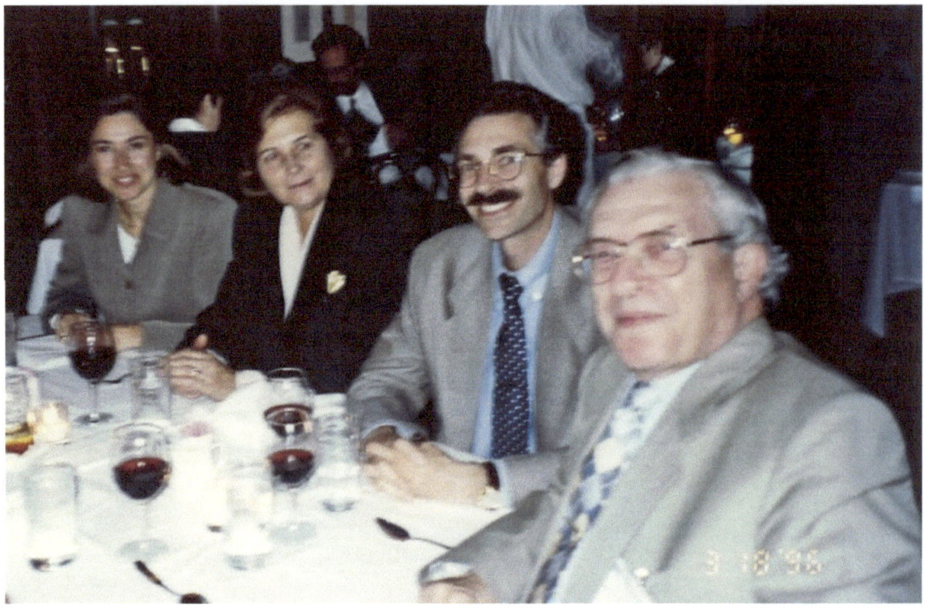

Left to right: Mrs. Albert G. Oehling; Mrs. Albert K. Oehling; Albert G. Oehling Jr., MD (Visiting Research Scholar, 1996); Albert K. Oehling, MD; 1997.

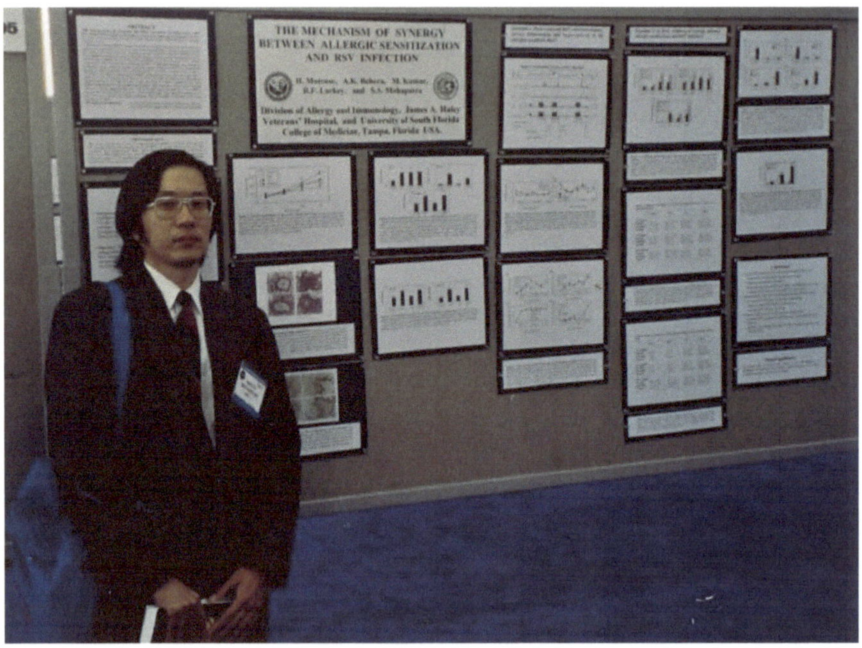

Hiroto Matsuse, MD (Exchange Visitor, May, 1997 – May, 1999). Poster: "The Mechanism of Synergy Between Allergic Sensitization and RSV Infection"; 1999 American Thoracic Society International Conference.

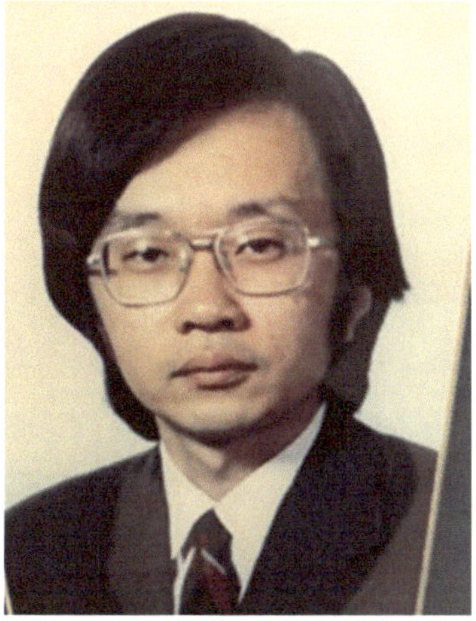

Hiroto Matsuse, MD (Exchange Visitor, May 1997 – May 1999)

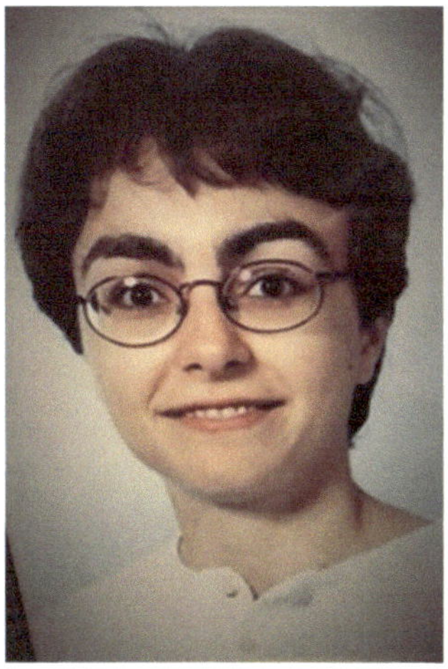

Cristina Jaen, BS (Exchange Visitor, 1998 - 1999)

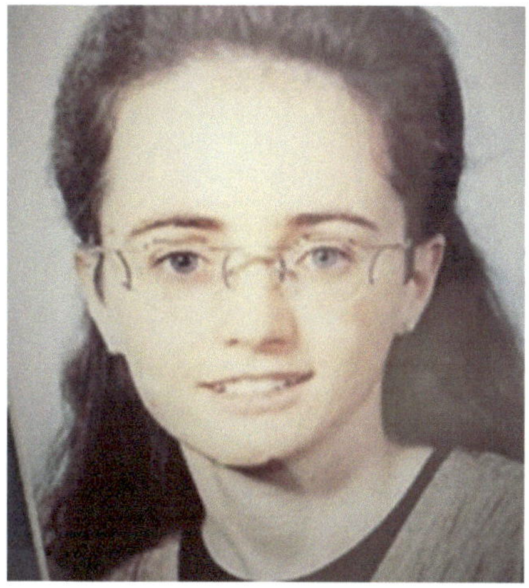

Nicole N. Kuderer (Exchange Visitor, 1998 – 2000)

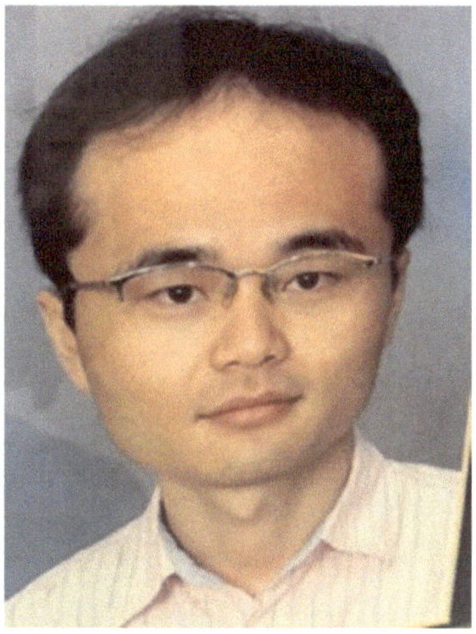

Dong-Won Lee, PhD (Exchange Visitor, 2004 – 2006)

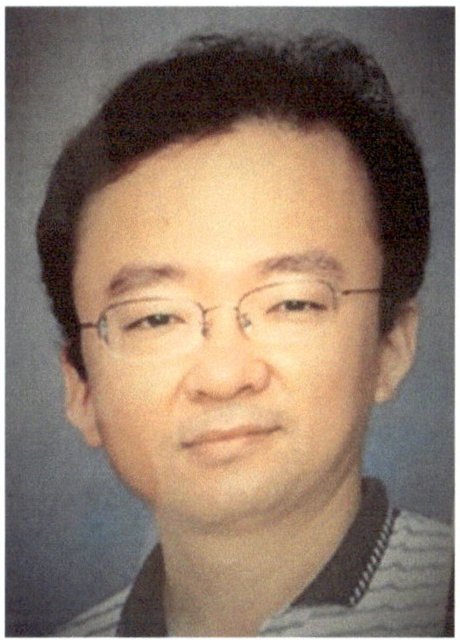

Sang-Joon Park, PhD (Visiting Research Scholar, 2006 – 2008)

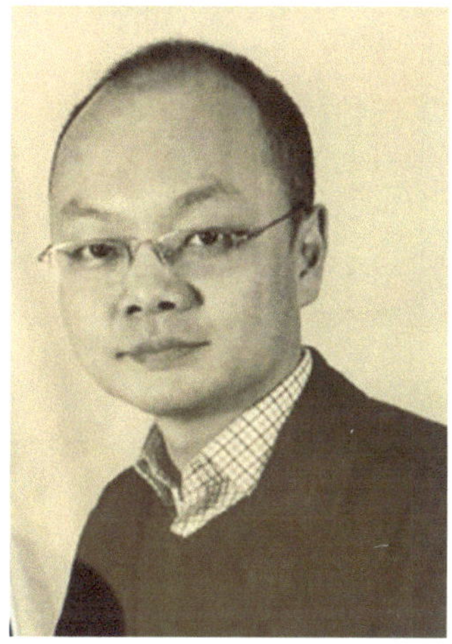

Jianjun Chen, MD (Visiting Research Scholar, 2015-2016)

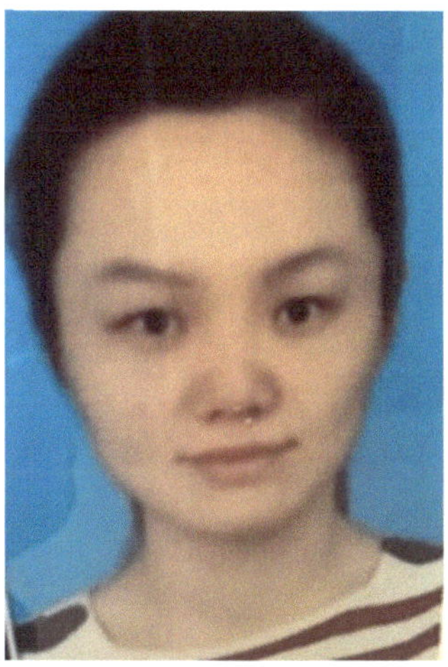

Wenjing Li, MD (Exchange Visitor, 2016 – 2017)

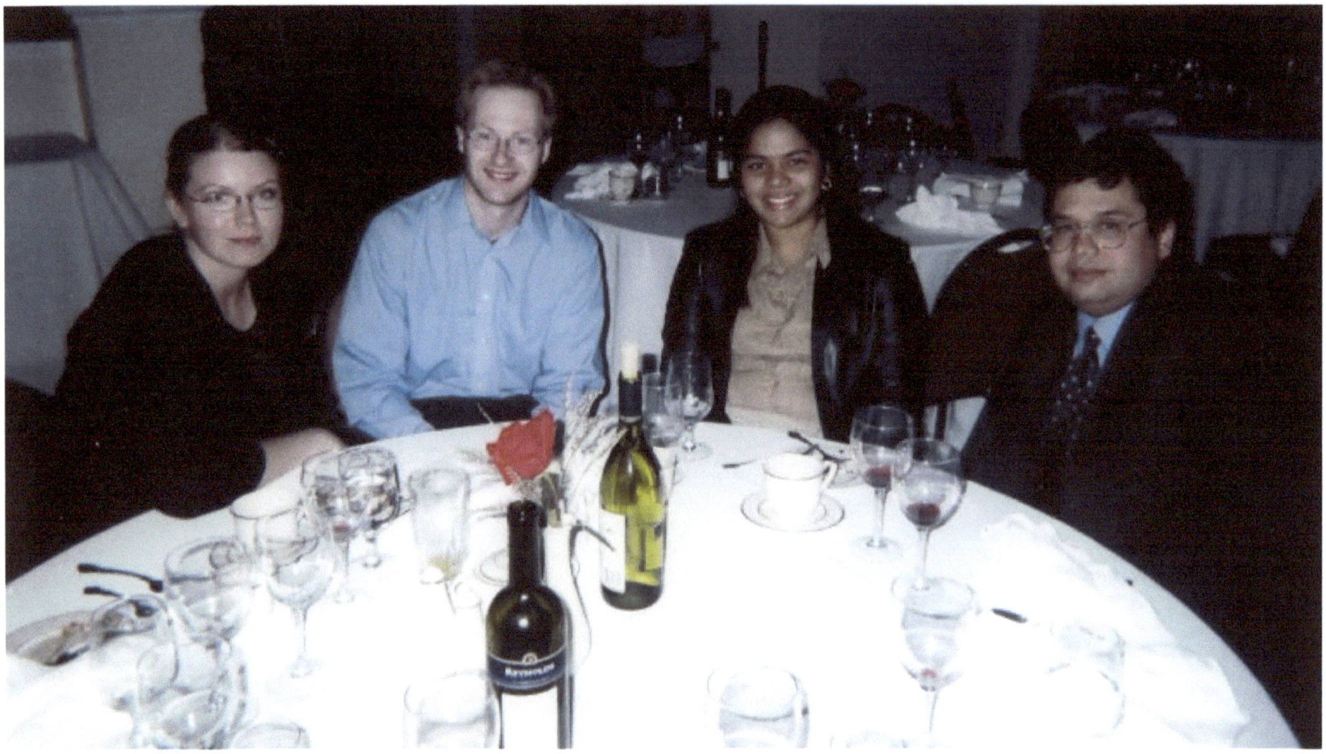

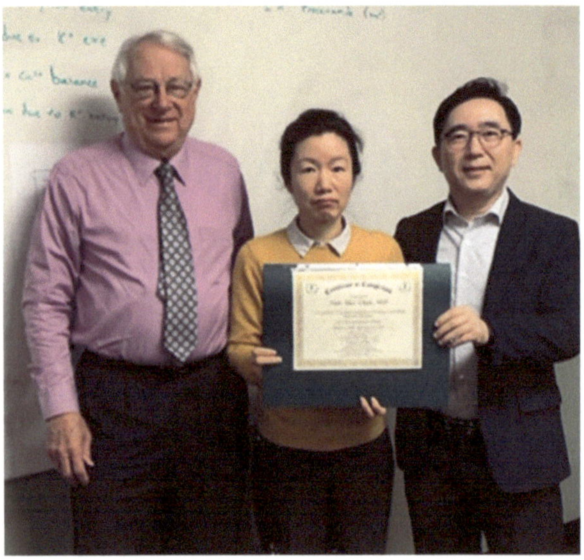

Above, left to right: guests; Dr. and Mrs. Homero San Juan (Visiting Research Scholar, August 1999 – August 2004).

Left, left to right: Richard F. Lockey, MD, MS; Sun-Hee Choi, MD, PhD (Visiting Research Scholar, March 2019 – February 2020); Seong

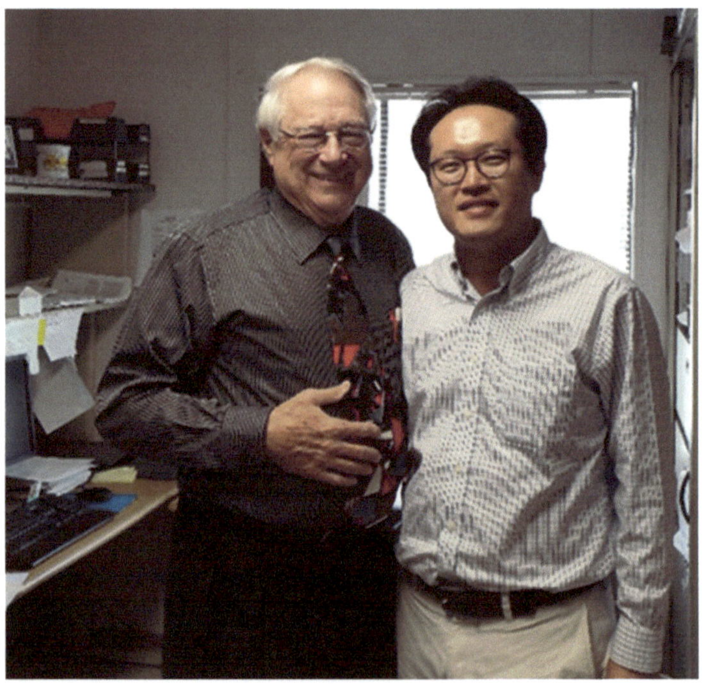

Left to right: Richard F. Lockey, MD, MS; Sun-Hee Choi, MD, PhD (Visiting Research Scholar, March 2019 – February 2020); Seong Cho, MD.

Chapter 11: USF Research Personnel

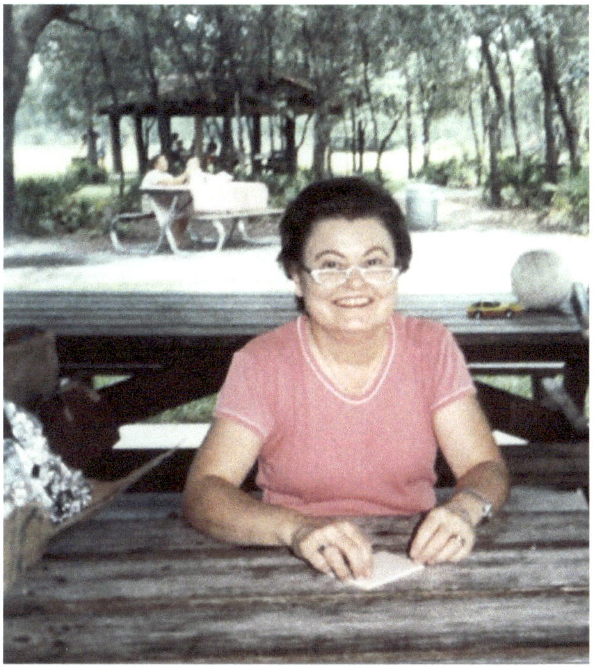

Lolita R. F. Binford, circa 1980.

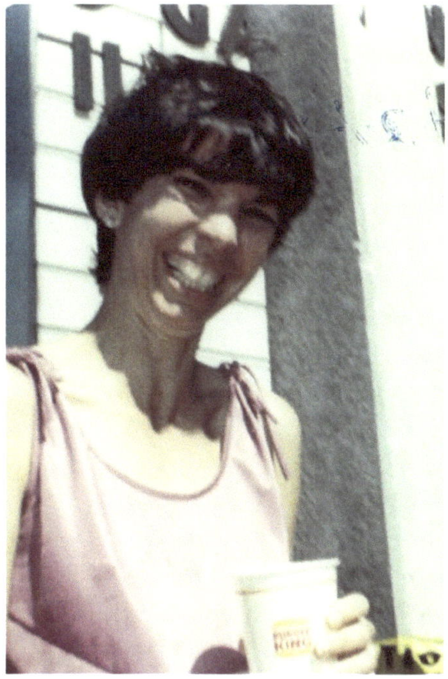

Debbie Serbousek; circa 1985.

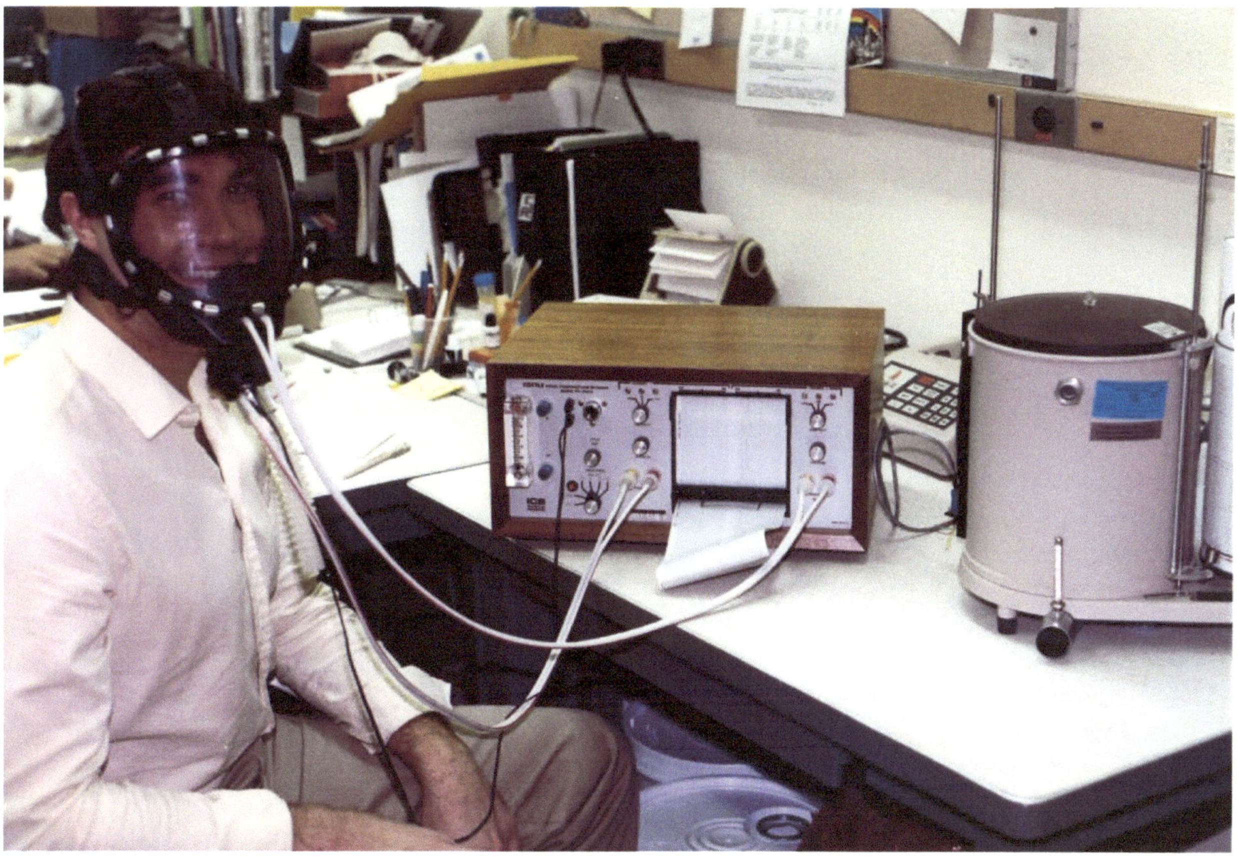

Robert P. Nelson, MD (1985-1987); circa 1987.

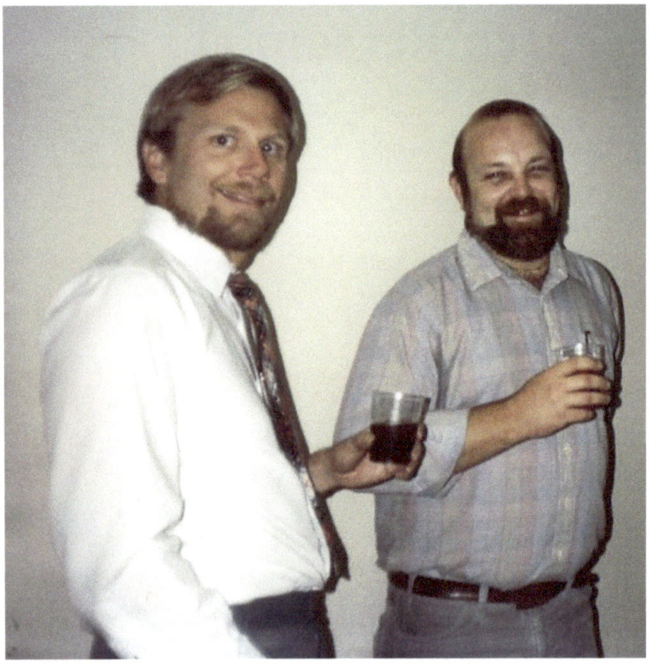

Left to right: Roger W. Fox, MD and Walter L. Trudeau III, MS; circa 1990.

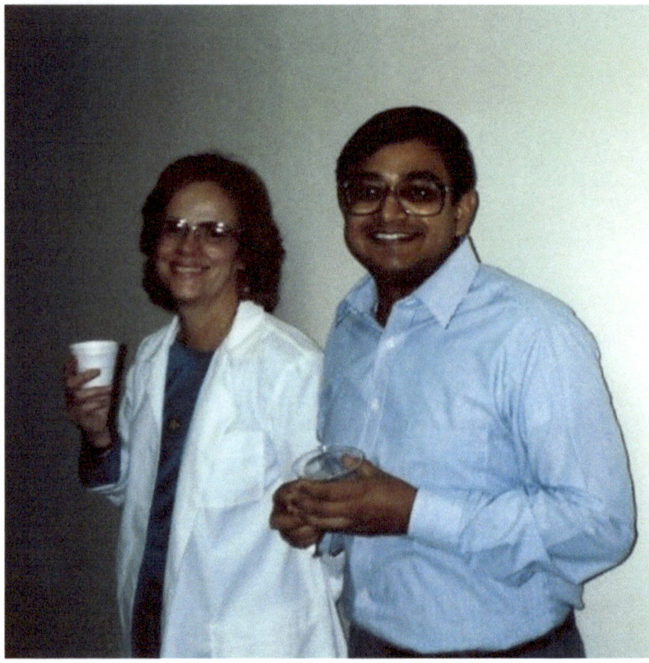

Left to right: Irene Baird-Warren and Donnie Banerji, MD; circa 1985.

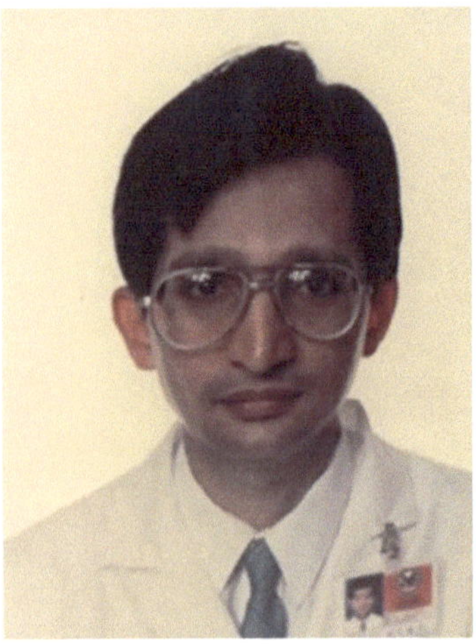

Khalid Ali, MD
1991-1992

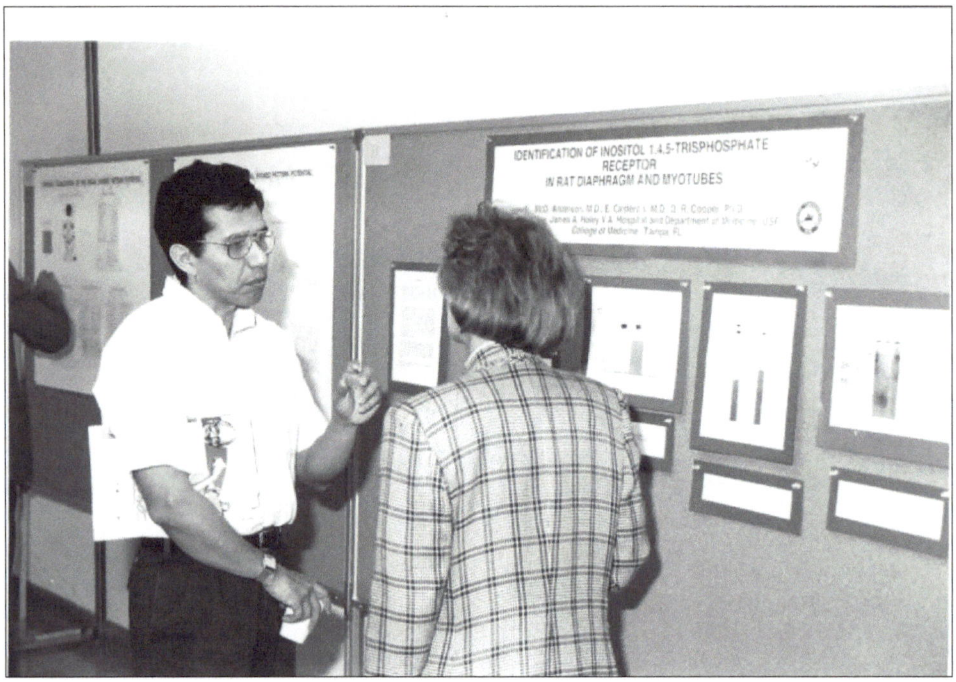

Left to right: Eduardo Calderon, MD (1988-1993) and Denise Cooper, PhD (Endocrinology); VA Research Day, circa 1990.

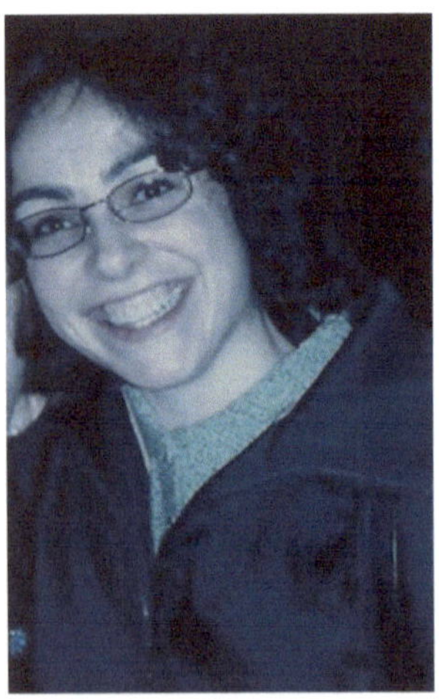

Cristina Jaen, MS,
circa 1999.

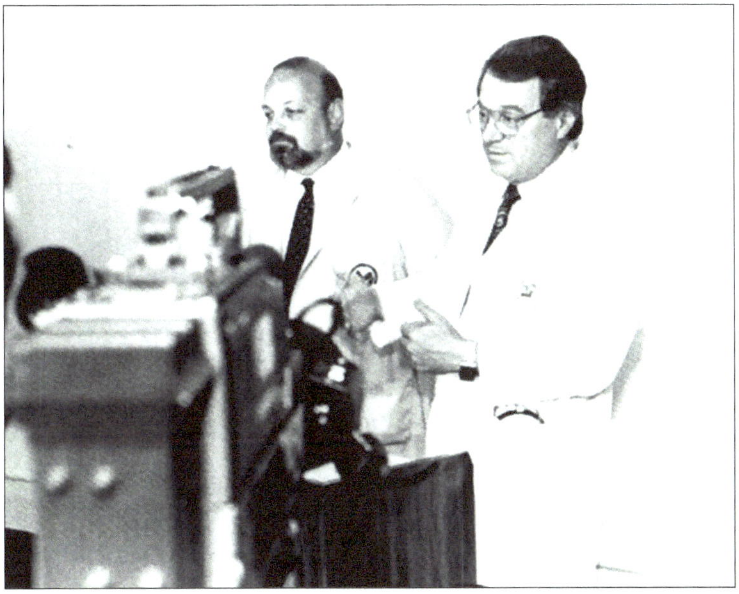

Left to right: Walter L. Trudeau III, MS and Richard F. Lockey, MD, MS speaking to the press, 1993.

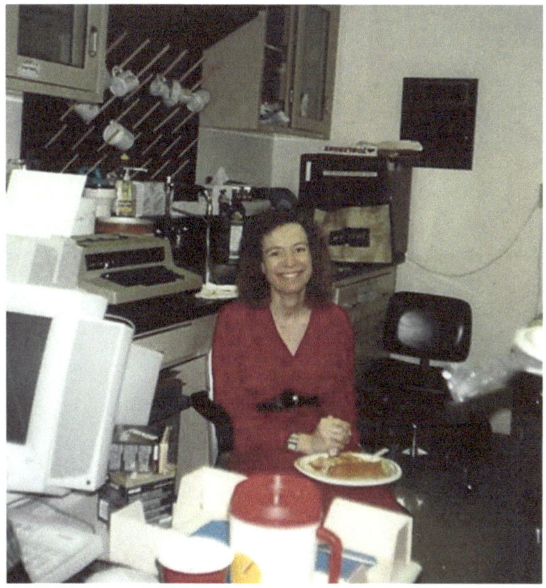

Linda Bergen-Losee, MS; circa 1996.

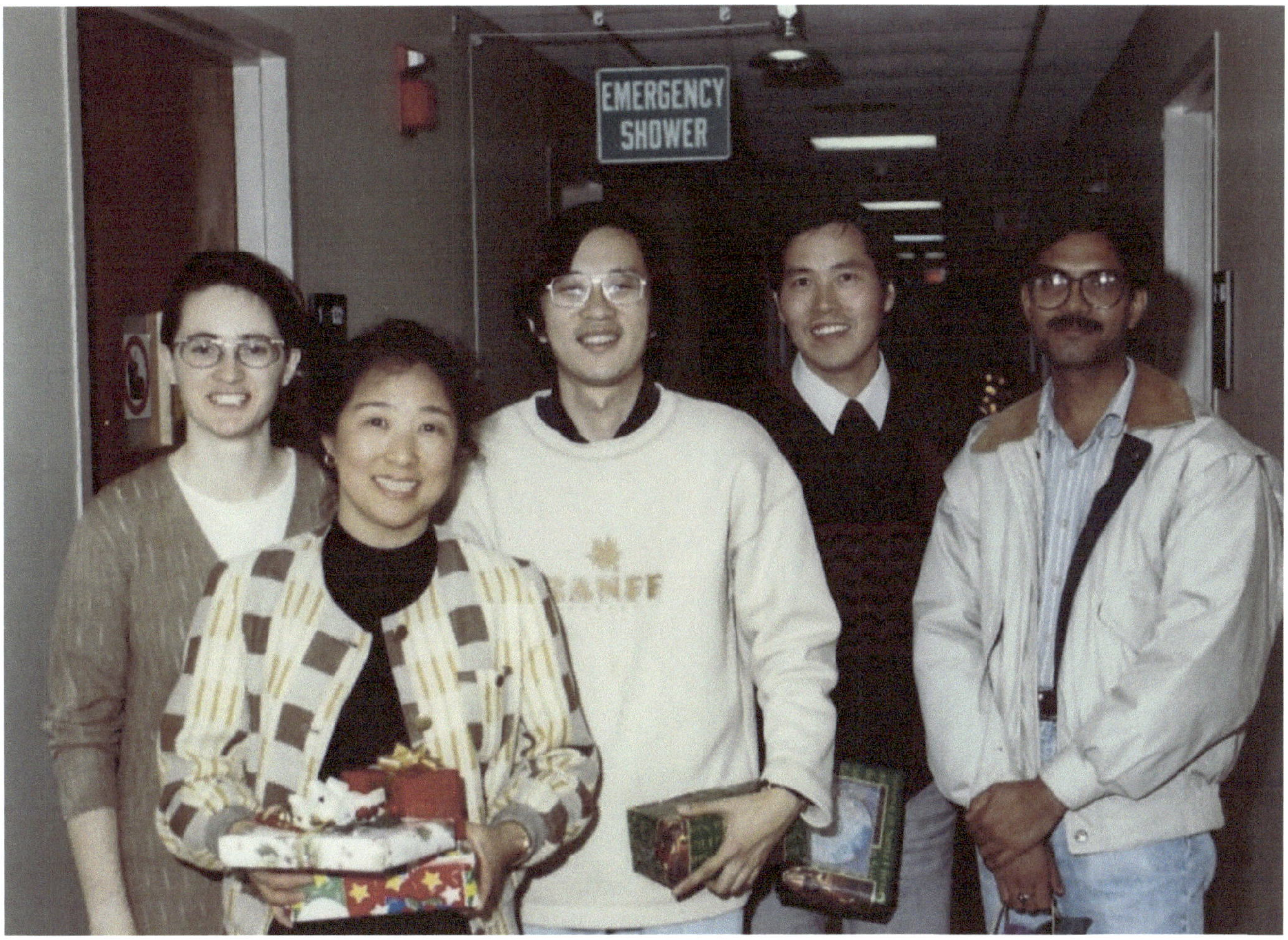

Left to right: Nicole Kuderer; Xiaoyuan (Sonya) Kong, MD; Hiroto Matsuse, MD; Jianan Hu, MD; Mukesh Kumar, PhD; circa 1999.

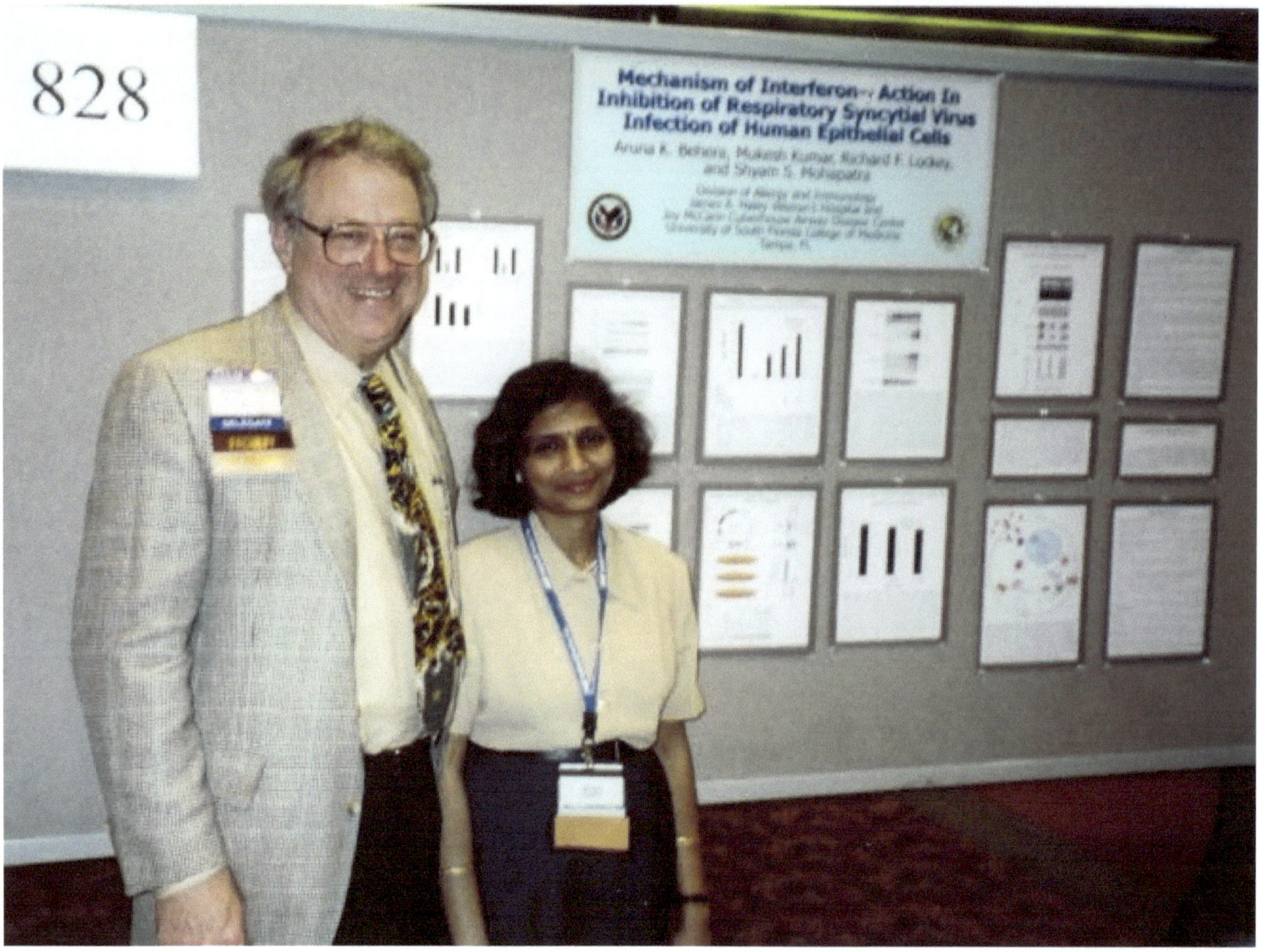

Left to right: Richard F. Lockey, MD, MS and Aruna Behera, PhD. Poster: "Mechanisms of Interferon-y Action in Inhibition of Respiratory Syncytial Virus Infection of Human Epithelial Cells". American Academy of Allergy Asthma and Immunology 56th Annual Meeting, San Diego, California, March 3 – March 8, 2000.

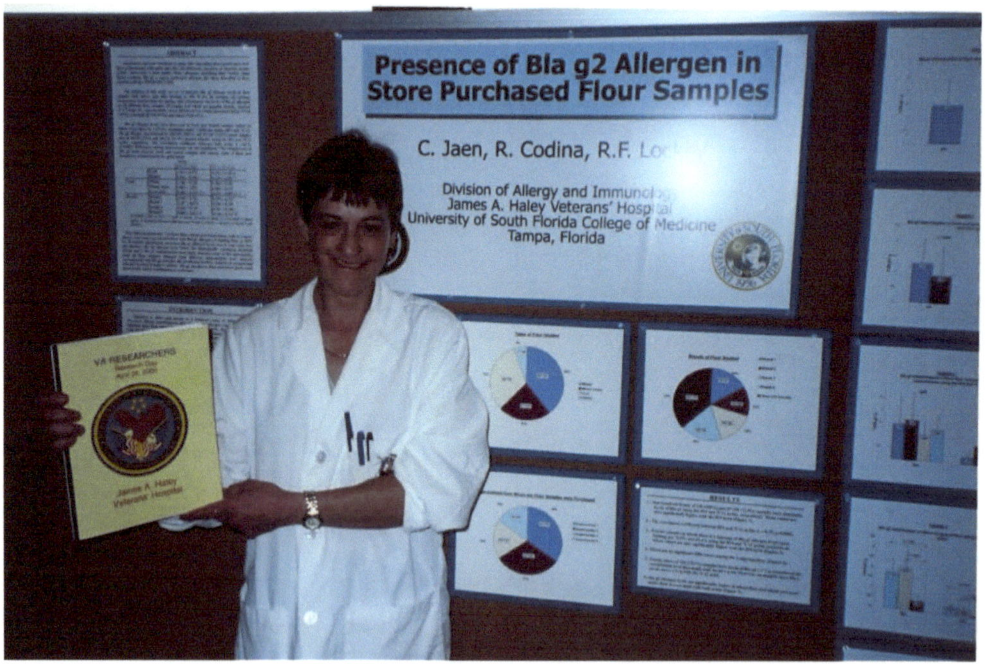

Rosa Codina, PhD; VA Research Day, April 2000.

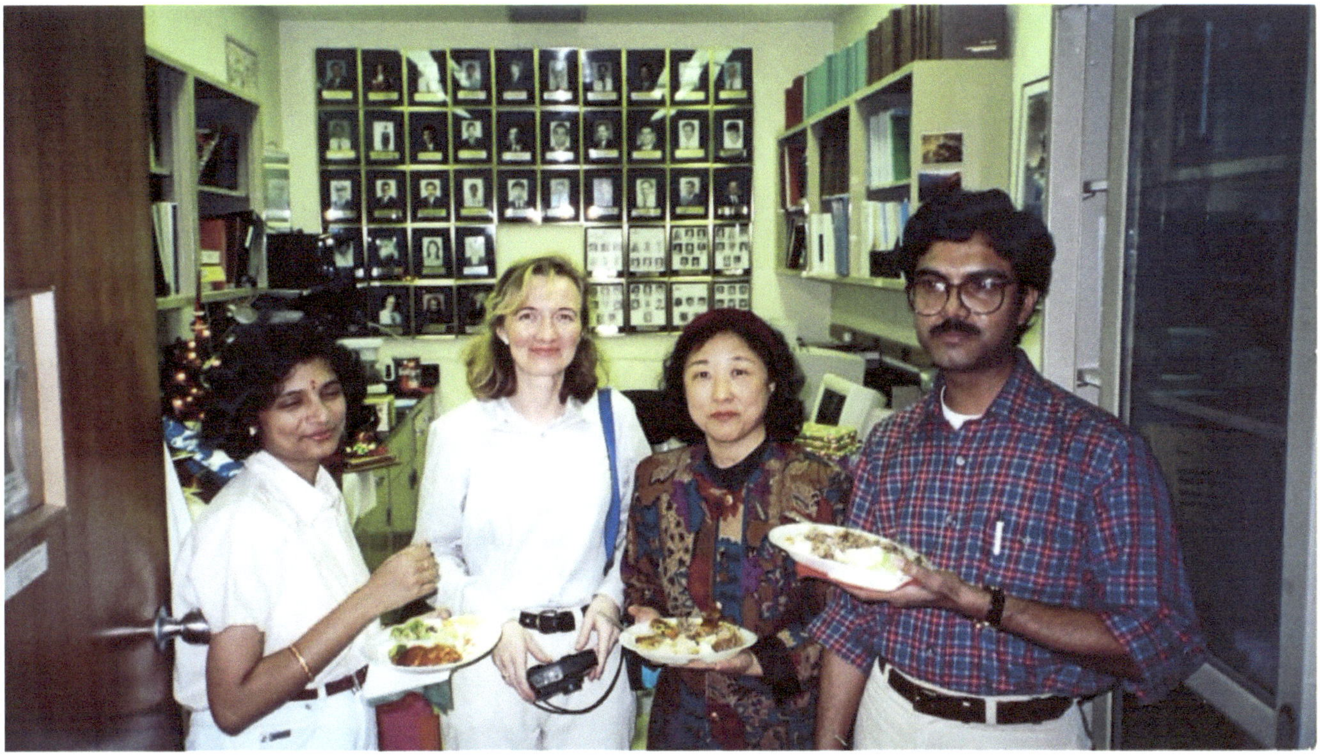

Left to right: Aruna Behera, PhD; Szilvia Nagy, MD, PhD; Xiaoyuan (Sonya) Kong, MD; Mukesh Kumar, PhD; (picture gallery of Division graduates in the background), circa 2000.

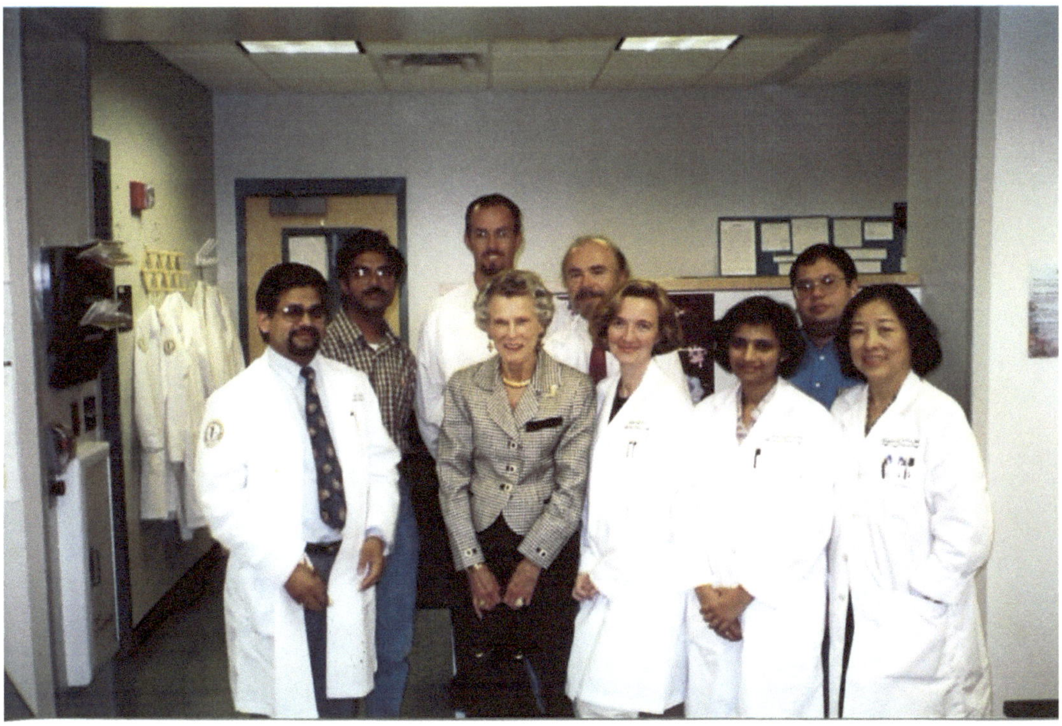

Joy McCann Culverhouse Airway Disease Research Center 2001. Front row (left to right): Shyam S. Mohapatra, PhD; Joy McCann Culverhouse; Szilvia Nagy, MD, PhD; Aruna Behera, PhD; Xiaoyuan (Sonya) Kong, MD. Back row (left to right): Mukesh Kumar, MD; Tim Randall; Gary Hellermann, PhD; Homero San Juan, MD.

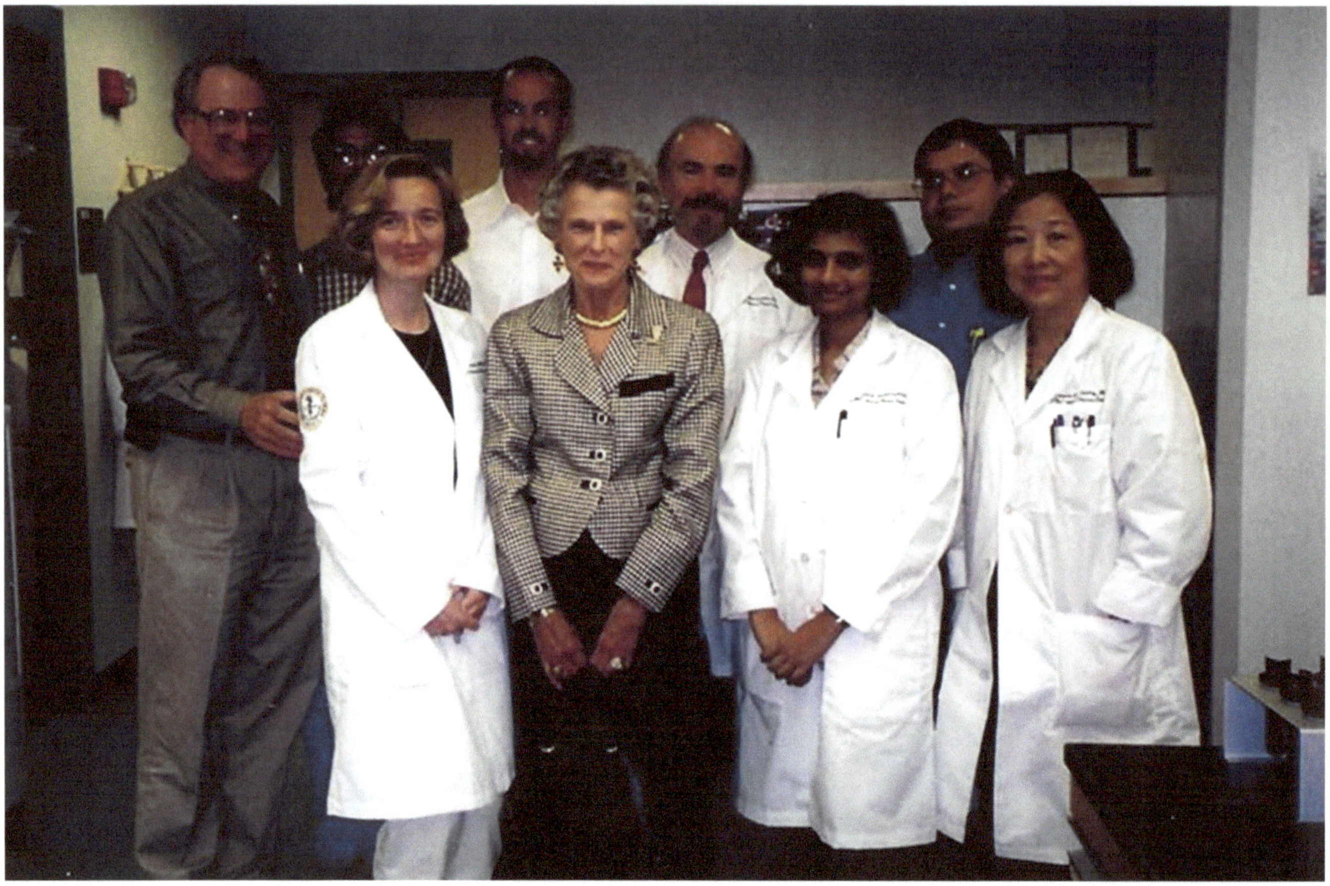

Joy McCann Culverhouse Airway Disease Research Center 2001. Front row (left to right): Szilvia Nagy, MD, PhD; Joy McCann Culverhouse; Aruna Behera, PhD; Xiaoyuan (Sonya) Kong, MD. Back row (left to right): Richard F. Lockey, MD; Mukesh Kumar, MD; Tim Randall; Gary Hellermann, PhD; Homero San Juan, MD.

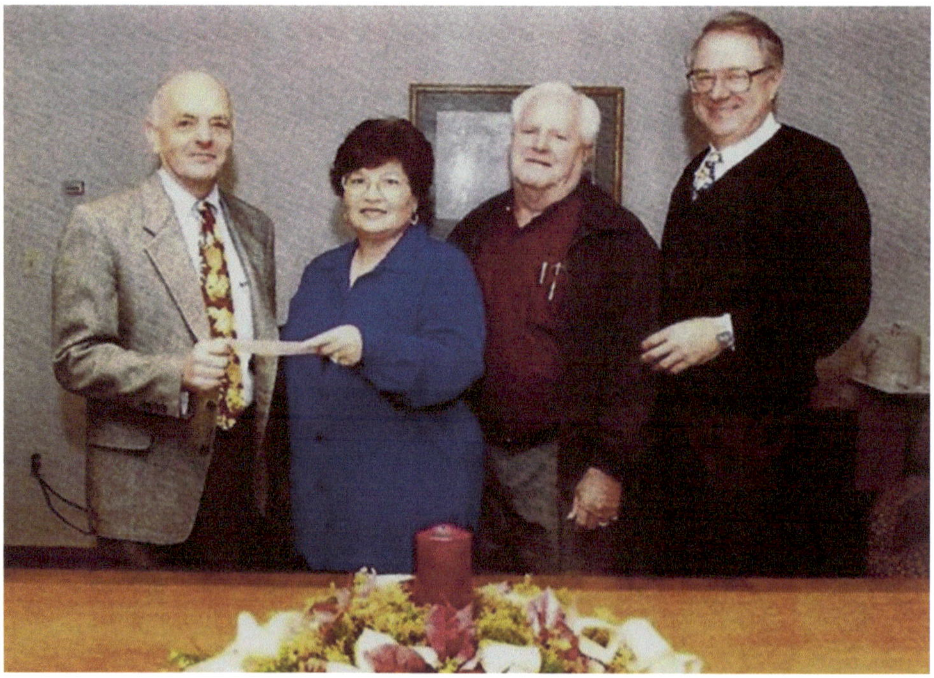

Awarding the Mabel and Ellsworth Simmons endowment to the Division of Allergy and Immunology in 2001. Left to right: Dean Martin Silbiger, MD; Sandy Simmons; George Simmons; Richard F. Lockey, MD, MS.

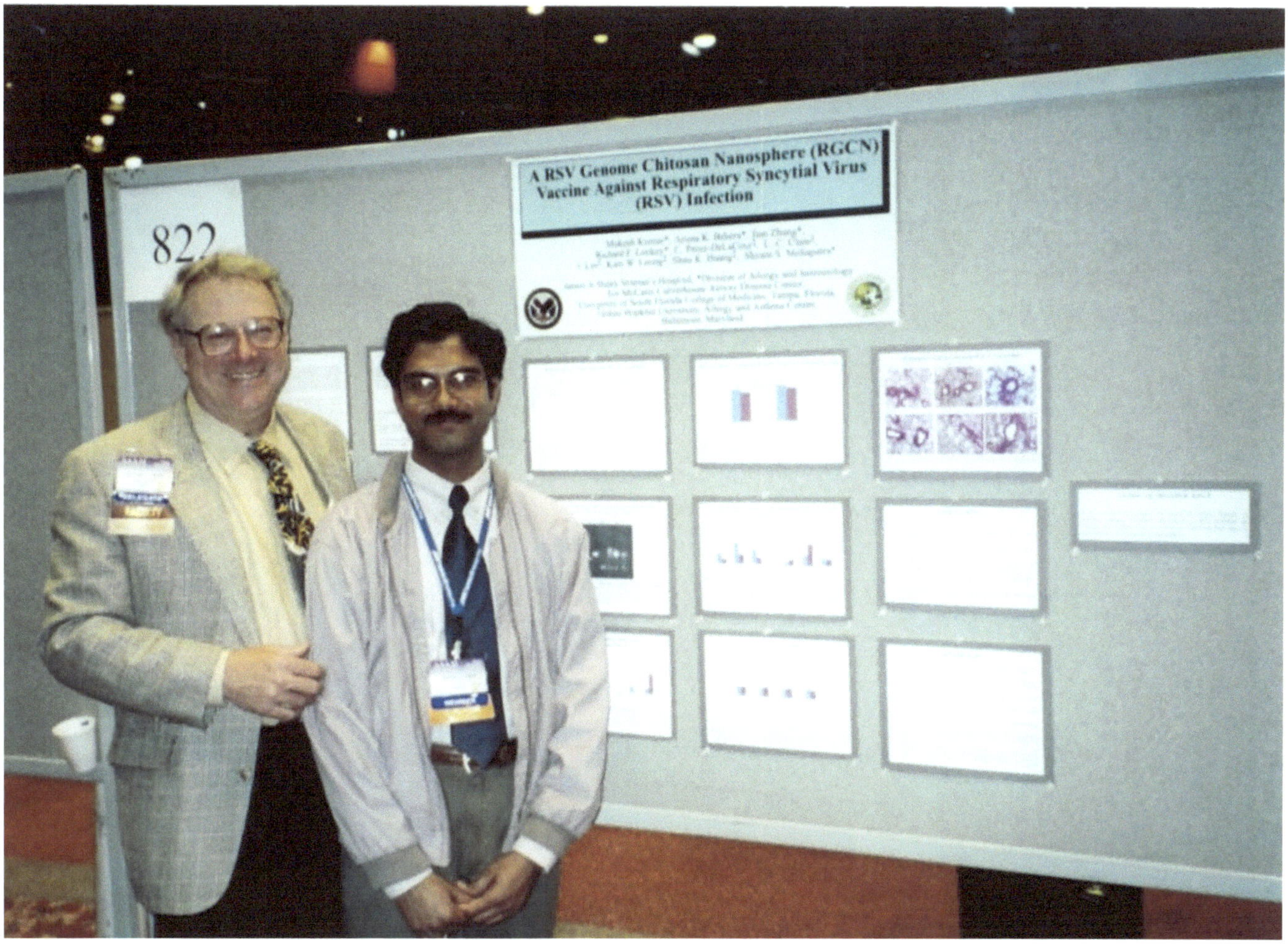

Left to right: Richard F. Lockey, MD and Mukesh Kumar, PhD. Poster: "A RSV Genome Chitosan Nanosphere (RGCN) Vaccine Against Respiratory Syncytial Virus (RSV) Infection". American Academy of Allergy Asthma and Immunology 57th Annual Meeting, New Orleans, Louisiana, March 16 – 21, 2001.

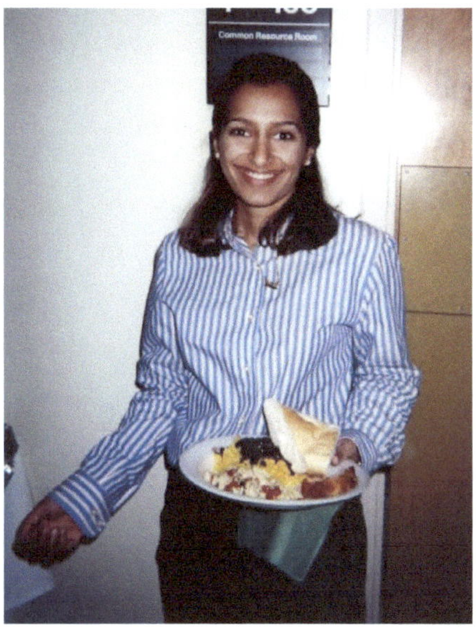

Runa Diwadkar, circa 2002.

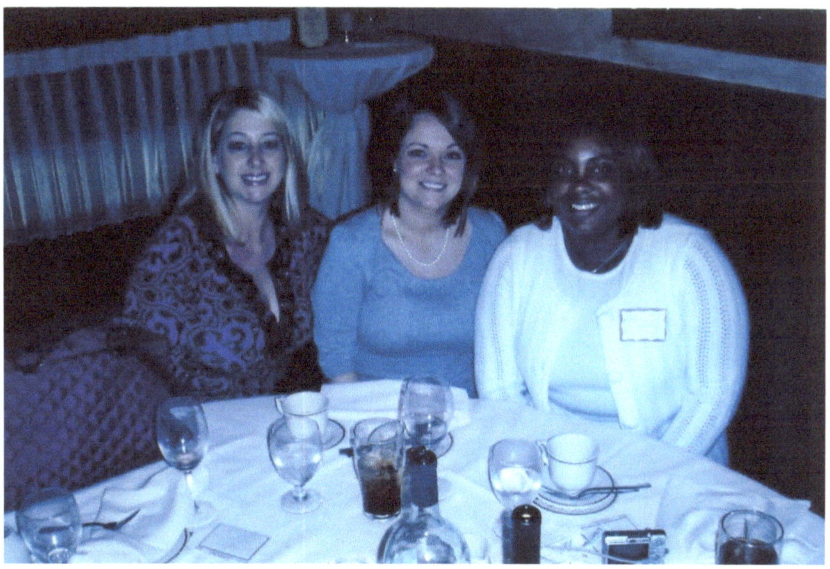

Left to right: Michelle Grandstaff-Singleton; Alison Jones; Shawna Shirley, circa 2006.

Left to right: Dongqing Chen, MD; Xiaoqin Wang, MD; Arun Kumar, PhD; circa 2006.

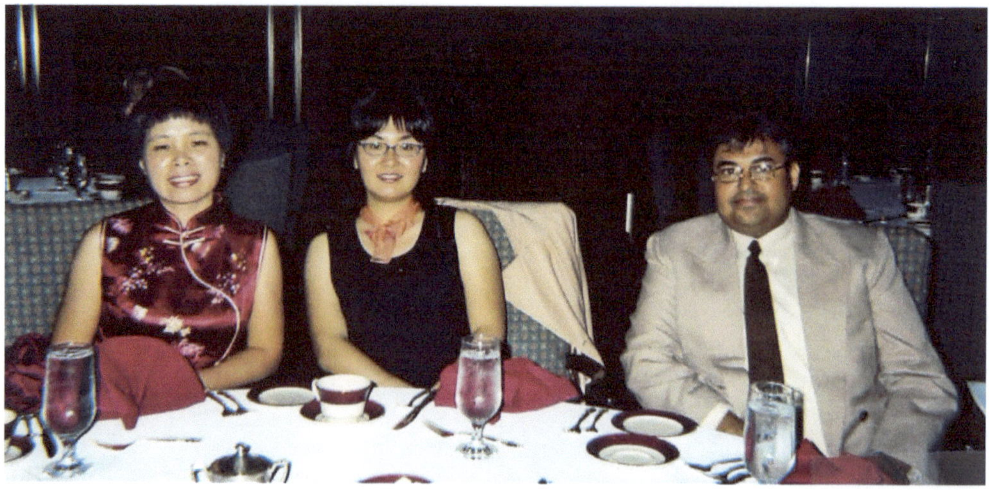

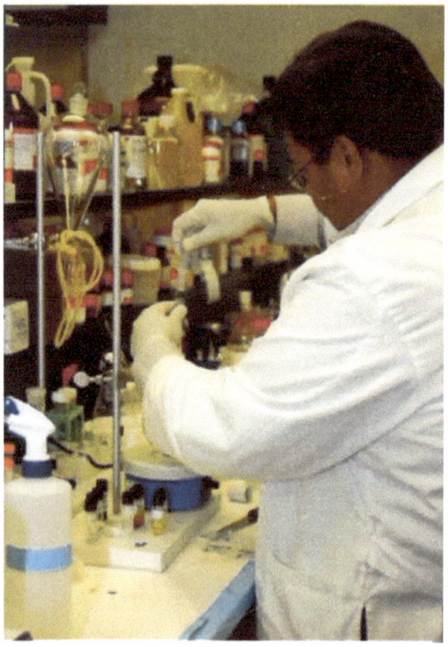

Arun Kumar, PhD; 2007.

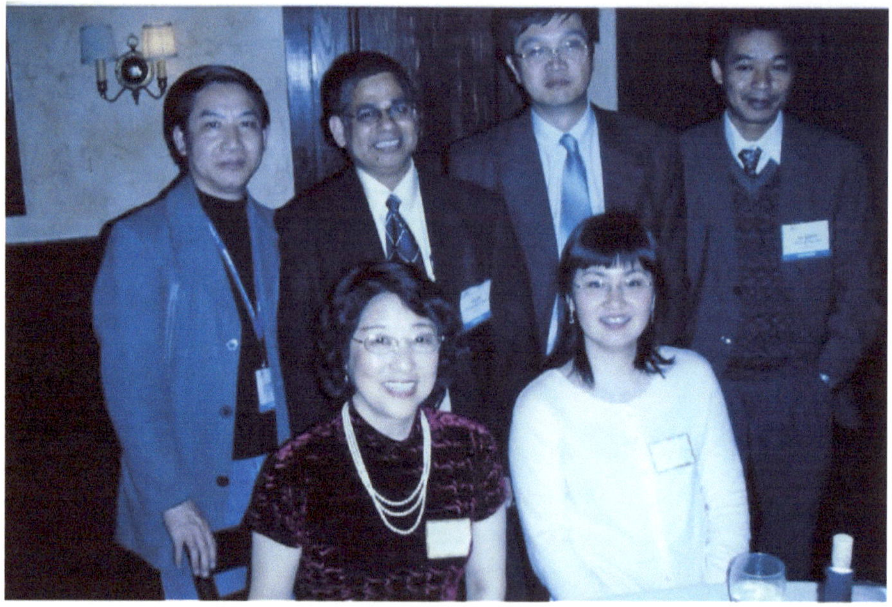

Front row (left to right); Xiaoyuan (Sonya) Kong, MD; Xiaoqin Wang, MD. Back row (left to right): Guoqing Liu, PhD; Shyam S. Mohapatra, PhD; Weidong Zhang, MD; Jia-Wang Wang, PhD, 2006.

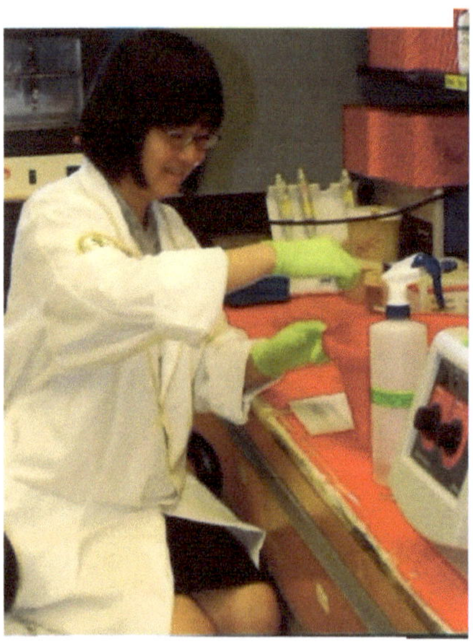

Xiaoqin Wang, MD; 2007.

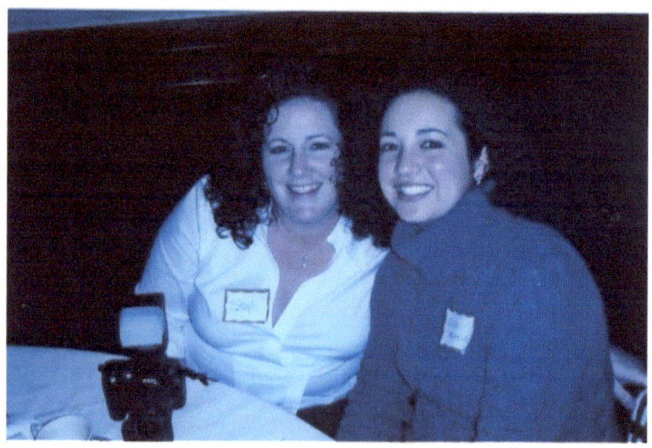

Left to right: Stephanie Medley and Sylvia Montalvo, circa 2008.

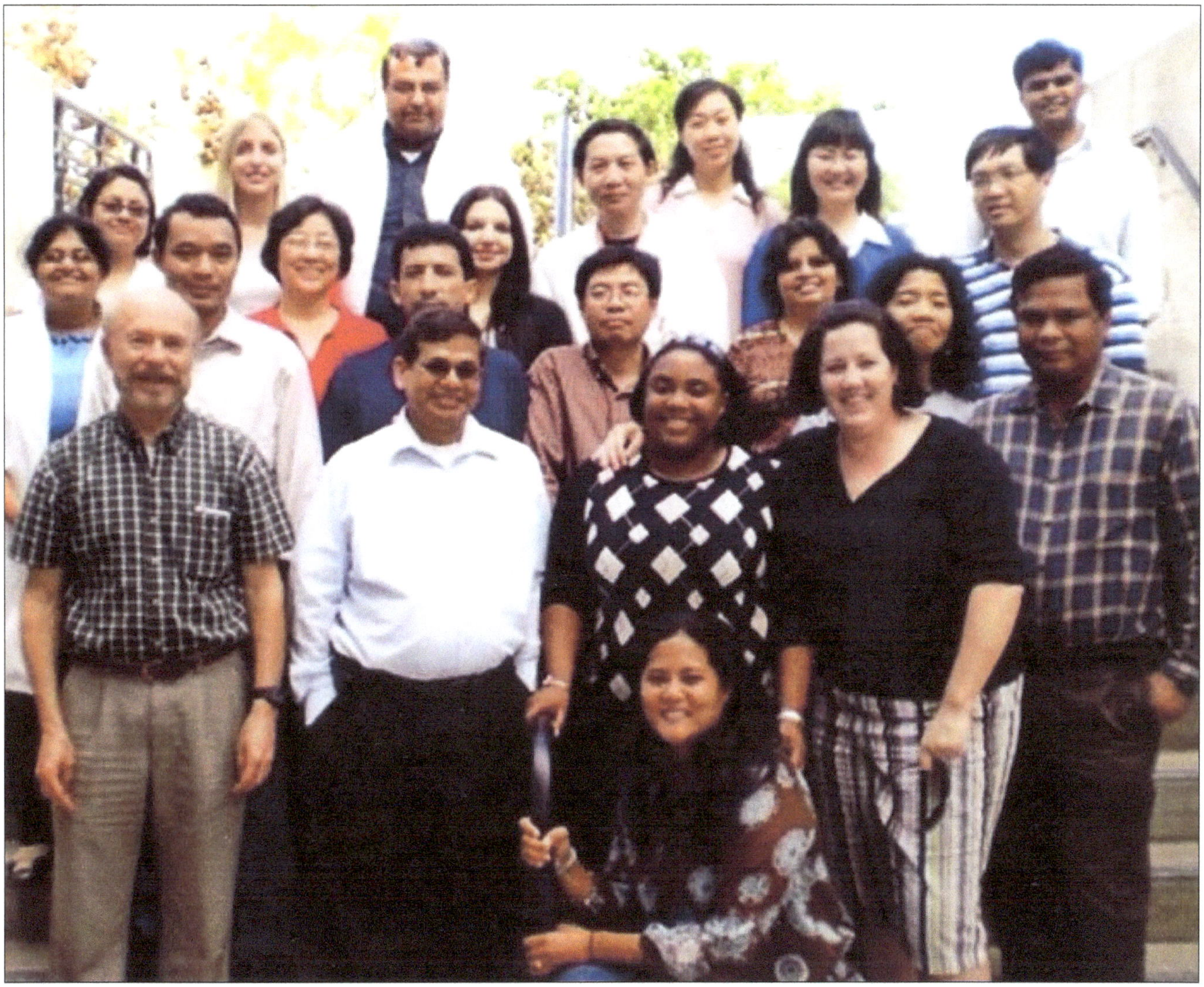

Taken 2007. Row 1 (bottom row): Liotta Dowdy. Row 2 (left to right): Gary Hellermann, PhD; Shyam S. Mohapatra, PhD; Shawna Shirley; Stephanie Medley; Prasanna Jena, PhD. Row 3 (left to right): Sandhya Boyapalle, PhD; Jia-Wang Wang, PhD; Julio Garay, PhD; Weidong (Wilson) Xu, PhD; Yvonne Davis. Row 4 (left to right): Mahasweta Das, PhD; Xiaoyuan (Sonya) Kong, MD; Brittany Caddick, Subhra Mohapatra, PhD. Row 5 (left to right): Leigh Nattkemper; Guoqing Liu, PhD; Xiaoqin Wang, MD; Weidong Zhang, MD, PhD. Row 6 (left to right): Arun Kumar, PhD; Hongyu Zheng, Murali Kanakanalli.

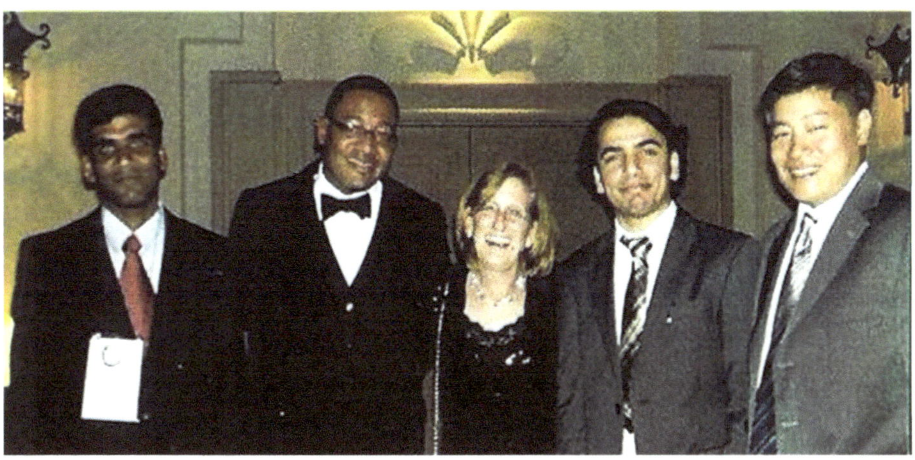

Left to right: Narasaiah Kolliputi, PhD; Ruan Cox; Peggy Hales; Salman Aljubran, MD; Michael Teng, PhD; 2011.

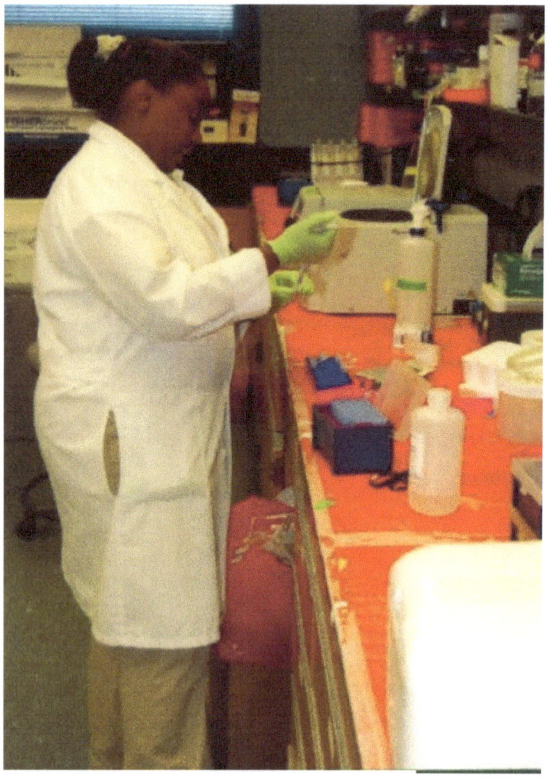

Shawna Shirley, MS; 2007.

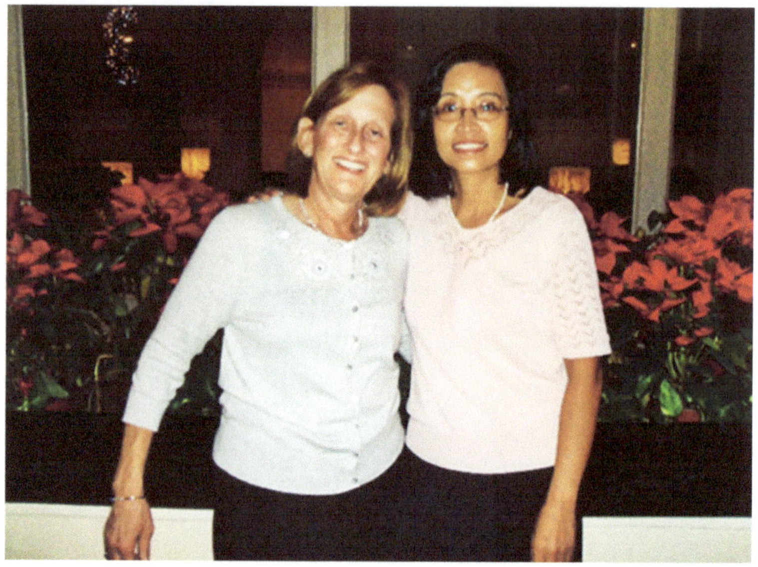

Left to right: Peggy Hales and Kunyu Li, 2011.

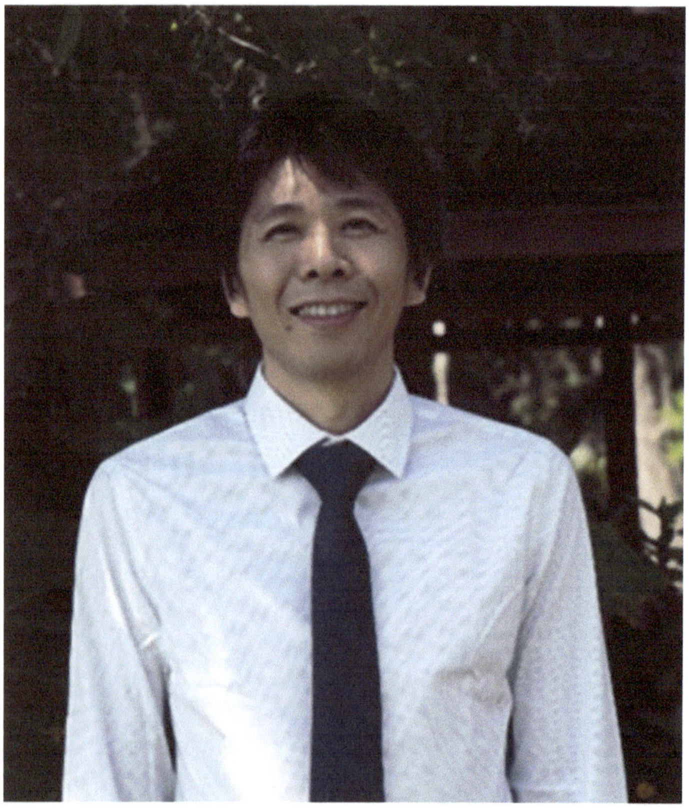

Jutaro Fukumoto, MD, PhD; circa 2014.

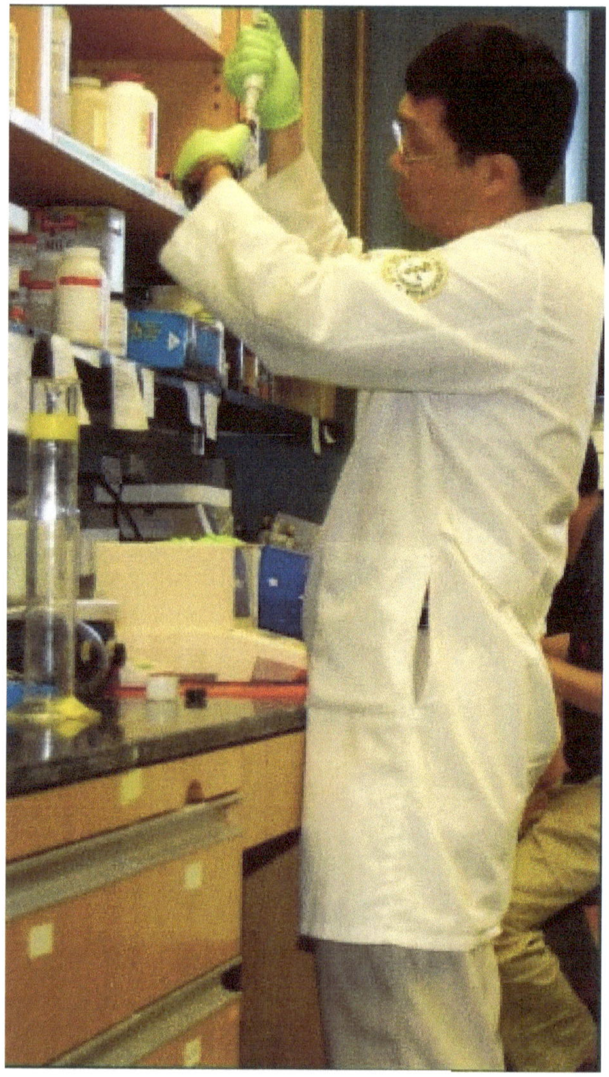

Weidong Zhang, MD, PhD; 2007.

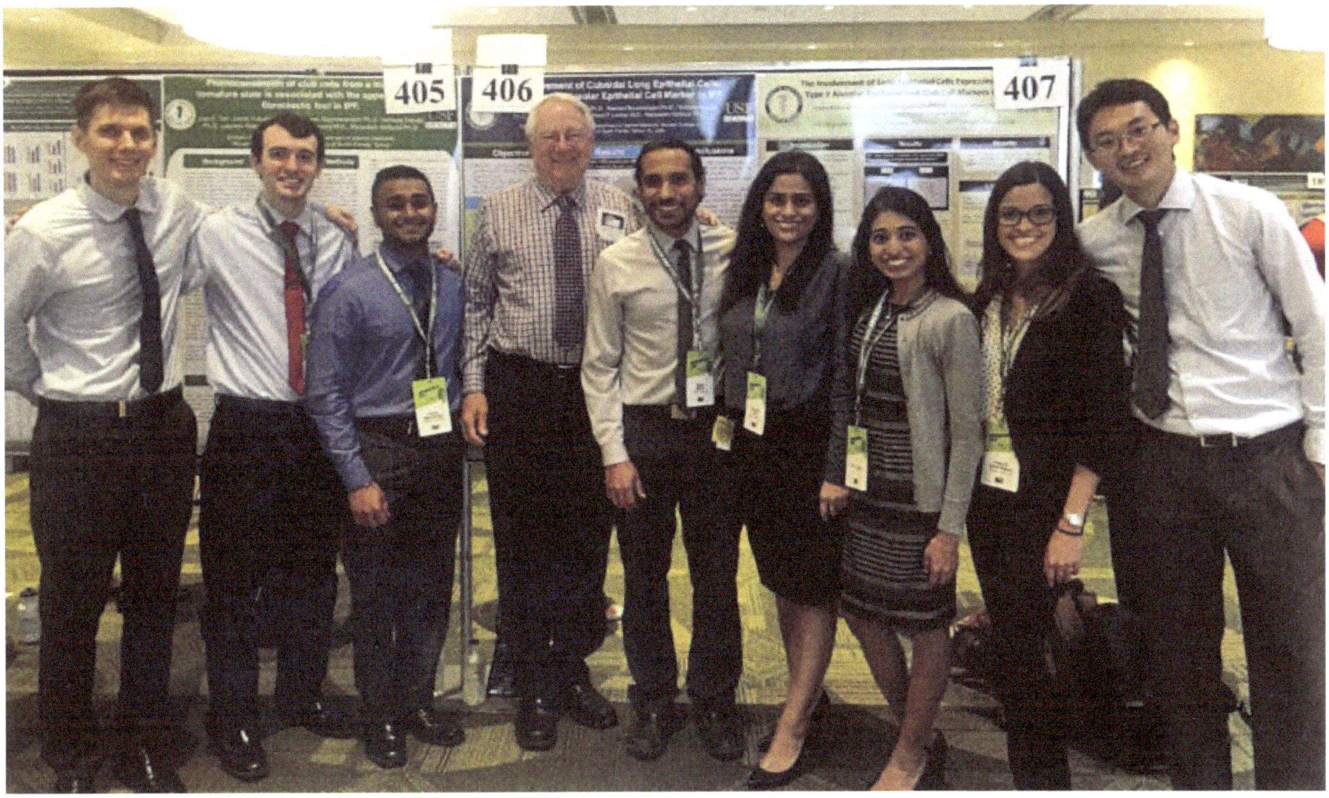

Left to right: Alex Czachor; Travis Herrin; Sanjay Mahendrasah; Richard F. Lockey, MD, MS; Adeeb Bulkhi, MD (2014-2017); Bhumika Patel, MD (ACH 2015-2017); Sonia Joychan, MD (ACH 2016-2018); Johana Castro-Wagner, MD (ACH 2015-2017); Chen Lin, MD (2015-2017). 2017 USF Health Research Day.

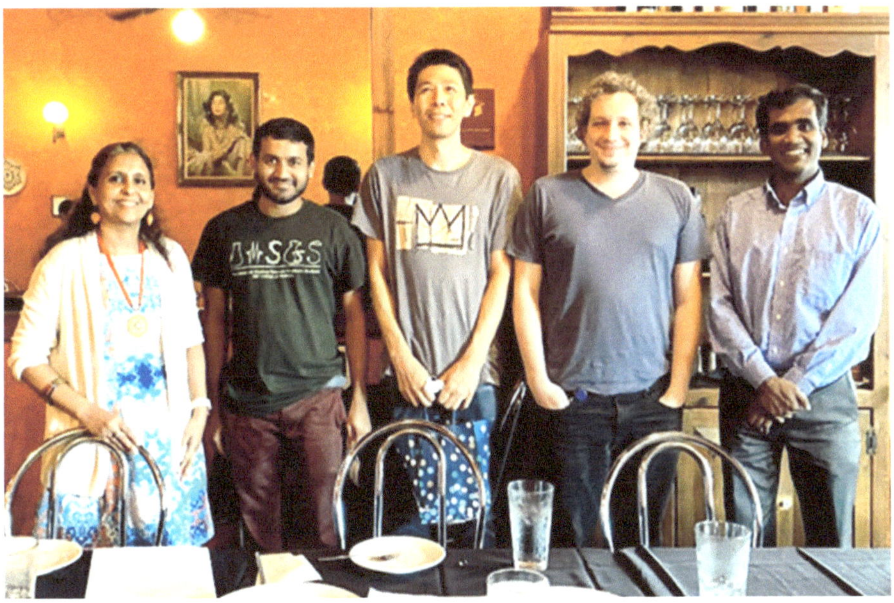

Left to right: Ramani Soundararajan, PhD; Sahebgowda Sidramagowda Patil, MS; Jutaro Fukumoto, MD, PhD; Matthew Allen; Narasaiah Kolliputi, PhD; 2020.

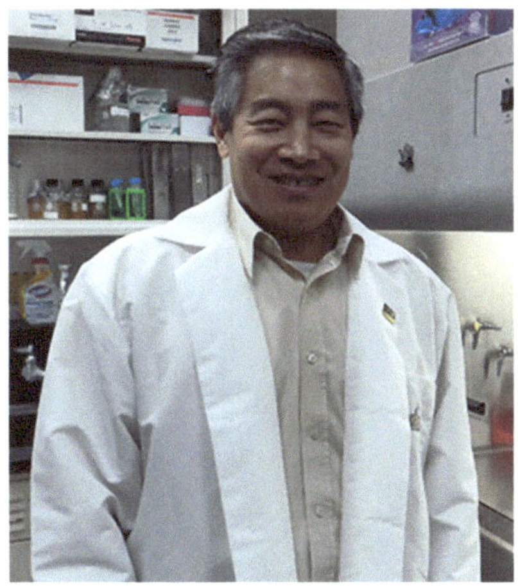

Michael Teng, PhD; 2020.

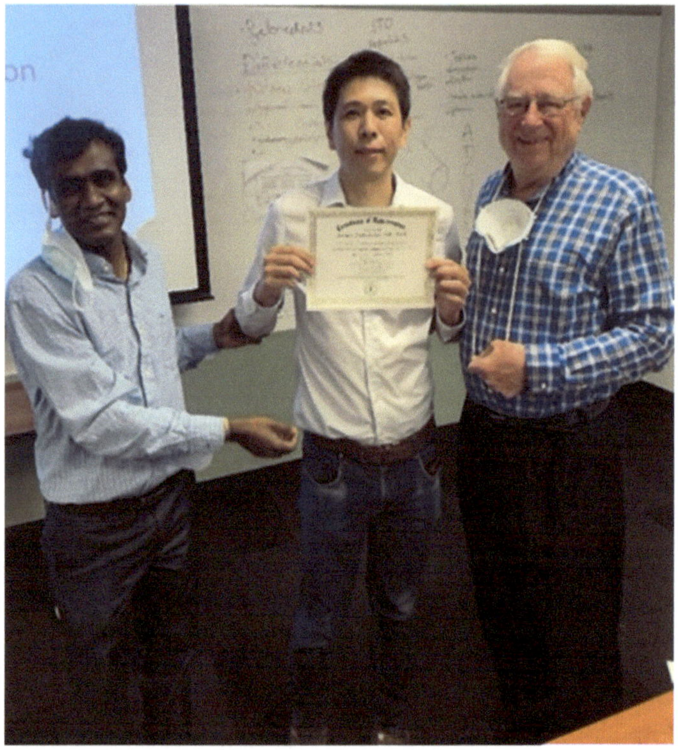

Right, left to right: Narasaiah Kolliputi, PhD; Jutaro Fukumoto, MD, PhD; Richard F. Lockey, MD, MS. Presentation of farewell certificate to Jutaro Fukumoto, MD, PhD; September 23, 2020.

Below: Narasaiah Kolliputi, PhD; member, USF National Academy of Inventors; 2021.

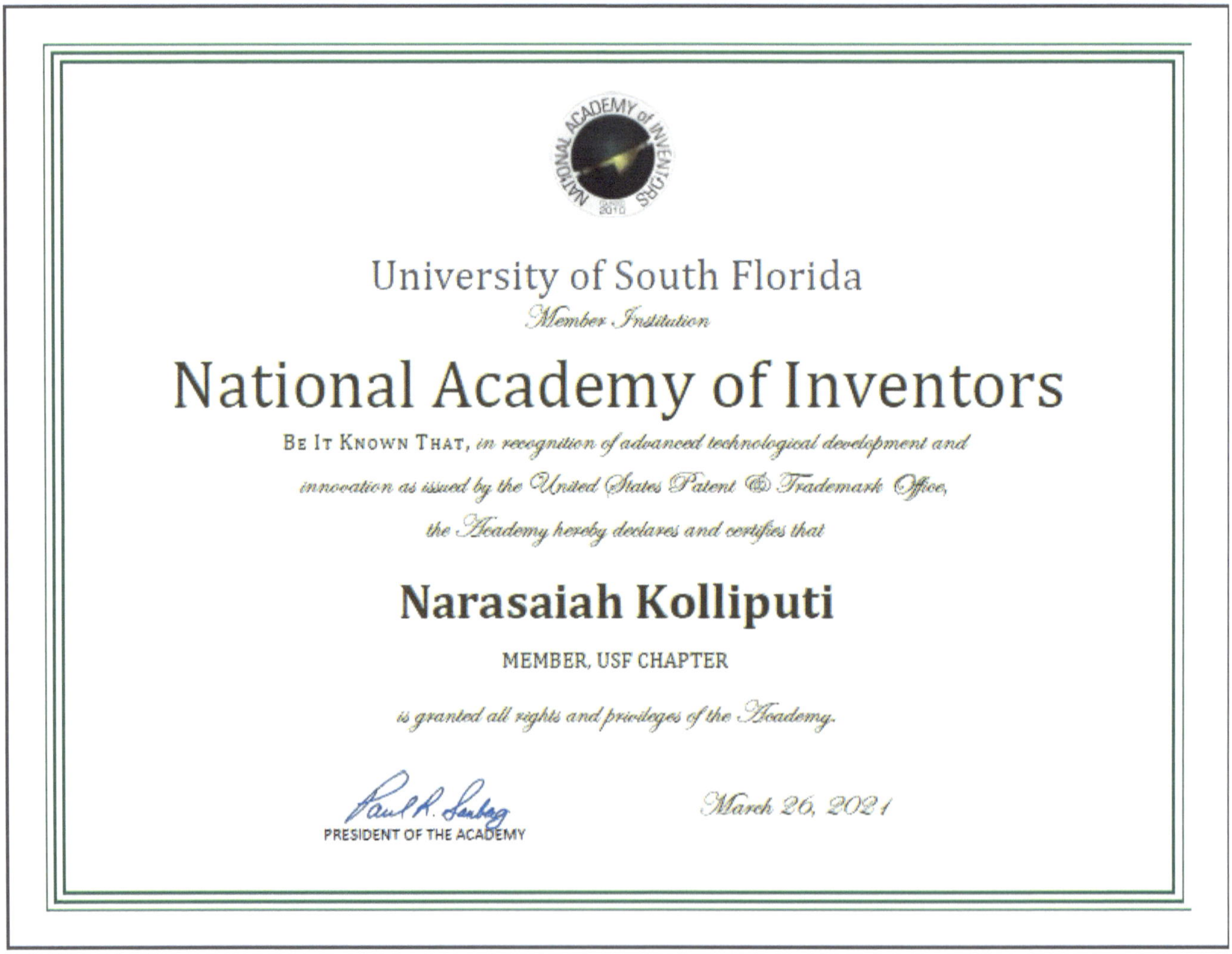

NATIONAL ACADEMY of INVENTORS

University of South Florida

Member Institution

National Academy of Inventors

BE IT KNOWN THAT, *in recognition of advanced technological development and innovation as issued by the United States Patent & Trademark Office, the Academy hereby declares and certifies that*

Narasaiah Kolliputi

MEMBER, USF CHAPTER

is granted all rights and privileges of the Academy.

PRESIDENT OF THE ACADEMY

March 26, 2021

Chapter 12: VA and USF Research Personnel

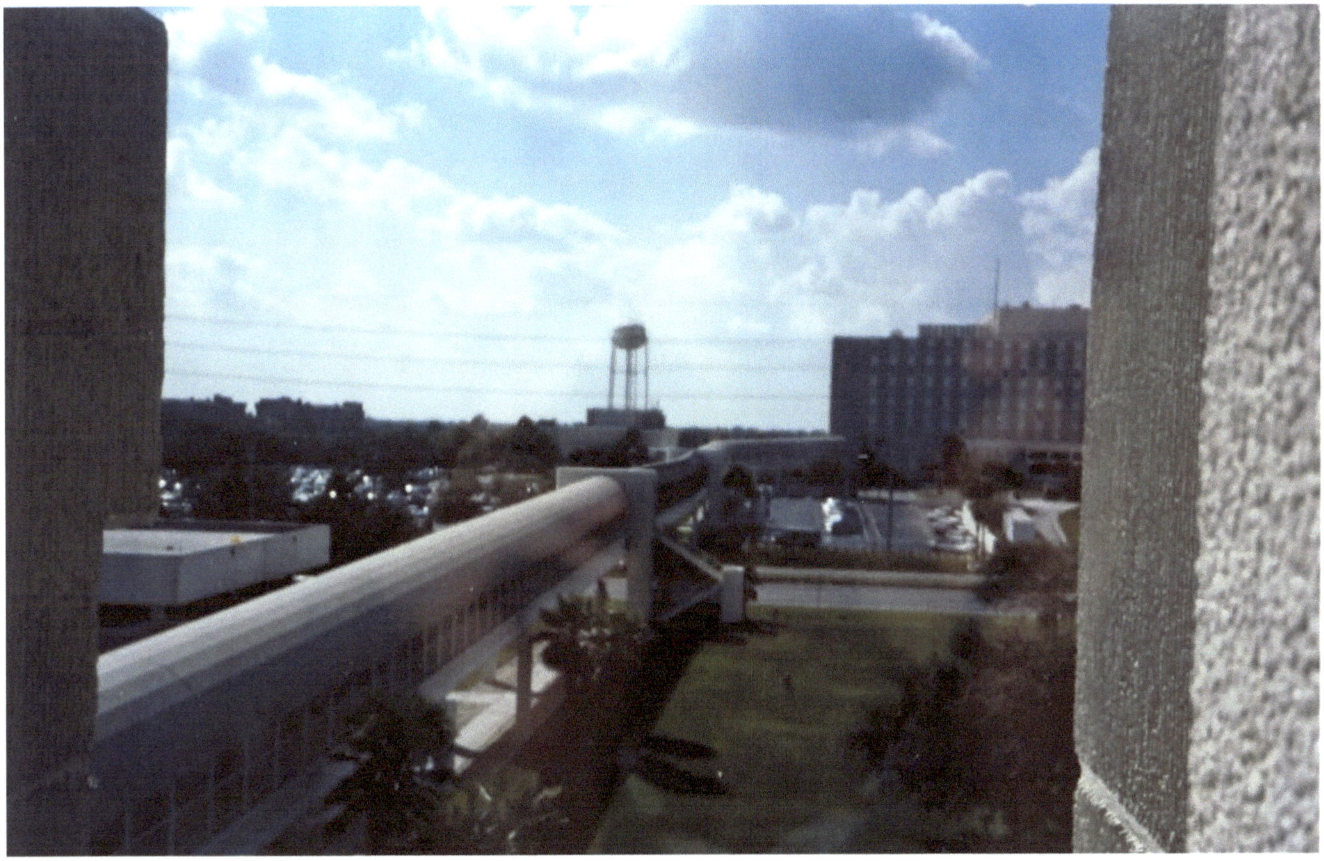

Walkway from USF Health Sciences Center to VA Hospital.

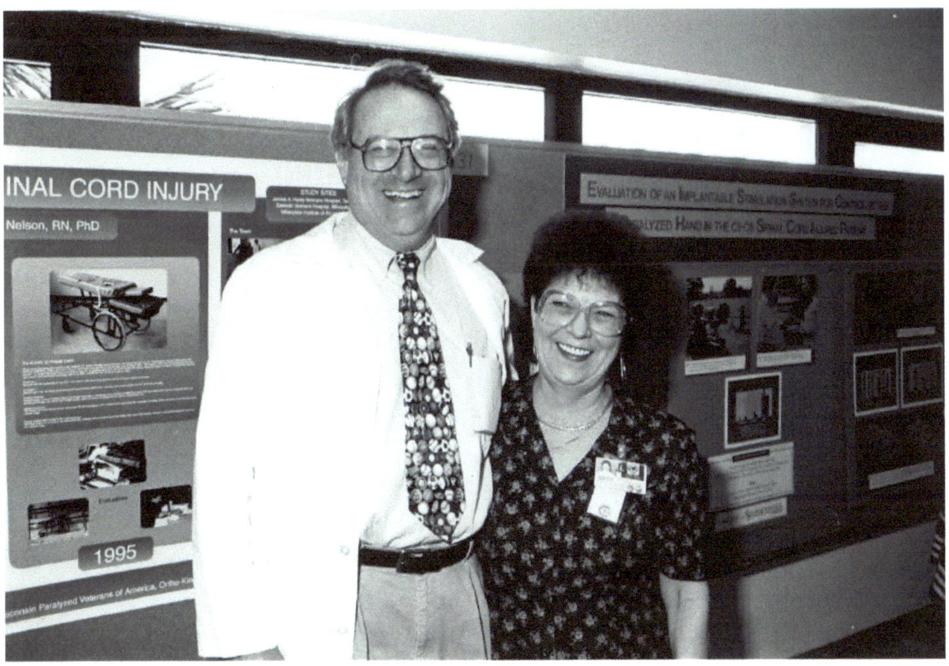

Left to right: Richard F. Lockey, MD, MS and Barbara Godwin (Medical Media), circa 1995.

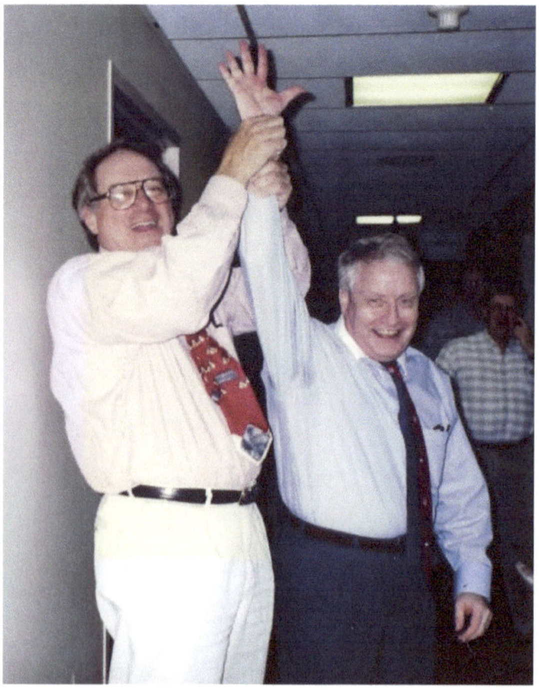

Left to right: Richard F. Lockey, MD, MS and David L. Vesely, MD (Endocrinology); 1997.

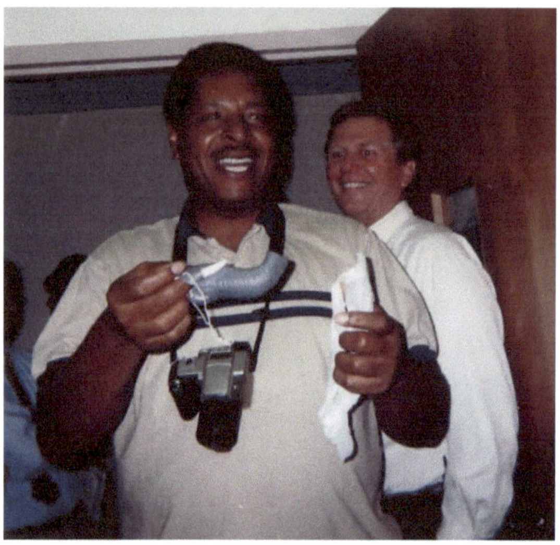

Left to right: Art Nelson (Medical Media); Roger W. Fox, MD; 2000.

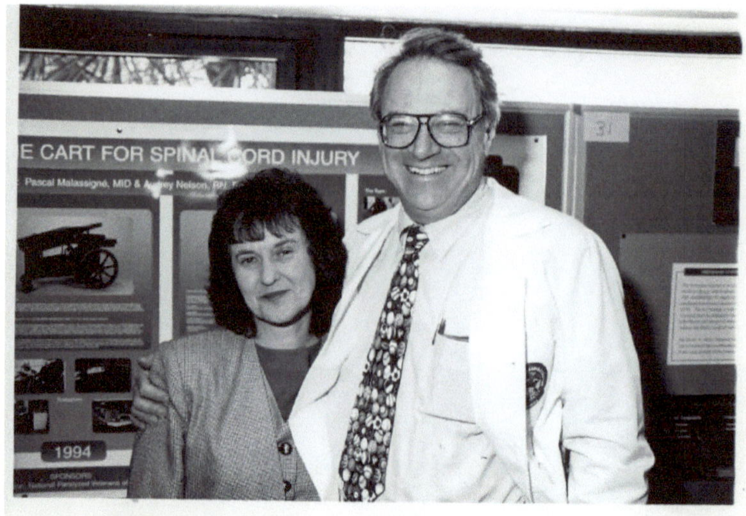

Left to right: Mary Standaert, PhD (Endocrinology) and Richard F. Lockey, MD, MS; 1995.

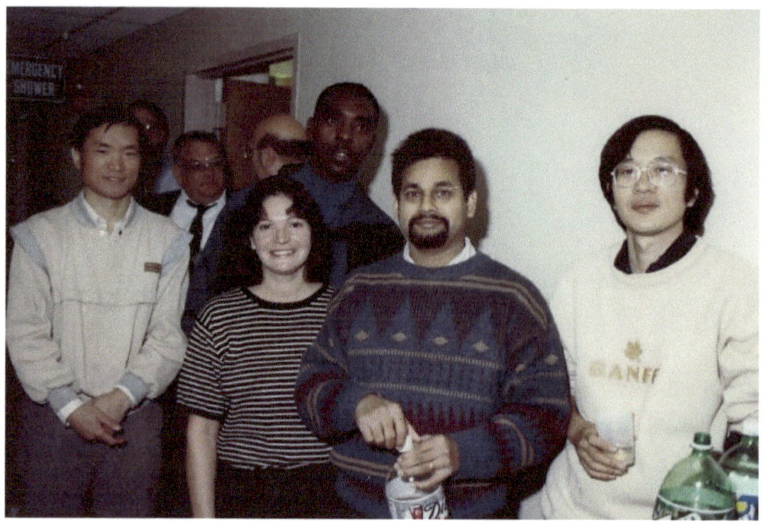

Front row (left to right): Mildred Acevedo-Duncan, PhD (Chemistry); Shyam S. Mohapatra, PhD; Hiroto Matsuse, MD. Back row (left to right): Jian Zhang, MD; Michael (surname unknown) (Medical Media). 1999.

Left to right: Ehon Hall (Chief, Medical Media); David L. Vesely, MD (Endocrinology); Tracy (surname unknow) (Medical Media); 2000.

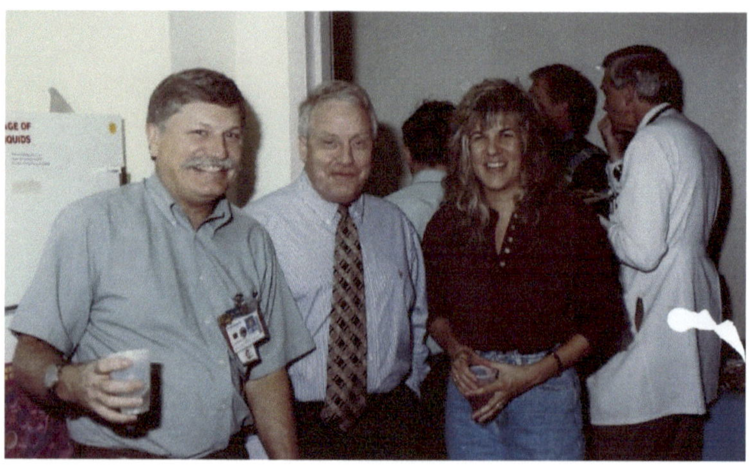

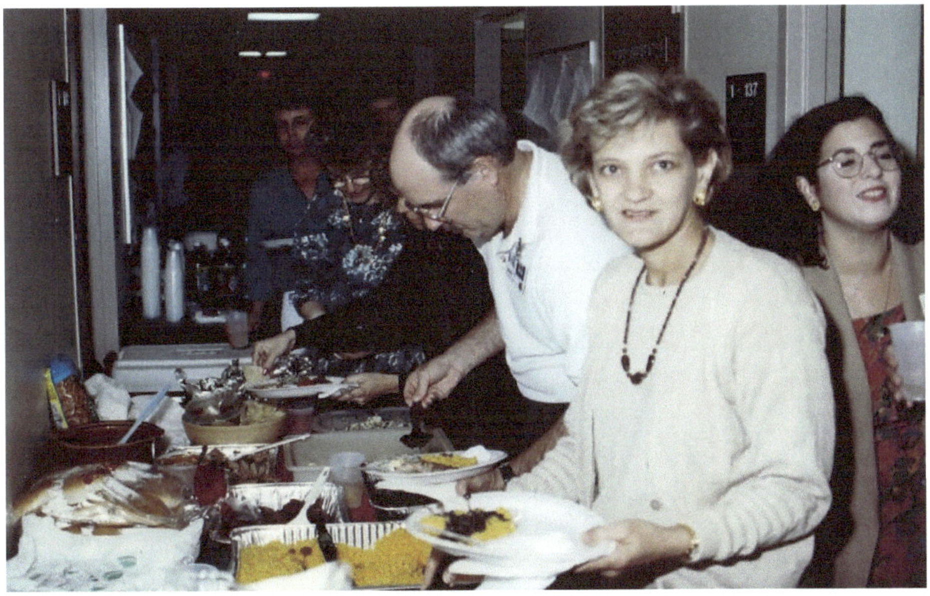

Left to right: William Gower, PhD (Surgery; Molecular Pharmacology & Physiology; Pathology & Cell Biology); Denise Cooper, PhD (Endocrinology); Dona Pecoraro (USF Health Clinic); circa 2000.

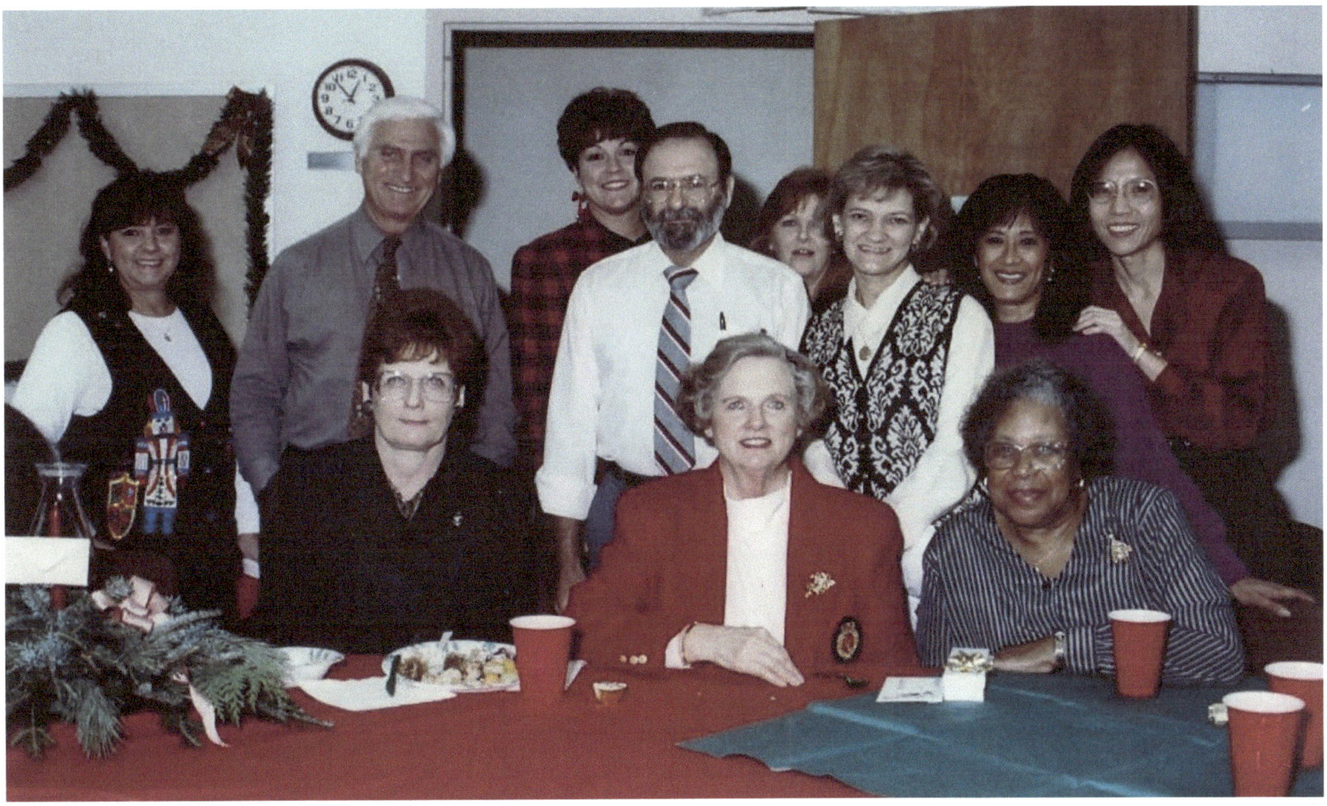

Front row (left to right): Doris Lukus; Vera Yelverton; Gladys Whaley. Second row (left to right): Frank DiPaola; Denise Cooper, PhD; Linda Sagun; Weimei Jenq. Third row (left to right): Benny Hilton; Robert Farese, MD; Sara Busquets; Charlene Pennington.

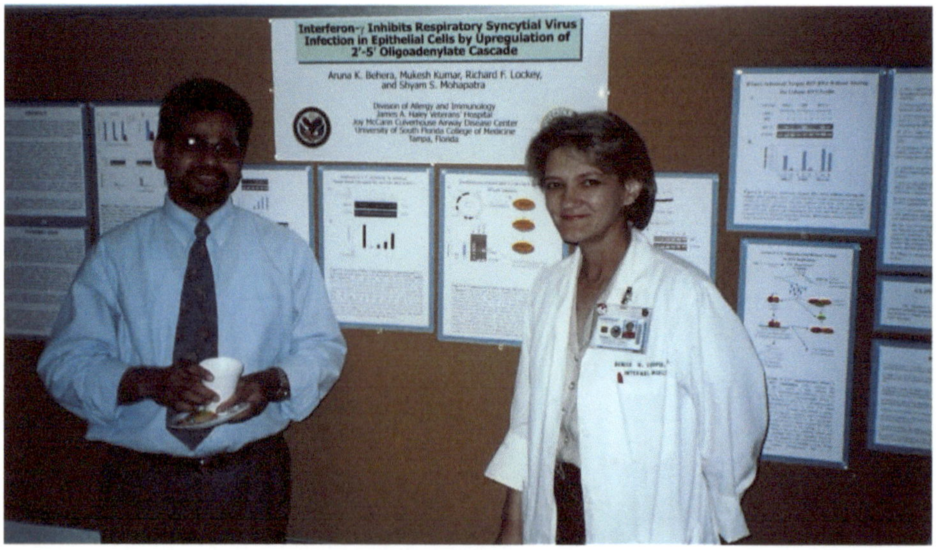
Interferon-γ Inhibits Respiratory Syncytial Virus Infection in Epithelial Cells by Upregulation of 2'-5' Oligoadenylate Cascade
Aruna K. Behera, Mukesh Kumar, Richard F. Lockey, and Shyam S. Mohapatra
Division of Allergy and Immunology
James A. Haley Veterans' Hospital
Joy McCann Culverhouse Airway Disease Center
University of South Florida College of Medicine
Tampa, Florida

Left to right: Shyam S. Mohapatra, PhD and Denise Cooper, PhD (Endocrinology); 2000.

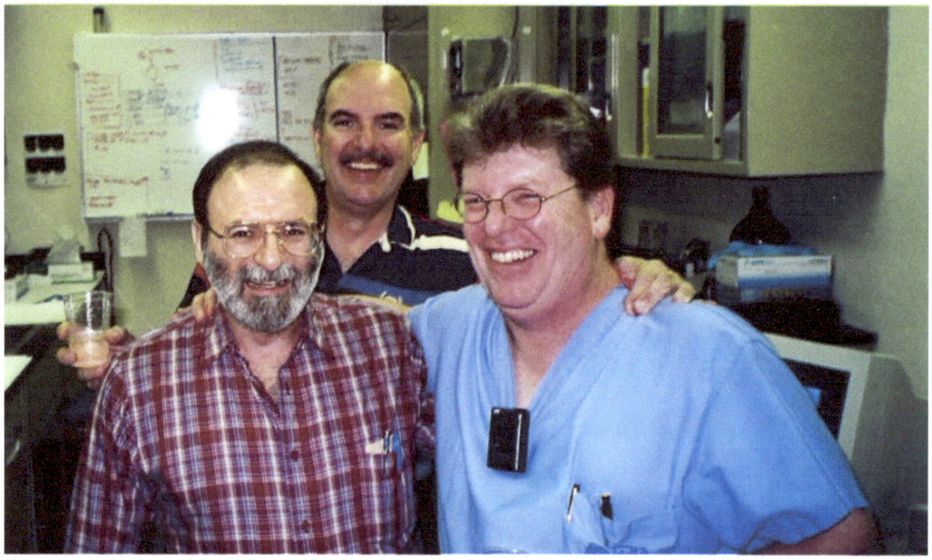

Front (left to right): Frank DiPaola (Administrative Officer, Research & Development); Jim Patterson (Pathology). Back: William Gower, PhD (Surgery; Molecular Pharmacology & Physiology; Pathology & Cell Biology) circa 2002.

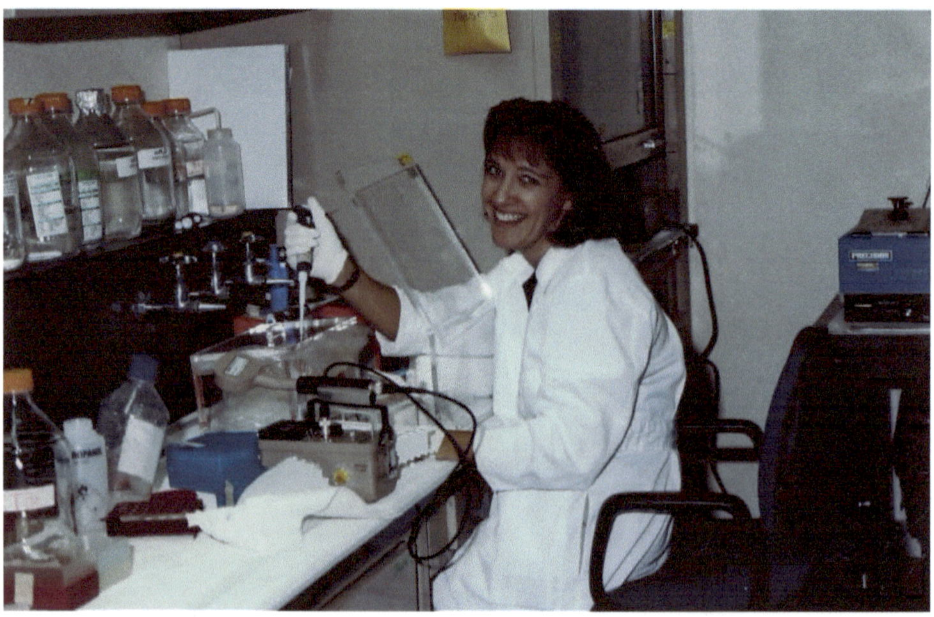

Gay Carter; Research Biologist, Research Service; circa 2010.

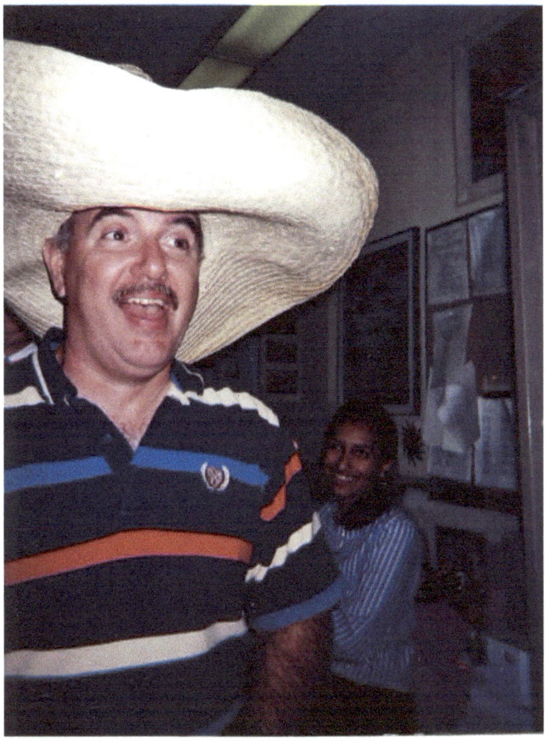

William Gower, PhD; 2002.

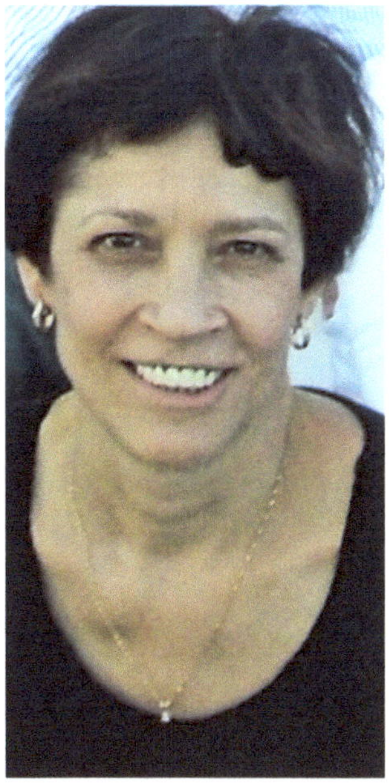

Debbie Houyou; Research Biologist, lab of Dr. William Gower, located across the hall from Allergy & Immunology; circa 2011.

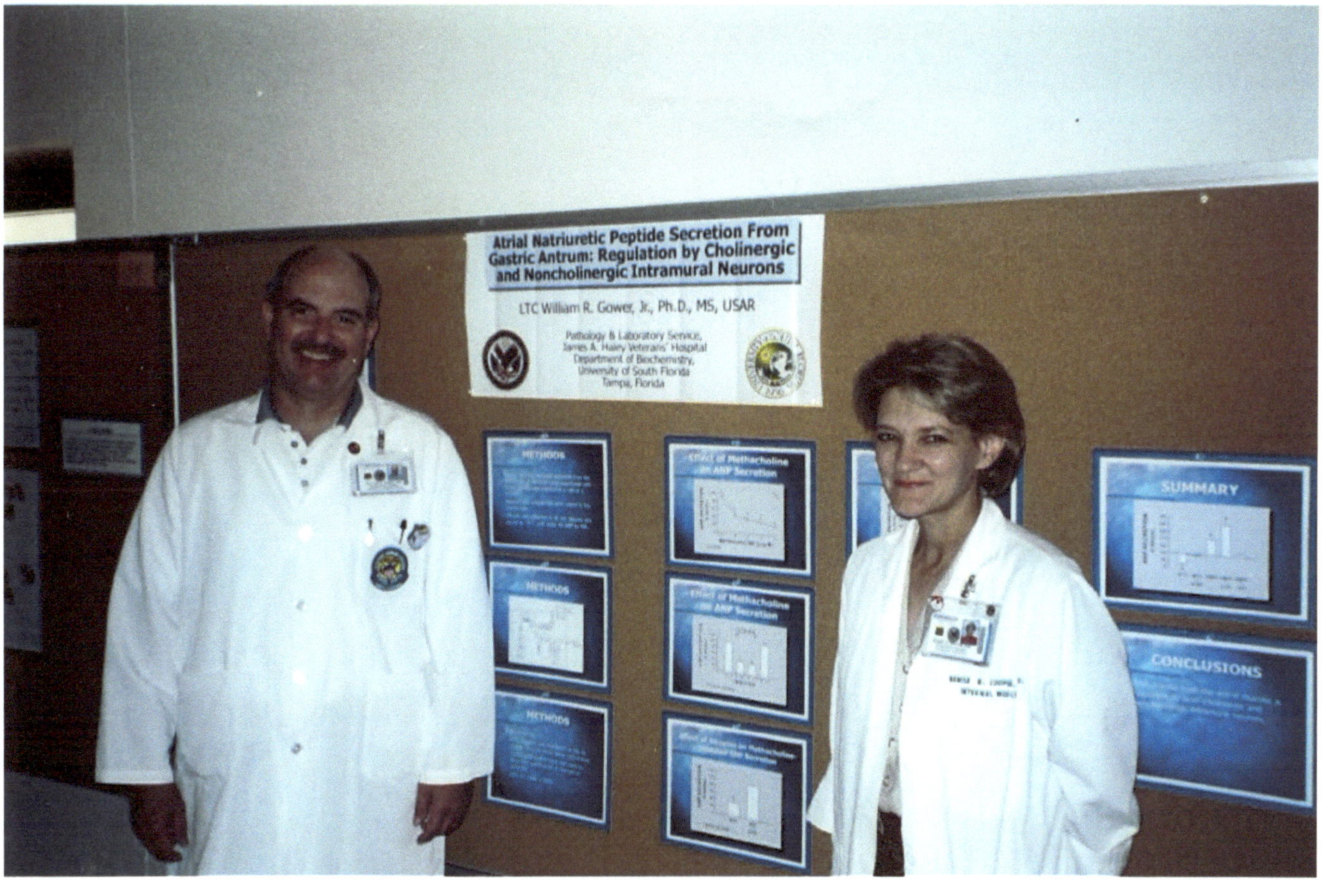

William Gower, PhD and Denise Cooper, PhD; circa 2003.

Chapter 13: Allergy and Immunology Postgraduate Programs Sponsored by the Division

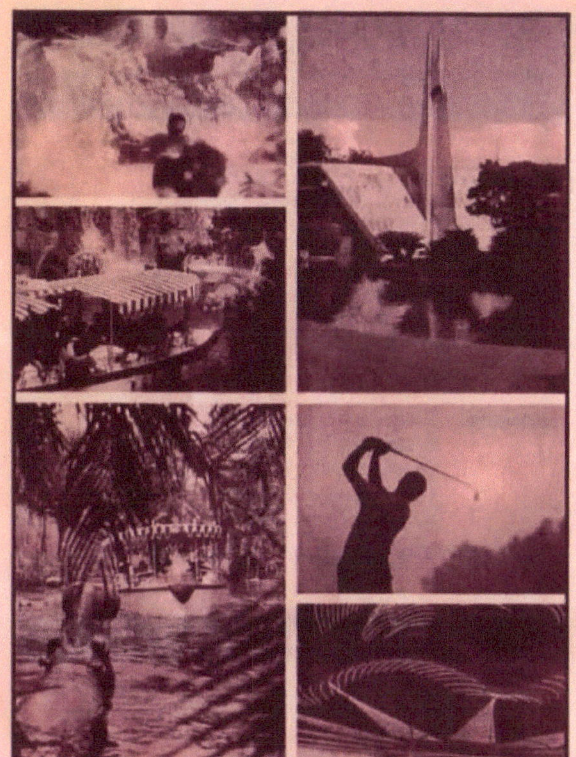

CLINICAL ALLERGY and IMMUNOLOGY for the PRACTICING PHYSICIAN

SPONSORED BY:
The UNIVERSITY of SOUTH FLORIDA COLLEGE of MEDICINE, DIVISION of ALLERGY and IMMUNOLOGY
The AMERICAN ACADEMY of ALLERGY and IMMUNOLOGY

American Academy of Allergy and Immunology

BUENA VISTA PALACE
DECEMBER 5, 6 AND 7, 1985
1900 Buena Vista Drive, Lake Buena Vista, Florida 32830

LOCAL FACULTY

From the University of South Florida College of Medicine and James A. Haley Veterans Administration Hospital, Tampa, Florida.

Loren J. Bartels, M.D.
Assistant Professor of Surgery
Division of Otolaryngology

Samuel C. Bukantz, M.D.
Professor of Medicine and Emeritus Chief
Division of Allergy/Immunology

Phillip W. DeVoe, M.D.
Assistant Professor of Pediatrics and Medicine
Division of Allergy/Immunology

Luis R. Espinoza, M.D.
Professor of Medicine
Divisions of Rheumatology and Allergy and Immunology

Roger W. Fox, M.D.
Assistant Professor of Medicine
Division of Allergy/Immunology

Dennis K. Ledford, M.D.
Assistant Professor of Medicine
Division of Allergy/Immunology

Richard F. Lockey, M.D.
Professor of Medicine and Pediatrics
Director; Division of Allergy/Immunology

Robert P. Nelson, M.D.
Instructor of Medicine
Division of Allergy/Immunology

David A. Solomon, M.D.
Associate Professor of Medicine
Division of Pulmonary & Critical Care Medicine

John J. Stablein, M.D.
Assistant Professor of Medicine
Division of Allergy/Immunology

William E. Stewart II, Ph.D.
Professor of Medical Microbiology/Immunology
Department of Medical Microbiology/Immunology

Avery H. Weiss, M.D.
Assistant Professor of Ophthalmology
Department of Ophthalmology

Clinical Allergy and Immunology for the Practicing Physician. Continuing Medical Education Conference sponsored by the Division. Lake Buena Vista, Florida.

REQUEST FOR ACCOMMODATIONS

(Mail direct to Buena Vista Palace)

CLINICAL ALLERGY AND IMMUNOLOGY
for the PRACTICING PHYSICIAN
DECEMBER 5-7, 1985

BUENA VISTA PALACE
1900 BUENA VISTA DRIVE
LAKE BUENA VISTA, FLORIDA 32830
(305) 827-2727

Contact the Buena Vista Palace directly, for room accommodations.

Convention rate per room, plus applicable taxes. (Convention rates apply 3 days prior and 3 days after meeting dates, subject to availability). Deposits are refundable if cancelled, 5 days prior to and not including the arrival date.

To guarantee a reservation, please forward a one-night room deposit of $96.30 (includes tax) by November 4, 1985.

Confention Rate $90.00
Single thru Quad

__________ # of rooms __________ # of persons

Please list names of additional members in your party and include children's ages.

____

____

NAME ______________________________

ADDRESS ______________________________

CITY ______________________________

STATE ______________ ZIP __________

ARRIVAL DATE __________ TIME __________ AM/PM

DEPARTURE DATE ______________________________

Circle card name and fill in the following to guarantee your reservation by credit card:

VISA | DINERS CLUB | MASTER CARD | AMERICAN EXPRESS

\# ______________________________

Expiration Date ______________________________

____
Signature   Date

Cut Here

PREREGISTRATION FORM

CLINICAL ALLERGY and IMMUNOLOGY
FOR THE PRACTICING PHYSICIAN

WALT DISNEY WORLD
BUENA VISTA PALACE

Please Print or Type:

NAME ______________________________

ADDRESS ______________________________

CITY ______________________________

STATE ______________ ZIP __________

PHONE NO. (____) ______________________________

SPECIALTY ______________________________

Registration Fee: (Check one)

Regular	— $250.00
Resident or Intern	— $100.00
(U.S. Currency only)	

Return form with registration fee made payable to The American Academy of Allergy and Immunology at the following address:

American Academy of Allergy and Immunology
ATTENTION: Mary Fogarty
611 East Wells Street
Milwaukee, Wisconsin 53202

For questions call Mary Fogarty at 414/272-6071.

Refunds for cancellations made prior to November 4, 1985 will be made less a $50.00 administration fee.

CLINICAL ALLERGY and IMMUNOLOGY for the PRACTICING PHYSICIAN

DATE: December 5, 6 and 7, 1985
(Early Registration December 4)

PLACE: Walt Disney World
The EPCOT Center
(Experimental Prototype Community of Tomorrow)
Buena Vista Palace
1900 Buena Vista Drive
Lake Buena Vista, Florida 32830
(305) 827-2727

SPONSORS: University of South Florida
College of Medicine
Division of Allergy and Immunology
The American Academy of Allergy and Immunology (A.A.A.I.)

COURSE DIRECTOR: Richard F. Lockey, M.D.

ACCREDITATION

The University of South Florida College of Medicine is accredited by the Accreditation Council for Continuing Medical Education to sponsor continuing medical education for physicians.

The University of South Florida College of Medicine certifies that this continuing medical education program meets the criteria for 13 hours of credit in Category I for the Physician's Recognition Award of the American Medical Association.

This program has been reviewed and is acceptable for 13 prescribed hours by the American Academy of Family Physicians.

FINANCIAL SUPPORT

We wish to express our appreciation to the following pharmaceutical companies for their generous support:

Ciba-Geigy
Glaxo
Greer Laboratories, Inc.
Key Pharmaceuticals
Diacom & Medical Equipment Designs
Merrell Dow
Miles Pharmaceuticals
Parke-Davis
Winthrop-Breon
Wyeth Laboratories

COURSE DESCRIPTION

Welcome to Disneyworld, EPCOT and Lake Buena Vista. This course is designed for **all** practicing physicians interested in asthma and allergic and immunologic problems as they relate to general practice, internal medicine, pediatrics and other specialties. The faculty includes world experts who will speak on a variety of timely subjects such as conjunctivitis, the role of allergy in the pathogenesis of otitis media, eosinophilia, urticaria, insect allergy, eczema, drug allergy, reactions to local anesthetics, nasal polyps, asthma (its classification and update on treatment) and the diagnosis and treatment of COPD. In addition, four talks on basic immunology as it relates to clinical medicine will also be included. Interesting case reports will add to the excitement of the daily morning conferences.

Audience participation will be encouraged and the meeting will adjourn promptly at 1:00 PM so everyone can enjoy the "Wonderful World of Disney" and the Experimental Prototype Community of Tomorrow "EPCOT" Center.

THE BUENA VISTA PALACE LAKE BUENA VISTA, FLORIDA

Welcome to the Palace at Lake Buena Vista . . . the area's tallest hotel and from every point of view the most spectacular. Imagine four spires of reflective glass glittering like crystal in their reach for the sun. Below, a lake surrounds the resort like a medieval moat. Turrets and courtyards call to mind the enchangment of another era. Yet this is 20th century splendor. A 12-story atrium welcomes you to this regal setting. Nature's own wealth of greenery fills every nook and corner and a glass elevator whisks you through a splashing waterfall to restaurants, convention facilities and private accommodations that are indeed palatial. Three elegant restaurants and four lounges invite you to gracious dining, exotic drinks, and top entertainment. The wide choice of on-site recreation allows any group to set its own pace. Facilities include tennis, indoor/outdoor swimming, health spa with hot tub, sauna, and jacuzzi, and nearby are 54 holes of championship golf.

A short stroll across the Boulevard takes you to the Walt Disney Shopping Village, a picturesque lakefront collection of specialty shops, restaurants, and one-of-a-kind lounges. A casual elegance and a leisurely pace characterize the Village, and promise hours of browsing.

PROGRAM

ANNUAL CONFERENCE CLINICAL ALLERGY AND IMMUNOLOGY FOR THE PRACTICING PHYSICIAN

December 5 - 7, 1985

WEDNESDAY, DECEMBER 4

7:00 - 8:00 p.m. Preregistration

THURSDAY, DECEMBER 5

7:00 - 8:00	REGISTRATION
7:30 - 7:55	CONTINENTAL BREAKFAST
	SESSION I
7:55 - 8:00	MODERATOR Samuel C. Bukantz, M.D.
8:00 - 8:05	WELCOME Richard F. Lockey, M.D.
8:05 - 8:35	Basic Immunology and Clinical Significance 1) Antibodies. Samuel C. Bukantz, M.D.
8:35 - 9:05	2) Lymphocytes (B and T Cells) Dennis K. Ledford, M.D.
9:05 - 9:35	3) Complement: Classical and Alternate Pathways John J. Stablein, M.D.
9:35 - 10:05	4) Interferon William E. Stewart II, Ph.D.
10:05 - 10:30	BREAK
10:30 - 11:00	Conjunctivitis, Differential Diagnosis & Therapy Avery H. Weiss, M.D.
11:00 - 11:30	Otitis Media: a) Diagnosis and Treatment Loren J. Bartels, M.D.
11:30 - 12:00	b) Role of Allergy Phillip W. DeVoe, M.D.
12:00 - 1:00	PANEL DISCUSSION Moderator: Samuel C. Bukantz, M.D. Discussants: Dennis K. Ledford, M.D. John J. Stablein, M.D. William E. Stewart II, Ph.D. Avery H. Weiss, M.D. Loren J. Bartels, M.D. Phillip W. DeVoe, M.D.

PROGRAM

ANNUAL CONFERENCE
CLINICAL ALLERGY AND IMMUNOLOGY FOR THE PRACTICING PHYSICIAN

December 5 - 7, 1985

WEDNESDAY, DECEMBER 4
7:00 - 8:00 p.m. Preregistration

THURSDAY, DECEMBER 5
7:00 - 8:00 REGISTRATION
7:30 - 7:55 CONTINENTAL BREAKFAST

SESSION I

7:55 - 8:00 MODERATOR
Samuel C. Bukantz, M.D.
8:00 - 8:05 WELCOME
Richard F. Lockey, M.D.
8:05 - 8:35 Basic Immunology and Clinical Significance
1) Antibodies.
Samuel C. Bukantz, M.D.
8:35 - 9:05 2) Lymphocytes (B and T Cells)
Dennis K. Ledford, M.D.
9:05 - 9:35 3) Complement: Classical and Alternate Pathways
John J. Stablein, M.D.
9:35 - 10:05 4) Interferon
William E. Stewart II, Ph.D.
10:05 - 10:30 BREAK
10:30 - 11:00 Conjunctivitis, Differential Diagnosis & Therapy
Avery H. Weiss, M.D.
11:00 - 11:30 Otitis Media:
a) Diagnosis and Treatment
Loren J. Bartels, M.D.
11:30 - 12:00 b) Role of Allergy
Phillip W. DeVoe, M.D.
12:00 - 1:00 PANEL DISCUSSION
Moderator:
Samuel C. Bukantz, M.D.
Discussants:
Dennis K. Ledford, M.D.
John J. Stablein, M.D.
William E. Stewart II, Ph.D.
Avery H. Weiss, M.D.
Loren J. Bartels, M.D.
Phillip W. DeVoe, M.D.

FRIDAY, DECEMBER 6
7:30 - 8:00 CONTINENTAL BREAKFAST

SESSION II

7:55 - 8:00 MODERATOR
Richard F. Lockey, M.D.
8:00 - 9:00 CASE REPORTS
1) Eosinophilia
Phillip W. DeVoe, M.D.
2) Common Variable Agammaglobulinemia
Dennis K. Ledford, M.D.
3) Fixed Drug Eruption
Samuel C. Bukantz, M.D.
9:00 - 10:00 Urticaria: Diagnosis and Treatment
Allen P. Kaplan, M.D.
10:00 - 10:30 Atopic Eczema
Roger W. Fox, M.D.
10:30 - 11:00 BREAK
11:00 - 12:00 Drug Allergy
N. Frank Adkinson, Jr., M.D.
12:00 - 1:00 PANEL DISCUSSION
Moderator:
Richard F. Lockey, M.D.
Discussants:
Phillip W. DeVoe, M.D.
Dennis K. Ledford, M.D.
Samuel C. Bukantz, M.D.
Allen P. Kaplan, M.D.
Roger W. Fox, M.D.
N. Frank Adkinson, Jr., M.D.

SATURDAY, DECEMBER 7
7:30 - 8:00 CONTINENTAL BREAKFAST

SESSION III

7:55 - 8:00 MODERATOR
John J. Stablein, M.D.
8:00 - 9:00 CASE REPORTS
1) Nasal Polyposis
Richard F. Lockey, M.D.
2) Hereditary Angioedema (HAE)
Robert P. Nelson, M.D.
3) Reaction To Local Anesthetic
John J. Stablein, M.D.
9:00 - 10:00 Asthma - Classification and Treatment
Charles E. Reed, M.D.
10:00 - 10:30 BREAK
10:30 - 11:00 Significance of Autoantibodies
Luis R. Espinoza, M.D.
11:00 - 11:30 COPD - Diagnosis and Treatment Functional and/or Clinical Reversibility
David A. Solomon, M.D.
11:30 - 12:00 Insect Sting (Hymenoptera) Hypersensitivity
Richard F. Lockey, M.D.
12:00 - 1:00 PANEL DISCUSSION
Moderator:
John J. Stablein, M.D.
Discussants:
Richard F. Lockey, M.D.
Robert P. Nelson, M.D.
Charles E. Reed, M.D.
Luis R. Espinoza, M.D.
David A. Soloman, M.D.

GUEST FACULTY

N. Franklin Adkinson, Jr., M.D.
Associate Professor of Medicine
The Johns Hopkins University School of Medicine
Clinical Immunology Division
Baltimore, Maryland

Allen P. Kaplan, M.D.
Professor of Medicine and Division Head
Division of Allergy, Rheumatology and Clinical Immunology
Health Science Center
State University of New York at Stony Brook
Stony Brook, New York

Charles E. Reed, M.D.
Professor of Medicine
Mayo Medical School
Chairman of the Department of Allergic Diseases, Internal Medicine

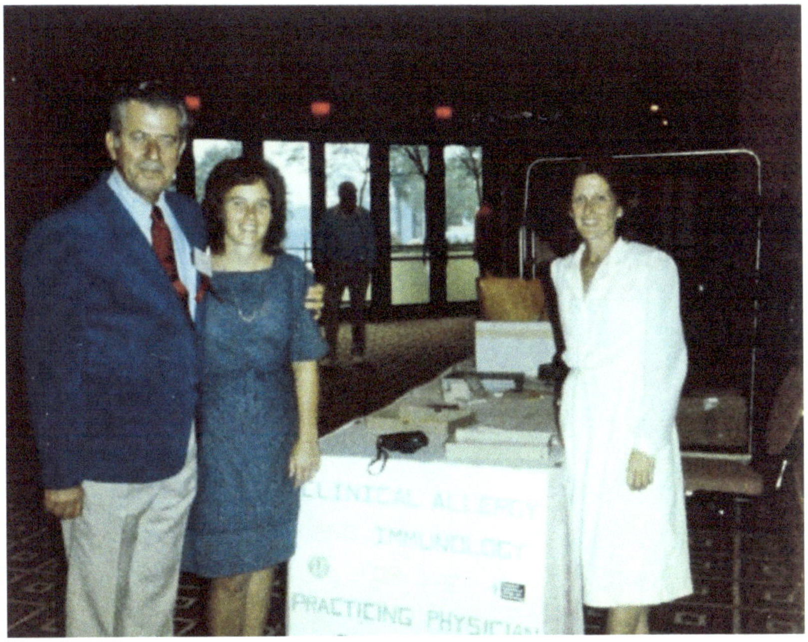

Left to right: Samuel C. Bukantz, MD; Pat Walsh; Peggy Hales. Registration desk, circa 1986.

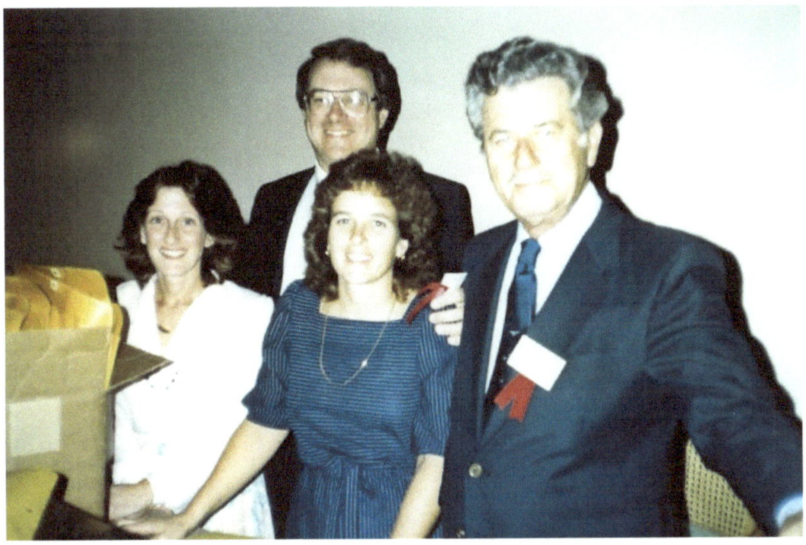

Left to right: Peggy Hales; Pat Walsh; Samuel C. Bukantz, MD. Back: Richard F. Lockey, MD, MS. Circa 1986.

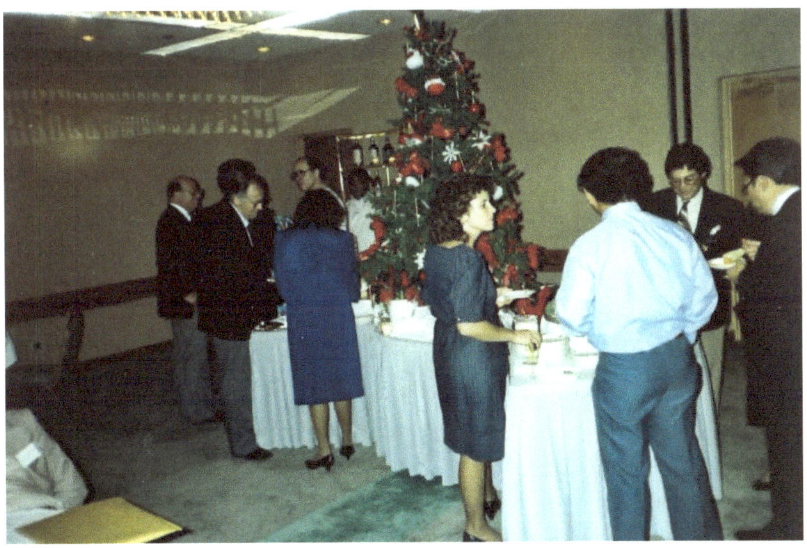

Mid-morning break, circa 1986.

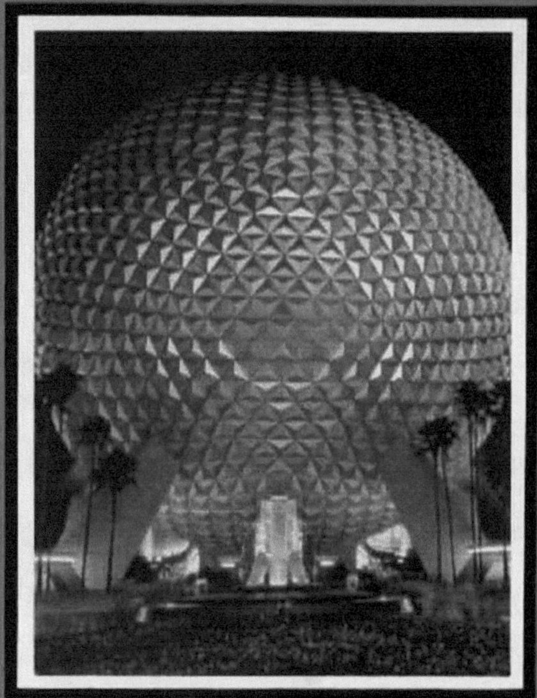

CLINICAL ALLERGY and IMMUNOLOGY for the PRACTICING PHYSICIAN

SPONSORED BY:
The AMERICAN ACADEMY OF ALLERGY and IMMUNOLOGY
AND
THE DIVISION OF ALLERGY and IMMUNOLOGY
UNIVERSITY OF SOUTH FLORIDA
COLLEGE OF MEDICINE

American Academy of Allergy and Immunology

DECEMBER 3-5, 1987
BUENA VISTA PALACE
Walt Disney World Village
P.O. Box 22206
Lake Buena Vista, FL 32830-2206

THE BUENA VISTA PALACE

From the first moment you arrive at the Buena Vista Palace, you begin to experience the excitement of a 21st Century resort that preserves the classic tradition of fine service and attention to detail. Towering 27 stories over EPCOT Center, the Buena Vista Palace provides regal accommodations with striking views of the Walt Disney World Vacation Kingdom. The service is impeccable, the value extraordinary - and each day is one of perfect enchantment.

Imagine four spires of reflective glass glittering like crystal in their reach for the sun. Below, a lake surrounds the resort like a medieval moat. Turrets and courtyards call to mind the enchantment of another era. A 12-story atrium welcomes you to this regal setting. Nature's own wealth of greenery fill every nook and corner and a glass elevator whisks you through a splashing waterfall to restaurants, convention facilities and private accommodations that are indeed palatial. Three elegant restaurants and four lounges invite you to gracious dining, exotic drinks, and top entertainment. The wide choice of on-site recreation allows any group to set its own pace. Facilities include tennis, swimming, health spa with hot tub, sauna and jacuzzi, and nearby are 54 holes of championship golf.

A short stroll across the Boulevard takes you to the Walt Disney Shopping Village, a picturesque lakefront collection of specialty shops, restaurants, and one-of-a-kind lounges. A casual elegance and a leisurely pace characterize the Village, and promise hours of browsing.

Right outside your Palace resort lies a whole world of enchantment in the Walt Disney World Vacation Kingdom. Mickey and the gang bring a lifetime of memories at the Magic Kingdom . . . at Epcot Center you experience the wonders of today and exciting visions of tomorrow. Complimentary Walt Disney World Shuttle transportation departs from the Palace every 15 minutes to take you throughout the Vacation Kingdom.

CLINICAL ALLERGY and IMMUNOLOGY for the PRACTICING PHYSICIAN

DATE: December 3, 4 and 5, 1987
[Early registration December 2, 1987]

PLACE: Buena Vista Palace
Walt Disney World Village
P.O. Box 22206
Lake Buena Vista, FL 32830-2206

SPONSORS: University of South Florida
College of Medicine
Division of Allergy and Immunology
The American Academy of Allergy and Immunology [AAAI]

COURSE DIRECTOR: Richard F. Lockey, M.D.

ACCREDITATION

As an organization accredited to provide Continuing Medical Education, the American Academy of Allergy and Immunology designates this activity as meeting the criteria for 13.5 credit hours in Category I of the Physician's Recognition Award of the American Medical Association.

This program has also been reviewed and is acceptable for 13.5 prescribed hours by the American Academy of Family Physicians.

FINANCIAL SUPPORT

We wish to express our appreciation to the following pharmaceutical companies for their generous support:

Becton-Dickinson [B-D]
Center Laboratories
DeVilbiss Company
Fisons Corporation
Fleming & Company, Inc.
Glaxo Inc.
Greer Laboratories, Inc.
Hollister-Stier
Janssen Pharmaceutica
Key Pharmaceuticals
Merrell Dow Pharmaceuticals Inc.
Muro Pharmaceutical, Inc.
Newtron Products, Co.
Parke-Davis
Pfizer Pharmaceuticals
Schering Corporation

PROGRAM

CLINICAL ALLERGY AND IMMUNOLOGY for the PRACTICING PHYSICIAN

WEDNESDAY, DECEMBER 2, 1987

6:30 - 7:30 a.m. PREREGISTRATION

THURSDAY, DECEMBER 3, 1987

7:00 - 8:00 a.m. REGISTRATION
7:30 - 7:55 a.m. CONTINENTAL BREAKFAST

SESSION I

7:55 - 8:00 a.m. WELCOME - Richard F. Lockey, M.D.
MODERATOR - Samuel C. Bukantz, M.D.

8:00 - 8:30 a.m. Occupational Lung Disease
Gerald A. Bucholtz, M.D.

8:30 - 9:00 a.m. AIDS in Children
Rajendra N. Pahwa, M.D.

9:00 - 9:30 a.m. Late Phase Allergic Reaction - Its Clinical Significance and Treatment
Samuel C. Bukantz, M.D.

9:30 - 10:00 a.m. Reactive Airway Dysfunction Syndrome (RADS)
Stuart M. Brooks, M.D.

10:00 - 10:30 a.m. CASE REPORTS
1) Vasculitis
Joseph D. Diaz, M.D.
2) Severe Asthma
Gerald A. Bucholtz, M.D.

10:30 - 11:00 a.m. **BREAK**

11:00 - 1:00 p.m. Meet the Professor Sessions
A. Occupational Lung Disease
Gerald A. Bucholtz, M.D.
B. AIDS in Children
Rajendra N. Pahwa, M.D.
C. Late Phase Allergic Reaction - Its Clinical Significance and Treatment
Samuel C. Bukantz, M.D.
D. Reactive Airway Dysfunction Syndrome (RADS)
Stuart M. Brooks, M.D.

PROGRAM (CONTINUED)

FRIDAY, DECEMBER 4, 1987

7:30 - 7:55 a.m. CONTINENTAL BREAKFAST

SESSION II

7:55 - 8:00 a.m. MODERATOR -
Richard F. Lockey, M.D.

8:00 - 8:30 a.m. Vasculitis
Dennis K. Ledford, M.D.

8:30 - 9:00 a.m. Use of Cholinergic Agents in COPD
Philip L. Lieberman, M.D.

9:00 - 9:30 a.m. Current Treatment of Asthma
Richard F. Lockey, M.D.

9:30 - 10:00 a.m. Food Allergy - Diagnosis and Treatment
John J. Condemi, M.D.

10:00 - 10:30 a.m. CASE REPORTS
1) Bee Sting Allergy
Joseph D. Diaz, M.D.
2) Atopic Eczema
Robert P. Nelson, M.D.

10:30 - 11:00 a.m. **BREAK**

11:00 - 1:00 p.m. Meet the Professor Sessions
A. Vasculitis
Dennis K. Ledford, M.D.
B. Use of Cholinergic Agents in COPD
Philip L. Lieberman, M.D.
C. Current Treatment of Asthma
Richard F. Lockey, M.D.
D. Food Allergy - Diagnosis and Treatment
John J. Condemi, M.D.

SATURDAY, DECEMBER 5, 1987

7:30 - 7:55 a.m. CONTINENTAL BREAKFAST

SESSION III

7:55 - 8:00 a.m. MODERATOR - Roger W. Fox, M.D.

8:00 - 8:30 a.m. Sampling Allergens in the Microenvironment
Enrique Fernandez-Caldas, Ph.D.

8:30 - 9:00 a.m. Fiberoptic Rhinolaryngoscopy
Roger W. Fox, M.D.

9:00 - 9:30 a.m. Laboratory Diagnosis of Autoimmune Disease
John J. Condemi, M.D.

9:30 - 10:00 a.m. Penicillin Allergy
Philip L. Lieberman, M.D.

10:00 - 10:30 a.m. **BREAK**

10:30 - 11:00 a.m. IgG Subclass Deficiency
Robert P. Nelson, M.D.

11:00 - 11:30 a.m. Connective Tissue Disease and Immune Deficiency
Luis R. Espinoza, M.D.

11:30 - 1:00 p.m. Question and Answer

LOCAL FACULTY

From the University of South Florida and James A. Haley Veterans Administration Hospital, Tampa, Florida.

College of Medicine:

Gerald A. Bucholtz, M.D.
Assistant Professor of Medicine
Division of Allergy and Immunology

Samuel C. Bukantz, M.D.
Professor of Medicine
Director Emeritus
Division of Allergy and Immunology

Joseph D. Diaz, M.D.
Advanced Subspecialty Resident
Division of Allergy and Immunology

Luis R. Espinoza, M.D.
Professor of Medicine
Divisions of Rheumatology and Allergy and Immunology

Enrique Fernandez-Caldas, Ph.D.
Assistant Professor of Medicine
Division of Allergy and Immunology

Roger W. Fox, M.D.
Assistant Professor of Medicine
Division of Allergy and Immunology

Dennis K. Ledford, M.D.
Assistant Professor of Medicine
Division of Allergy and Immunology

Richard F. Lockey, M.D.
Professor of Medicine and Pediatrics
Director, Division of Allergy and Immunology

Robert P. Nelson, M.D.
Advanced Subspecialty Resident
Division of Allergy and Immunology

Rajendra N. Pahwa, M.D.
Professor of Pediatrics
Head, Immunology Division and Bone Marrow Transplant Unit
All Children's Hospital, St. Petersburg, Florida

College of Public Health:

Stuart M. Brooks, M.D.
Chairman, Department of Environmental and Occupational Health
Professor of Medicine
Professor, College of Public Health

COURSE DESCRIPTION

Welcome to Disney World, EPCOT and Lake Buena Vista. This course is for all practicing physicians interested in allergic, pulmonary and immunologic diseases. It is designed as an update of current pathogenesis, precipitating factors and treatment of asthma; diagnosis and treatment of food allergy; and laboratory diagnosis and treatment of various types of autoimmune diseases. The program will also include timely lectures on fiberoptic rhinolaryngoscopy, sampling allergens in the microenvironment and IgG subclass deficiencies. Other topics of interest will be presented.

There will be a series of case reports and "Meet the Professor" conferences as well as concise formal presentations on subjects of interest to the clinician. The case reports are designed to complement the formal presentations. The "Meet the Professor" conference will be group sessions allowing active dialogue between the speakers and participants.

In summary, this conference is designed for clinicians who care for and treat patients in a practice setting. It allows the physician ample time for learning and for recreation in an environment conducive to both. The faculty of the Division of Allergy and Immunology at the University of South Florida College of Medicine and the American Academy of Allergy and Immunology invite your participation in the sixth annual conference entitled "Clinical Allergy and Immunology for the Practicing Physician".

GUEST FACULTY

John J. Condemi, M.D.
Clinical Professor of Medicine
University of Rochester Medical School
Rochester, New York

Philip L. Lieberman, M.D.
Clinical Professor of Medicine and Pediatrics
Allergy/Immunology Section
University of Tennessee
Memphis, Tennessee

American Academy of Allergy and Immunology

REQUEST FOR ACCOMMODATIONS

[Mail direct to Buena Vista Palace]

CLINICAL ALLERGY and IMMUNOLOGY
for the PRACTICING PHYSICIAN
DECEMBER 3-5, 1987
BUENA VISTA PALACE
WALT DISNEY WORLD VILLAGE
P.O. BOX 22206
LAKE BUENA VISTA, FLORIDA 32830-2206
(305) 827-2727

Contact the Buena Vista Palace directly, for room accommodations or mail in form.

Convention rate per room, plus applicable taxes. [Convention rates apply 3 days prior and 3 days after meeting dates, subject to availability]. Deposits are refundable if cancelled 5 days prior to and not including the arrival date.

To guarantee a reservation, please forward a one-night room deposit of $106.92 [includes tax] by November 1, 1987.

Convention Rate $99.00
Single thru Quad

_________# of rooms _________# of persons

Please list names of additional members in your party and include childrens' ages.

____

____

NAME ______________________________

ADDRESS ______________________________

CITY ______________________________

STATE ______________ ZIP ______________

ARRIVAL DATE __________ TIME __________ AM/PM

DEPARTURE DATE ______________________________

Circle card name and fill in the following to guarantee your reservation by credit card:

VISA DINERS CLUB MASTER CARD AMERICAN EXPRESS

____

Expiration Date ______________________________

______________________________ ______________

Signature Date

PREREGISTRATION FORM

CLINICAL ALLERGY and IMMUNOLOGY for the PRACTICING PHYSICIAN

WALT DISNEY WORLD BUENA VISTA PALACE

Please Print or Type:

NAME ______________________________

ADDRESS ______________________________

CITY ______________________________

STATE ______________ ZIP ______________

PHONE NO. (   ) ______________________________

SPECIALTY ______________________________

Registration Fee: [Check one]
Regular —$250.00
Resident or Intern —$100.00
[U.S. Currency only]

The number of registrants will be limited, therefore, early registration is encouraged.

Return form with registration fee made payable to The American Academy of Allergy and Immunology at the following address:

American Academy of Allergy and Immunology
ATTENTION: Mary Fogarty
611 East Wells Street
Milwaukee, Wisconsin 53202

For questions call Mary Fogarty at 414/272-6071.

Refunds for cancellations made prior to November 3, 1987 will be made less a $50.00 administration fee.

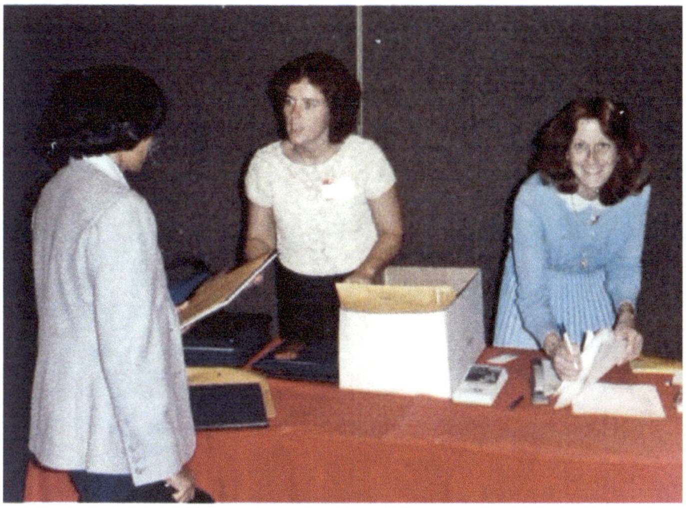

Left to right: Pat Walsh and Peggy Hales, registration desk, circa 1987.

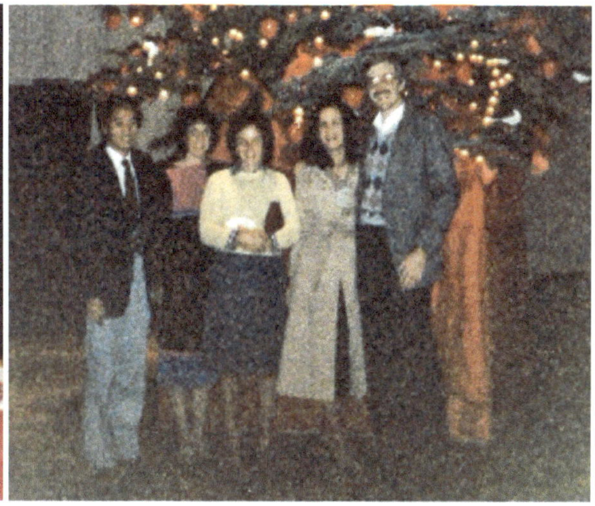

Left to right: Steven J. Louie, MD (1981-1983); Barbara Louie; Pat Walsh; Jennifer Ledford; Dennis K. Ledford, MD (1983-1985). Buena Vista Palace lobby, circa 1987.

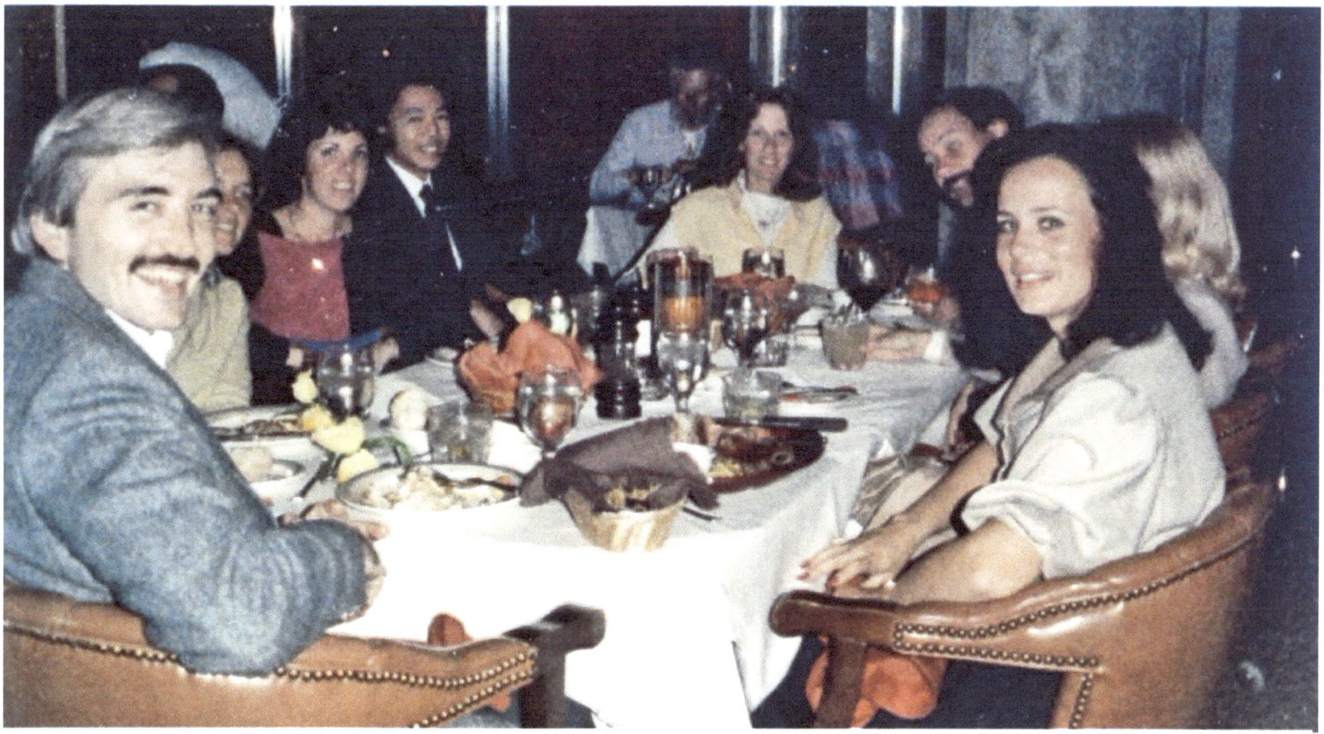

Clockwise from the left: Dennis K. Ledford, MD (1983-1985); Pat Walsh; arbara Louie; Steven J. Louie, MD (1981-1983); Peggy Hales; Gerald A. Bucholtz, MD (1980-1982); Randi Bucholtz; Jennifer Ledford; dinner, circa 1987.

CLINICAL ALLERGY and IMMUNOLOGY for the PRACTICING PHYSICIAN

This annual conference is intended for all practicing physicians interested in allergic, pulmonary and immunologic disease.

DECEMBER 8 - 10, 1988

BUENA VISTA PALACE, WALT DISNEY WORLD VILLAGE BUENA VISTA, FLORIDA

TOPICS INCLUDE:

- Precipitating Factors and Treatment of Asthma
- Pulmonary Function Studies
- Occupational Lung Disease
- AIDS Update
- Chronic EB Virus Syndrome

SPONSORED BY:

THE AMERICAN ACADEMY OF ALLERGY and IMMUNOLOGY

THE DIVISION OF ALLERGY and IMMUNOLOGY
DEPARTMENT OF INTERNAL MEDICINE
UNIVERSITY OF SOUTH FLORIDA, COLLEGE OF MEDICINE

COURSE DESCRIPTION

The faculty of Division of Allergy and Immunology at the University of South Florida College of Medicine and the American Academy of Allergy and Immunology welcome your participation in the 7th Annual Conference "Clinical Allergy and Immunology for the Practicing Physician".

This course is for all practicing physicians interested in allergic and immunologic diseases. There are lectures covering the precipitating factors and treatment of asthma as well as the laboratory diagnosis and treatment of various immunologic diseases. The program will also include timely lectures on occupational lung disease, monitoring the indoor environment, in vivo and in vitro testing of the allergic patient and anaphylaxis. Other topics of interest, such as the chronic EB viral syndrome, will also be presented.

There will be a series of case reports and "Meet the Professor" conferences. Case reports are designed to complement the formal lectures. The "Meet the Professor" conferences will enable active dialogue between the speakers and participants.

In summary, the conference is designed for clinicians who care for and treat patients in a practice setting. It allows the physician ample time for learning and for recreation in an environment conducive to both.

ACCREDITATION

The University of South Florida College of Medicine is accredited by the Accreditation Council for Continuing Medical Education to sponsor continuing medical education for physicians.

The University of South Florida College of Medicine certifies that this continuing medical education program meets the criteria for 14 hours of credit in Category I for the Physician's Recognition Award of the American Medical Association.

This program has also been reviewed and is acceptable for 13½ prescribed hours by the American Academy of Family Physicians.

THE BUENA VISTA PALACE

From the first moment you arrive at the Buena Vista Palace, you begin to experience the excitement of a 21st Century resort that preserves the classic tradition of fine service and attention to detail. Towering 27 stories over EPCOT Center, the Buena Vista Palace provides regal accommodations with striking views of the Walt Disney World Vacation Kingdom. The service is impeccable, the value extraordinary - and each day is one of perfect enchantment.

Imagine four spires of reflective glass glittering like crystal in their reach for the sun. Below, a lake surrounds the resort like a medieval moat. Turrets and courtyards call to mind the enchantment of another era. A 12-story atrium welcomes you to this regal setting. Nature's own wealth of greenery fill every nook and corner and a glass elevator whisks you through a splashing waterfall to restaurants, convention facilities and private accommodations that are indeed palatial. Three elegant restaurants and four lounges invite you to gracious dining, exotic drinks, and top entertainment. The wide choice of on-site recreation allows any group to set its own pace. Facilities include tennis, swimming, health spa with hot tub, sauna and jacuzzi, and nearby are 54 holes of championship golf.

A short stroll across the Boulevard takes you to the Village Market Place, a picturesque lakefront collection of specialty shops, restaurants, and one-of-a-kind lounges. A casual elegance and a leisurely pace characterize the Village, and promise hours of browsing.

Right outside your Palace resort lies a whole world of enchantment in the Walt Disney World Vacation Kingdom. Mickey and the gang bring a lifetime of memories at the Magic Kingdom . . . at Epcot Center you experience the wonders of today and exciting visions of tomorrow. Complimentary Walt Disney World Shuttle transportation departs from the Palace every 15 minutes to take you throughout the Vacation Kingdom.

BUENA VISTA PALACE
Walt Disney World Village

PROGRAM

WEDNESDAY, DECEMBER 7, 1988

6:30 - 7:30 p.m.	PREREGISTRATION

THURSDAY, DECEMBER 8, 1988

7:00 - 7:55 a.m.	REGISTRATION
7:30 - 7:55 a.m.	CONTINENTAL BREAKFAST
	SESSION I
7:55 - 8:00 a.m.	WELCOME - **Richard F. Lockey, M.D.**
	MODERATOR: Gerald A. Bucholtz, M.D.
8:00 - 8:30 a.m.	Occupational Lung Disease - **Stuart M. Brooks, M.D.**
8:30 - 9:00 a.m.	Allergic Rhinitis - **Gerald A. Bucholtz, M.D.**
9:00 - 9:30 a.m.	All That Wheezes is Not Asthma - **Roy H. Behnke, M.D.**
9:30 - 10:00 a.m.	Treatment of Severe Asthma - **Richard F. Lockey, M.D.**
10:00 - 10:30 a.m.	CASE REPORTS
	1) Sulfite Sensitive Asthmatics - **Donald W. Russell, M.D.**
	2) Occupational Asthma - **Gerald A. Bucholtz, M.D.**
10:30 - 11:00 a.m.	*BREAK*
11:00 - 1:00 p.m.	MEET THE PROFESSOR SESSIONS
	1) Occupational Lung Disease - **Stuart M. Brooks, M.D.**
	2) Allergic Rhinitis - **Gerald A. Bucholtz, M.D.**
	3) All That Wheezes is Not Asthma - **Roy H. Behnke, M.D.**
	4) Treatment of Severe Asthma - **Richard F. Lockey, M.D.**

FRIDAY, DECEMBER 9, 1988

7:00 - 7:55 a.m.	CONTINENTAL BREAKFAST
	SESSION II
7:55 - 8:00 a.m.	**MODERATOR:** Dennis K. Ledford, M.D.
8:00 - 8:30 a.m.	AIDS Update - **James M. Oleske, M.D.**
8:30 - 9:00 a.m.	Clinical Evaluation of the Patient with Suspected Chronic Fatigue Syndrome (Chronic EB Virus Syndrome) - **Dennis K. Ledford, M.D.**
9:00 - 9:30 a.m.	In Vivo Testing to Diagnose Allergic Diseases - **Samuel C. Bukantz, M.D.**
9:30 - 10:00 a.m.	Laboratory Diagnosis of Allergic and Immunologic Diseases - **Richard D. deShazo, M.D.**
10:00 - 10:30 a.m.	Monitoring the Indoor Environment and Its Relationship to Respiratory Disease - **Enrique Fernandez-Caldas, Ph.D.**
10:30 - 11:00 a.m.	*BREAK*
11:00 - 1:00 p.m.	MEET THE PROFESSOR SESSIONS
	1) AIDS Update - **James M. Oleske, M.D.**
	2) Clinical Evaluation of the Patient with Suspected Chronic Fatigue Syndrome (Chronic EB Virus Syndrome) - **Dennis K. Ledford, M.D.**
	3) In Vivo Testing to Diagnose Allergic Diseases - **Samuel C. Bunkantz, M.D.**
	4) Laboratory Diagnosis of Allergy and Immunologic Diseases - **Richard D. deShazo, M.D.**
	5) Monitoring the Indoor Environment and Its Relationship to Respiratory Disease - **Enrique Fernandez-Caldas, Ph.D.**

SATURDAY, DECEMBER 10, 1988

7:30 - 7:55 a.m.	CONTINENTAL BREAKFAST
	SESSION III
7:55 - 8:00 a.m.	**MODERATOR:** - Robert P. Nelson, M.D.
8:00 - 8:30 a.m.	Anaphylaxis - **Roger W. Fox, M.D.**
8:30 - 9:00 a.m.	The Proper Use of IV Gammaglobulin by the Practicing Physician - **James M. Oleske, M.D.**
9:00 - 9:30 a.m.	Vaccination of the Adult Patient - **Rama Ganguly, Ph.D.**
9:30 - 10:00 a.m.	Immunologic Lung Diseases - **Richard D. deShazo, M.D.**
10:00 - 10:30 a.m.	*BREAK*
10:30 - 11:00 a.m.	Bone Marrow Transplantation - When is It Indicated? - **Robert P. Nelson, M.D.**
11:00 - 11:30 a.m.	CASE REPORTS
	1) Nasal Polyposis - **David N. Wright, M.D.**
	2) Allergic Bronchopulmonary Aspergillosis - **Richard P. Silton, M.D.**
11:30 - 1:00 p.m.	Questions and Answers

COURSE DIRECTOR

RICHARD F. LOCKEY, M.D.	University of South Florida College of Medicine, Professor of Medicine, Pediatrics and Public Health Director, Division of Allergy and Immunology

LOCAL FACULTY

University of South Florida College of Medicine

ROY H. BEHNKE, M.D.	Professor and Chairman, Department of Internal Medicine
STUART M. BROOKS, M.D.	Chairman, Department of Environmental & Occupational Health, Professor of Medicine, Division of Allergy and Immunology Professor, College of Public Health
GERALD A. BUCHOLTZ, M.D.	Assistant Professor of Medicine, Division of Allergy and Immunology
SAMUEL C. BUKANTZ, M.D.	Professor of Medicine - Director Emeritus, Division of Allergy and Immunology
ENRIQUE FERNANDEZ-CALDAS, PH.D.	Assistant Professor of Medicine, Division of Allergy and Immunology
ROGER W. FOX, M.D.	Associate Professor of Medicine, Division of Allergy and Immunology
RAMA GANGULY, PH.D.	Professor of Medicine, Divisions of Allergy and Immunology & Infectious Diseases
DENNIS K. LEDFORD, M.D.	Assistant Professor of Medicine Divisions of Allergy and Immunology & Rheumatology
ROBERT P. NELSON, M.D.	Assistant Professor of Medicine and Pediatrics, Division of Allergy and Immunology
DONALD W. RUSSELL, M.D.	Advanced Subspecialty Resident, Division of Allergy and Immunology
RICHARD P. SILTON, M.D.	Advanced Subspecialty Resident, Division of Allergy and Immunology
DAVID N. WRIGHT, M.D.	Advanced Subspecialty Resident, Division of Allergy and Immunology

GUEST FACULTY

JAMES M. OLESKE, M.D.	Professor of Pediatrics, Medicine and Pathology, UMDNJ - New Jersey Medical School Newark, New Jersey
RICHARD D. deSHAZO, M.D.	Professor of Medicine and Pediatrics, Tulane University School of Medicine New Orleans, Louisiana

FINANCIAL SUPPORT

We wish to express our appreciation to the following pharmaceutical companies for their generous support:

Allergy Control Products, Inc.
Becton-Dickinson [B-D]
Center Laboratories
Dura Pharmaceuticals, Inc.
Fisons Corporation
Glaxo, Inc.
Greer Laboratories, Inc.
Janssen Research Foundation, Inc.
Merrell Dow Pharmaceuticals Inc.
Muro Pharmaceutical, Inc.
Parke-Davis
Purdue Frederick Co.
Roerig (Pfizer Pharmaceuticals)
Rorer (Dermik Laboratories, Inc.)
Sandoz Pharmaceuticals
Schering Corporation
Searle
Storz Instrument Company
Wallace Laboratories

PREREGISTRATION FORM

CLINICAL ALLERGY and IMMUNOLOGY for the PRACTICING PHYSICIAN
WALT DISNEY WORLD - BUENA VISTA PALACE

Please Print or Type:

NAME ______________________________

ADDRESS ______________________________

CITY ______________ STATE ______________ ZIP ______

PHONE NO. ( ) ______________________________

SPECIALTY ______________________________

Registration Fee: (Check one)
Regular — $250.00
Resident or Intern — $100.00
(U.S. Currency only)

The number of registrants will be limited, therefore, early registration is encouraged.

Return form with registration fee made payable to The American Academy of Allergy and Immunology at the following address:

American Academy of Allergy and Immunology
ATTENTION: Donna Kaczmarek
611 East Wells Street, Milwaukee, Wisconsin 53202

For questions call Donna Kaczmarek at 414/272-6071.

Refunds for cancellations made prior to November 8, 1988 will be made less a $50.00 administration fee.

REQUEST FOR ACCOMMODATIONS (Mail direct to Buena Vista Palace)

CLINICAL ALLERGY and IMMUNOLOGY for the PRACTICING PHYSICIAN
DECEMBER 8-10, 1988
BUENA VISTA PALACE, WALT DISNEY WORLD VILLAGE
P.O. BOX 22206, LAKE BUENA VISTA, FLORIDA 32830-2206 • Phone (305) 827-2727

Contact the Buena Vista Palace directly for room accommodations or mail in form.

Convention rate per room, plus applicable taxes. (Convention rates apply 3 days prior and 3 days after meeting dates, subject to availability). Deposits are refundable if cancelled 5 days prior to and not including the arrival date.

To guarantee a reservation, please forward a one-night room deposit of $114.45 (includes tax) by November 1, 1988.

Convention Rate $105.00 Single thru Quad

______________ # of rooms ______________ # of persons

Please list names of additional members in your party and include childrens' ages.

____

____

NAME ______________________________

ADDRESS ______________________________

CITY ______________ STATE ______ ZIP ______

ARRIVAL DATE ______________ TIME ______________ AM ______ PM ______

DEPARTURE DATE ______________________________

Circle card name and fill in the following to guarantee your reservation by credit card. Credit card will process first night's room deposit:

VISA   DINERS CLUB   MASTER CARD   AMERICAN EXPRESS

______________________________ Expiration Date ______________

____

Signature   Date

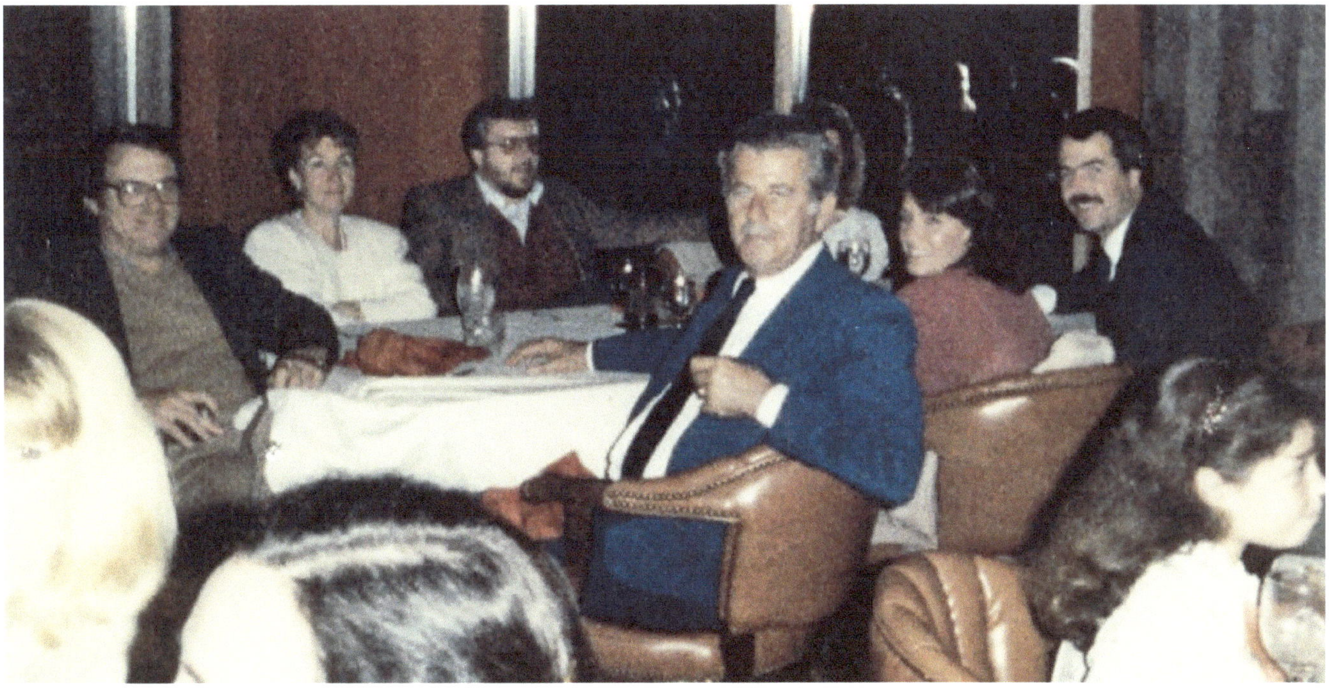

Left side of table (left to right): Richard F. Lockey, MD, MS; Carol Lee Lockey, James E. Lockey, MD (University of Cincinnati; Division of Environmental and Occupational Medicine; guest speaker). Right side of table (left to right): Samuel C. Bukantz, MD; Diane Stablein; John J. Stablein, MD (1979-1981). Dinner, Lake Buena Vista Palace, circa 1989.

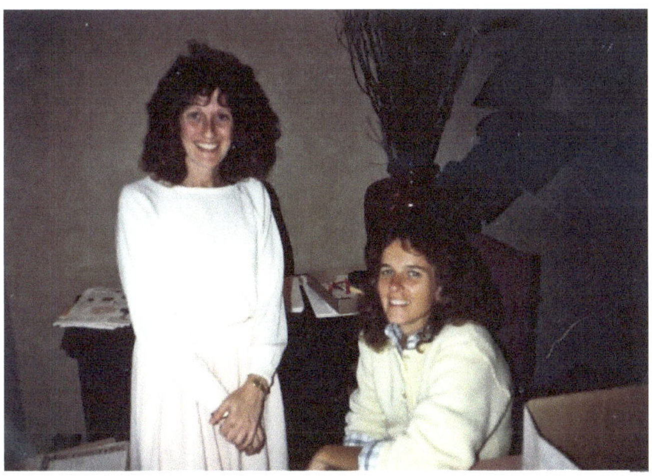

Left to right: Peggy Hales and Pat Walsh. Registration desk, circa 1989.

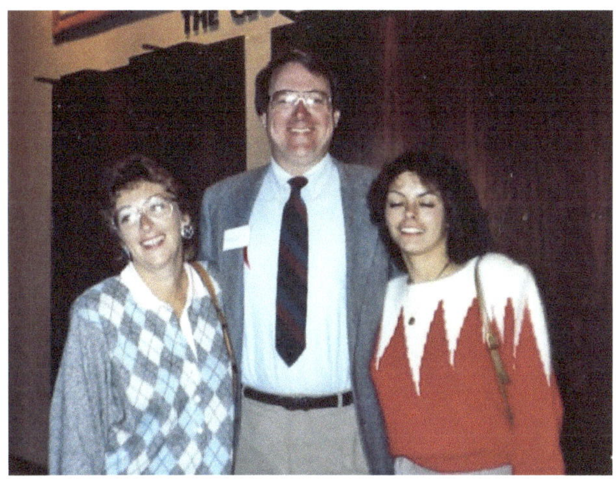

Left to right: Dona Shearer (office manager, clinical office of Drs. Lockey, Fox, Ledford); Richard F. Lockey, MD, MS; Robin Crabb

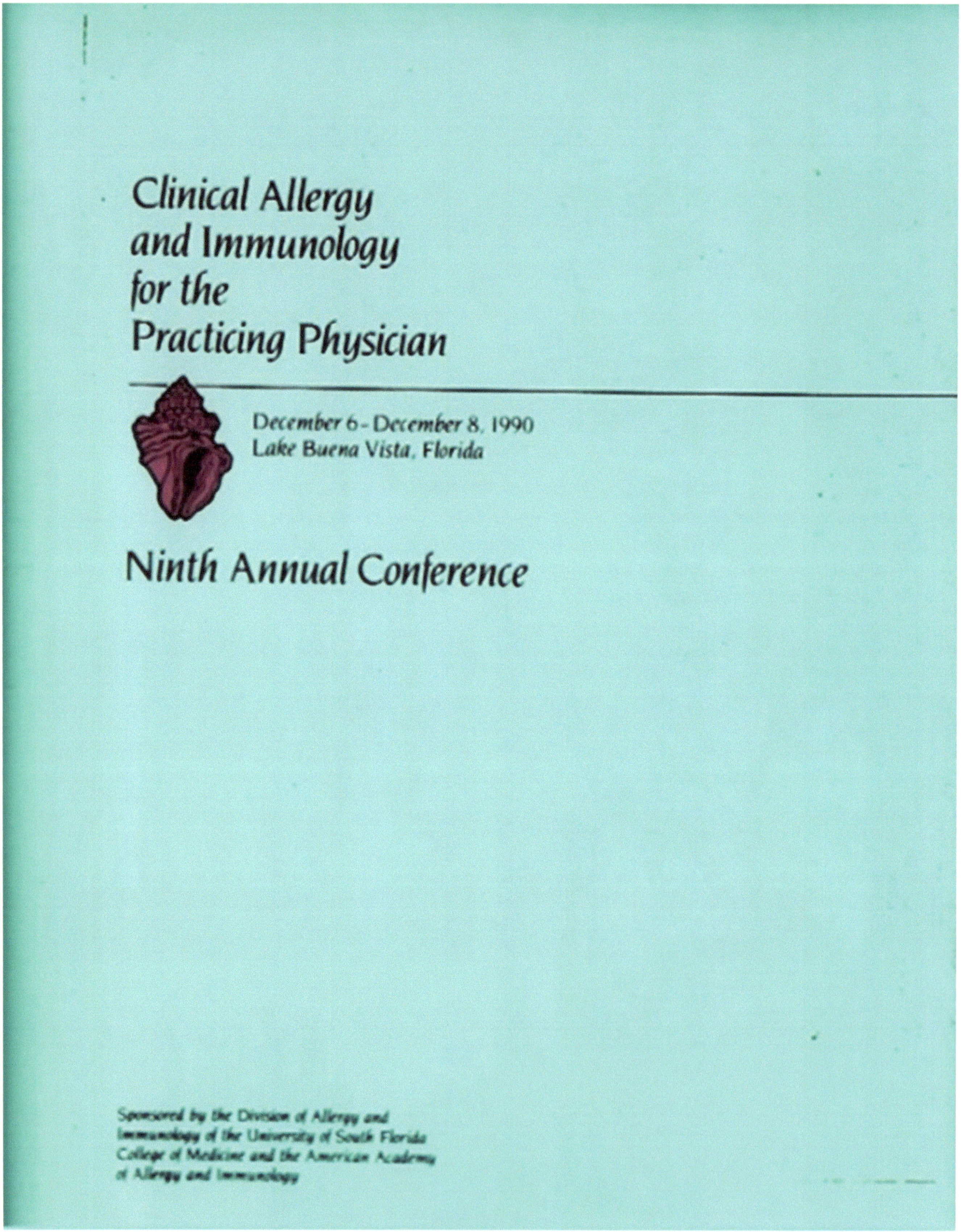

1990 Conference folder/notepad compliments of Parke-Davis.

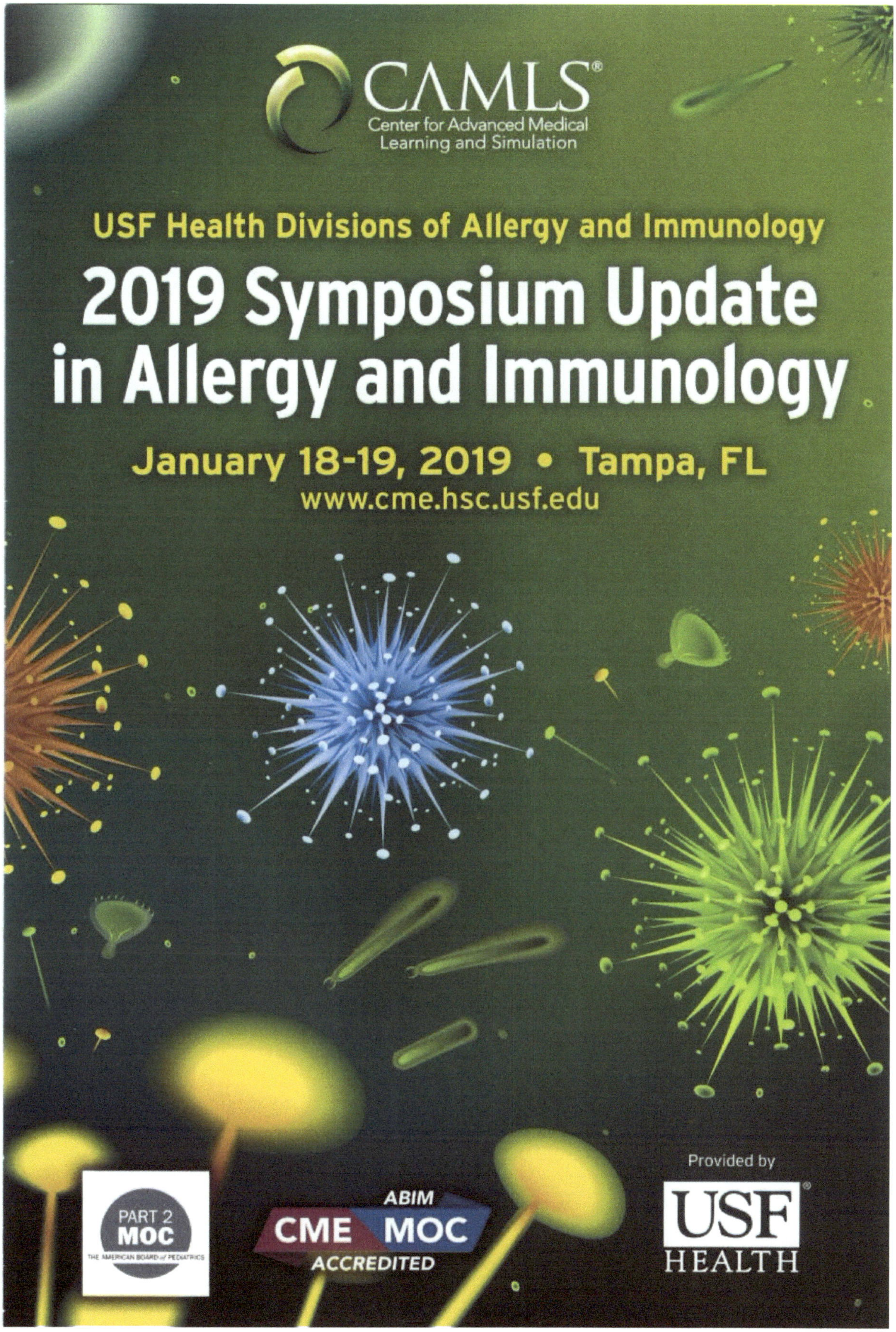
CAMLS®
Center for Advanced Medical Learning and Simulation
USF Health Divisions of Allergy and Immunology
2019 Symposium Update in Allergy and Immunology
January 18-19, 2019 • Tampa, FL
www.cme.hsc.usf.edu
PART 2 MOC
THE AMERICAN BOARD of PEDIATRICS
ABIM
CME MOC
ACCREDITED
Provided by
USF® HEALTH

The conference will focus on the latest breakthroughs and recommendations to evaluate and manage asthma, its pathogenesis, diagnosis, and treatment; food allergy, its diagnosis and treatment; and current and future treatments of primary immunodeficiency diseases. Other subjects include: comorbid conditions of asthma; mechanisms, efficacy, substitution, and proper use of asthma inhalers; nasal polyps; common allergic and nonallergic dermatologic problems and a gastroenterologist's versus an allergist/immunologist's perspective of eosinophilic esophagitis. **A rhinoscopy breakout skills session is available the first morning for 20 physicians.**

Concurrent Sessions

New this year - the full conference will begin for all learners on the morning of the first day with two concurrent sessions. One session will be the rhinoscopy skills workshop which is limited to 20 physicians (Preregistration is required for the rhinoscopy workshop). The other concurrent session, on Severe Asthma and its Comorbid Conditions, will be for all other conference attendees. The Asthma session is included in the registration as part of the full activity.

Target Audience

This activity is designed to meet the educational needs of Internal Medicine physicians, (ABIM MOC Points available) and Pediatric physicians (ABP MOC Part 2 credit available), Family Medicine, Emergency Medicine, and Allergy/Immunology physician specialists. The target audience also includes Physician Assistants, Advanced Practice Nurses, Registered Nurses, Residents, Medical Students and any other healthcare practitioners who care for patients with allergic and immunologic disorders.

Learning Objectives

As a result of participating in this activity, participants should be able to:

1. **Perform** a diagnostic examination of the upper airway with a flexible rhinoscope (for those participating in the Rhinoscopy workshop only)
2. **Recognize** and treat acute and severe asthma
3. **List** the co-morbid conditions associated with asthma
4. **Recognize** the evolution of asthma during a lifetime and the infectious diseases, which exacerbate or are associated with asthma
5. **Explain** how practice-based learning will enhance the understanding, diagnosis, and treatment of acute asthma and co-morbid conditions of asthma.
6. **Describe** spirometry; peak flow and how to perform and interpret results
7. **Identify** the main dermatologic problems in any medical practice
8. **Identify** the difference between food intolerance versus allergy
9. **Summarize** eosinophilic esophagitis, its diagnosis and treatment

Competencies

The competencies being addressed are patient care and procedural skills, medical knowledge, interpersonal and communication skills, and professionalism.

ABIM MOC Points

This entire activity has been approved for ABIM MOC Points for Internal Medicine. In order to obtain ABIM MOC Points, the Internal Medicine participant must:

- Provide their ABIM Number during registration
- Provide permission during registration for USF Health to share their completion data with the ACCME, to be transmitted on behalf of the participant to the ABIM
- Attend the entire session (No partial MOC points are being offered)
- Post-course: complete the activity evaluation
- Pass the course post-test with a score of ≥ 80%

This entire activity has been approved for ABP MOC Part 2 credits. In order to obtain ABP MOC credits, the Pediatrician must:

- Provide their ABP Number during registration
- Provide permission during registration for USF Health to share their completion data with the ACCME, to be transmitted on behalf of the participant to the ABP
- Attend the entire session (No partial MOC points are being offered)
- Post-course: complete the activity evaluation
- Pass the course post-test with a score of ≥ 80%

This program does not require prerequisites. Learning objectives apply to all professions in the target audience.

Agenda

Day One: Friday, January 18, 2019 (6:45am - 6:00pm)	
Concurrent Sessions	
6:45-7:35am	**Symposium Registration and Breakfast**
Concurrent Session: Rhinoscopy Skills *(Limited to 20 physician participants; pre-registration required)*	
7:35-8:30am	Didactic Session - Rhinoscopy, Key Diagnostic Tool for Upper Airway Diseases ~ Mark C. Glaum, M.D., Ph.D.
8:30am-12:00pm	Rhinoscopy Skills: Cadaver and Live Subjects
Concurrent Session: Severe Asthma and Comorbid Conditions	
7:35-9:30am	Severe Asthma ~ Thomas B. Casale, M.D.
9:30-10:00am	Break
10:00am-12:00pm	Comorbid Conditions of Asthma ~ Dennis K. Ledford, M.D.
Plenary Sessions Asthma and Dermatology	
12:00-1:00pm	**Lunch and Exhibits**
1:00-1:25pm	Spirometry and Peak Flow: How are They Performed and What Do They Mean? ~ Farnaz Tabatabaian, M.D.
1:25-1:50pm	Acute Asthma: Diagnosis and Treatment ~ Richard F. Lockey, M.D.
1:50-2:15pm	Mechanisms and Efficacy of Asthma Inhalers ~ Shiven Patel, M.D.
2:15-2:40pm	Inhalers: Techniques for Proper Use ~ Amber N. Pepper, M.D.
2:40-3:10pm	**Break**
3:10-3:35pm	Pruritus: Diagnosis and Treatment ~ Roger W. Fox, M.D.
3:35-4:00pm	Atopic Dermatitis, Urticaria and Angioedema ~ Panida Sriaroon, M.D.
4:00-4:30pm	Top 10 Dermatologic Diseases in Any Medical Practice ~ Lucia Seminario Vidal, M.D., Ph.D.
4:30-5:30pm	Case Presentation and Discussion on Therapy for Primary Immunodeficiency, Now and in the Future ~ Jolan E. Walter, M.D., Ph.D., Moderator ~ Mark Ballow, M.D. ~ Jennifer Leiding, M.D.
5:30-6:00pm	**Questions and Answers**
6:00pm	**Adjourn**

Day Two: Saturday Morning, January 19, 2019 (7:00am-1:00pm)	
Asthma, Food Allergy, and Nasal Polyps	
7:00-8:00am	**Symposium Registration and Breakfast**
8:00-8:30am	Lifetime Evolution of Asthma ~ Robert F. Lemanske Jr., M.D.
8:30-9:00am	Viral, Bacterial, and Fungal Infections and Asthma ~ Robert F. Lemanske Jr., M.D.
9:00-9:30am	Phenotypes and Endotypes of Asthma ~ Juan Carlos Cardet, M.D., M.P.H.
9:30-10:00am	Nasal Polyposis: Pathogenesis and Treatment ~ Seong Cho, M.D.
10:00-10:30am	**Break**
10:30-11:00am	Food Intolerance Versus Allergy ~ Mark C. Glaum, M.D., Ph.D.
11:00-11:30am	Oral Immunotherapy: Is It Ready for Prime Time? ~ Thomas B. Casale, M.D.
11:30am-12:00pm	Eosinophilic Esophagitis: GI Perspective ~ Joel Richter, M.D.
12:00-12:30pm	Eosinophilic Esophagitis: Allergist/Immunologist Perspective ~ Dennis K. Ledford, M.D.
12:30-1:00pm	**Questions and Answers**
1:00pm	**Adjourn**

USF Health Divisions of Allergy and Immunology

2019 Symposium Update in Allergy and Immunology

January 18-19, 2019 Tampa, FL

Accreditation

ACCME: USF Health is accredited by the Accreditation Council for Continuing Medical Education (ACCME) to provide continuing medical education for physicians.

USF Health designates this live activity for a maximum of 12.50 *AMA PRA Category 1 Credits*™. Physicians should claim only the credit commensurate with the extent of their participation in the activity.

AAFP: Application for CME credit has been filed with the American Academy of Family Physicians (AAFP). The application number is: 81355.

ABIM MOC Points: Successful completion of this CME activity, which includes participation in the evaluation component, enables the participant to earn up to 12.50 MOC points in the American Board of Internal Medicine's (ABIM) Maintenance of Certification (MOC) program. Participants will earn MOC points equivalent to the amount of CME credits claimed for the activity. It is the CME activity healthcare professional's responsibility to submit participant completion information to the ACCME for granting ABIM MOC credit.

ABP MOC Credits: Successful completion of this CME activity, which includes participation in the activity, with individual assessments of the participant and feedback to the participant, enables the participant to earn 12.50 MOC points in the American Board of Pediatrics (ABP) Maintenance of Certification (MOC) program. It is the CME activity provider's responsibility to submit participant completion information to ACCME for the purpose of granting ABP MOC credit.

Nurses (Florida Board of Nurses): USF Health is an approved provider of continuing education for nurses through FBN 50-2970. This program has been approved for 12.50 contact hours.

One Easy Way to Register, Two Easy Ways to Pay

ONE EASY WAY TO REGISTER:

Go to www.cme.hsc.usf.edu and click on "Course Calendar"

TWO EASY WAYS TO PAY:

Pay by Credit Card Online: A payment confirmation will be emailed to the participant

Pay by Check: After registering online, a payment voucher with instructions will be emailed to the participant. Registration will not be confirmed until payment is received.

PLEASE NOTE: *Payment will not be accepted onsite.*

Friday A.M. Rhinoscopy Workshop (Limited to 20 physicians)	
Physician Workshop only	$400.00
Physicians Workshop and Main Conference	$500.00
Main Conference	
Physicians Main Conference only	$400.00
PA's and ARNP's	$300.00
Nurses	$200.00
Residents and Fellows	$100.00

Fees include the course content, hands-on experience (where applicable), syllabus, certificate of attendance, and food & beverage functions. No registration will be confirmed without full payment. Cancellations must be received in writing by December 15, 2018 and will be subject to a $50.00 processing fee. No refunds will be given for cancellations after December 15, 2018, but you may transfer your registration to a colleague.

The Office of Continuing Professional Development at USF Health reserves the right to cancel this program due to unforeseen circumstances. In the event of such cancellation, the full enrollment fee will be returned to the registrant.

EQUAL OPPORTUNITY

USF is an Equal Opportunity/Affirmative Action/Equal Access Institution. For disability accommodations contact the Office of Continuing Professional Development

AE2019112/1115

Faculty

USF Health Morsani College of Medicine

Divisions of Allergy and Immunology
Departments of Internal Medicine & Pediatrics
Tampa/St. Petersburg, FL

Director

Farnaz Tabatabaian, M.D.
Assistant Professor of Medicine

Co-Director

Richard F. Lockey, M.D.
University Distinguished Health Professor
Professor of Medicine, Pediatrics and Public Health
Director, Division of Allergy and Immunology
Department of Internal Medicine,
Joy McCann Culverhouse Chair of Allergy and Immunology

Faculty

Mark Ballow, M.D.
Professor of Pediatrics and Medicine

Juan Carlos Cardet, M.D., M.P.H.
Assistant Professor of Medicine and Pediatrics

Thomas B. Casale, M.D.
Professor of Medicine and Pediatrics

Seong H. Cho, M.D.
Associate Professor of Medicine and Pediatrics

Roger W. Fox, M.D.
Professor of Medicine, Pediatrics and Public Health

Mark C. Glaum, M.D., Ph.D.
Associate Professor of Medicine and Pediatrics

Dennis K. Ledford, M.D.
Professor of Medicine and Pediatrics
Mabel & Ellsworth Simmons Professor

Jennifer Leiding, M.D.
Associate Professor of Pediatrics and Medicine

Shiven Patel, M.D.
Chief Resident

Amber N. Pepper, M.D.
Associate Professor of Medicine and Pediatrics

Joel E. Richter, M.D., FACP, MACG
Professor of Medicine
Hugh F. Culverhouse Chair for Esophageal Disorders, Director, Division of Digestive Diseases & Nutrition, Director, Joy McCann Culverhouse Center for Swallowing Disorders
University Distinguished Health Professor

Panida Sriaroon, M.D.
Associate Professor of Pediatrics and Medicine

Jolan Walter, M.D., Ph.D.
Associate Professor of Pediatrics and Medicine
Robert A. Good Endowed Chair in Pediatric Immunology
Chief, Division of Allergy and Immunology
Department of Pediatrics

Lucia Seminario Vidal, M.D., Ph.D.
Associate Professor of Dermatology

Visiting Faculty

Robert F. Lemanske, Jr., M.D.
Professor of Pediatrics and Medicine
Associate Dean for Clinical and Translational Research
University of Wisconsin School of Medicine and Public Health, Madison, WI

Faculty Disclosure

USF Health adheres to the ACCME and FBN standards regarding commercial support of continuing medical education. It is the policy of USF Health that the faculty and planning committee disclose real or apparent conflicts of interest relating to the topics of this educational activity, that relevant conflicts of interest are resolved, and also that speakers will disclose any unlabeled or unapproved use of drugs or devices during their presentation. Detailed disclosure will be made in the course syllabus.

Disclaimer

The information provided at this CME/CE activity is for continuing education purposes only and is not meant to substitute for the independent medical/clinical judgment of a healthcare provider relative to diagnostic and treatment options of a specific patient's medical condition.

Meeting Location:

Center for Advanced Medical Learning and Simulation (CAMLS)
124 S. Franklin Street • Tampa, FL 33602
(813) 224-7860 • **www.camls-us.org**

Directions: Directions to CAMLS are available at: www.camls-us.org

Accommodations:

1. **Embassy Suites Downtown Convention Center**
2. **Marriott Waterside Downtown Tampa**
3. **Hilton Downtown Tampa**
4. **Marriott Courtyard**

All hotels are conveniently located in the heart of downtown Tampa and are within a 5-minute walking distance from USF Health CAMLS.

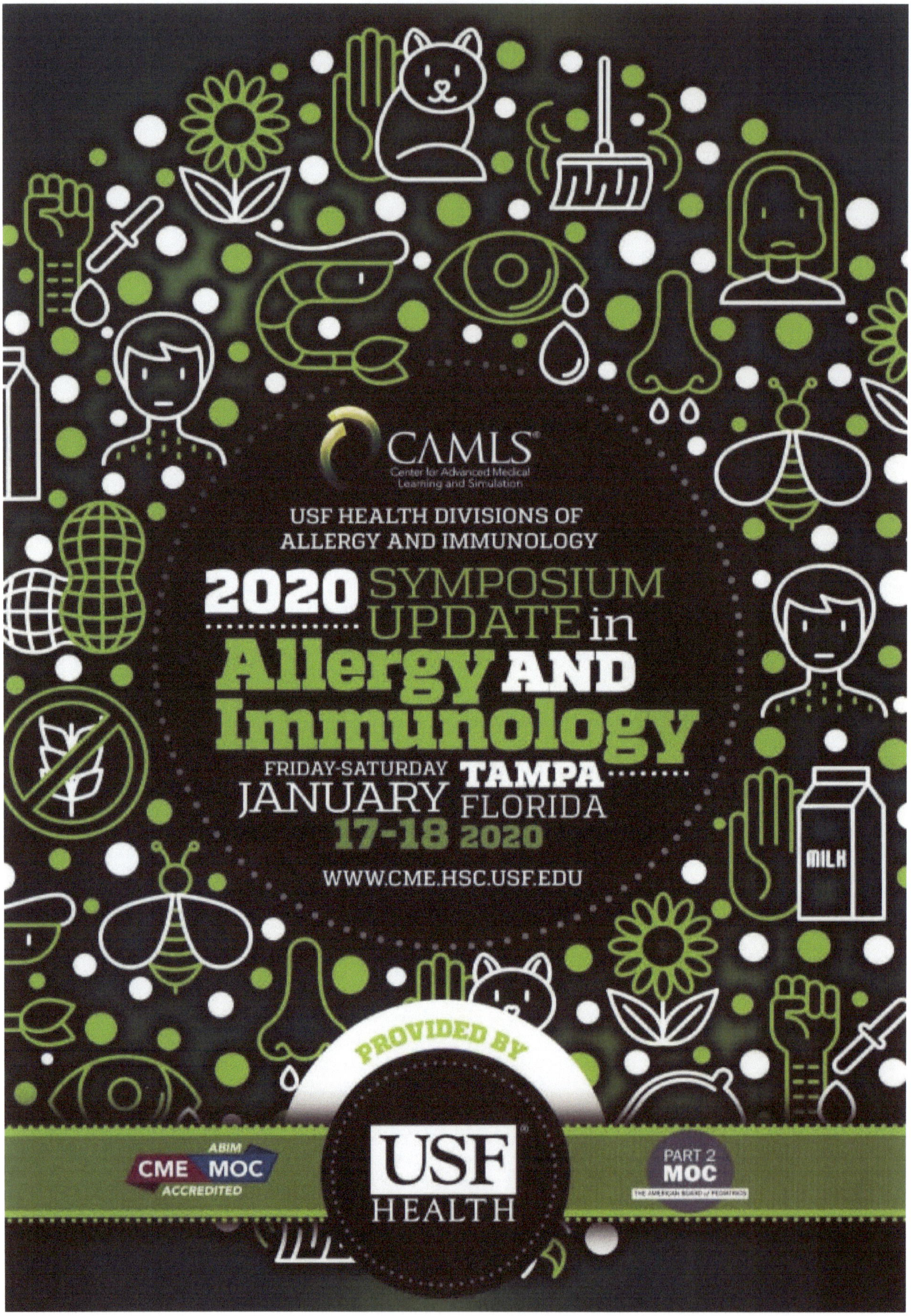
CAMLS
Center for Advanced Medical Learning and Simulation
USF HEALTH DIVISIONS OF
ALLERGY AND IMMUNOLOGY
2020 SYMPOSIUM
UPDATE in
Allergy AND
Immunology
FRIDAY-SATURDAY
JANUARY
17-18
TAMPA
FLORIDA
2020
WWW.CME.HSC.USF.EDU
MILK
PROVIDED BY
USF
HEALTH
ABIM
CME MOC
ACCREDITED
PART 2
MOC

FACULTY

Course Directors

DIRECTOR
Farnaz Tabatabaian, MD, MS
Assistant Professor of Medicine and Pediatrics

CO- DIRECTOR
Amber N. Pepper, MD
Assistant Professor of Medicine & Pediatrics

Senior Advisor
Richard F. Lockey, MD
University Distinguished Health Professor, Professor of Medicine, Pediatrics and Public Health; Director, Division of Allergy and Immunology, Department of of Internal Medicine; Joy McCann Culverhouse Chair of Allergy and Immunology

Faculty

Mark Ballow, MD
Professor of Pediatrics and Medicine

Karel Calero, MD
Assistant Professor of Pulmonary, Critical Care and Sleep Medicine

Jaun Carlos Cardet, MD, MPH
Assistant Professor of Medicine and Pediatrics

Thomas B. Casale, MD
Professor of Medicine and Pediatrics

Seong H. Cho, MD
Associate Professor of Medicine and Pediatrics

Roger W. Fox, MD
Professor of Medicine and Pediatrics

Mark C. Glaum, MD, PhD
Associate Professor of Medicine and Pediatrics

Dennis K. Ledford, MD
Professor of Medicine and Pediatrics, Mabel &Ellsworth Simmons Professor

Jennifer Leiding, MD
Associate Professor of Pediatrics and Medicine

Sagarika Nallu, MD
Assistant Professor of Pediatric Neurology, Epilepsy and Sleep Medicine

Tara V. Saco, MD
Graduate Fellow Allergy and Immunology

Mandel Sher, MD
Professor of Pediatrics and Medicine

Panida Sriaroon, MD
Associate Professor of Pediatrics and Medicine

Michael N. Teng, PhD
Associate Professor of Medicine and Pediatrics; Associate Dean, PhD and Postdoctoral, Programs: Graduate and Postdoctoral Affairs

Jolan Walter, MD, PhD
Associate Professor of Pediatrics and Medicine; Robert A. Good Endowed Chair in Pediatric Immunology; Chief, Division of Allergy and Immunology, Department of Pediatrics.

Hugh H. Windom, MD
Clinical Professor of Medicine and Pediatrics

Visiting Faculty

Mariana C. Castells, MD, PhD
Director, Drug Hypersensitivity and Desensitization Center; Director, Mastocytosis Center; Brigham and Women's Hospital; Professor in Medicine, Harvard Medical School

Joy Gaziano, MA, CCC-SLP, BCS-S
Director, Swallowing Rehabilitation Section, Joy McCann Culverhouse Center for Swallowing Disorders

AGENDA

THURSDAY, JANUARY 16, 2020

5:30 pm - 7:00 pm	**Welcome Reception (NON CE Lecture provided by AstraZeneca)** FESENRA TM (benralizumab) Subcutaneous Injection 30 mg: A Targeted Approach to Severe Eosinophilic Asthma	Dennis K. Ledford, MD

DAY 1: FRIDAY, JANUARY 17, 2020

06:45 - 7:35am	Symposium Registration and Breakfast	

CONCURRENT SESSIONS

RHINOSCOPY SKILLS WORKSHOP *(Limited to 20 physician participants only; pre-registration required)*

07:35 - 08:30 am	Didactic Session – Rhinoscopy, Key Diagnostic Tool for Upper Airway Diseases	Mark C. Glaum, MD, PhD & Seong Cho, MD
08:30 - 12:00 pm	Rhinoscopy Skills: Cadaver and Live Subjects	Mark C. Glaum, MD, PhD & Seong Cho, MD

PROBLEM-BASED LEARNING (PBL), CASE PRESENTATIONS, AND SLEEP APNEA

07:35 - 09:00 am	Severe Asthma: With or Without Monoclonals? (PBL)	Richard F. Lockey, MD, Dennis K. Ledford, MD and Thomas B. Casale, MD
09:00 - 09:30 am	Vocal Cord Dysfunction: Diagnosis and Treatment	Joy Gaziano, PhD
09:30 - 10:00 am	**Break**	
10:00 - 10:30 am	Sleep Apnea in Pediatrics: Diagnosis and Treatment	Sagarika Nallu, MD
10:30 - 11:00 am	Sleep Apnea in Adults: Diagnosis and Treatment	Karel Calero, MD
11:00 - 11:30 am	Exercise-Induced Brochospasm	Juan Carlos Cardet, MD
11:30 - 12:00 pm	Temporomandibular Joint (TMJ) Dysfunction and Headaches, Case Presentation and Discussion	Richard F. Lockey, MD and Fellow

PLENARY SESSIONS

12:00 - 1:00 pm	**Lunch**	
01:00 - 3:00 pm	IgE-Mediated vs. Non-IgE-Mediated Food Reactions: (PBL)	Mark C. Glaum, MD, PhD, Hugh Windom, MD, Amber Pepper, MD and Paninda Sriaroon, MD
3:00 - 3:30 pm	**Break**	
3:30 - 4:30 pm	Innate Immunity and Associated Diseases (PBL)	Dennis K. Ledford, MD Michael Teng, PhD, and Roger W. Fox, MD
4:30 - 5:30 pm	Adaptive Immunity and Immunodeficiency (PBL)	Jolan Walter MD, PhD Jennifer Leiding, MD, Emma Westermann-Clark, MD and Mark Ballow, MD
5:30 - 6:00 pm	**Questions and Answers**	

DAY 2: SATURDAY, JANUARY 18, 2020

7:00 - 8:00 am	**Symposium Registration and Breakfast**	
8:00 - 9:30 am	Drug Allergy (PBL)	Mariana C. Castells, MD,PhD
9:30 - 10:00 am	Mastocytosis	Tara Saco, MD and Fellow
10:00 - 10:30 am	**Break**	
10:30 - 11:00 am	Aeroallergens: What Are They and Clinical Importance	Mark C. Glaum, MD, PhD
11:00 - 11:30 am	Fungi (Molds) and Health in the Indoor Environment	Farnaz Tabatabaian MD, MS
11:30 - 12:00 pm	Urticaria and Angioedema: Diagnosis and Treatment	Roger Fox, MD and Fellow
12:00 - 12:30 pm	Contact Dermatitis: Diagnosis and Treatment	Mandel Sher, MD and Fellow
12:30 - 1:00 pm	**Questions and Answers**	
1:00 pm	**Adjourn**	

Faculty Disclosure

USF Health adheres to the ACCME and FBN standards regarding commercial support of continuing medical education. It is the policy of USF Health that the faculty and planning committee disclose real or apparent conflicts of interest relating to the topics of this educational activity, that relevant conflicts of interest are resolved, and also that speakers will disclose any unlabeled or unapproved use of drugs or devices during their presentation. Detailed disclosure will be made in the course syllabus.

Disclaimer

The information provided at this CME/CE activity is for continuing education purposes only and is not meant to substitute for the independent medical/clinical judgment of a healthcare provider relative to diagnostic and treatment options of a specific patient's medical condition.

Meeting Location:

Center for Advanced Medical Learning and Simulation (CAMLS)

124 S. Franklin Street
Tampa, FL 33602
813-224-7860
www.camls-us.org
Directions to CAMLS are available at:
www.camls-us.org

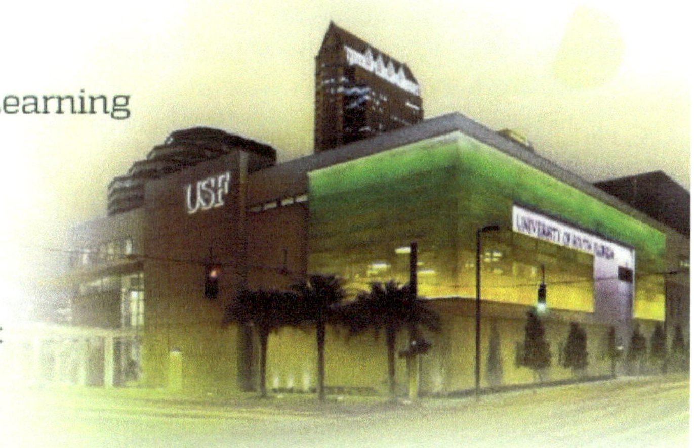

Parking:

Parking is available within one block of CAMLS at the Fort Brooke Garage off Whiting Street (107 S. Franklin Street) for $1.60 per hour or a maximum of $10 per day. There is a pedestrian walkway from the garage to CAMLS. The main entrance to CAMLS is located at the corner of Franklin Street & Brorein Street.

Accommodations:

1. **Embassy Suites Tampa Downtown Convention Center**
2. **Marriott Waterside Downtown Tampa**
3. **Hilton Downtown Tampa**
   * Referrence name CAMLS when making reservations
4. **Marriott Courtyard**

All hotels are conveniently located in the heart of downtown Tampa and are within a 5-minute walking distance from USF Health CAMLS.

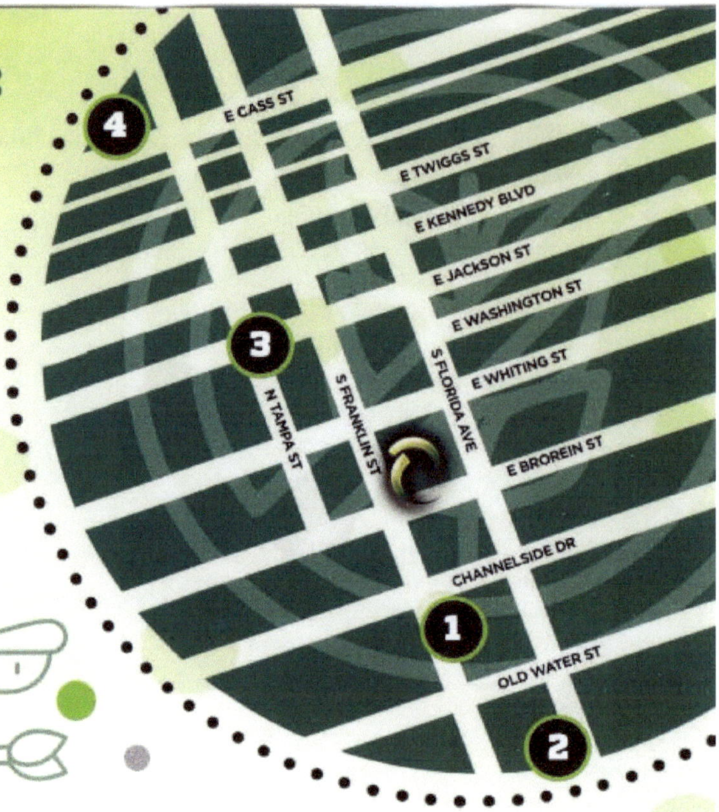

Registration

ONE EASY WAY TO REGISTER:

Go to www.cme.hsc.usf.edu and click on "Course Calendar"

TWO EASY WAYS TO PAY:

Pay by Credit Card Online: A payment confirmation will be emailed to the participant.

Pay by Check: After registering online, a payment voucher with instructions will be emailed to the participant.

Registration will not be confirmed until payment is received.

Fees include the course content, hands-on experience (where applicable), syllabus, certificate of attendance, and food & beverage functions. No registration will be confirmed without full payment. Cancellations must be received in writing by December 13, 2019 and will be subject to a $50.00 processing fee. No refunds will be given for cancellations after December 13, 2019, but you may transfer your registration to a colleague.

Friday A.M. Rhinoscopy Workshop (Physicians Only- limited to 20 physicians)	$400.00
Rhinoscopy Workshop and Main Conference	$500.00
Physicians Main Conference only	$400.00
PA's and ARNP's	$300.00
Nurses	$200.00
Residents and Fellows	$100.00

PLEASE NOTE: Cash or check payment will not be accepted onsite.

The Office of Continuing Professional Development at USF Health reserves the right to cancel this program due to unforeseen circumstances. In the event of such cancellation, the full enrollment fee will be returned to the registrant.

USF is an Equal Opportunity/Affirmative Action/Equal Access Institution. For disability accommodations contact the Office of Continuing Professional Developemnt.

Accreditation

Physicians

ACCME: USF Health is accredited by the Accreditation Council for Continuing Medical Education (ACCME) to provide continuing medical education for physicians.

USF Health designates this live activity for a maximum of 13.00 *AMA PRA Category 1 Credits*™. Physicians should claim only the credit commensurate with the extent of their participation in the activity.

AAFP: This Live activity, USF Health Allergy and Immunology 2020 Symposium Update in Allergy and Immunology, with a beginning date of 01/17/2020, has been reviewed and is acceptable for up to 13.25 Prescribed credit(s) by the American Academy of Family Physicians. Physicians should claim only the credit commensurate with the extent of their participation in the activity.

ABIM MOC Points: Successful completion of this CME activity, which includes participation in the evaluation component, enables the participant to earn up to 13.00 MOC points in the American Board of Internal Medicine's (ABIM) Maintenance of Certification (MOC) program. Participants will earn MOC points equivalent to the amount of CME credits claimed for the activity. It is the CME activity healthcare professional's responsibility to submit participant completion
information to the ACCME for granting ABIM MOC credit.

ABP MOC Credits: Successful completion of this CME activity, which includes participation in the activity, with individual assessments of the participant and feedback to the participant, enables the participant to earn 13.00 MOC points in the American Board of Pediatrics' (ABP) Maintenance of Certification (MOC) program. It is the CME activity provider's responsibility to submit participant completion information to ACCME for the purpose of granting ABP MOC credit.

Pharmacists

Day One: USF Health is accredited by the Accreditation Council for Pharmacy Education as a provider of continuing pharmacy education. This live program has been approved for 8.5 contact hours (0.85 CEUs). Universal program number is as follows: (0230-0000-20-001-L01-P).

Day Two: USF Health is accredited by the Accreditation Council for Pharmacy Education as a provider of continuing pharmacy education. This live program has been approved for 4.5 contact hours (0.45 CEUs). Universal program number is as follows: 0230-0000-002-L01-P.

Pharmacy Credit Disclosure: To receive continuing education credit, a pharmacist must attend the accredited sessions, actively participate in questions and answers, and must return the program evaluation instrument. In order to receive full credit, registrants must register no later than 10 minutes after the start of the meeting and must attend the entire meeting.

It is the responsibility of the pharmacy participant to ensure the provider has the learner's birthday and ePID/NABP number; it is the responsibility of the provider to submit to CPE Monitor participant information within 60 days of the activity for all participants who have attended, attested to their participation and provided their ePID/NABP number and birthdate.

ACPE indicates it is the responsibility of the pharmacy professional to confirm the status of their NABP contact hours before 60 days past the activity. If there are any discrepancies, contact the provider immediately. You may contact USF Health through cpdsupport@health.usf.edu.

Nurses (Florida Board of Nurses): USF Health is an approved provider of continuing education for nurses through FBN 50-2970. This program has been approved for 13.00 contact hours.

Course Description

The conference will focus on the breakthrough advances in allergy and immunology. A rhinoscopy breakout skills session is available the first morning.

Learning Objectives

As a result of participating in this activity, participants should be aable to:

Perform a diagnostic examination of the upper airway with a flexible rhinoscope (for those participating in the rhinoscopy workshop only)

Recognize and manage severe asthma

Recognize and treat tempomandibular joint (TMJ) dysfunction and headaches

List the important aeroallergens, including fungi, which cause allergic disease

Recognize different drug reactions

Discuss diagnosis and/or treatment guidelines of obstructive sleep apnea in children and adults

Describe the diagnosis and treatment of vocal cord dysfunction and mastocytosis

Discuss the difference between food intolerance and food allergy

Discuss innate and adaptive immunity and associated diseases

Target Audience

This activity is designed to meet the educational needs of internal medicine, (ABIM, MOC Points available) pediatrics (ABP MOC Part 2 credit available), family medicine, emergency medicine, allergy/immunology specialists and other physicians. The target audience also includes pharmacists, physician assistants, advanced practice nurses, registered nurses, residents, medical students and any other healthcare practitioner who cares for patients with allergic and immunologic disorders.

Competencies The competencies being addressed are patient care and procedural skills, medical knowledge, interpersonal and communication skills, and professionalism.

This entire activity has been approved for ABIM MOC Points for Internal Medicine. In order to obtain ABIM MOC Points, the Internal Medicine participant must:

- Provide their ABIM Number during registration
- Provide permission during registration for USF Health to share their completion data with the ACCME, to be transmitted on behalf of the participant to the ABIM
- Post-course: complete the activity evaluation
- Pass the course post-test with a score of ≥ 80%

ABIM CME MOC ACCREDITED

This entire activity has been approved for ABP MOC Part 2 credits. In order to obtain ABP MOC credits, the Pediatrician must:

- Provide their ABP Number during registration
- Provide permission during registration for USF Health to share their completion data with the ACCME, to be transmitted on behalf of the participant to the ABP
- Attend the entire session (No partial MOC points are being offered)
- Post-course: complete the activity evaluation
- Pass the course post-test with a score of ≥ 80%

PART 2 MOC THE AMERICAN BOARD of PEDIATRICS

Chapter 14: Select Commemorative Publications

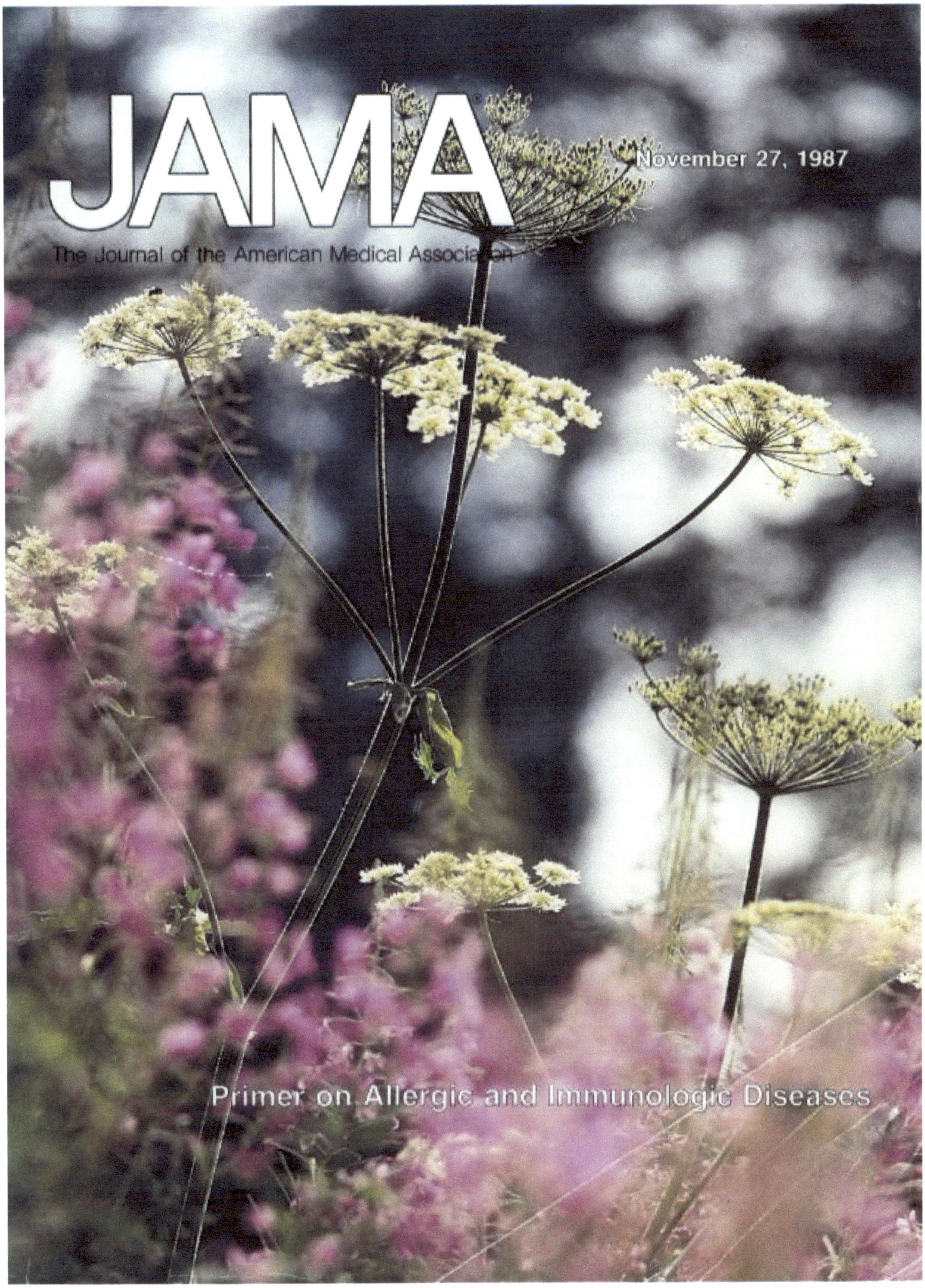

The Journal of the American Medical Association, JAMA Primer on Allergic and Immunologic Diseases, November 27, 1987, Vol. 258, No. 20. Richard F. Lockey, MD, MS and Samuel C. Bukantz, MD (Editors).

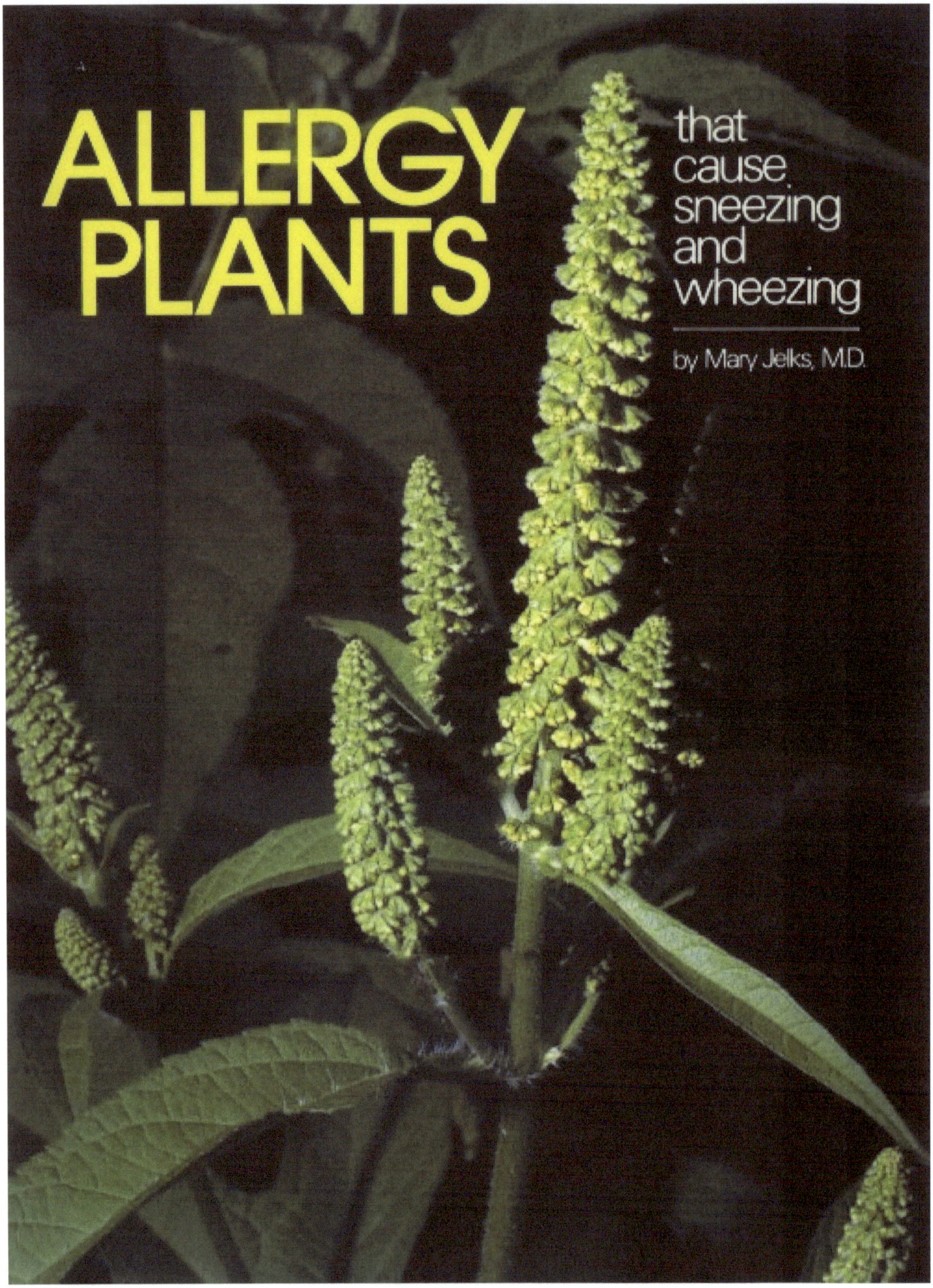

Allergy Plants That Cause Sneezing and Wheezing. Mary Jelks, MD; 1987.

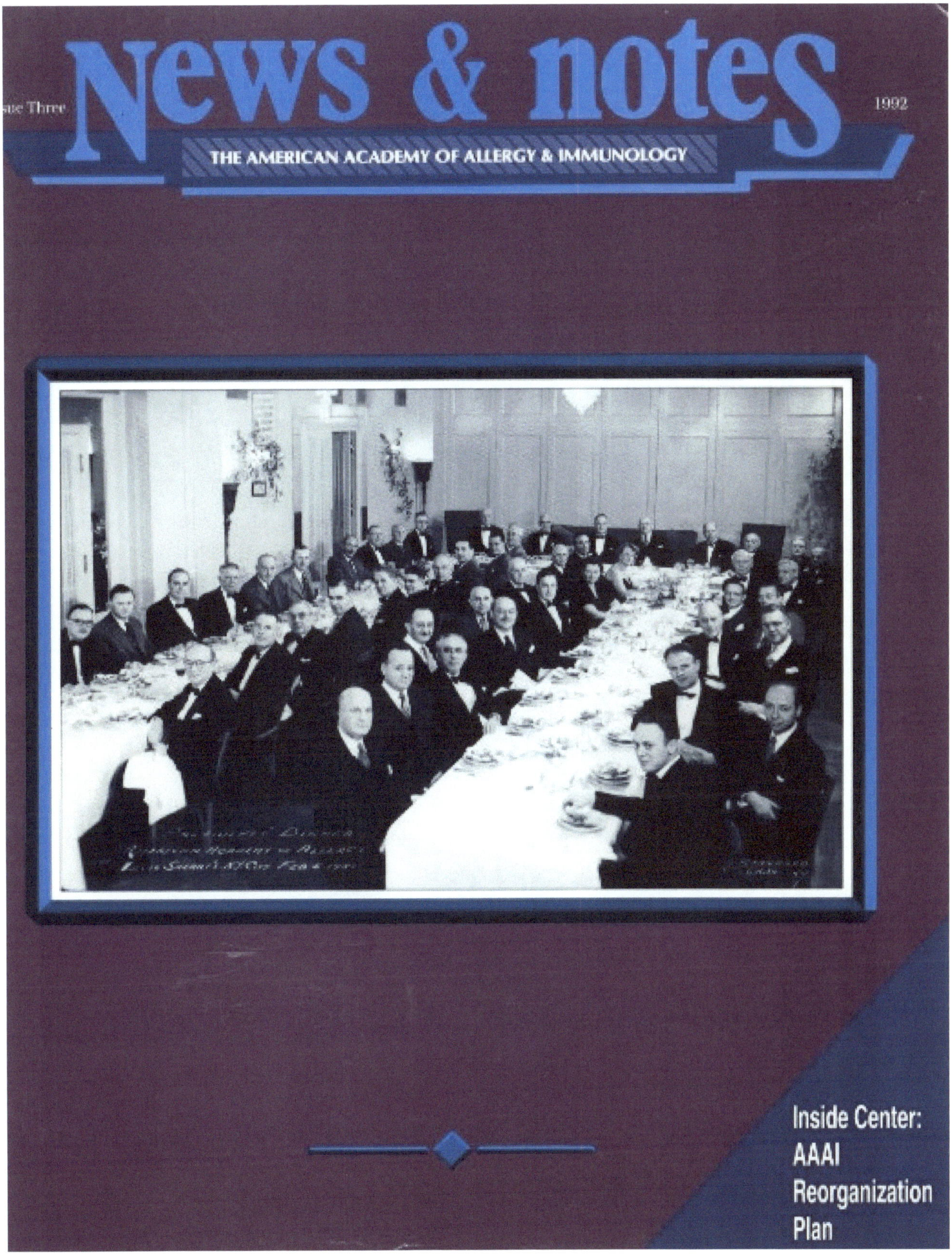

The American Academy of Allergy & Immunology, News & Notes, Vol. 92, Issue Three; 1992. AAAI Reorganization Plan led by Richard F. Lockey, MD, MS.

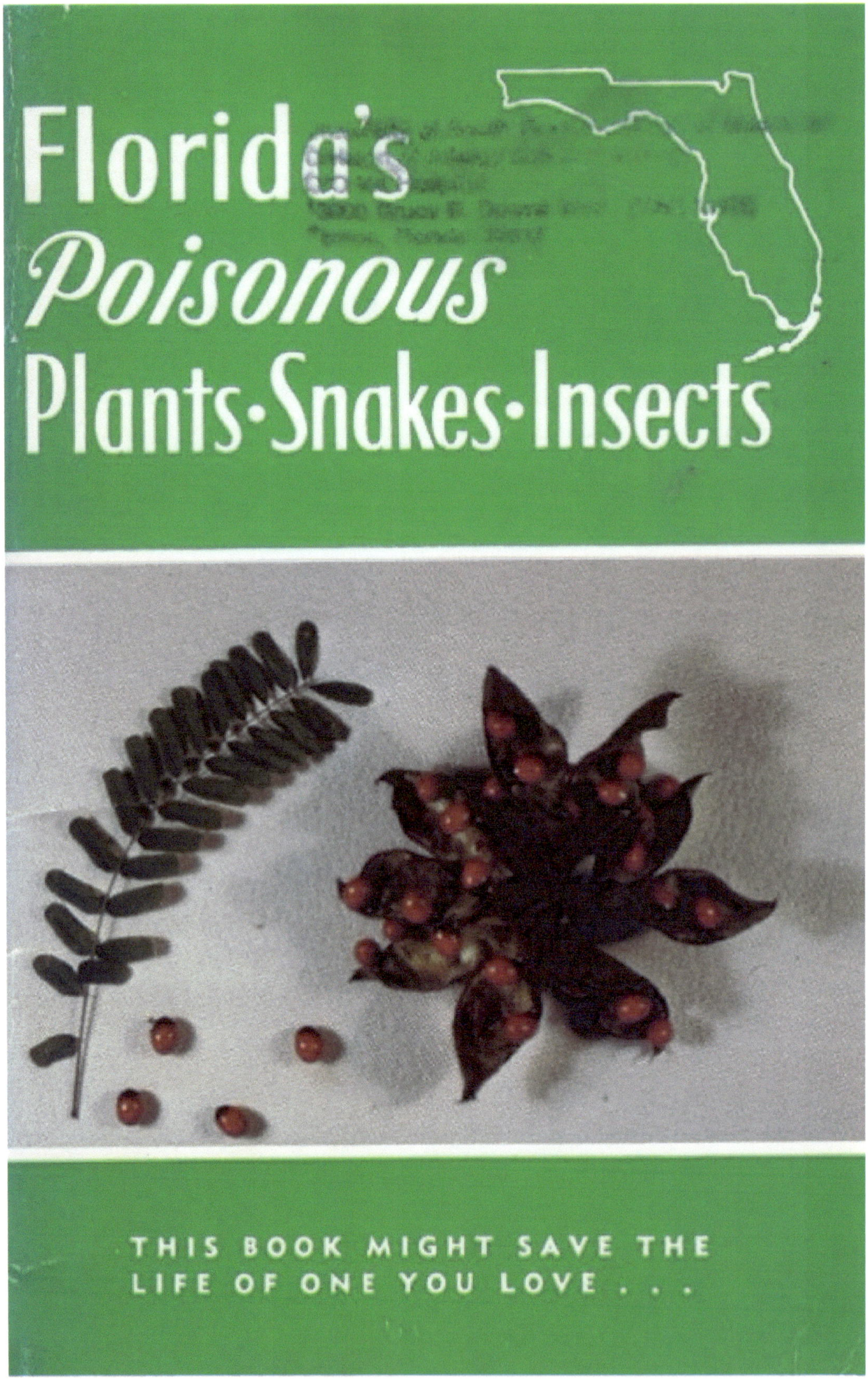

Florida Poisonous Plants, Snakes, Insects. Lockey RF, Stewart II GE, Maxwell LS. Lewis S. Maxwell, Publisher; Tampa, FL, 1992.

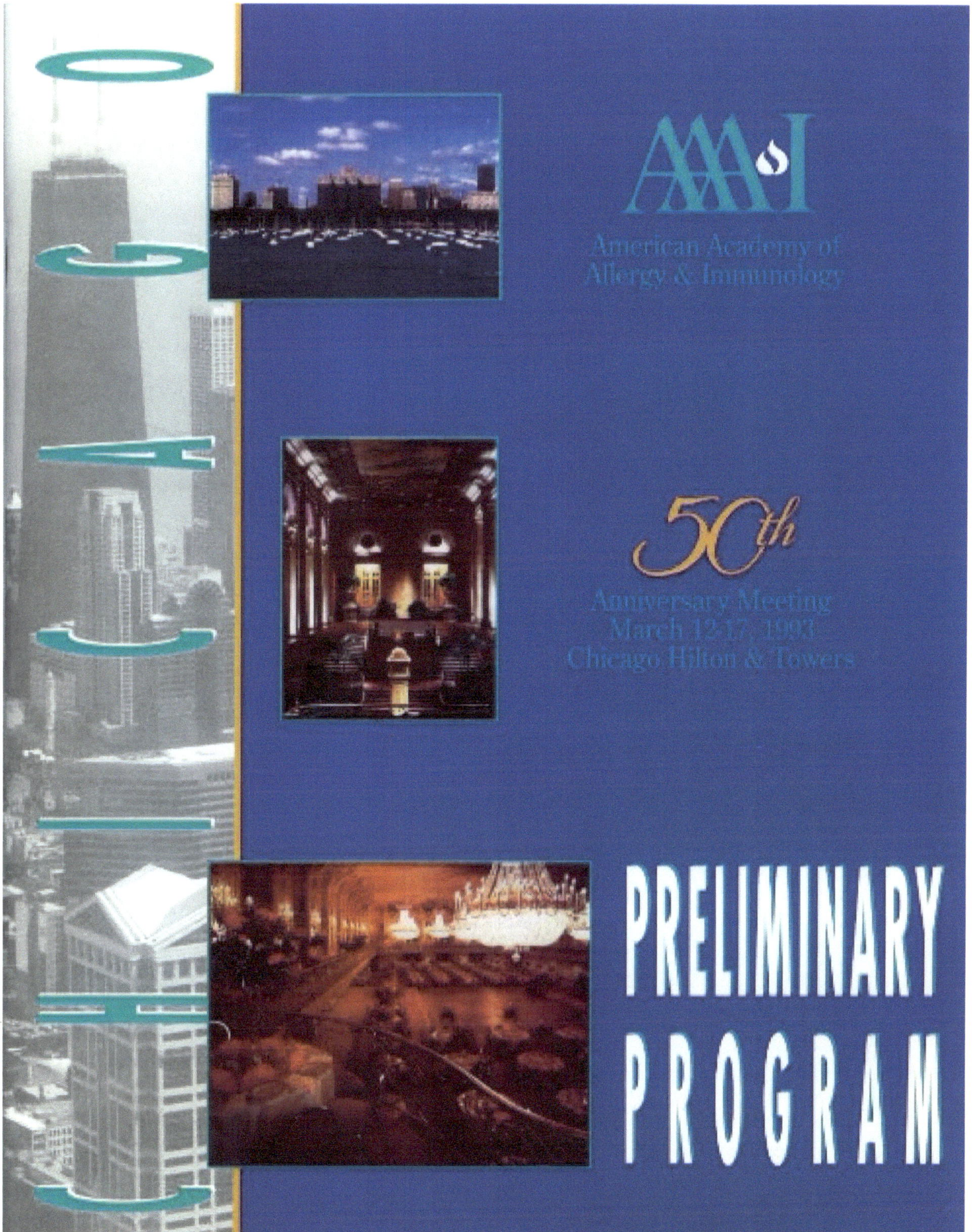

American Academy of Allergy & Immunology 50th Anniversary Meeting. Chicago Preliminary Program, Annual Meeting, American Academy of Allergy & Immunology, Hilton & Towers, March 12-17, 1993. Richard F. Lockey, MD, MS; President, 1992-1993.

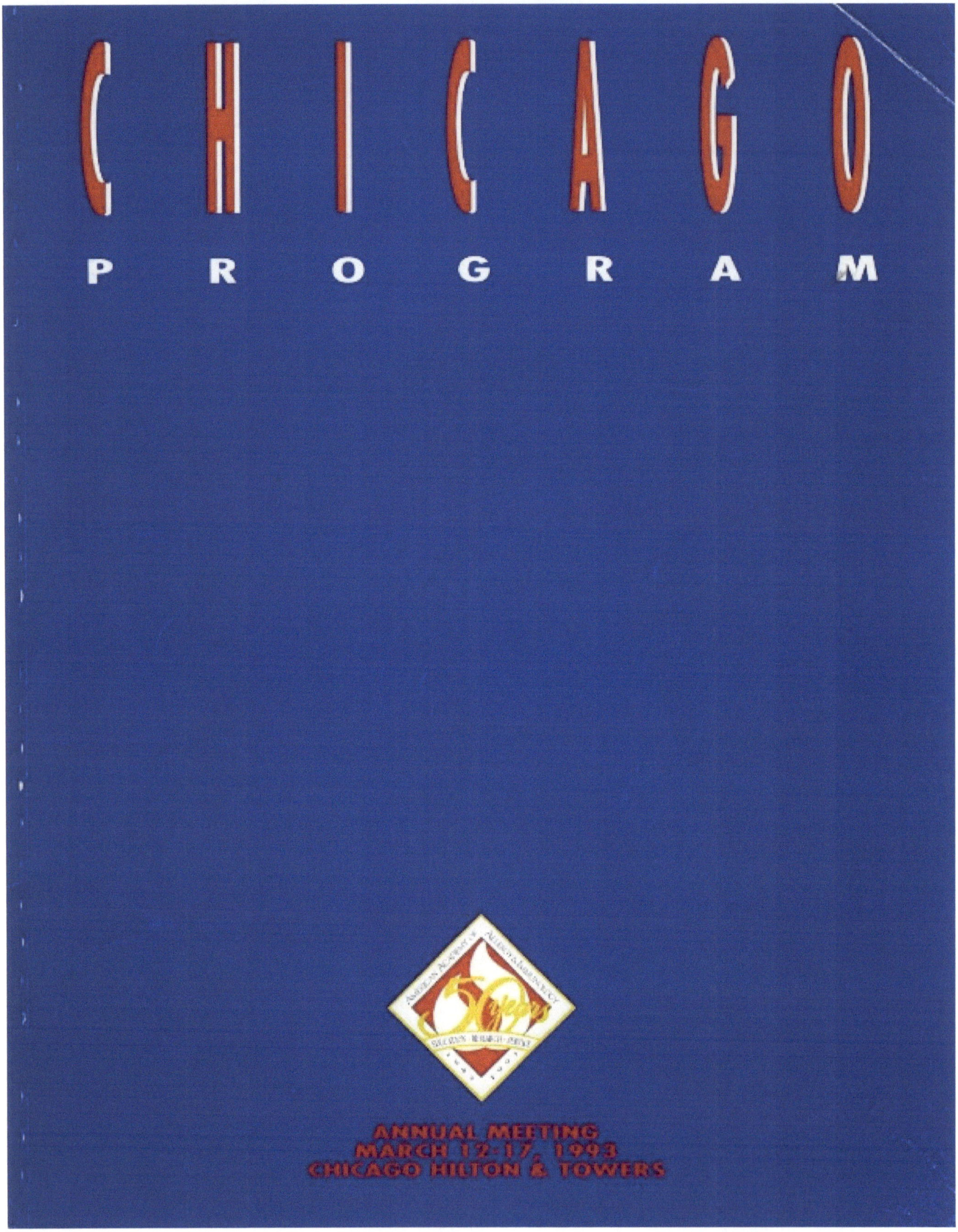

Chicago Program, Annual Meeting, American Academy of Allergy & Immunology, Chicago Hilton & Towers, March 12-17, 1993. Richard F. Lockey, MD, MS; President, 1992-1993.

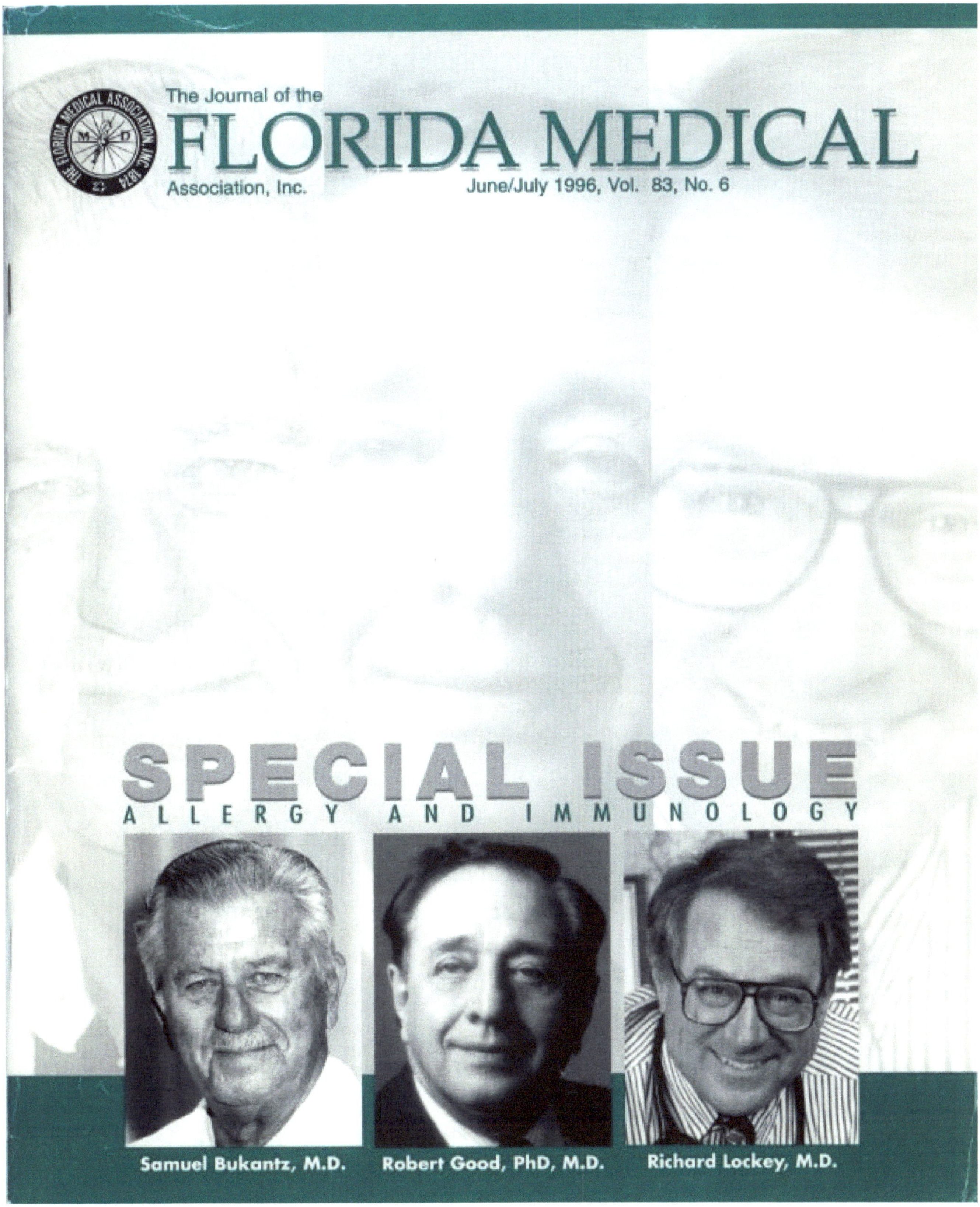

The Journal of the Florida Medical Association, Inc., Special Issue: Allergy and Immunology, June/July 1996, Vol. 83, No. 6. Special issue dedicated to Samuel C. Bukantz, MD; Robert A. Good, MD, PhD, DSc; and Richard F. Lockey, MD, MS.

Appreciation and Contributions

It is historically fitting that an issue of *The Journal of the Florida Medical Association* be devoted at this time to a review of allergy and immunology within the state of Florida. The growth of scientific information has been exponential during the past three decades. This is not unique to allergy and immunology, as all of the fields of medicine are dramatically changing.

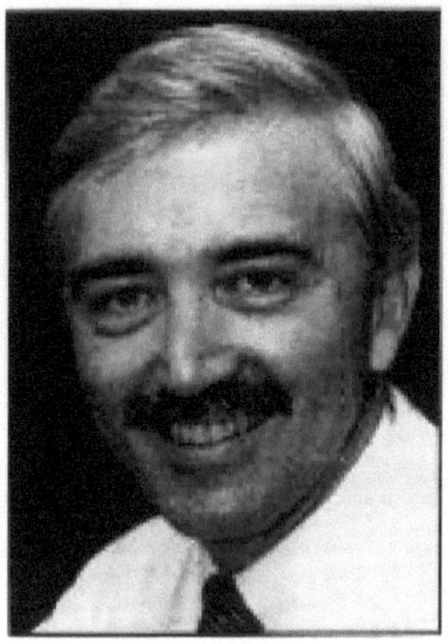

Dr. Ledford

The changes in allergy and immunology are particularly challenging because there is no single organ of the immune system to provide an anatomical structure to study and understand. Rather the immune system, much like the endocrine system, is an amorphous, mobile network of interacting cells which are continually changing. The regulation of the system via cytokines is extraordinarily complex, the genetic elements that permit immunologic specificity are unique and the effects of this system influence all other organ systems and tissue. Thus, every clinician should have some understanding of the immune system.

As the 21st century approaches, it is difficult to predict the impact of allergy and immunology on the future of medicine. The centennial of the death of the father of immunology, Louis Pasteur, was last year and in six years will be the centennial anniversary of the description of anaphylaxis by Charles Richet and Paul Portier. The past century of immunology has brought an intimidating bulk of scientific knowledge that is poised to move rapidly from the laboratory to the bedside. The application of this knowledge will require clinician-scientists who are aware of the questions needing answers. Florida fortunately is positioned to participate in the immunology explosion that will occur as the 21st century approaches.

This issue honors three of the individuals in Florida who epitomize the clinician-scientist-teacher, the classical triple threat of medicine.

Dr. Samuel Bukantz founded the training program in allergy and immunology at the University of South Florida approximately 25 years ago. He has contributed to the discipline for over four decades by unique scientific and clinical investigation, mentoring of students, medical writing and editing and always looking ahead. He continues to be an active member of the University faculty and presented an abstract of new research this year, demonstrating his lifelong commitment to the advancement of the specialty.

Dr. Robert Good's contributions to medicine in general and immunology in particular defy brief summary. Dr. Good, director of the allergy and immunology training program at All Childrens' Hospital, was the first to perform a bone marrow transplantation and cure an incurable disease in humans. His prodigious energy, scientific insight and contribution to the world's literature is intimidating and inspiring. Despite his being a veritable giant in the scientific arena, he prides himself on bedside teaching and looking for the "experiments of nature" that teach us the mysteries of biology. His many students will testify to the influence of this bedside-scientist.

Dr. Richard Lockey, current director of the allergy and immunology training program at the University of South Florida and James A. Haley VA Hospital in Tampa, completes the Florida triumvirate of clinician-scientist-teachers. Dr. Lockey has made major contributions in the local, national and international arena. He has advanced the understanding of immunotherapy, both its effectiveness and risks. His leadership has been one to always look to the future and not cling to the past. He also finds

finds great satisfaction and stimulation from patient care, using his clinical experience to ask the questions that need to be answered.

These three are among many notable immunologists in Florida, and they are exceptional in combining science with hands-on patient care.

I have tried to utilize the numerous outstanding allergist and immunologists within the state to provide an update of the field in this issue. Space would not permit a contribution from everyone who should be represented. Nevertheless, I hope the information in *The Journal* provides the reader a clinical update, an appreciation of the contributions of physicians within the state and an anticipation of the future.

Dennis K. Ledford, M.D.
Guest Editor

Dr. Ledford is Associate Professor of Medicine and Director, Clinical and Laboratory Immunology Training Program, University of South Florida College of Medicine, and the James A. Haley VA Hospital, Tampa.

Guest Editorial: Appreciation and Contributions. Dennis K. Ledford, MD. The Journal of the Florida Medical Association, Inc., Special Issue: Allergy and Immunology, June/July 1996, Vol. 83, No. 6, pp 367-368.

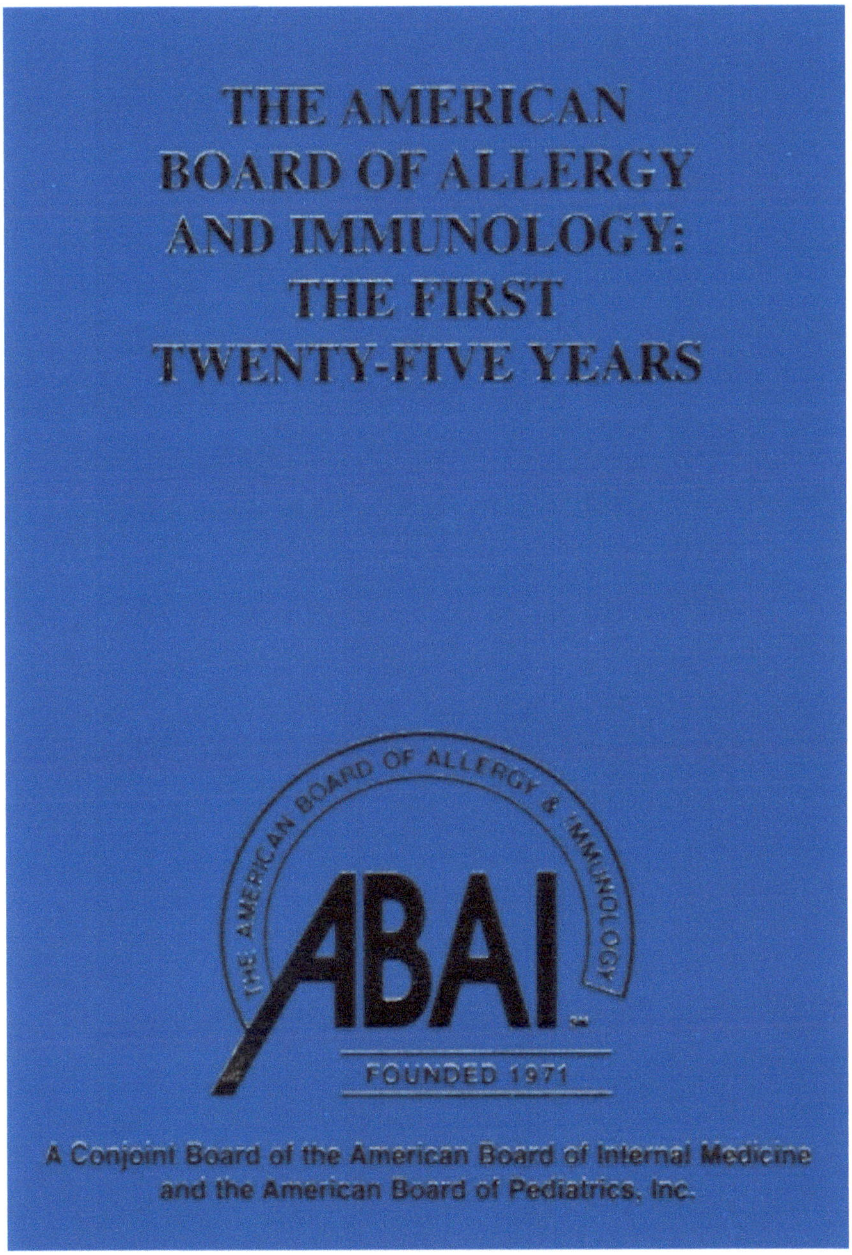

The American Board of Allergy and Immunology: The First Twenty-Five Years. Charles E. Reed, MD; Paul M. Seebohm, MD; Lynn De Prez, 1996.

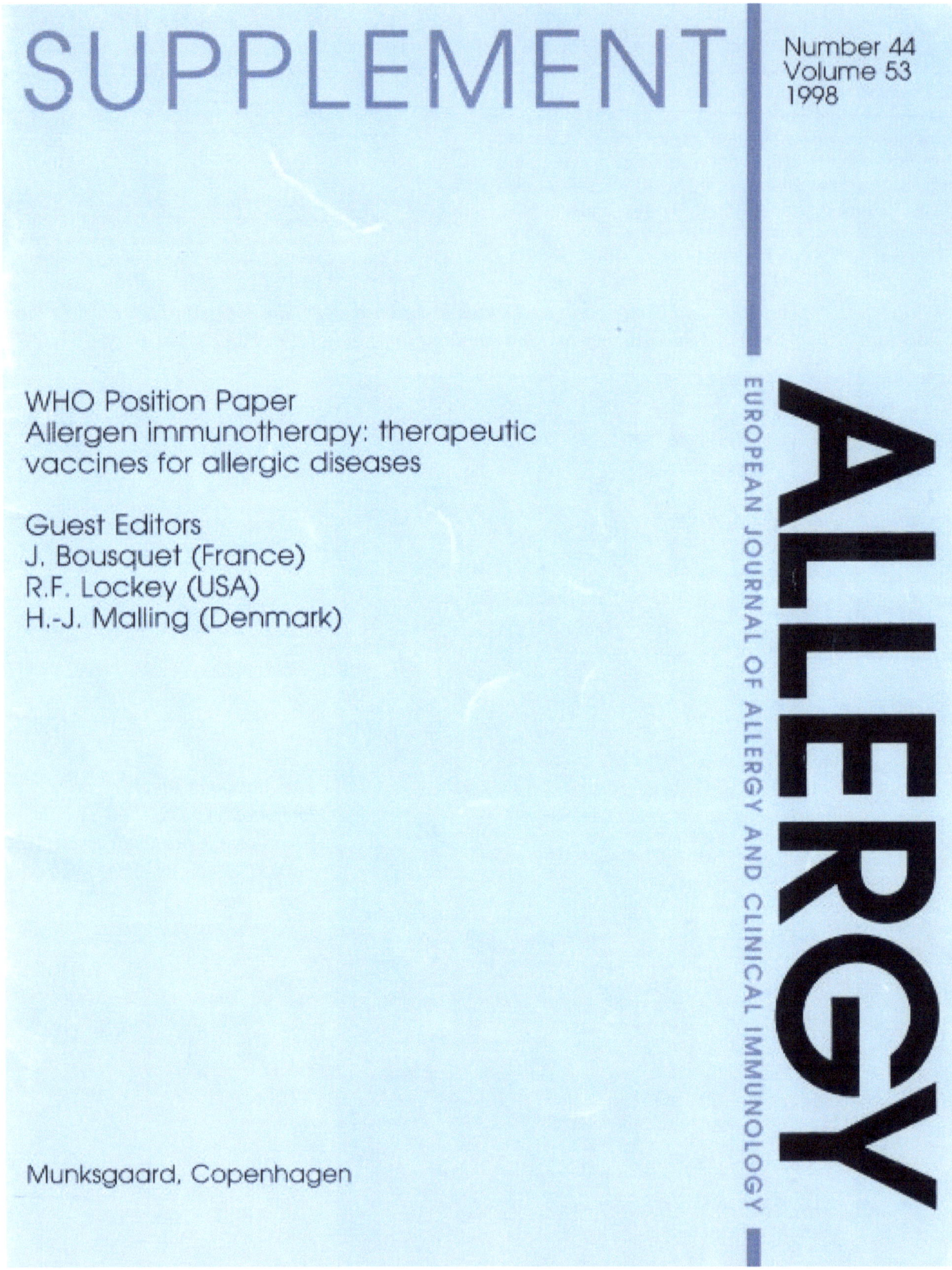

SUPPLEMENT

Number 44
Volume 53
1998

ALLERGY

EUROPEAN JOURNAL OF ALLERGY AND CLINICAL IMMUNOLOGY

WHO Position Paper
Allergen immunotherapy: therapeutic vaccines for allergic diseases

Guest Editors
J. Bousquet (France)
R.F. Lockey (USA)
H.-J. Malling (Denmark)

Munksgaard, Copenhagen

Allergy, European Journal of Allergy and Clinical Immunology, Supplement, Number 44, Vol. 53, 1998. WHO Position Paper: Allergen Immunotherapy: therapeutic vaccines for allergic diseases. Guest Editors: J Bousquet (France), RF Lockey (USA), H-J Malling (Denmark).

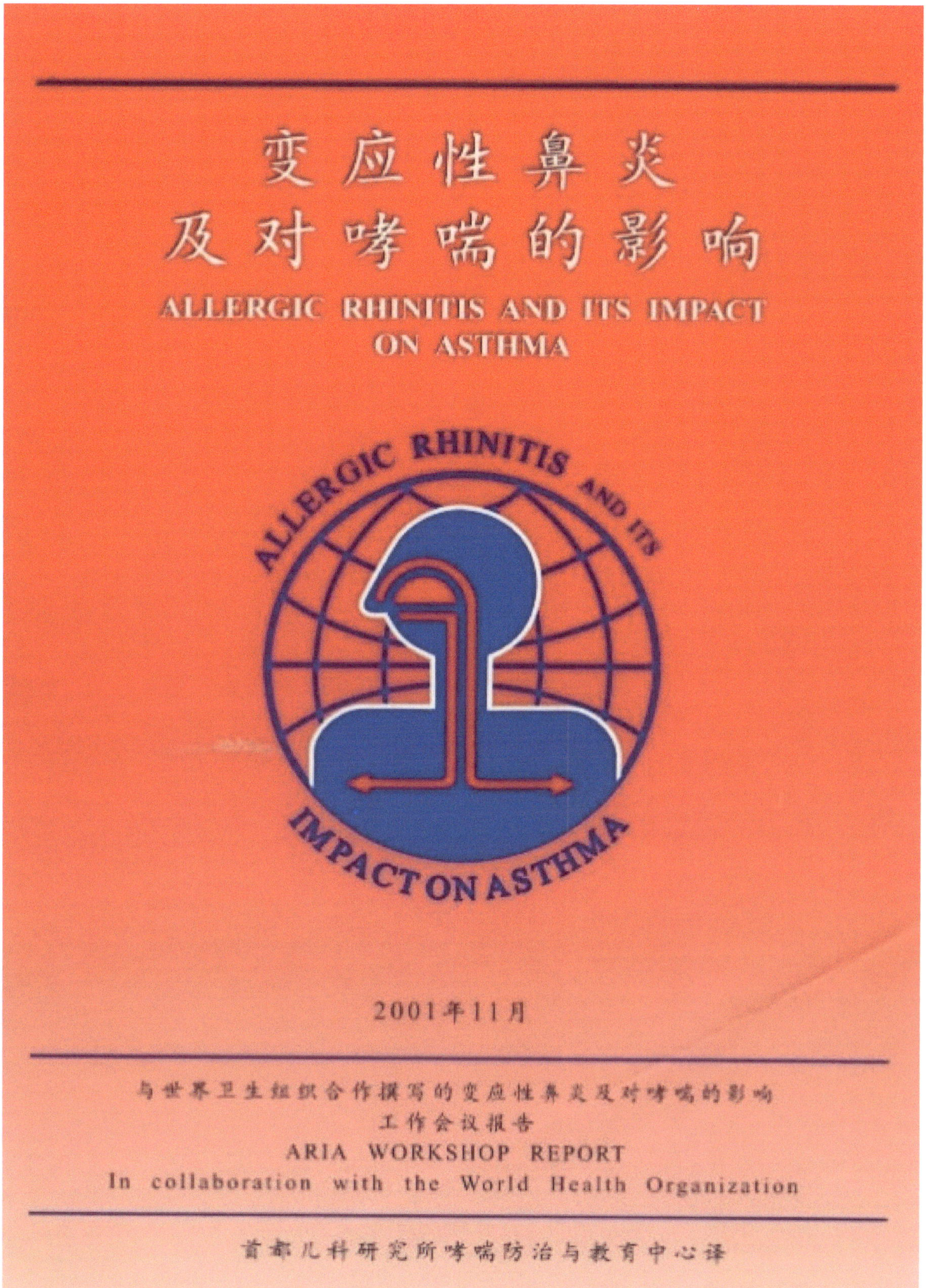

Allergic Rhinitis and Its Impact on Asthma; ARIA Workshop Report in Collaboration with the World Health Organization, 2001. Richard F. Lockey, MD, MS, contributor.

AAAAI Business Meeting 2008

Letter from the President of the AAAAI

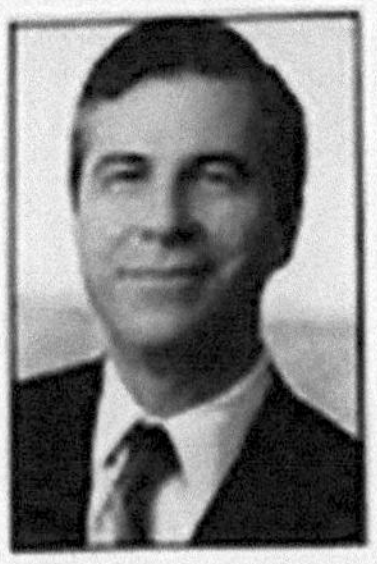

Dear Colleagues:

Welcome to the 2008 Business Meeting of the American Academy of Allergy, Asthma & Immunology (AAAAI). As has been for the past 63 years, this meeting is an opportunity to present an overview of current activities, highlight future initiatives and introduce you to the new AAAAI leadership. During this meeting, members will also vote on a number of Bylaws changes that are direct results of strategic planning and member feedback.

We are also here to honor some of our members for their dedication to the AAAAI and to the specialty, and to take note of the accomplishments of the past year. These achievements were made possible through the teamwork and dedication of our members, and by reaching out to partner with other professional and lay organizations. The allergy/immunology specialty faces many challenges, yet we continue to support important initiatives and implement new ones that respond to an everchanging environment and secure the future for our specialty.

Thank you for giving me the privilege to serve as your president. Today, I pass this leadership role on to Dr. Hugh Sampson. I look forward to working with him and with you to advance the knowledge and practice of allergy, asthma and immunology for optimal patient care.

Thomas B. Casale

Thomas B. Casale, MD, FAAAAI
President, 2007-2008

2008 AAAAI Business Meeting

Letter from the President of the American Academy of Allergy Asthma & Immunology, 2008. Thomas B. Casale, MD; President.

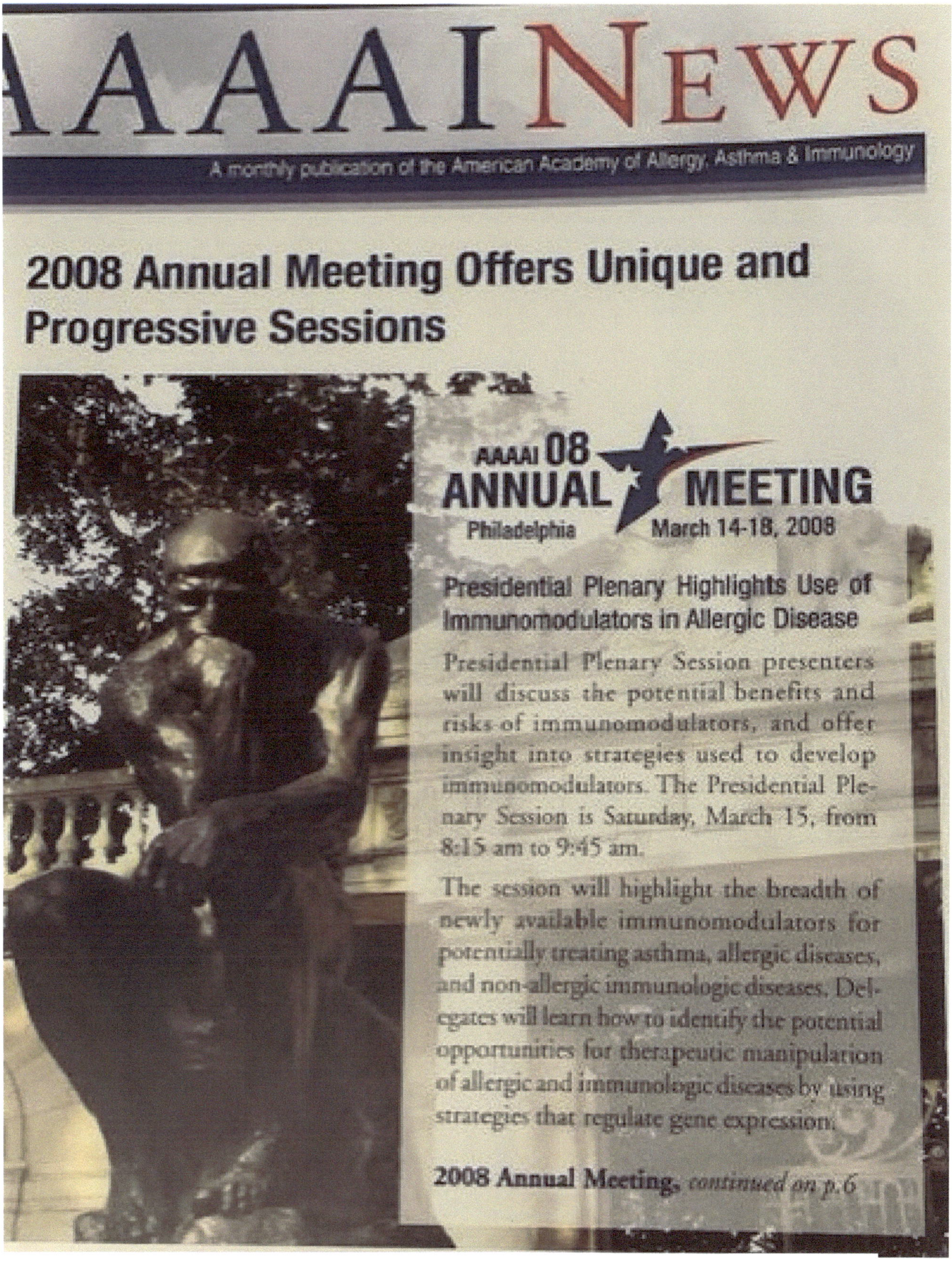

AAAAI NEWS

A monthly publication of the American Academy of Allergy, Asthma & Immunology

2008 Annual Meeting Offers Unique and Progressive Sessions

Presidential Plenary Highlights Use of Immunomodulators in Allergic Disease

Presidential Plenary Session presenters will discuss the potential benefits and risks of immunomodulators, and offer insight into strategies used to develop immunomodulators. The Presidential Plenary Session is Saturday, March 15, from 8:15 am to 9:45 am.

The session will highlight the breadth of newly available immunomodulators for potentially treating asthma, allergic diseases, and non-allergic immunologic diseases. Delegates will learn how to identify the potential opportunities for therapeutic manipulation of allergic and immunologic diseases by using strategies that regulate gene expression.

2008 Annual Meeting, *continued on p.6*

2008 American Academy of Allergy Asthma & Immunology Annual Meeting. Thomas B. Casale, MD; President.

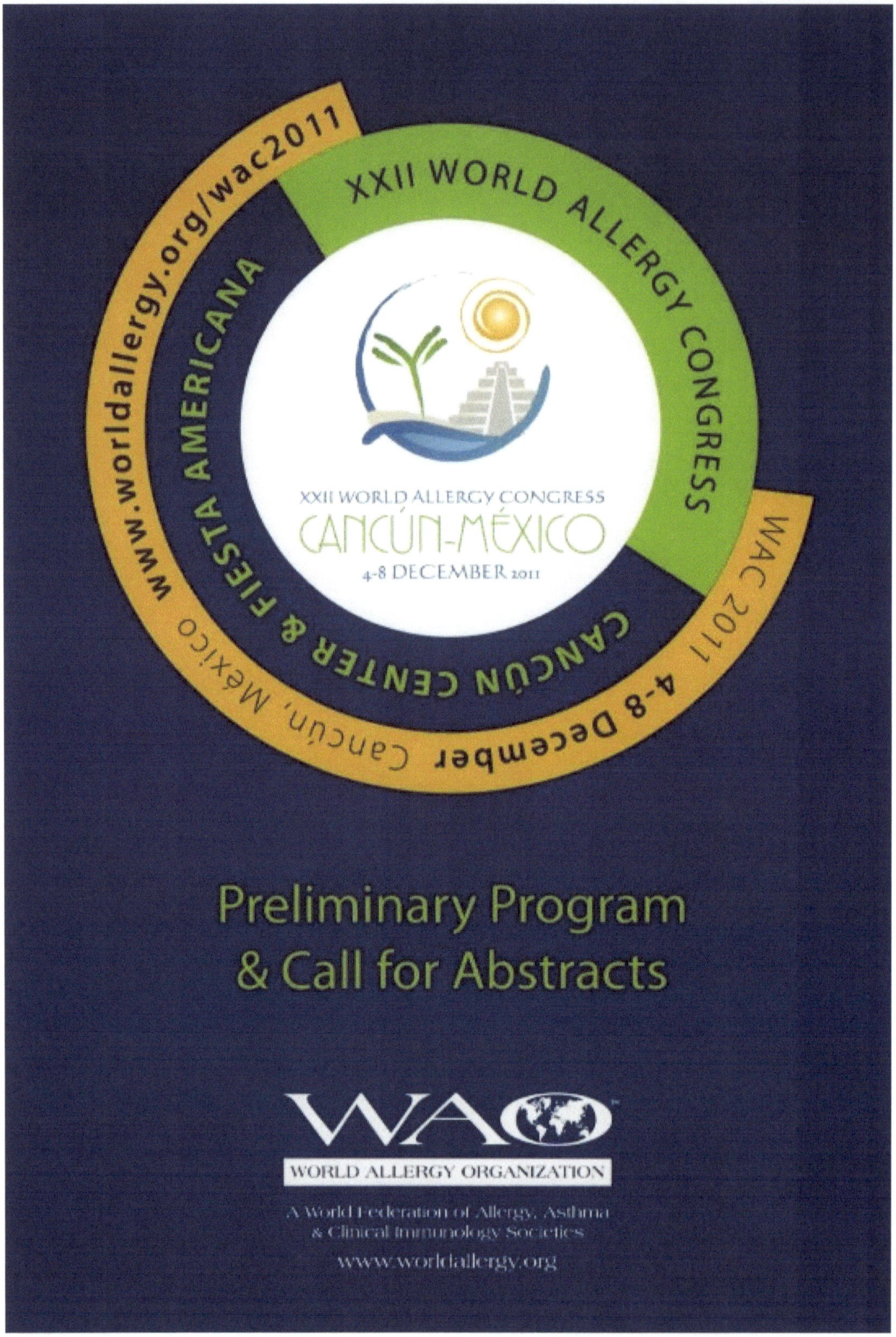

Preliminary Program & Call for Abstracts, World Allergy Organization, XXII World Allergy Congress, Cancún Center & Fiesta Americana, December 4-8, 2011. Richard F. Lockey, MD; President, World Allergy Organization, 2010-2011.

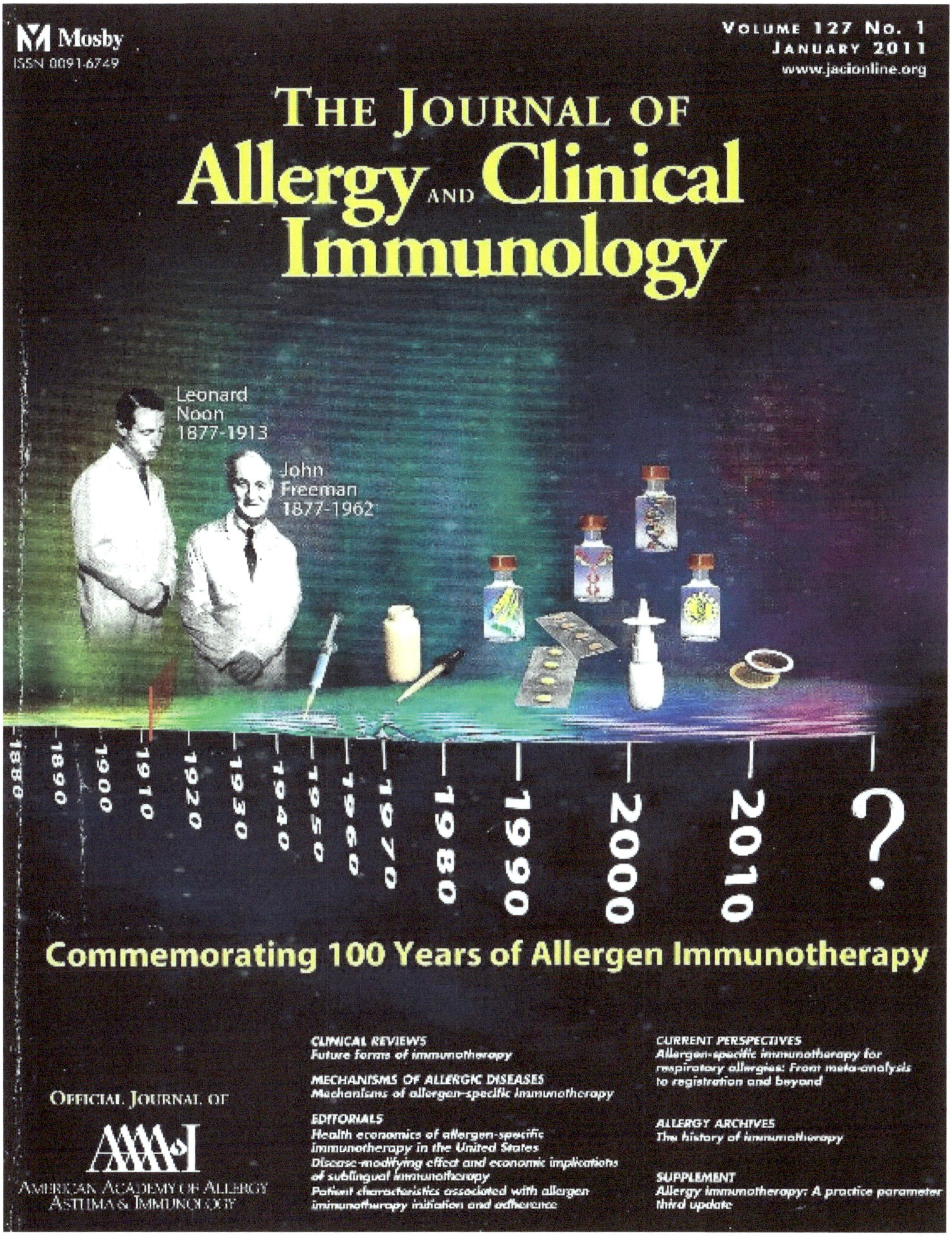

The Journal of Allergy and Clinical Immunology, Commemorating 100 Years of Allergen Immunotherapy, Vol. 127 No. 1, January 2011.

footNOTES[1] from the AAAAI American Academy of Allergy Asthma & Immunology

In Person

During the 2010 Annual Meeting in New Orleans, Mark Ballow, MD, FAAAAI, began his year as AAAAI President. This month, Ballow took time to answer a few questions.

Q You have a special interest in immunodeficiencies. What are the most exciting scientific inroads in this area? A It has been almost 40 years since I finished my clinical immunology fellowship under Robert A. Good at the University of Minnesota. Dr. Good performed the first bone marrow transplant in a patient with Severe Combined Immunodeficiency Disease. Fortunately, the donor was an HLA, MLC matched sibling. The patient is now alive and well and has a family of his own.

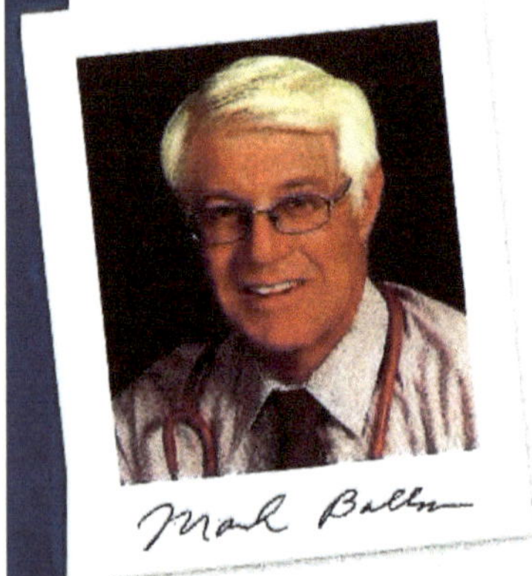

Dr. Good, along with Dr. Fred Rosen in Boston, laid the groundwork for many advances in clinical immunology and in the care of patients with primary immunodeficiency disease. Today, there are over 150 genetic defects associated with PIDD. Accurate diagnosis is important not only for genetic counseling and potential clinical outcome, but also in the development of treatment modalities.

Over the past 15 years, delineating the molecular defects in PIDD has led to a stream of information on how the immune system works, particularly host defense mechanisms that protect us from bacterial and viral pathogens that lead to serious infections. Our understanding of the pathogenesis and etiology of these PIDD have been facilitated by development of new tools that make possible the analysis for mutations in the host genome and the immunobiology of altered immune regulation.

In 1981, one of the most important treatment modalities was the approval of intravenous immunoglobulin (IGIV) as replacement therapy in patients with PIDD for abnormalities in the production of immunoglobulins and specific antibodies. Since that time, we have seen an evolution in this plasma product to make it not only a more highly purified IgG product with greater stability for intravenous use and enhanced tolerability, but also safer against the potential transmission of certain viral pathogens. Related to this advance is the extension in the use of IGIV to a variety of patients with autoimmune processes.

One exciting area for future discovery is the delineation of the mechanisms by which IGIV modulates the immune system. Hopefully, this will make it possible to develop "designer" IgG molecules, which will have an enhanced and perhaps even a selective immune modulating capability in these autoimmune and inflammatory diseases.

Because IVIG is derived from human plasma, it is a very limited and precious "commodity." With a better understanding of how IGIV modulates the immune system, it may be possible to use molecular biology and bioengineering to manufacture products which will have the same immune modulating capabilities as the native IgG molecule.

Q What advice would you give AAAAI members regarding the scope of practice of allergist/immunologists? A The scope of practice for all allergists/immunologists should extend beyond asthma and allergic disorders. The evaluation and treatment of patients with immune disorders, especially patients with immune deficiency diseases, must happen in order to preserve and advance the specialty. This is one of my Presidential initiatives.

Through educational programs at the AAAAI Annual Meeting and within the pages of the JACI, we will continue to offer the latest translational research and educational programs on the evaluation and diagnosis of patients with immune deficiency disorders.

My goal is to help members become more comfortable with and capable of at least the initial recognition and assessment of patients with potential underlying immune deficiency disease.

Q What are you most looking forward to during your year as AAAAI President? A As we enter the second decade of the new millennium, I look forward to working with AAAAI leadership, staff and AAAAI members in implementing the AAAAI 2010-2012 Strategic Plan. This plan ensures that the AAAAI is positioned as a global leader in discovering, identifying, enabling and translating basic and clinical research and the knowledge of allergy, asthma and immunology to optimize patient care.

Q Will there be challenges for the AAAAI during your Presidency? A Our biggest challenges are financial. The changing environment–particularly the relationship between industry, academia and continuing medical education–has put a strain on our ability to provide our membership with some ancillary services. Many of you may have noticed this during the Annual Meeting.

However, I want to assure members that the Academy will not compromise on activities related to our core values. We will do everything possible to maintain the highest standards of "cutting-edge" science and clinical knowledge to allow our membership to provide the best possible care to our patients with asthma, allergies and immunologic disorders.

[1]Notes of interest from the American Academy of Allergy, Asthma & Immunology. Footnotes: Vol. 125, No. 3

We have engaged a task force to make sure we preserve these ideals in the face of financial changes. I consider this an opportunity, rather than a diminutive exercise. It is always healthy to examine processes to optimize goals.

Also, with the changing landscape, we will rely more heavily on members' support to preserve our educational objectives and protect the future of the specialty through contributions to the AR Trust.

Q As U.S. healthcare initiatives move forward, patient access to A/I and other specialty care is becoming increasingly volatile. Are there measures the AAAAI and our members can take? A The AAAAI, JCAAI and the ACAAI, are collaborating on proactive measures to ensure that the specialty "has a seat at the table" during this challenging time of healthcare reform. Additionally, we are forming partnerships with other medical specialty societies. Hopefully, this "strength in numbers" will allow us to be better heard and have a participatory approach as healthcare reform unfolds.

Also, we encourage our members, as individual citizens, to make certain their congressional leaders are aware of the importance of patient access to specialty care.

Q How do you cope with the amount of snow you receive in Buffalo, New York? A Buffalo always gets a bad rap regarding snow. A little known fact is that Syracuse gets almost twice the amount of snow that Buffalo does. Yet, we probably have been on the Weather Channel more than any other city in the nation because of occasional large snowstorms. This snow phenomenon in Western New York hits particularly hard south of Buffalo. That's why I chose to live north of the city!

Notes of interest from the American Academy of Allergy Asthma & Immunology. Mark Ballow, MD; President. Footnotes: Vol 126, No 3, 2010; published in The Journal of Allergy and Clinical Immunology, March 2010.

news&notes from the AAAAI American Academy of Allergy Asthma & Immunology

Special Annual Meeting Issue

Highlighting Immune Deficiency at the Presidential Plenary

Make sure your itinerary in San Francisco includes the Presidential Plenary Session at the 2011 Annual Meeting, scheduled for Saturday, March 19 from 8:15 to 9:45 am.

This year's Presidential Plenary topic is Immune Therapy for Immunodeficiency, moderated by Jordan Orange, MD, PhD, FAAAAI. President Mark Ballow, MD, FAAAAI, is set to discuss the mechanisms by which IVIG modulates the immune system.

Joining Ballow as speakers are Jennifer M. Puck, MD, and Luigi D. Notarangelo, MD. Puck will present early diagnosis of primary immune deficiency, including new molecular approaches in the early diagnosis of severe combined immunodeficiency.

Notarangelo will close the session by focusing on the identification of patients with primary immune deficiency as potential candidates for bone marrow transplantation.

More Immune Deficiency Sessions in San Francisco

Aside from the Presidential Plenary, a variety of sessions at the 2011 Annual Meeting in San Francisco revolve around the topic of immune deficiency. This supports a key initiative of President Ballow to promote the scope of practice of immunology.

> "The evaluation, diagnosis and care of patients with immune deficiency is not easy. In order to ensure optimal care for these patients, the AAAAI Annual Meeting provides a menu of educational programs on this and related topics." Mark Ballow, MD, FAAAAI

Session Number	Session Title
1207	Basic Immunology Update for the Practicing Allergist
1607	Outpatient Recognition of Primary Immunodeficiency
2504	Primary Immunodeficiencies Discovered in the Last Five Years
3003	TH17 Cells in Primary Immunodeficiency Diseases
3504	Use of Pneumococcal Vaccination in Immunodeficiency Diagnosis and Management
3702	BCI Interest Section Forum
4004	Immunodeficiency Screening in Newborns
5002	Pulmonary Diseases That Can Mimic Immunodeficiency
5014	Evaluating Immunodeficiency in Adults

Find more details on all of these sessions in the Final Program, which is posted as a downloadable PDF at annualmeeting.aaaai.org.

Additional Plenary Sessions to Explore Immune Tolerance, Hygiene Hypothesis

Along with the Presidential Plenary, there will be plenary sessions from 8:15 to 9:45 am on Sunday, Monday and Tuesday.

Immune Dysregulation and Immunomodulation of Chronic Rhinosinusitis

Sunday, March 20

Moderator: Katharine M. Woessner, MD, FAAAAI

Speakers: Robert P. Schleimer, PhD, FAAAAI; Pradeep K. Singh, MD; Claus Bachert, MD, PhD

Induction of Immune Tolerance to Allergic Disease: Benchside Finally Reaches Bedside

Monday, March 21

Moderator: Joshua A. Boyce, MD, FAAAAI

Speakers: Judith A. Woodfolk, MBChB, PhD, FAAAAI; Gideon Lack, MD; Stacie M. Jones, MD

Evolution of the Hygiene Hypothesis: Understanding New Pathways in Immune Deviation

Tuesday, March 22

Moderator: Kathleen C. Barnes, PhD, FAAAAI

Speakers: Graham A. Rook, BA, MB, BChir, MD; Susan V. Lynch, PhD; Harald E. Renz, MD

Special Annual Meeting Issue News & Notes, 2011 American Academy Allergy Asthma & Immunology Annual Meeting, Mark Ballow, MD; President.

34A Notes of interest from the American Academy of Allergy, Asthma & Immunology. News & Notes: Vol. 127, No. 2

3. Secure the future of our organization and the specialty

I've always taken a strong interest in the underserved and in diversity. The practice of allergy/immunology is a nonprocedural, cognitive specialty that relies upon education of the patient for effective outcomes. Communication is enhanced by reducing barriers (perceived or real) of ethnicity and/or language between patient and physician.

Nurture prior AAAAI efforts to increase diversity of the AAAAI and within our specialty by working to maintain and increase funding for the Odyssey Program and the Fellowship of Excellence Award. To accomplish this, we need to build a better pipeline. This requires a financial as well as philosophical commitment. The impact could be tremendous, but is long term.

(Accountable to the core values of "Inclusion" and "Service" within the 2010-2014 Strategic Plan.)

I recently participated in a leadership "school" within my institution. It taught me that the ability to lead isn't reflective of age or viewpoint. What matters are confidence, leadership tools and commitment, plus access to routes of involvement. Combined, these attributes build strong leaders who can guide others in strategizing for success.

Although we may start on a small scale during my presidency, my long term goal is to develop an AAAAI leadership program. This can be accomplished by exploring additional ways of including more candidates for nomination to positions of leadership and providing interactive forums to allow members to gain insight into the views of candidates for leadership prior to the election.

(Accountable to the core value of "Leadership" within the 2010-2014 Strategic Plan.)

4. Impact $10 Million

ARTrust's current endowment is approximately $8.1 million. I want our community to strive to reach an impact of $10 million to support the future of our specialty.

This is significant, but it would open new doors to available funding streams for junior faculty, supporting research and enhancing visibility of our specialty. The symbolism of the "perfect 10" resonates with the progress of the JACI toward reaching an impact factor of 10. Research and science secures our place in health care. Dedicated support through the ARTrust as well as publishing this research in high impact journals allows us to sustain these efforts. That is why I am committed to raising $1 million for the ARTrust during my presidency.

(Accountable to the core value of "Stewardship" within the 2010-2014 Strategic Plan.)

Dennis K. Ledford, MD; President, American Academy of Allergy Asthma & Immunology. News & Notes in The Journal of Allergy & Clinical Immunology, March 2011.

news&notes from the AAAAI American Academy of Allergy Asthma & Immunology

In Person

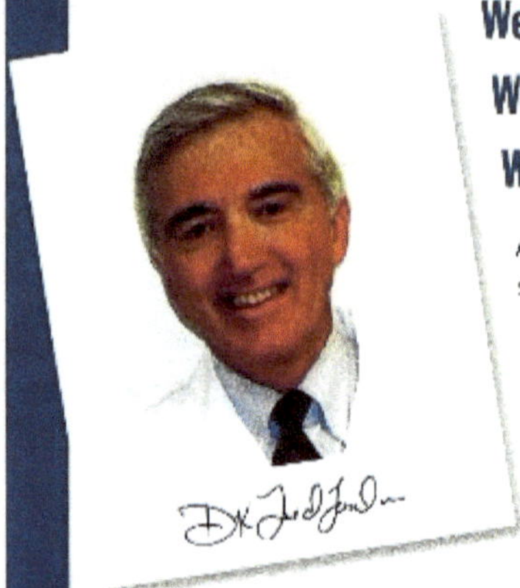

We are Many.
We are One.
We are Allergy/Immunology.

As Dennis K. Ledford, MD, FAAAAI, steps into his role as AAAAI president, he will focus on a set of initiatives that uses the strengths and diversity of the membership to keep the AAAAI focused on the future of the specialty.

"The AAAAI represents members with a variety of viewpoints, talents, interests and demographics. Yet, we are focused on a unified goal: sustaining the specialty for optimal patient care," said Ledford. "Together we are allergy/immunology."

1. Enhance collaborations on issues management

We may not always agree on issues, but it is important to have respect for each other's position. Respect develops and flourishes when barriers are removed so that ideas can be exchanged and synergies created.
I envision collaborating with the ACAAI on further development of a practice community. This community or counsel would bring together members of the RSLs and the HODs to communicate with a common voice. We cannot fix everything. We likely will not achieve 100% consensus on any decision, but we can make sure everyone is heard.

We must embrace diversity and maximize input among membership categories. In particular, I would like to energize the International Assembly through the creation of recognition awards for international young investigators. Additionally, we will explore new ways leadership can communicate with the international community.

(Accountable to the core value of "Inclusion" within the 2010-2014 Strategic Plan.)

2. Utilize technology to enhance scientific development as well as professional learning experiences

As the demands of MOC change, and to focus on self-assessment and performance improvement modules, the AAAAI will need to change its programming processes and the types of activities it offers. An LMS will provide capabilities for members to complete these activities and document them for MOC purposes, and for the AAAAI to report these completions directly to the ABAI.

(Accountable to the core value of "Professionalism & Integrity" within the 2010-2014 Strategic Plan.)

Our specialty is distinguished by our knowledge and understanding of the environment and immunotherapy. The National Allergy Bureau™ (NAB) is a unique resource that can be leveraged to benefit medical science, our specialty and patients/consumers.

In cooperation with the AAAAI's NAB community, I want us to develop a methodology to use molecular biology to facilitate and automate allergen identification on a nationwide basis. This is a long range project that will move allergen identification into the 21st century and ideally increase the number of counting stations.

(Accountable to the core value of "Leadership" within the 2010-2014 Strategic Plan.)

Notes of interest from the American Academy of Allergy Asthma & Immunology; News & Notes; Vol 132, No. 6, December 2013.

news&notes from the AAAAI American Academy of Allergy Asthma & Immunology

In Person

With: Dennis K. Ledford, MD, FAAAAI

This month, we interviewed Dennis K. Ledford, MD, FAAAAI, Chair of the Allergy, Asthma & Immunology Education and Research Organization, Inc. (ARTrust™) Steering Committee. The mission of the ARTrust is to find treatments and cures for the millions of people suffering from allergies, asthma and other immunologic diseases by supporting education and research.

Dr. Ledford, who served as AAAAI President from 2011 to 2012, is Professor of Medicine and Pediatrics and the Mabel and Ellsworth Simmons Professor of Allergy and Immunology at the University of South Florida College of Medicine.

Q Can you explain the work that the ARTrust does? A The work of the ARTrust revolves around investing together in our future. Each contribution to the ARTrust builds the reserve from which investment proceeds support research and education in our specialty.

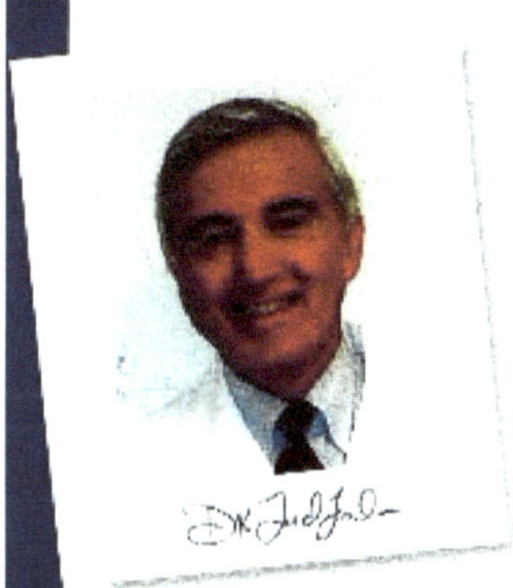

Allergy/immunology spans a complex array of diseases and the ARTrust is committed to sustaining research and education in all of these diseases. The ARTrust supports the best research ideas and the best investigators to ultimately improve patient care for those with allergies, asthma and immunologic diseases.

Our remarkable membership is replete with ideas so the AAAAI and ARTrust have identified our best and brightest investigators and supported their early work through ARTrust awards. For every dollar of support awarded to AAAAI member scientists, more than $35 dollars of additional funding has come into the discipline.

Any way you look at it, investing in ARTrust is a wise decision. We are building a legacy for today and tomorrow.

Q Why would you encourage new allergist/immunologists to become involved in supporting the ARTrust? A A new allergist/immunologist has worked hard to reach an important goal in their career. Sometimes we focus on our own accomplishments, sacrifices and successes and lose sight of the role of those before us who made it possible for our individual success. All of us are in various communities, but we all share the fact that we're part of the allergy/immunology community.

The allergy/immunology community will not grow unless we all do our part. Clinicians take pride in the care of their patients, research scientists in the strength of their ideas, and new developments and educators in the success of their students. But all components in this community must thrive if the community is to be sustained. Effective patient care is not possible without new discovery, new physicians, new faculty and new students. ARTrust helps to make all of this possible.

Q The First Annual Race for Allergy & Asthma Research 5K Run/Walk was a resounding success at the 2013 Annual Meeting. How did the idea for this event come about, and why would you urge members and others to register for the Second Annual Race for Allergy & Asthma Research 5K Run/Walk in San Diego? A The San Antonio Race for Allergy & Asthma Research 5K Run/Walk was an amazing success due to the interest of our members and the hard work of a team lead by Joseph D. Diaz, MD. A single telephone call to this busy physician resulted in his assembling a team of our best staff, our friends in industry and other AAAAI members to develop the idea and make it happen.

This successful event all came from one member saying "yes." I know we are busy in a profession we love, but we should never be too busy to say "yes" and make a difference.

I am confident the second event at the 2014 Annual Meeting in San Diego will be bigger and better under the leadership of John Kelso, MD, FAAAAI, who is currently serving on the AAAAI Board of Directors. I encourage everyone to join us and celebrate the ARTrust, the beauty of San Diego and the opportunity to come together. The Second Annual ARTrust 5K Run/Walk will be held on Sunday, March 2 at 5:30 pm with runners and walkers of all ages looping through the lights of the San Diego Embarcadero. I hope each of you will be there to help us Light Up the Night.

Q Who (or what) influenced you to choose a career in allergy/immunology? A Never underestimate the power of having fun and enjoying your work. I was impressed by the excitement and fun I witnessed when I worked with Phillip L. Lieberman, MD, FAAAAI, at the University of Tennessee Center for Health Sciences when I was a medical resident.

Dr. Lieberman has contributed to the careers of many of our members and he has contributed to the ARTrust. This man is an amazing ambassador for our specialty and I am proud to say he launched my career. I am grateful for the example he provides in scholarship, patient care, leadership, contribution to the common good and joy of living.

24A Notes of interest from the American Academy of Allergy, Asthma & Immunology. News & Notes: Vol. 132, No. 6

(continued) Dennis K. Ledford, MD; President, American Academy of Allergy Asthma & Immunology. News & Notes in The Journal of Allergy & Clinical Immunology, March 2011.

AAAAI
American Academy of Allergy Asthma & Immunology

Q What is your favorite memory from your time as AAAAI President? A The year is a blur of memories and it is difficult to recall or identify my favorite. I think the last Board of Directors meeting I had in Orlando was one of the best. The AAAAI has a remarkable and dedicated group of volunteer leaders who work tirelessly for the specialty. All of these men and women are major donors to the ARTrust and major contributors to our success. Their acknowledgment at our last meeting will remain near or at the top of the list of my favorite memories.

Q We know that you are very proud of your family. What important lessons have your children and grandchildren taught you? A I am grateful and proud of the blessing of my family. I certainly cannot take much credit for the three incredible young men I am privileged to call son, as my wife Jennifer was the major influence in their development and growth as human beings. I always encouraged them to pursue a life's calling that brings them joy, just as I saw joy in the work of Dr. Lieberman.

And indeed, they each have taken their own direction in life and have succeeded. Along the way, these young men and the women who joined them have blessed us with ten grandchildren. I look forward with optimism to the next generation, just as I look forward with optimism to the next generation of faculty members, fellows-in-training, students and physicians who will grow the family of allergy/immunology with the help of the ARTrust.

I ask everyone to help us reach our next goal of $13 million by 2015. Our family will be strong if we all work together. To those whom much has been given, much is expected. Please help today, not tomorrow, and join the ARTrust in investing together in our future.

ARTrust™

INVESTING TOGETHER IN OUR FUTURE

Make a Donation to the ARTrust and Invest in Our Future

Since its inception, the ARTrust has given 77 awards totaling more than $4.65 million in funding, but there is still a great need for additional resources to continue its mission. With your help, the ARTrust will:

- Sustain and grow a network of academic faculty, educators and clinical specialists in allergy, asthma and immunology to optimally treat individuals with these diseases.
- Discover new knowledge and develop a better understanding of these diseases through the support of pivotal, ground-breaking research.
- Enhance public awareness of these diseases.

Large or small, each donation to the ARTrust assures a healthy future for our specialty and our patients. Visit aaaai.org/global/ARTrust or call (414) 272-6071.

You can also support the ARTrust by attending the ARTrust Benefit and 5K Run/Walk for Allergy & Asthma Research at the 2014 Annual Meeting.

ARTrust Events at the 2014 Annual Meeting in San Diego

ARTrust Benefit: A First Class Event

Saturday, March 1, 7:00 pm
Mark your calendar for this themed event at the San Diego Air & Space Museum.

Attend an adventurous evening exploring aviation and the history of flight. Try on your own set of wings in the flight simulators, indulge in fine dining and cocktails, and enjoy live entertainment. Join your friends and colleagues for an exciting evening and help raise funds for the ARTrust.

ARTrust 5K Run/Walk for Allergy & Asthma Research: Light Up the Night

Sunday, March 2, 5:30 pm
Tighten up your laces and start your training now for the Light Up the Night 5K Run/Walk. As the sun sets on Sunday, March 2, attention will be on the 5K participants running and walking to raise funds for the ARTrust.

This glowing event will be hard to miss. The race will begin at 5:30 pm with runners and walkers of all ages looping through the twinkling lights of the San Diego Embarcadero.

Ticket and registration information for both events is available at annualmeeting.aaaai.org.

(continued) Notes of interest from the American Academy of Allergy Asthma & Immunology; News & Notes; Vol 132, No. 6, December 2013.

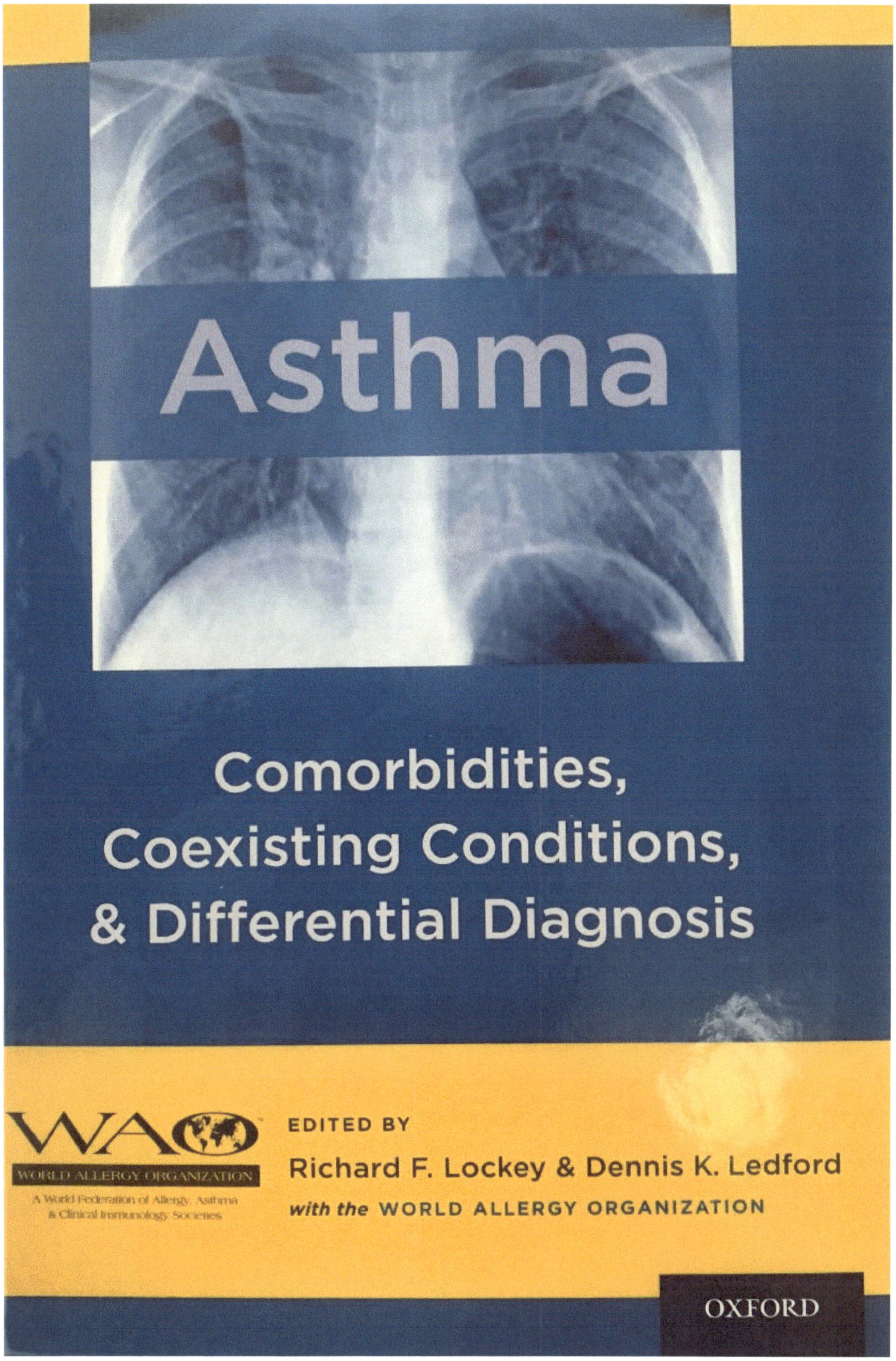

Lockey RF and Ledford DK and the World Allergy Organization (eds): Asthma: Comorbidities, Coexisting Conditions, & Differential Diagnosis. Oxford University Press, New York, NY, 2014. This book was the first of its kind documenting multiple comorbid or coexisting conditions associated with asthma.

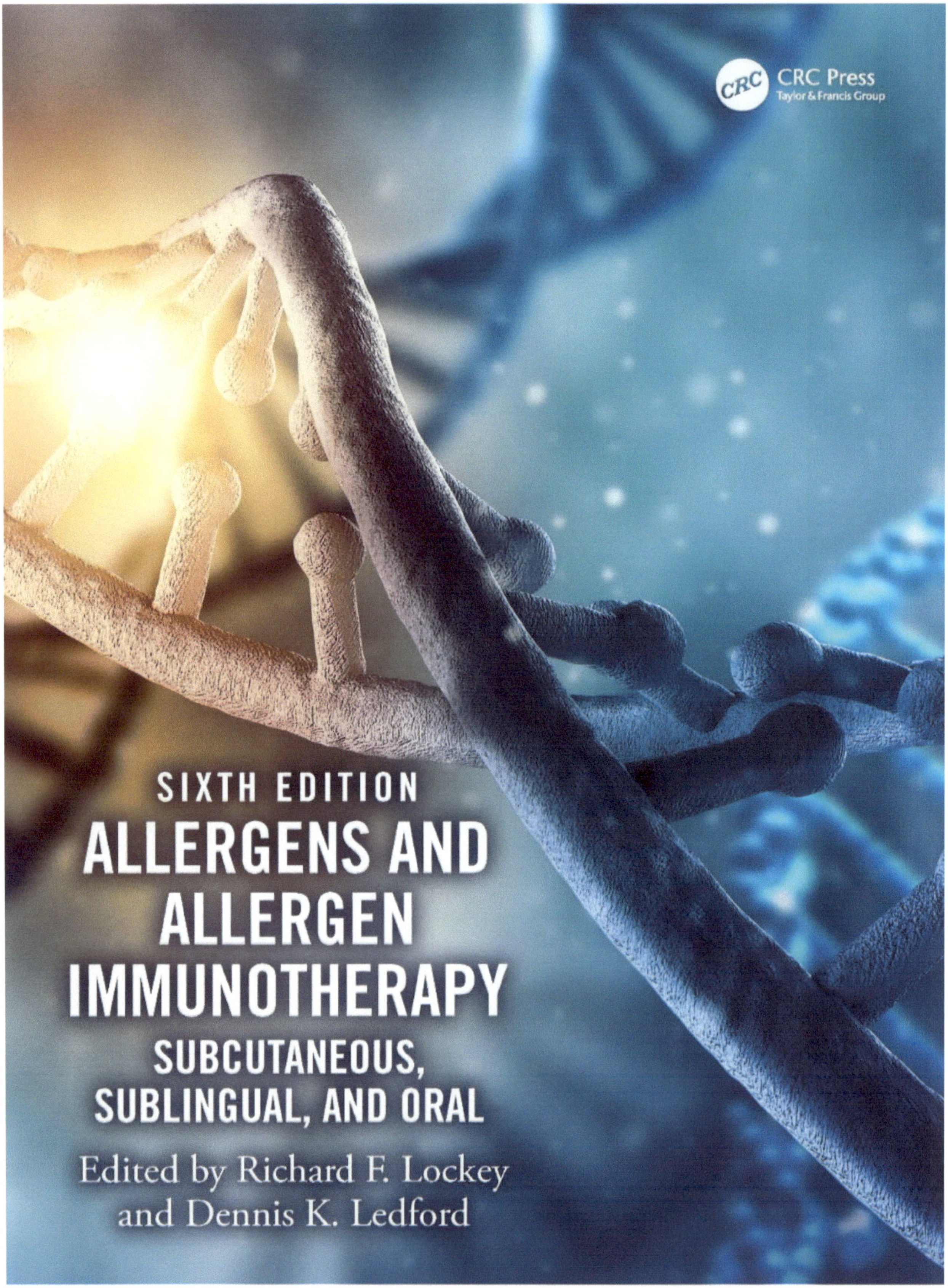

Lockey RF, Ledford DK (eds): Allergens and Allergen Immunotherapy for Allergic Diseases, Subcutaneous, Sublingual and Oral, 6th edition. CRC Press/Taylor & Francis Group, New York, NY, 2020.

Chapter 15: American Academy of Allergy Asthma & Immunology Meetings

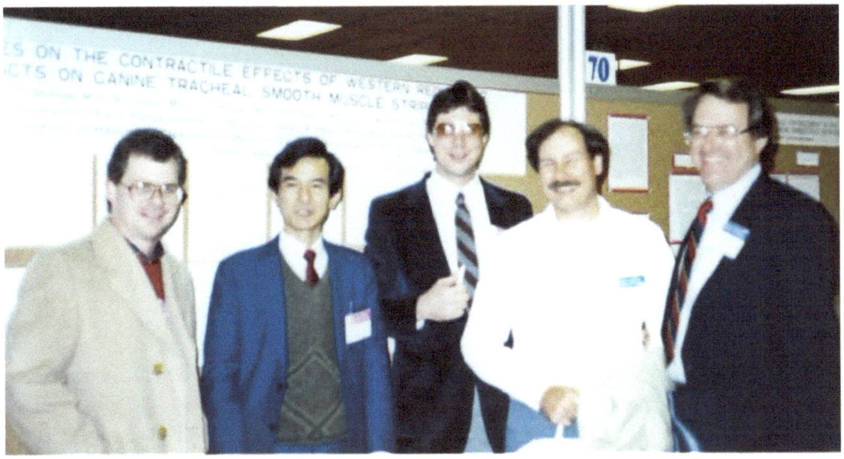

Left to right: Robert Duncan (Pharmacology and Therapeutics); Terufumi Shimoda, MD; Robert P. Nelson, MD (1985 – 1987); Gerald A. Bucholtz, MD (1980 – 1982); Richard F. Lockey, MD, MS, circa 1985.

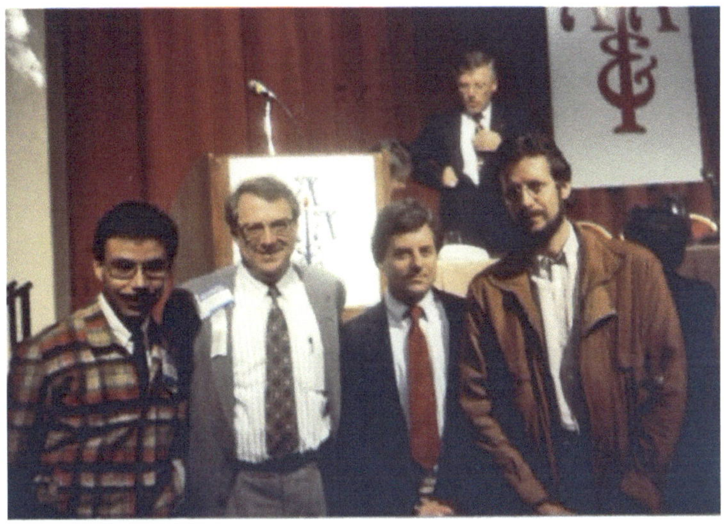

Left to right: Mohammed Askar, MD (visiting researcher from Egypt); Richard F. Lockey, MD, MS; Donald W. Russell, MD (1987 - 1990); Enrique Fernandez-Caldas, PhD. circa 1990.

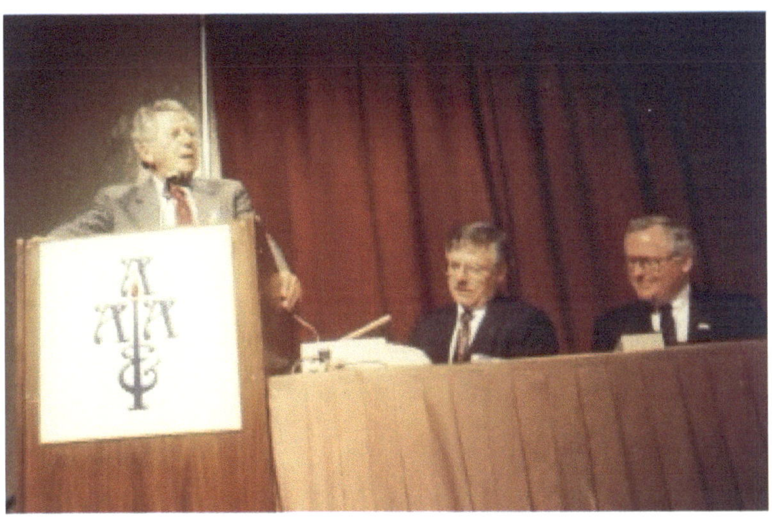

Left to right: Samuel C. Bukantz, MD; John Anderson, MD; William Pierson, MD, circa 1991. American Academy of Allergy & Immunology Annual Meeting, San Francisco, CA (Academy name has not yet been changed to American Academy of Allergy Asthma & Immunology).

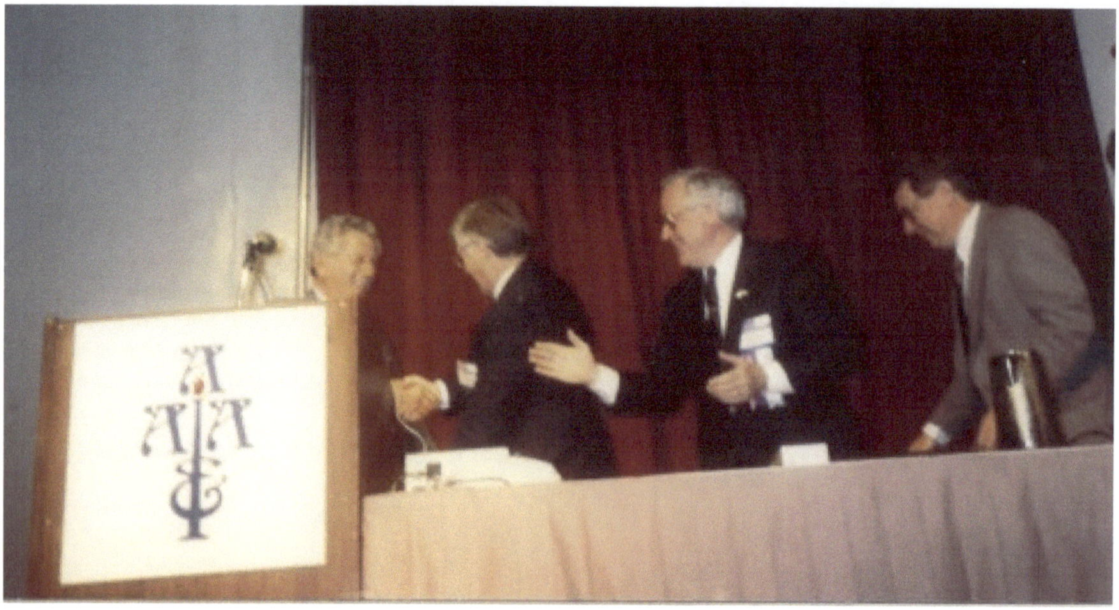

Left to right: Samuel C. Bukantz, MD; John Anderson, MD; William Pierson, MD; Richard F. Lockey, MD, MS; circa 1991.

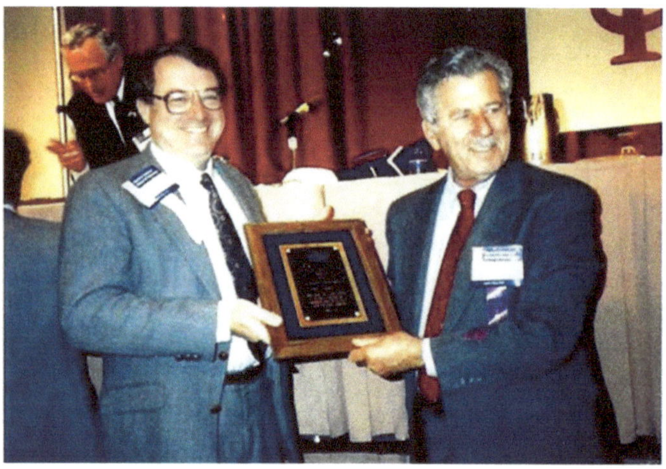

Left to right: Richard F. Lockey, MD, MS; Samuel C. Bukantz, MD. Dr. Bukantz, recipient of Distinguished Clinician Award, at the 1991 American Academy of Allergy & Immunology Annual Meeting, San Francisco, CA.

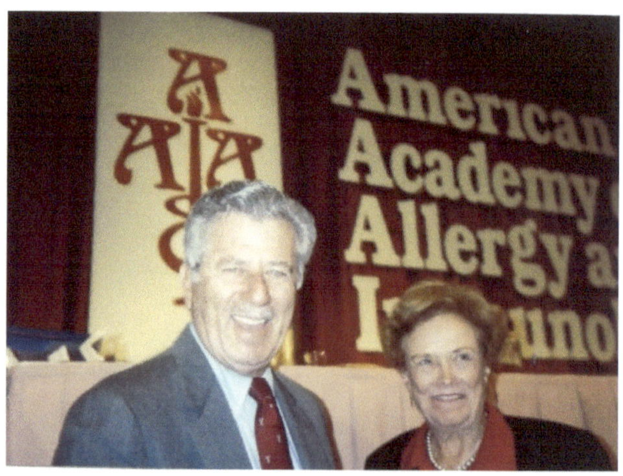

Dr. and Mrs. Samuel Bukantz (Jewell). American Academy of Allergy & Immunology Annual Meeting, San Francisco, CA, circa 1991.

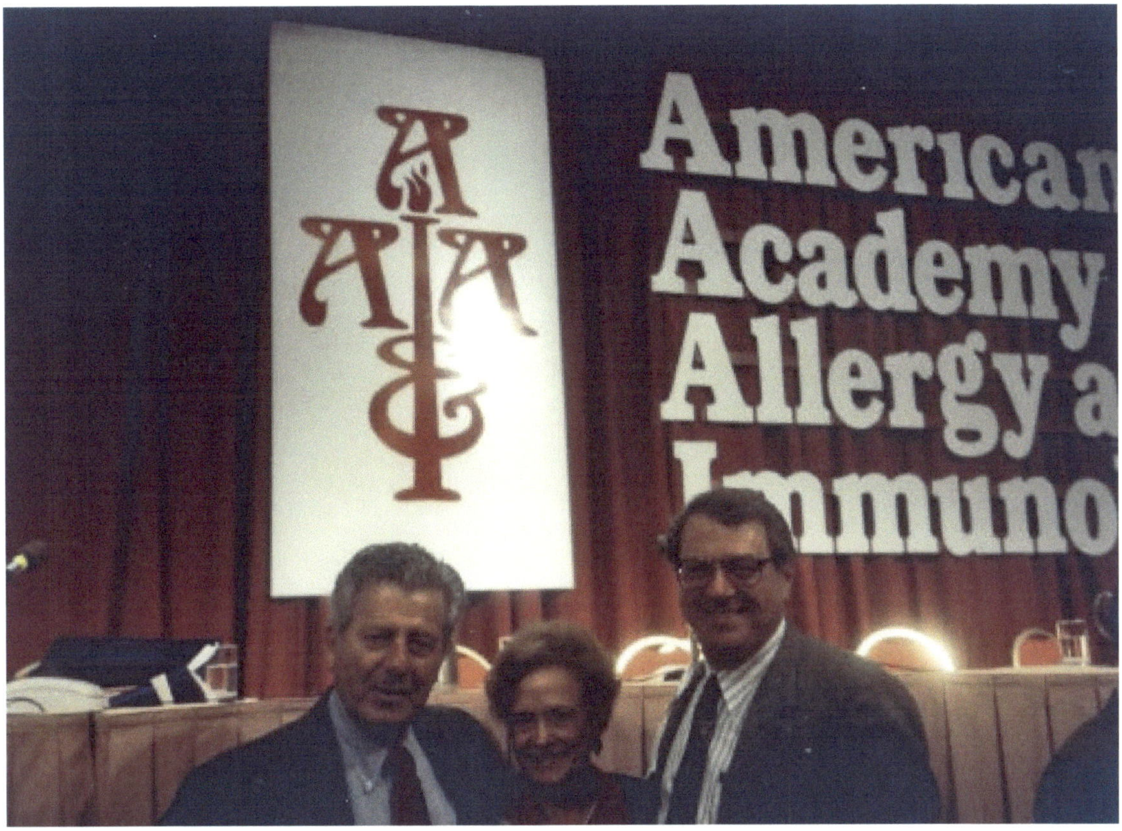

Left to right: Dr. and Mrs. Samuel Bukantz; Richard F. Lockey, MD, MS; circa 1991.

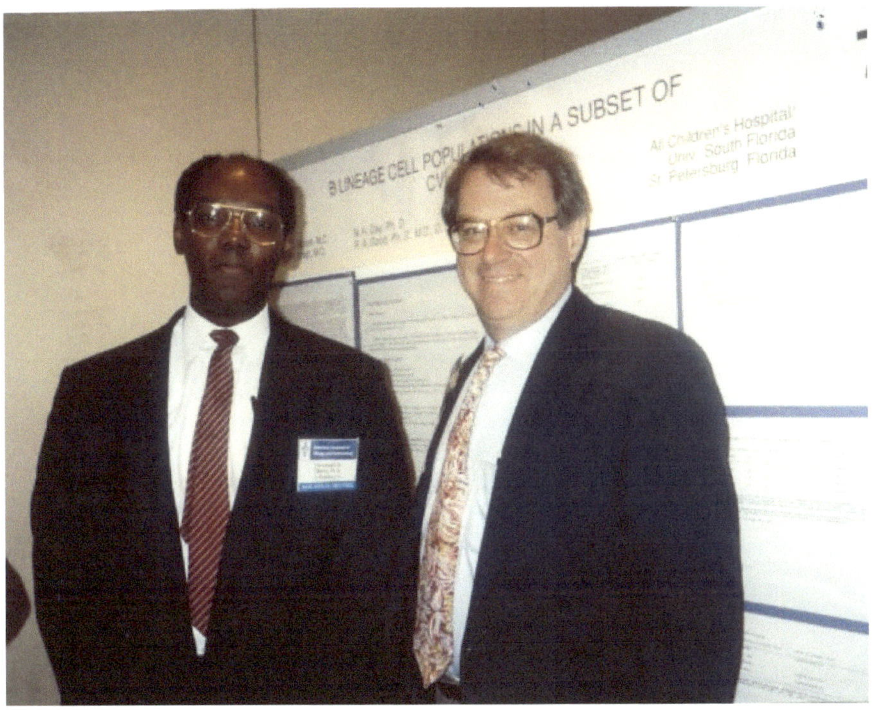

Left to right: Cleveland Moore, MD (ACH, 1990-1992) and Richard F. Lockey, MD, MS. 1991 American Academy of Allergy & Immunology Annual Meeting, San Francisco, CA. Poster: "B Lineage Cell Populations in a Subset of CVID Patients".

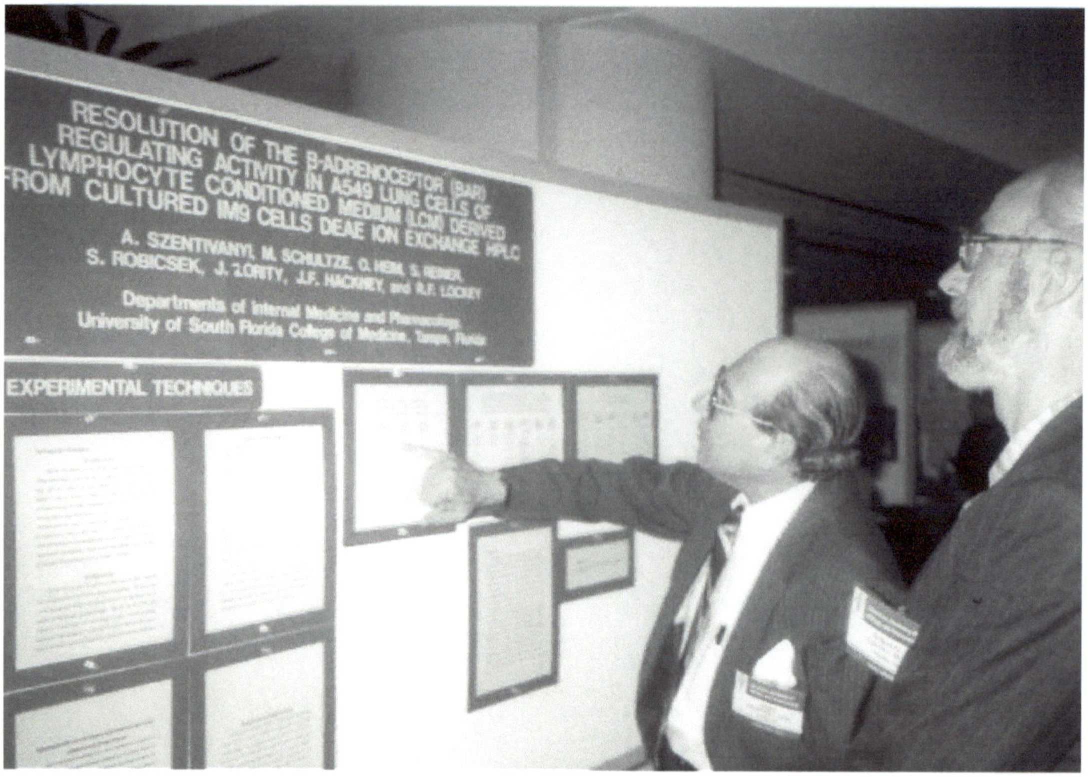

Andor Szentivanyi, MD. 1991 American Academy of Allergy & Immunology Annual Meeting, San Francisco, CA. Poster: "Resolution of the B Adrenoceptor (BAR) Regulating Activity in A549 Lung Cells of Lymphocyte Conditioned Medium (LCM) Derived from Cultured IM9 Cells with DEAE Ion Exchange HPLC".

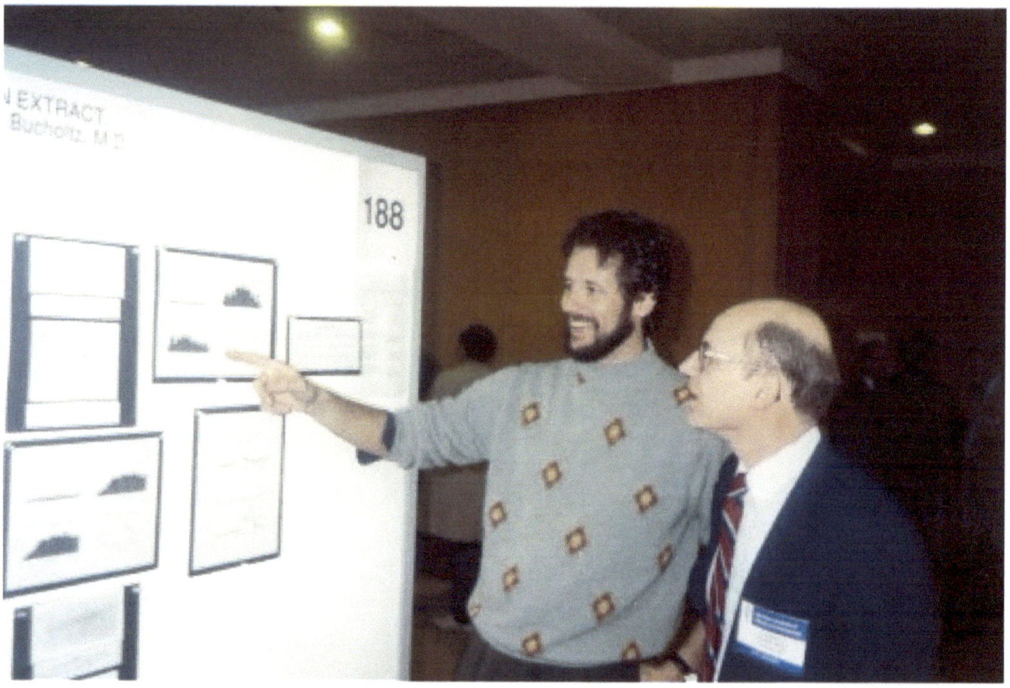

Left to right: Enrique Fernandez-Caldas, PhD; Gerald Gleich, MD. 1991 American Academy of Allergy & Immunology Annual Meeting, San Francisco, CA. Poster: "Immunochemical analysis of Bahia grass [Paspalum notation] pollen extract"

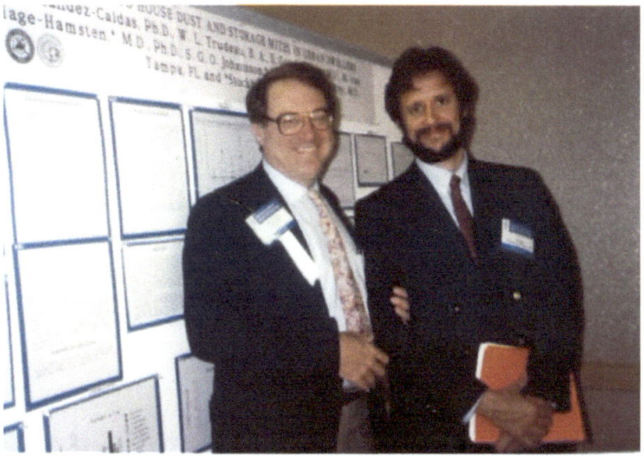

Left to right: Richard F. Lockey, MD, MS and Enrique Fernandez-Caldas, PhD. 1991 American Academy of Allergy & Immunology Annual Meeting, San Francisco, CA.

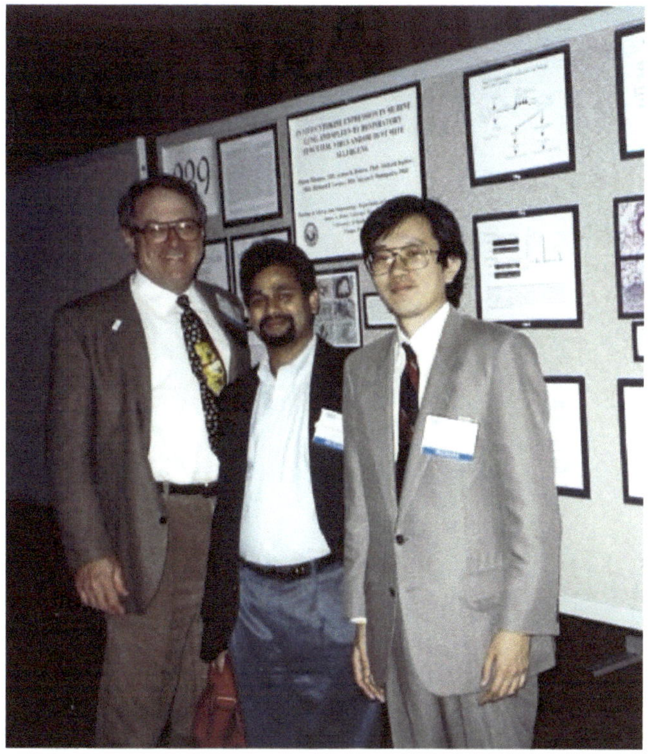

Above, left to right: Richard F. Lockey, MD, MS; Shyam S. Mohapatra, PhD; Hiroto Matsuse, MD. 1998 American Academy of Allergy Asthma & Immunology Annual Meeting, Washington, D.C. Poster: "In Vivo Cytokine Expression in Murine Lung and Spleen by Respiratory Syncytial Virus and/or Dust Mite Allergens".

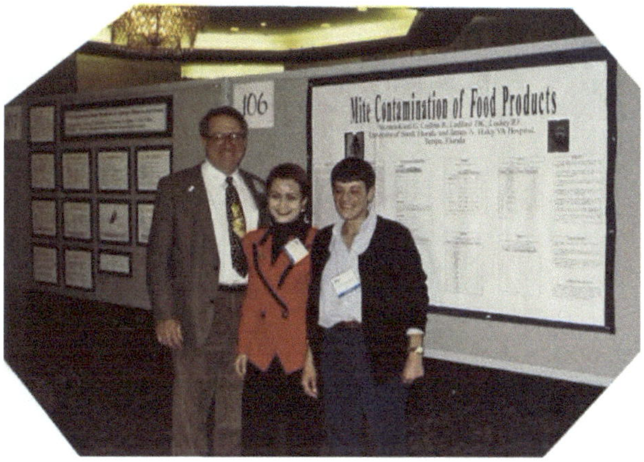

Left to right: Richrd F. Lockey, MD, MS; Giana L. Nicoara-Kasti, MD (1996-1998); Rosa Codina, PhD, at the 1998 American Academy of Allergy Asthma & Immunology Annual Meeting; Washington D.C. Poster: "Mite Contamination of Food Products".

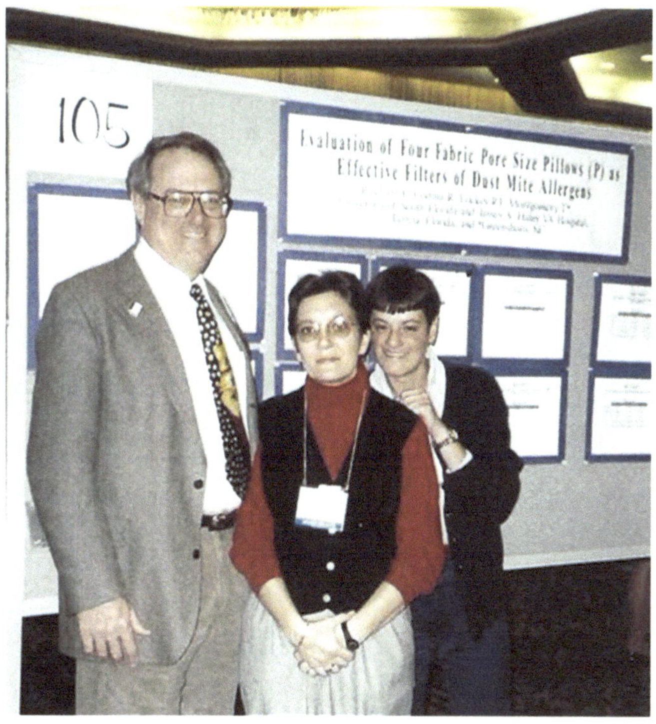

Left to right: Richard F. Lockey, MD, MS; Cindy Reichart; Rosa Codina, PhD. 1998 American Academy of Allergy Asthma & Immunology Annual Meeting, Washington, D.C. Poster: "Evaluation of Four Fabric Pore Size Pillows (P) as Effective Filters of Dust Mite Allergens".

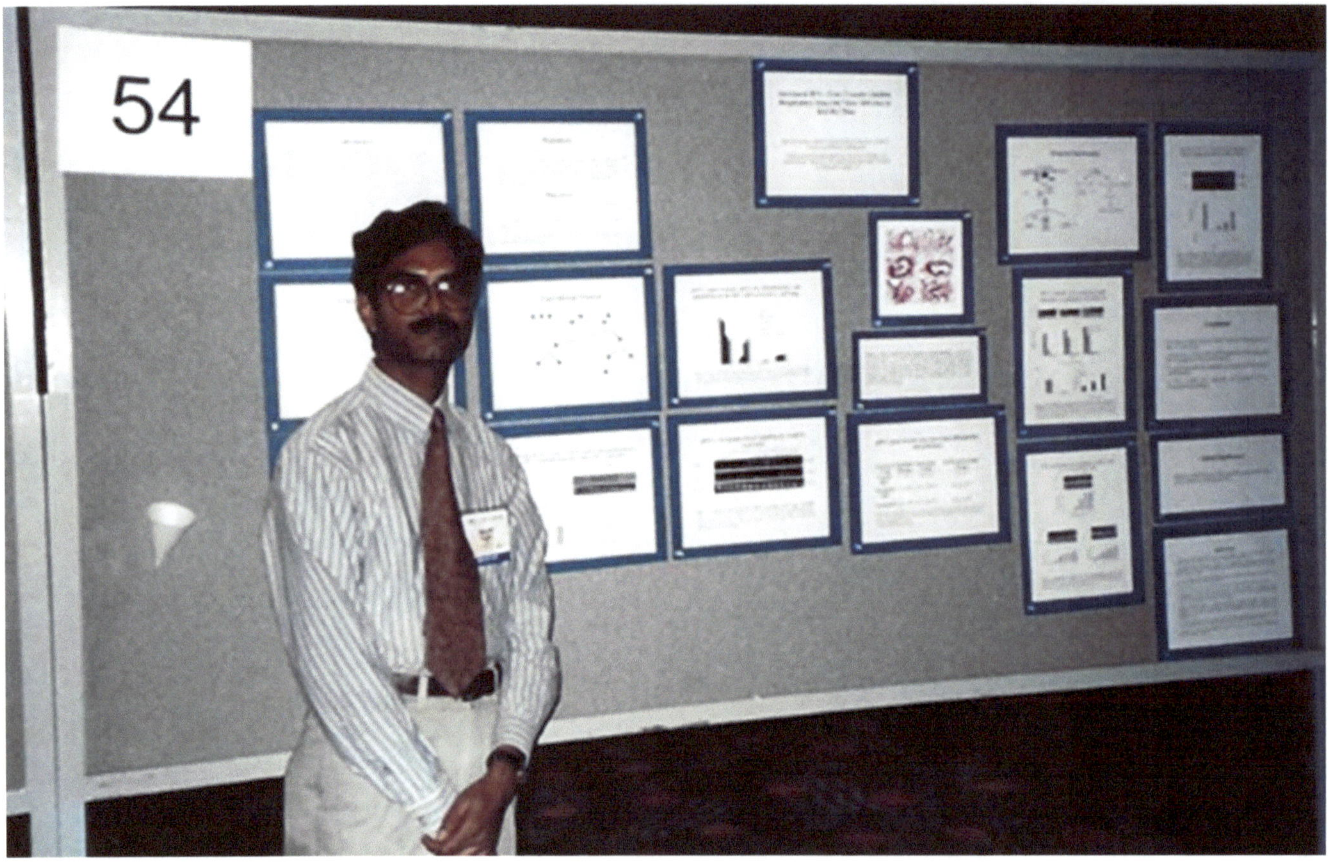

Mukesh Kumar, PhD. 1999 American Academy of Allergy Asthma & Immunology Annual Meeting, Orlando, FL. Poster: "An IFN-γ Plasmid DNA Vaccine Protects BALB/c Mice Against Respiratory Syncytial Virus Infection".

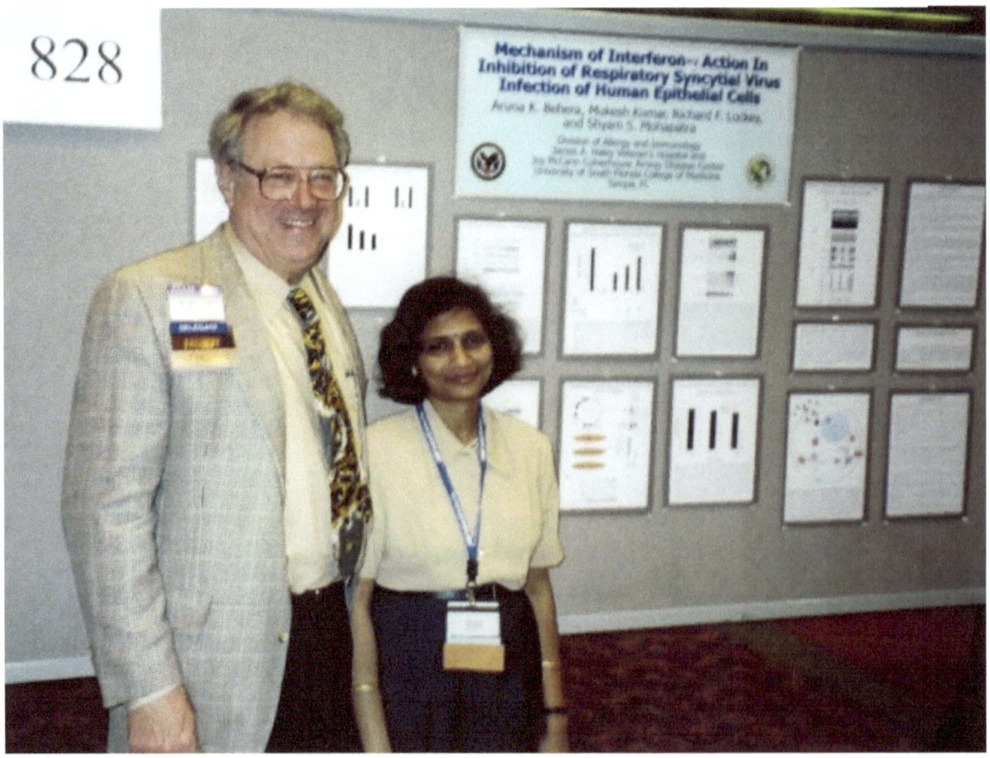

Left to right: Aruna Behera, PhD and Richard F. Lockey, MD, MS. 2001 American Academy of Allergy Asthma & Immunology Annual Meeting, New Orleans, LA. Poster: "Mechanism of Interferon-γ Inhibition of Respiratory Syncytial Virus Infection of Human Epithelial Cells".

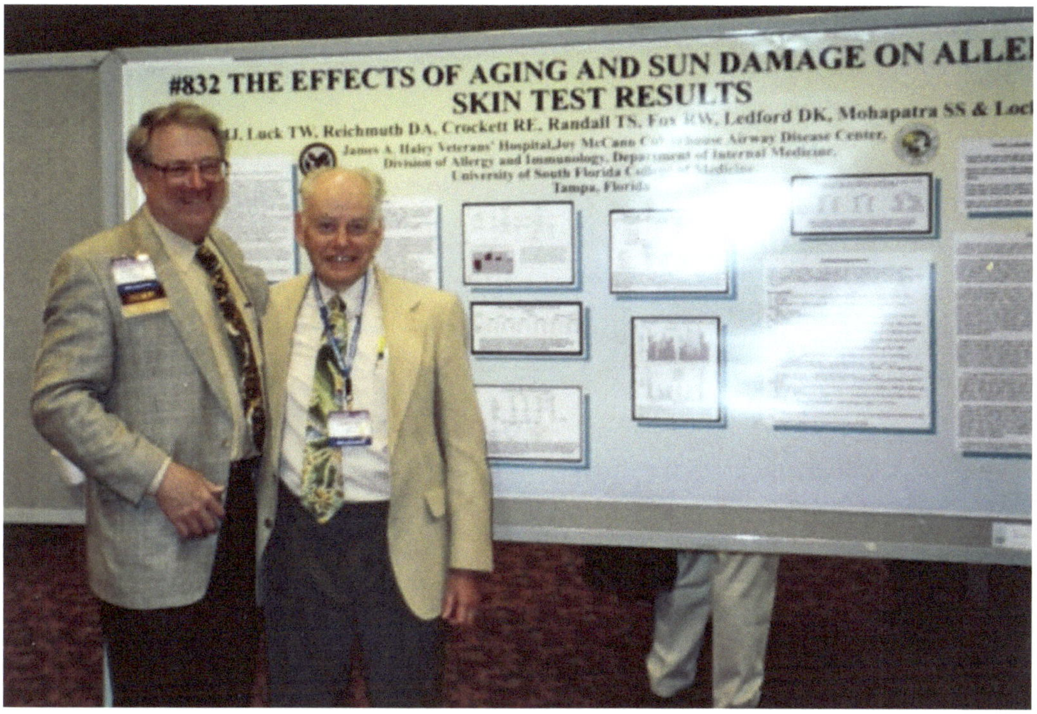

Left to right: Richard F. Lockey MD and Monroe J. King, DO. 2001 American Academy of Allergy Asthma & Immunology Annual Meeting, New Orleans, LA. Poster: "The Effects of Aging and Sun Damage on Allergy Skin Test Results".

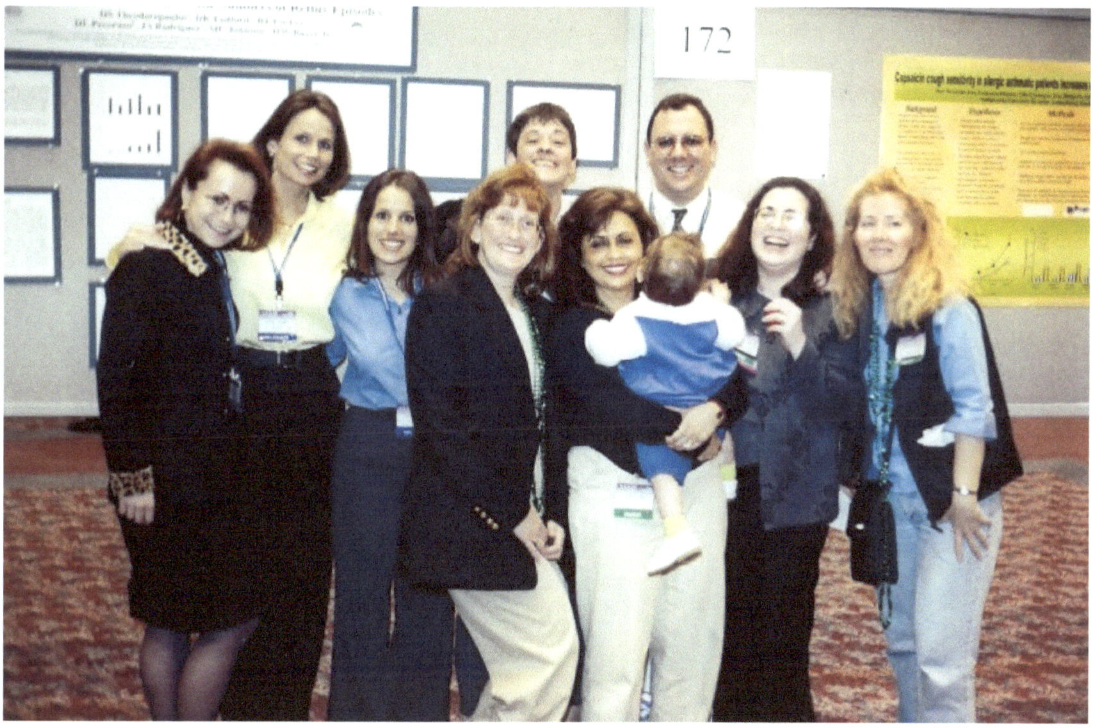

Front row (left to right): Peggy Hales; Geeta Gehi; Donna Pecoraro; Sandra Rocha. Back row (left to right): Giana L. Nicoara-Kasti, MD (1996-1998); Diana Miller; Alisa Diecidue; Rosa Codina, PhD; Demetrios Theodoropoulos, MD (1997-2000). 2001 American Academy of Allergy Asthma & Immunology Annual Meeting, New Orleans, LA. Poster: "Gastroesophageal Reflux Disease (GERD) Associated Symptom Scores Correlate with Numbers of Reflux EpisoSandes".

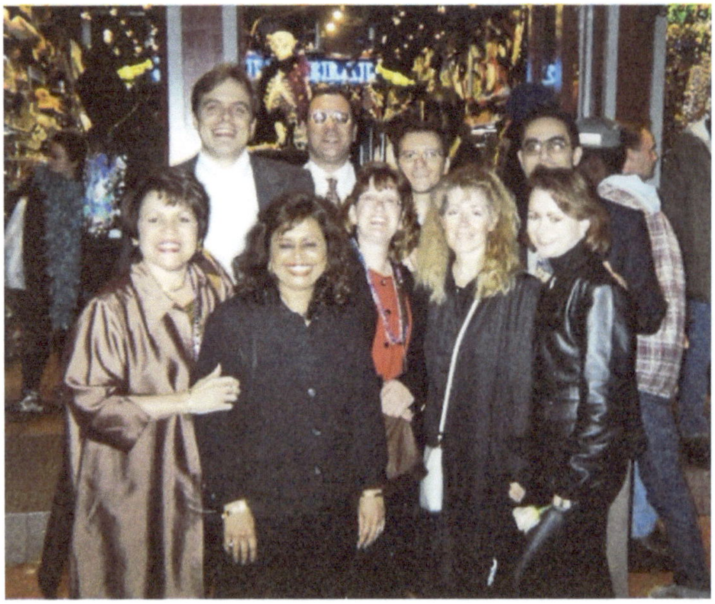

Front row (left to right): Nina Ramirez, MD (2000 – 2002); Geeta Gehi; Peggy Hales; Sandra Rocha; Giana L. Nicoara-Kasti, MD (1996-1998).
Back row (left to right): Richard Crockett, MD (2000 – 2003); Demetrios Theodoropoulos, MD (1997-2000); Pedro M. Ojeda, MD; Mo Kasti.
New Orleans, LA, 2001.

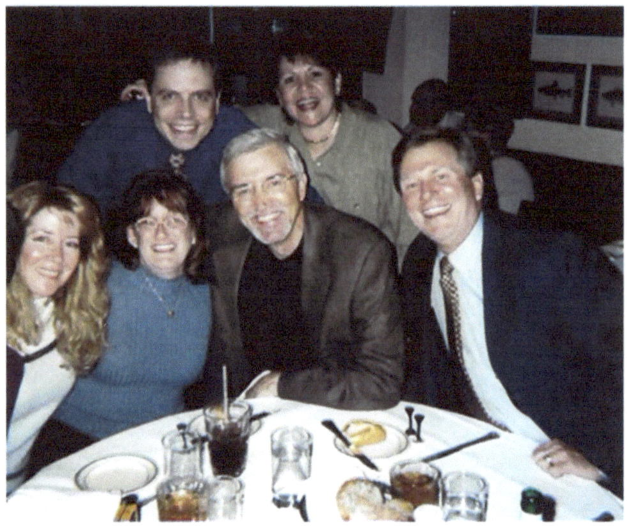

Front row (left to right): Sandra Rocha; Peggy Hales; Dennis K. Ledford, MD (1983-1986); Roger W. Fox, MD (1978-1980). Back row (left to right): Richard Crockett, MD (2000-2003); Nina Ramirez, MD (2000-2002). Dinner at the American Academy of Allergy Asthma & Immunology Annual Meeting, 2002 New York City, NY.

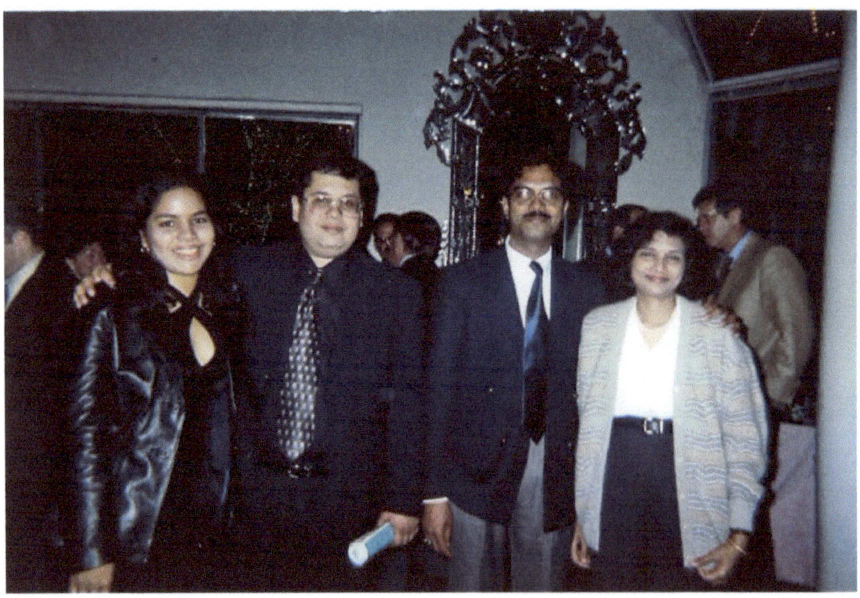

Left to right: Dr. and Mrs. Homero San Juan; Mukesh Kumar, PhD; Aruna Behera, PhD. 2002 USF Alumni Dinner, American Academy of Allergy Asthma & Immunology Annual Meeting, Tavern on the Green, New York City, NY.

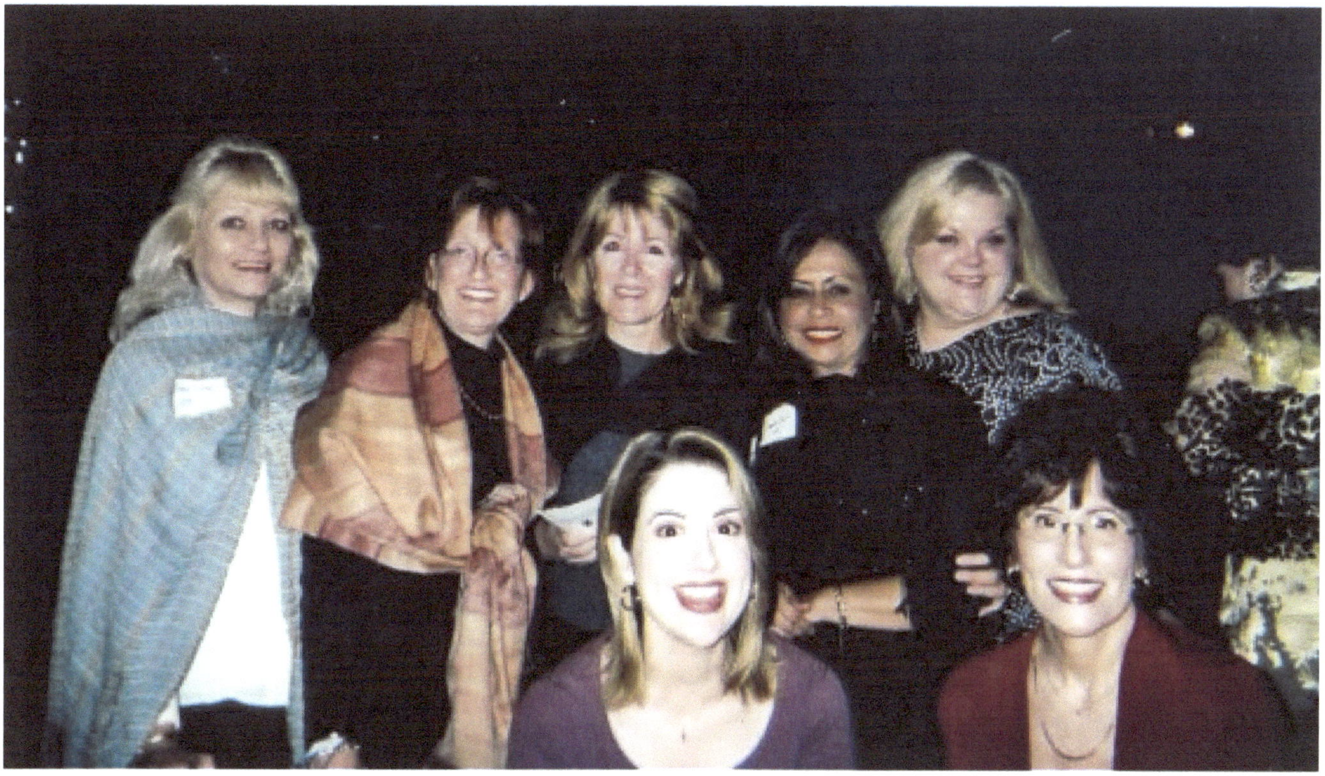

Front row (left to right): Lizette Hernandez, MD (1994-1997) and Sonia Hernandez. Back row (left to right): Rebecca Carter-Muncey; Peggy Hales; Sandra Rocha; Geeta Gehi; Anna Palles (nurse, USF Clinic). 2006 USF Alumni Dinner, American Academy of Allergy Asthma & Immunology Annual Meeting, Miami, FL.

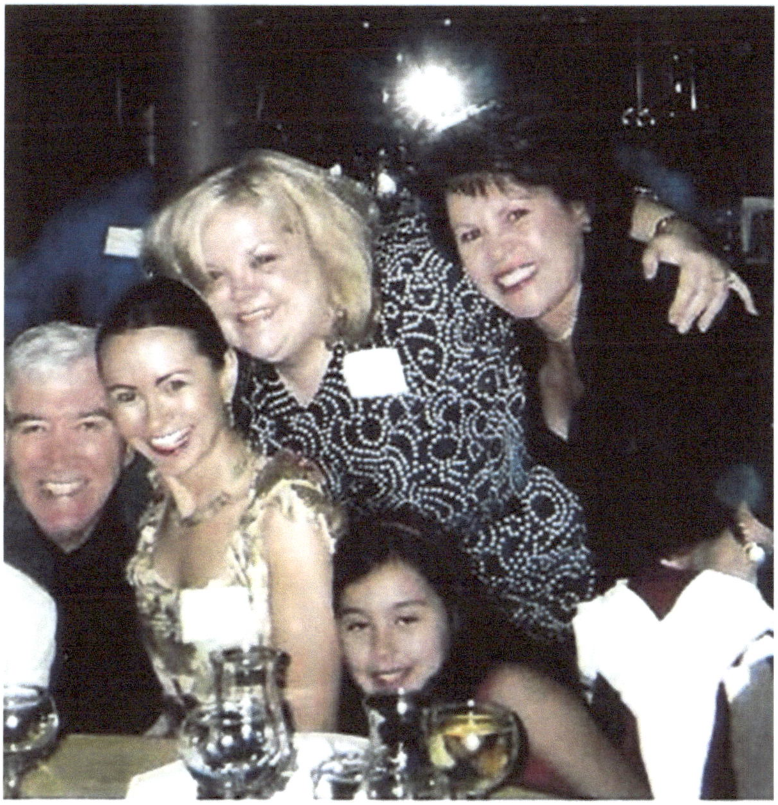

Front (left to right:) Giana L. Nicoara-Kasti, MD (1996-1998) and Ines Kasti. Back (left to right:) Dennis K. Ledford, MD (1983-1985); Anna Palles (nurse USF Clinic); Nina Ramirez, MD (2000 – 2002). 2006 USF Alumni Dinner, American Academy of Allergy Asthma & Immunology Annual Meeting, Miami, FL.

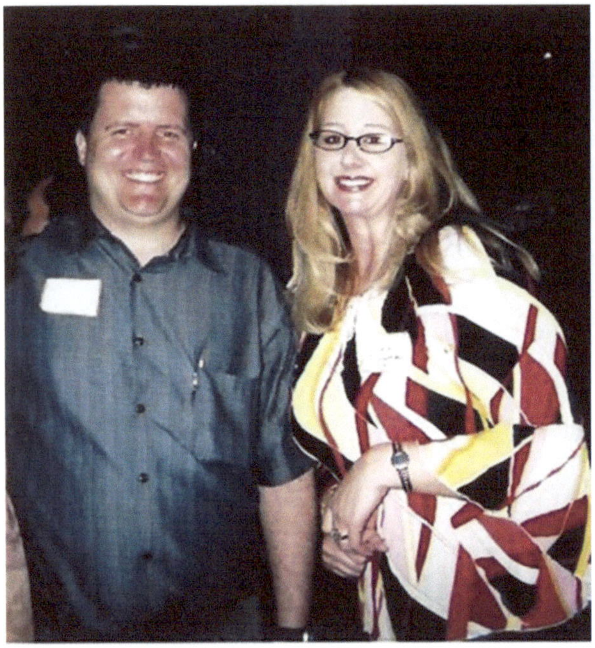

Sean McKnight, MD (2002-2004) and Michelle Grandstaff-Singleton. 2006 USF Alumni Dinner, American Academy of Allergy Asthma & Immunology Annual Meeting, Miami, FL.

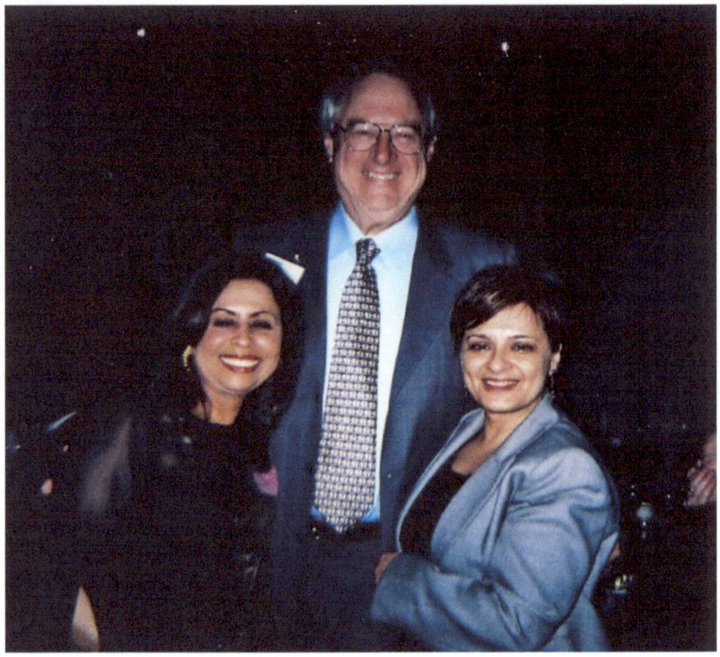

Left to right: Geeta Gehi; Richard F. Lockey, MD, MS; Charu Malik, PhD (World Allergy Organization Executive Director). 2009 American Academy of Allergy Asthma & Immunology Annual Meeting, Education and Research Trust Fund Dinner, Washington, D.C.

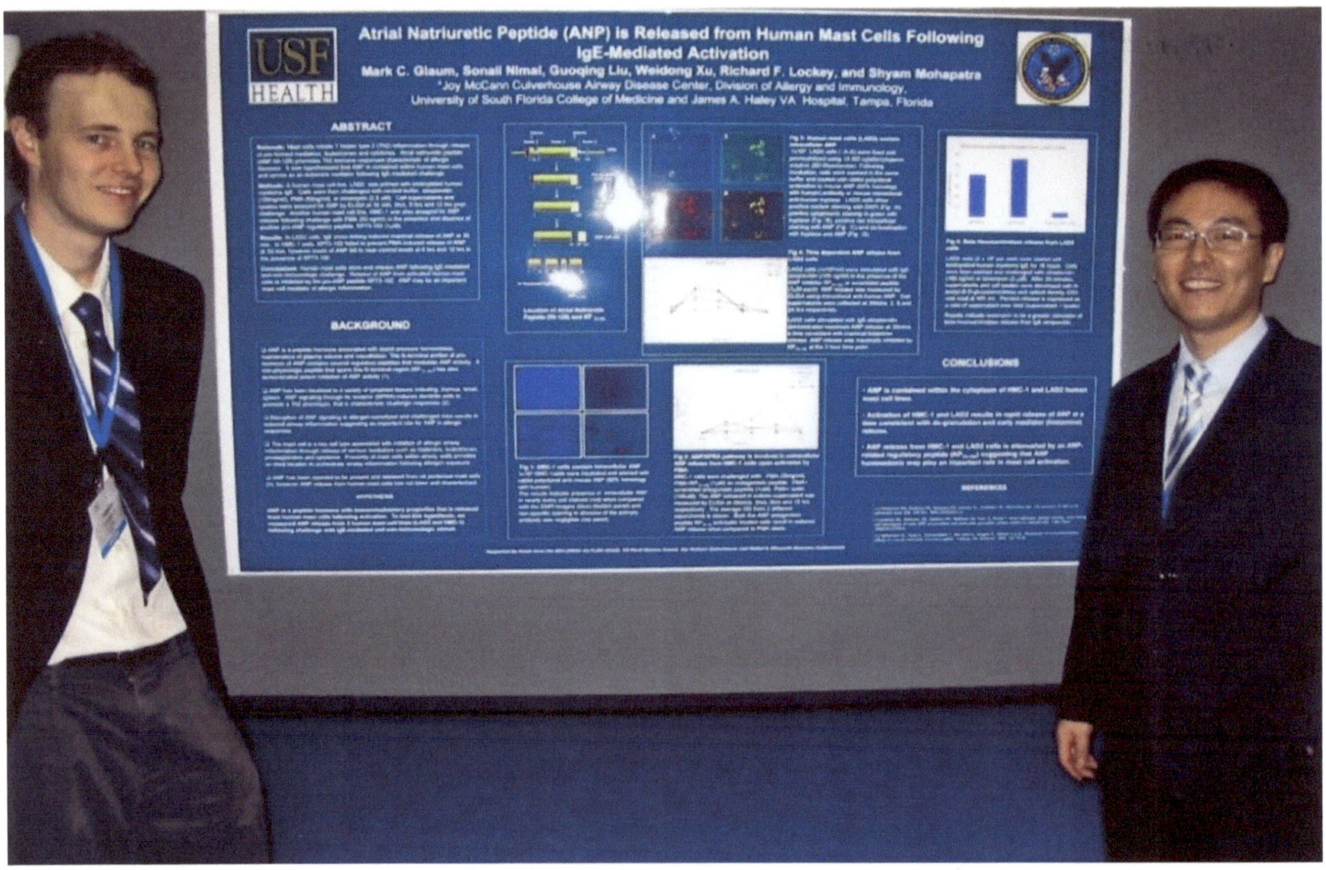
USF
HEALTH
Atrial Natriuretic Peptide (ANP) is Released from Human Mast Cells Following IgE-Mediated Activation
Mark C. Glaum, Sonali Nimal, Guoqing Liu, Weidong Xu, Richard F. Lockey, and Shyam Mohapatra
Joy McCann Culverhouse Airway Disease Center, Division of Allergy and Immunology,
University of South Florida College of Medicine and James A. Haley VA Hospital, Tampa, Florida
ABSTRACT
BACKGROUND
CONCLUSIONS
REFERENCES

Andrew Bagg, MD (2006-2008) and Byol Shin, DO (2006-2008). 2007 American Academy of Allergy, Asthma & Immunology Annual Meeting, San Diego, CA.

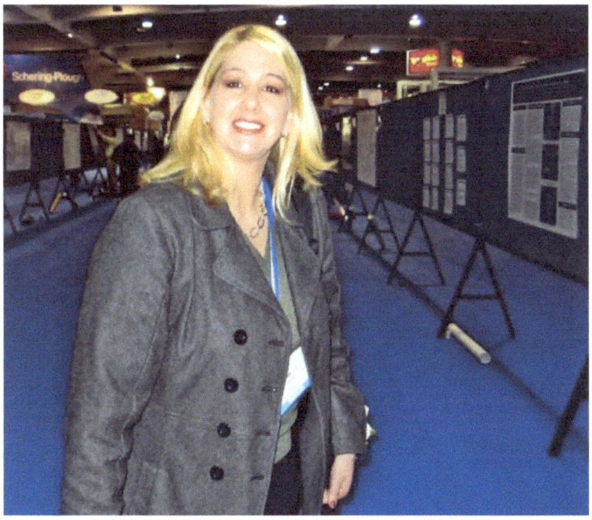

Michelle Grandstaff-Singleton. 2007 American Academy of Allergy Asthma & Immunology Annual Meeting exhibit hall, San Diego, CA.

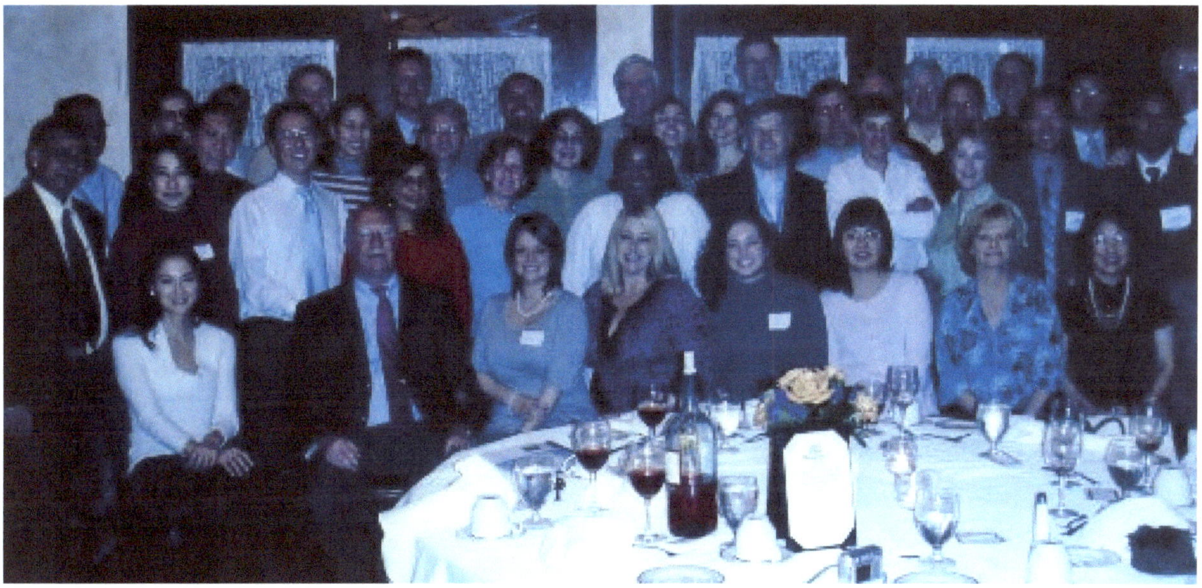

2008 USF Alumni Dinner; American Academy of Allergy Asthma & Immunology Annual Meeting, Philadelphia, PA.

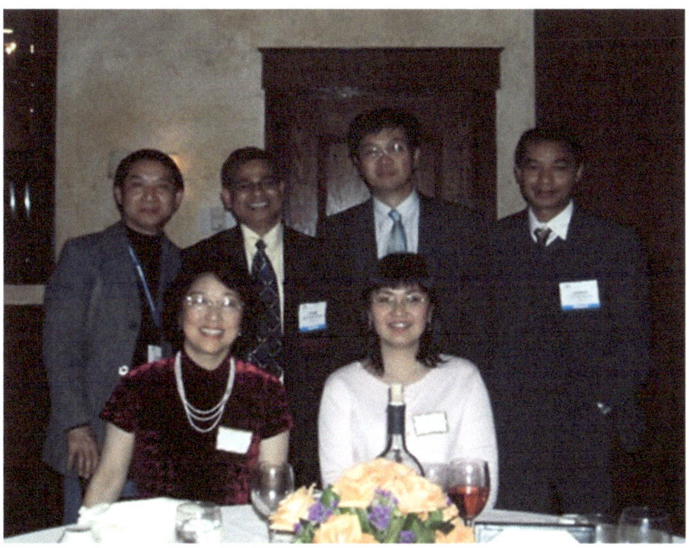

Front row (left to right); Xiaoyuan (Sonya) Kong, MD and Xiaoqin Wang. Back row (left to right): Guoqing Liu, PhD; Shyam S. Mohapatra, PhD; Weidong Zhang, MD, PhD; Jia-Wang Wang, PhD. 2008 USF Alumni Dinner; American Academy of Allergy Asthma & Immunology Annual Meeting, Philadelphia, PA.

Left to right: Cristina Jaen, PhD; Richard F. Lockey, MD, MS; Rosa Codina, PhD; Enrique Fernandez-Caldas, PhD; Maria Teresa de la Morena, MD (ACH, 1991-1995); Lionel V. Bonini, MD (ACH, 1986-1988). 2008 USF Alumni Dinner, American Academy of Allergy Asthma & Immunology Annual Meeting.*

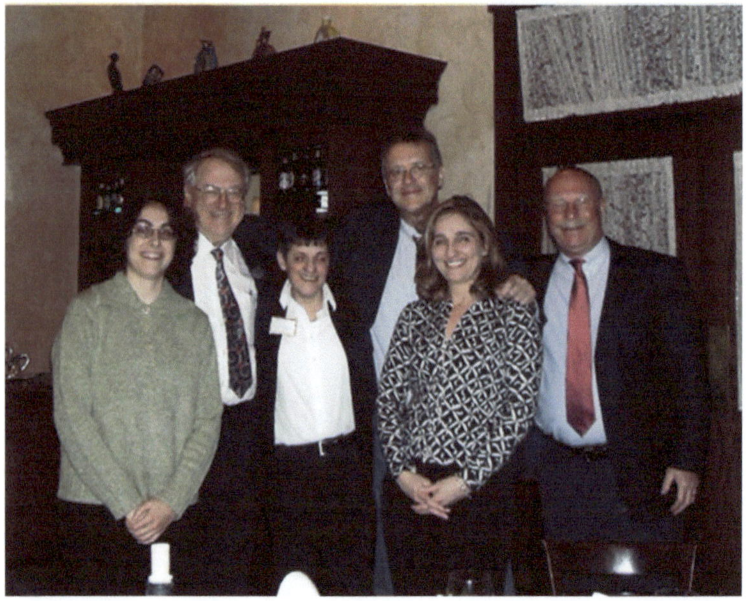

Left to right: Drs. Dennis (2008-2010) and Jenny Kim; Trace Adkins; Joshua Phillips, MD (2007-2009). Trace Adkins, country music artist, guest speaker, 2009 Education and Research Trust Fund Dinner, American Academy of Allergy Asthma & Immunology Annual Meeting, Washington, D.C.

Left to right: Suhail Dever (nurse, Drs. Lockey, Fox, Ledford, Glaum clinical practice); Richard F Lockey, MD, MS; Kathy O'Berry (nurse, Drs. Lockey, Fox, Ledford, Glaum clinical practice); 2009 Education and Research Trust Fund Dinner, American Academy of Allergy Asthma & Immunology Annual Meeting, Washington, D.C.

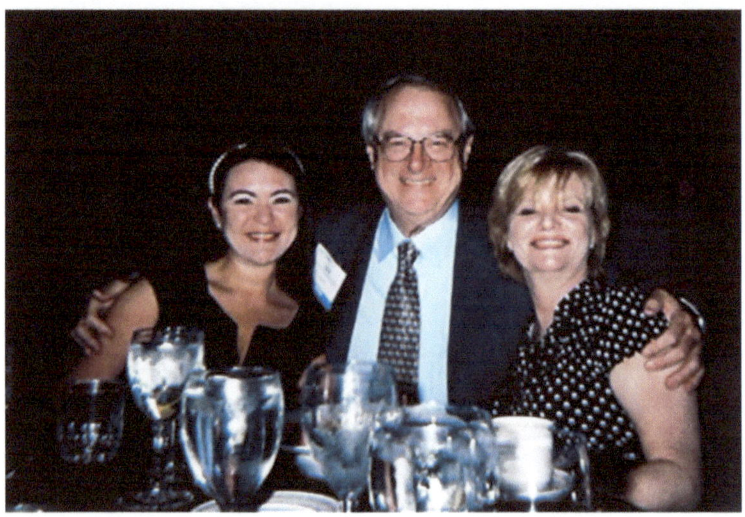

Left to right: Mr. and Mrs. Michael Ledford; Dennis K. Ledford, MD (1983-1986); and Thomas B. Casale, MD. 2009 American Academy of Allergy Asthma & Immunology Annual Meeting, Education and Research Trust Fund Dinner, Washington, D.C.

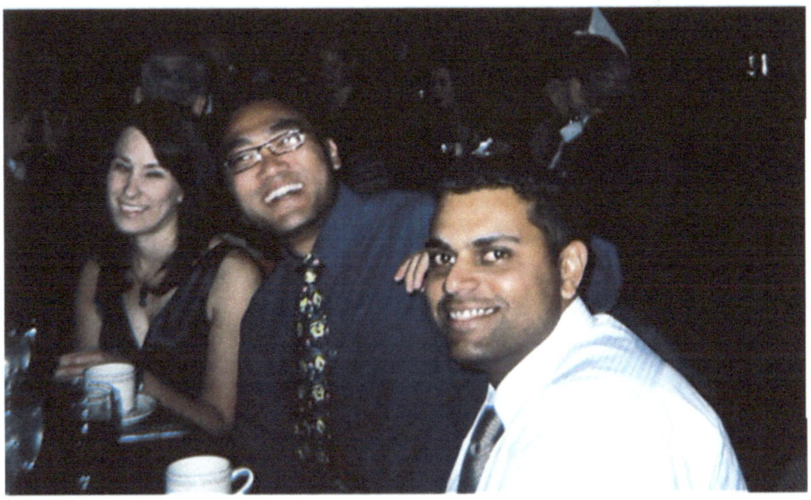

Left to right: Drs. Jenny and Dennis Kim (2008-2010) and Mathew Varghese, MD (2007-2009). 2009 American Academy of Allergy Asthma & Immunology Annual Meeting, Education and Research Trust Fund Dinner, Washington, D.C.

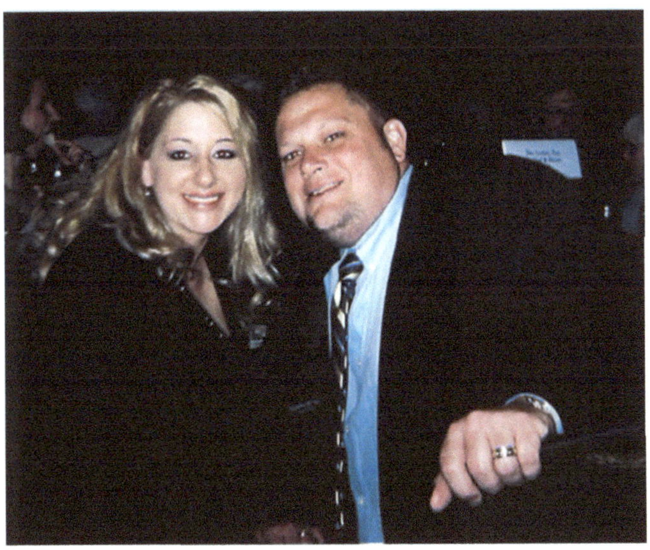

Left to right: Michelle Grandstaff-Singleton and Michael Singleton. 2009 Education and Research Trust Fund Dinner, American Academy of Allergy Asthma & Immunology Annual Meeting, Washington, D.C.

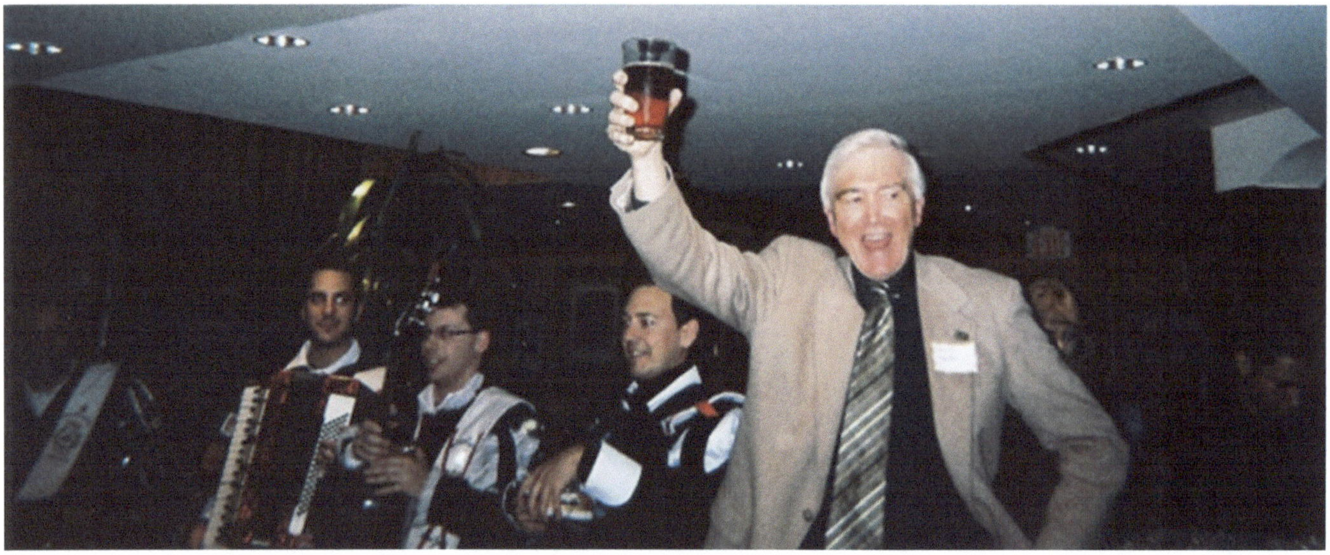

Dennis K. Ledford, MD (1983-1986) and mariachi band. 2009 USF Alumni Dinner, American Academy of Allergy Asthma & Immunology Annual Meeting, Washington, D.C.

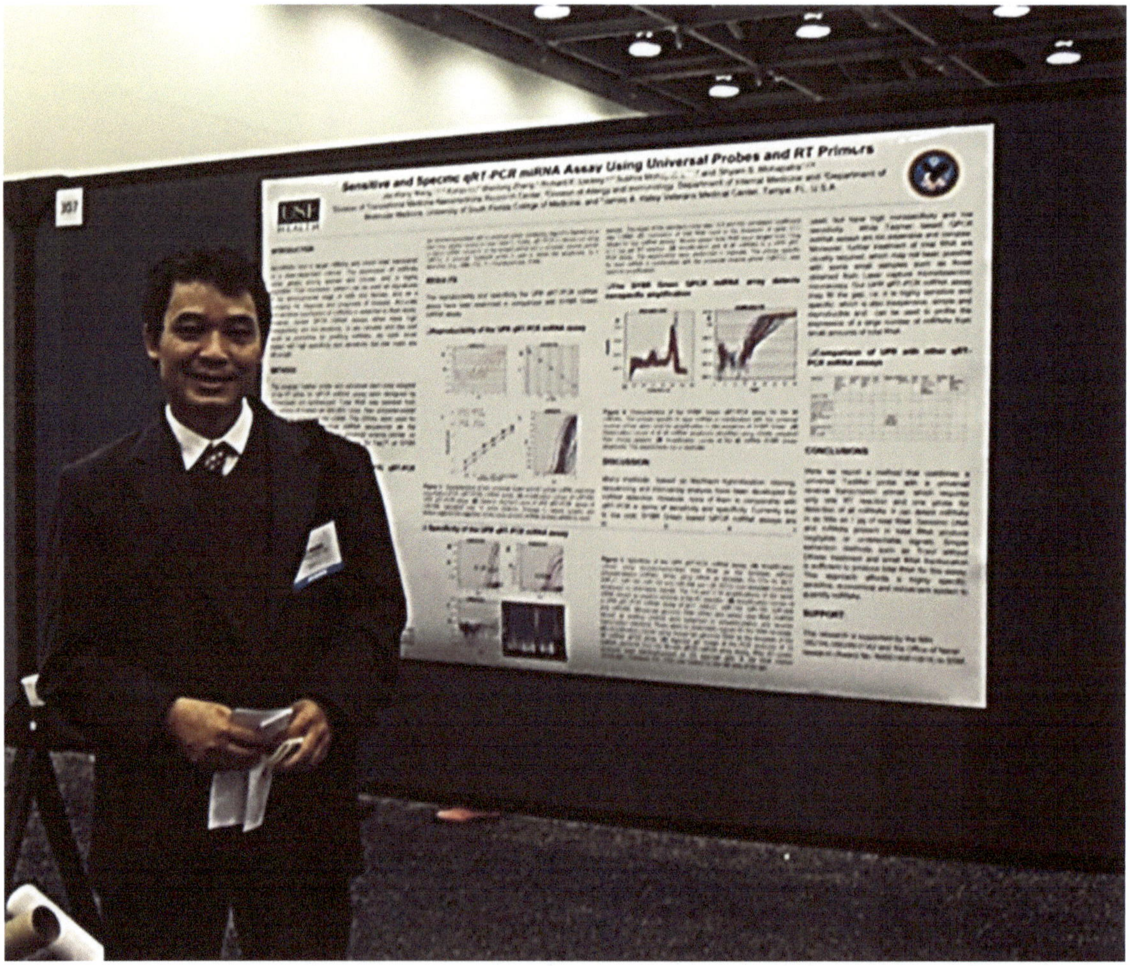

Jia-Wang Wang, PhD. 2011 Annual American Academy of Allergy Asthma & Immunology Annual Meeting, San Francisco, CA. Poster: "Sensitive and Specific qRT-PCR miRNA Assay Using Universal Probes and RT Primers".

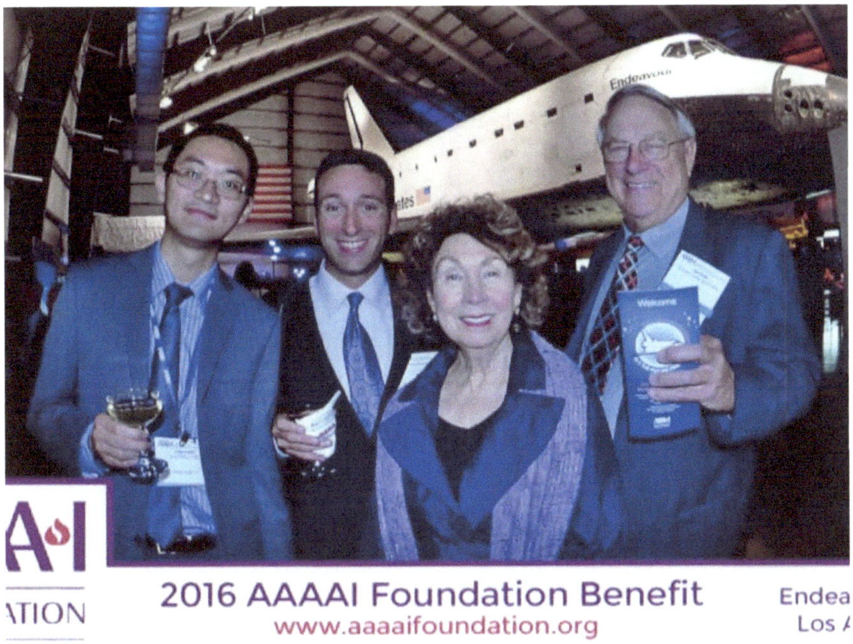

Left to right: Chen Hsing Lin, MD (2015 – 1027); Peter Ricketti, DO (2015 – 2017); Carol Lee Lockey; Richard F. Lockey, MD, MS. 2016 American Academy of Allergy Asthma & Immunology Foundation Benefit; Los Angeles, CA.

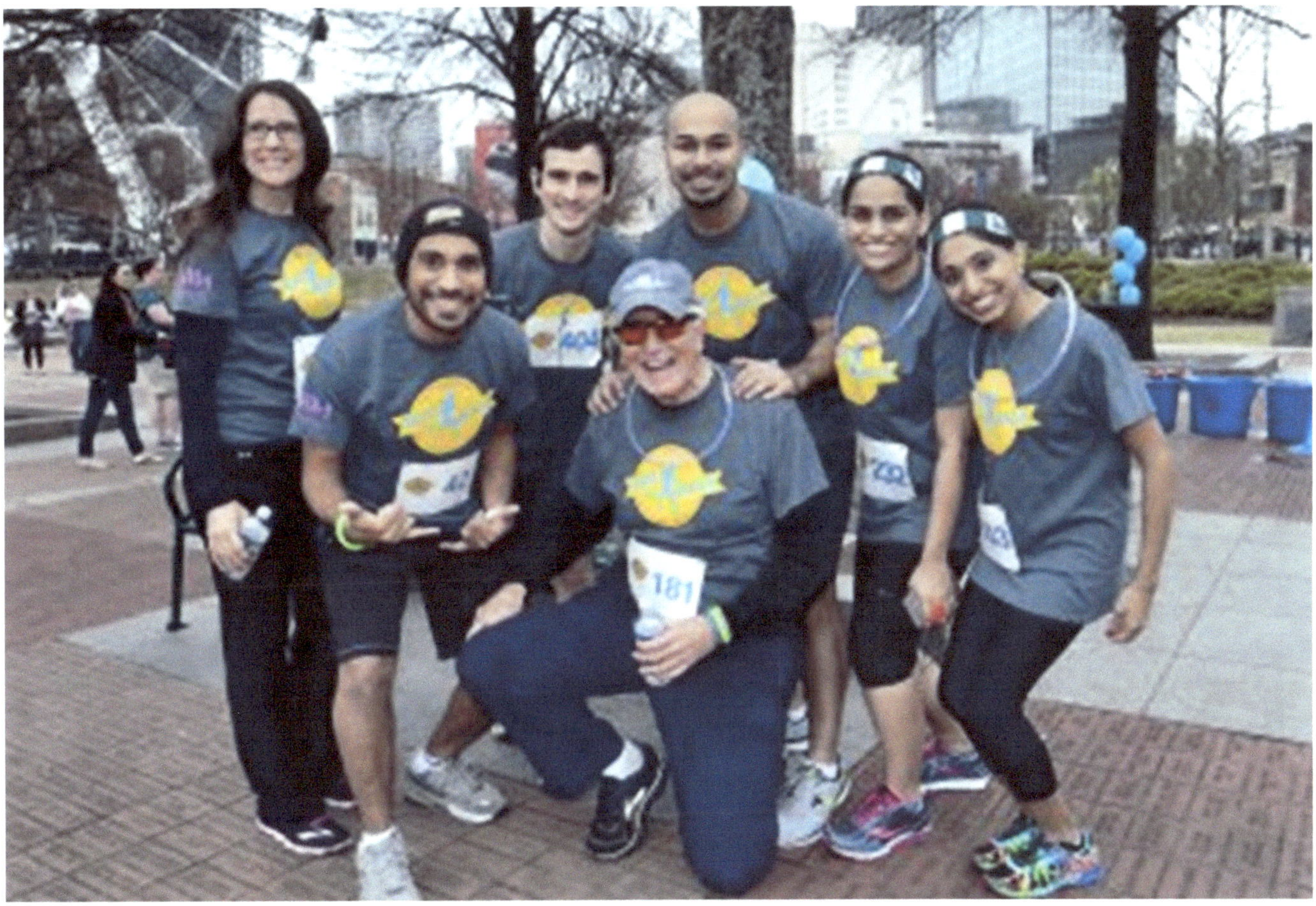

Front row (left to right): Adeeb Bulkhi, MD (2014-2017); Dennis K. Ledford, MD (1983-1985). Back row (left to right): Michelle Twitmyer; Andrew Cooke, MD (2014-2016); Sultan Alandijani, MD (2015-2017); Bhumika Patel, MD (ACH, 2015-2017); Sonia Joychan, MD (ACH, 2016-2018). 2017 American Academy of Allergy Asthma & Immunology Foundation 5K Run/Walk fund raiser, Atlanta, GA.

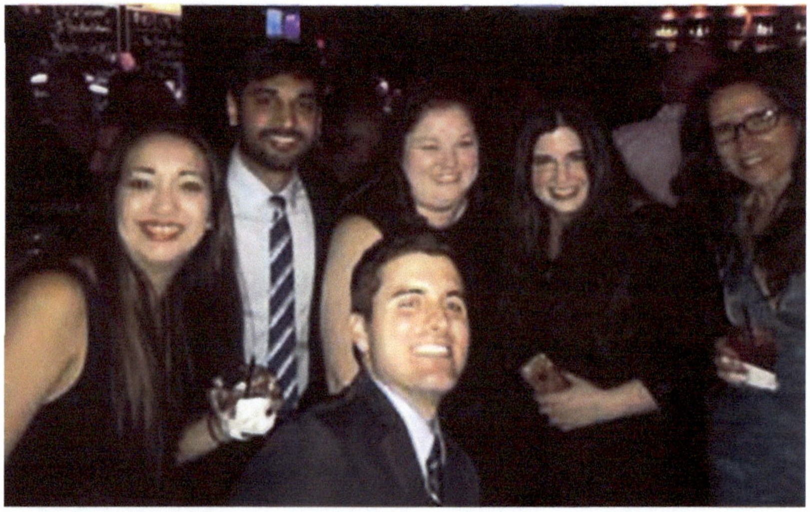

Front row: Kirk Shepard, MD (2017-2019). Back row (left to right): Tiffani Kaage; Shiven Patel, MD (2017-2019); Renee Smith; Tara V. Saco, MD (2017-2019); Michelle Twitmyer. 2017 American Academy of Allergy Asthma & Immunology Annual Meeting; Atlanta, GA.

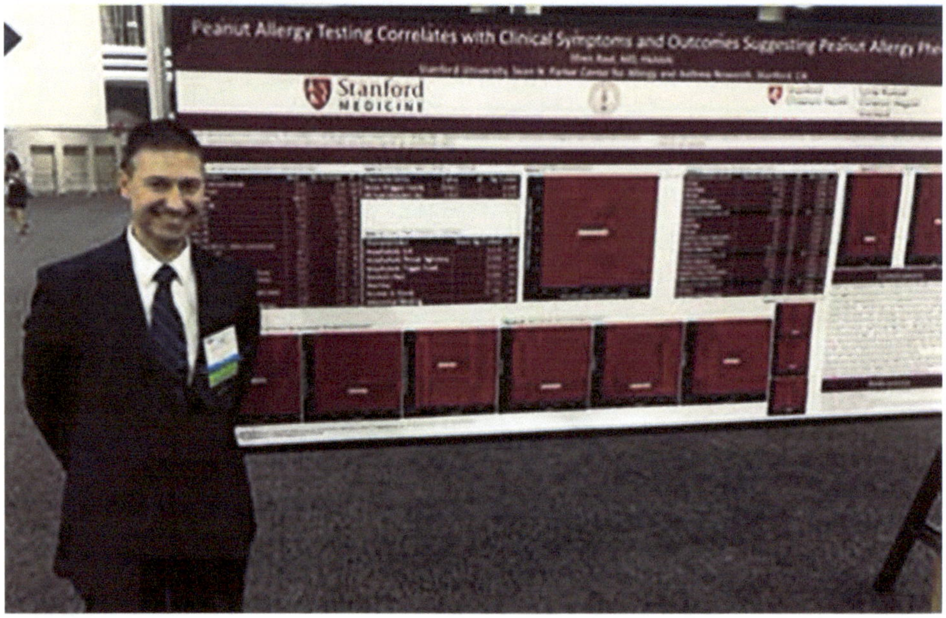
Peanut Allergy Testing Correlates with Clinical Symptoms and Outcomes Suggesting Peanut Allergy
Stanford MEDICINE

Efren Rael, MD (2008-2010). 2017 American Academy of Allergy Asthma & Immunology Annual Meeting, Atlanta, GA.

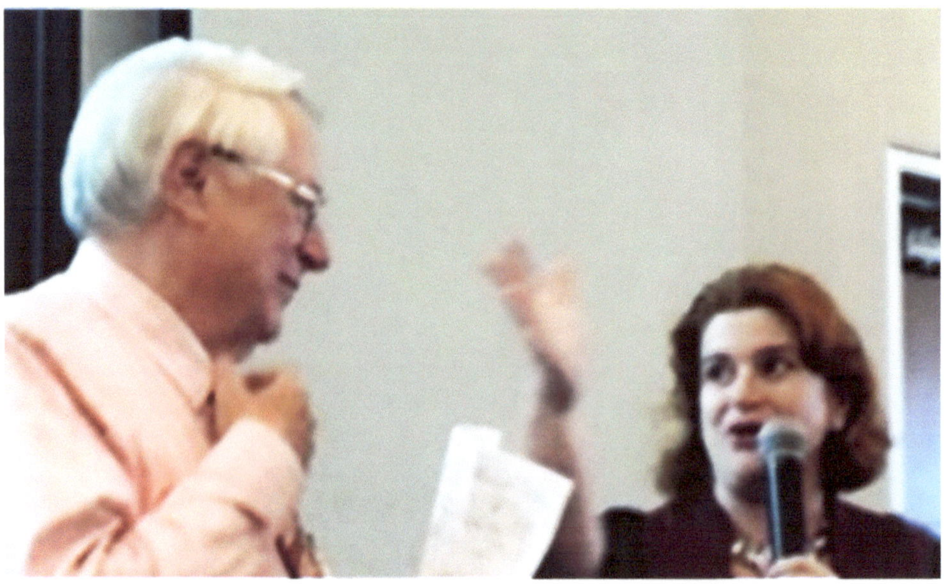

Left to right: Richard F. Lockey, MD, MS and Jolan Walter, MD, PhD. 2018 USF Alumni Dinner; American Academy of Allergy Asthma & Immunology Annual Meeting, Orlando, FL.

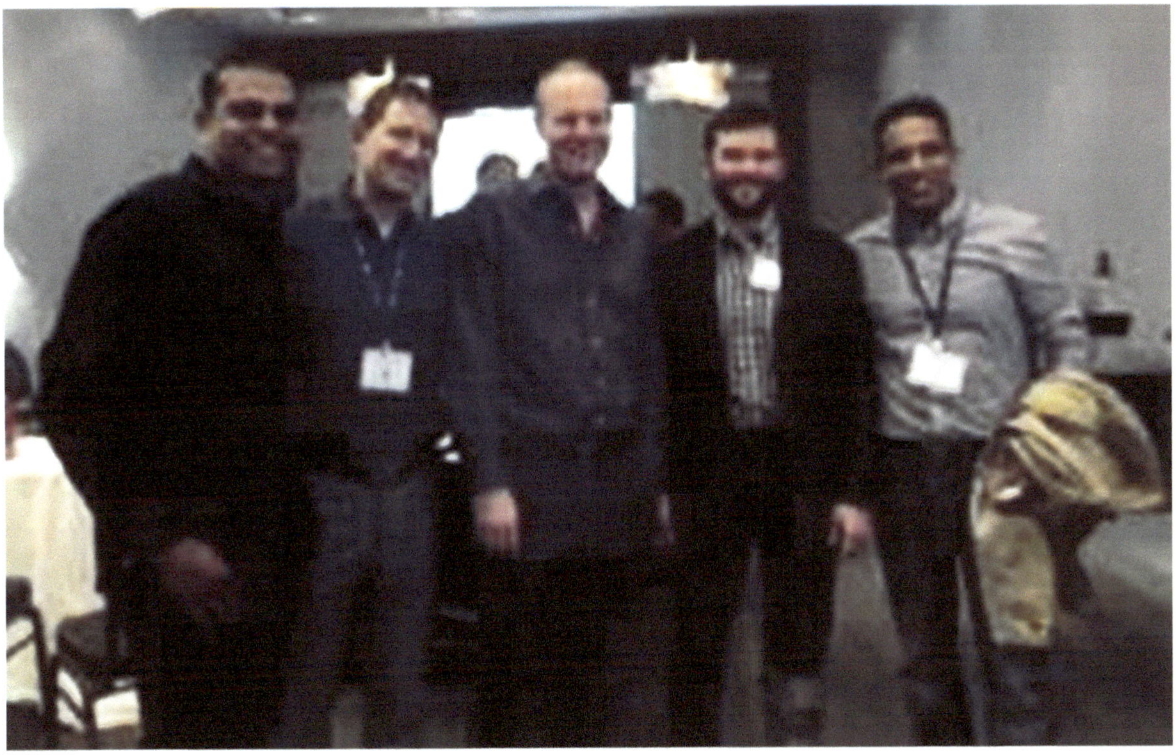

Left to right: Mathew Varghese, MD (2007-2009); Steven L. Cole, DO (2005-2007); Andrew Bagg, MD (2006-2008); Joshua Phillips, MD (2007-2009); Thomas Chacko, MD (2005-2007).2018 USF Alumni Dinner; American Academy of Allergy Asthma & Immunology Annual Meeting, Orlando, FL.

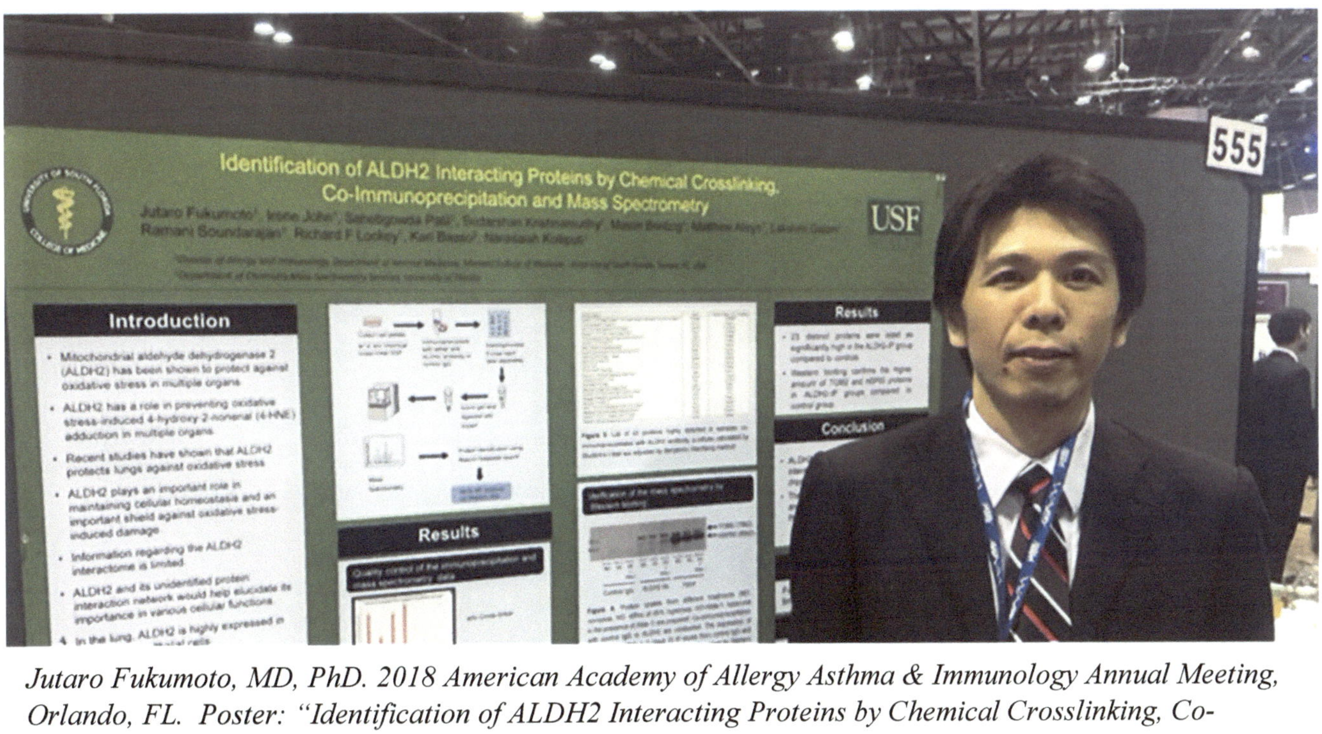

Jutaro Fukumoto, MD, PhD. 2018 American Academy of Allergy Asthma & Immunology Annual Meeting, Orlando, FL. Poster: "Identification of ALDH2 Interacting Proteins by Chemical Crosslinking, Co-Immunoprecipitation and Mass Spectrometry".

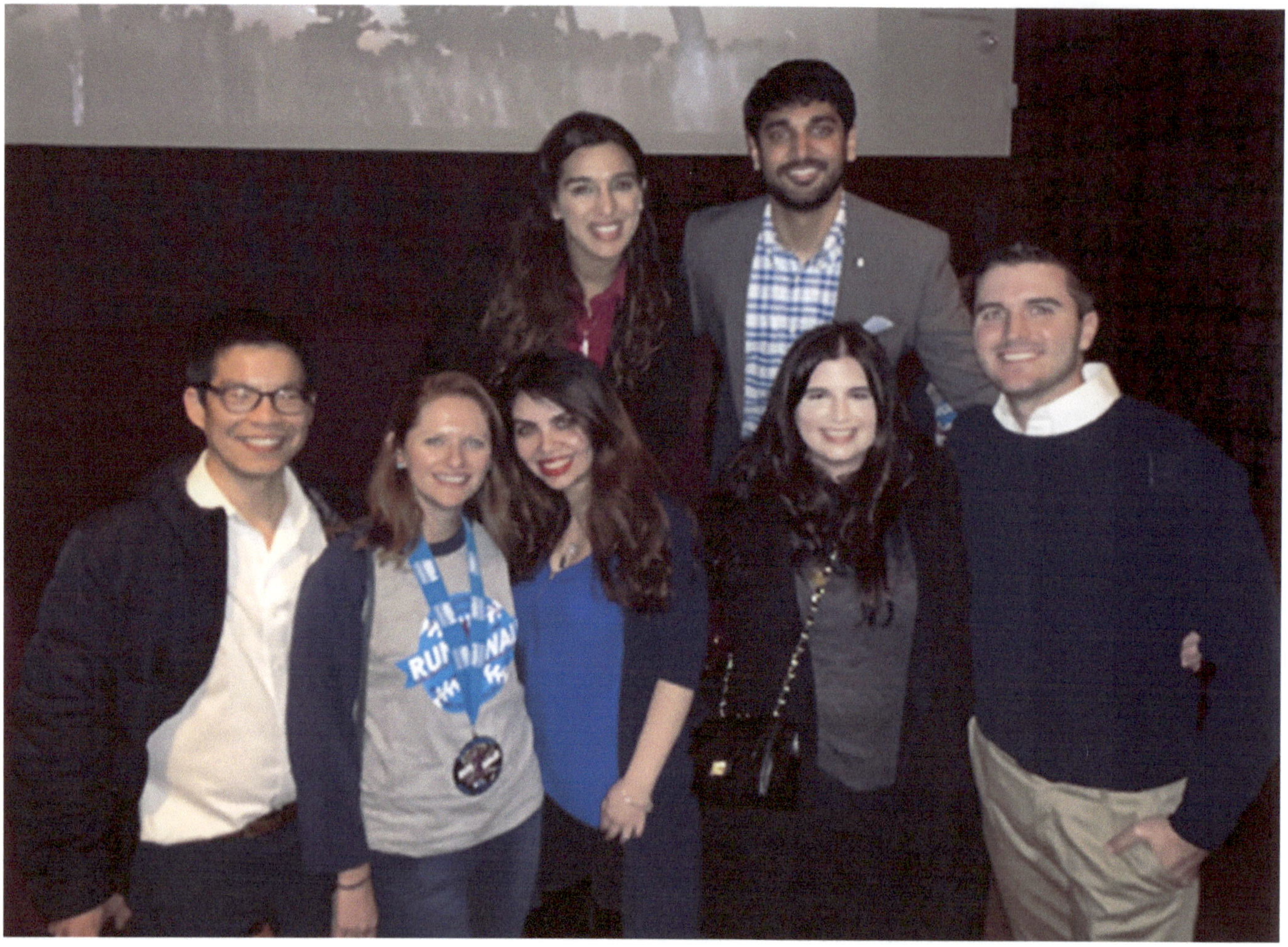

Front row (left to right): Warit Jithpratuck, MD (ACH, 2017-2019); Irina Dawson, MD (ACH, 2018-2020); Claudia Gaefke, MD (2018-2020); Tara V. Saco, MD (2017-2019); Kirk V. Shepard, MD (2017-2019). Back row (left to right): Fatima Khan, MD (ACH, 2017-2019); Shiven S. Patel, MD (2017-2019). 2019 American Academy of Allergy Asthma & Immunology Annual Meeting; San Francisco, CA.

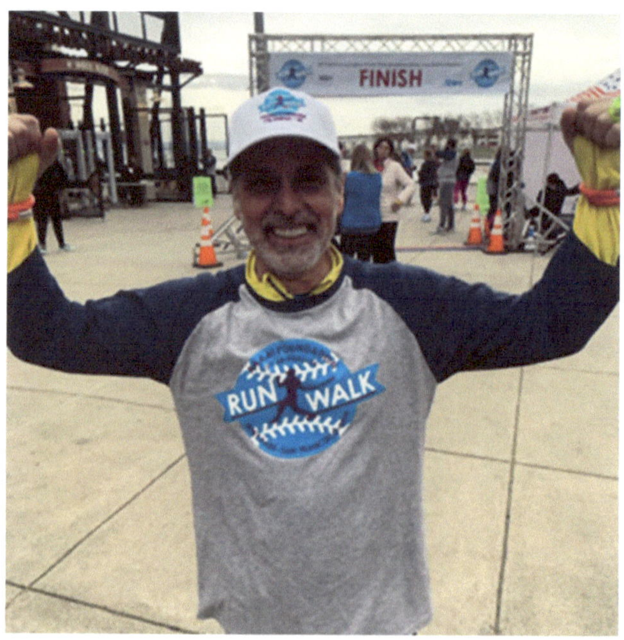

Joseph D. Diaz, MD (1986-1988). 2019 American Academy of Allergy Asthma & Immunology Foundation 7th Annual 5K Run/Walk, San Francisco, CA.

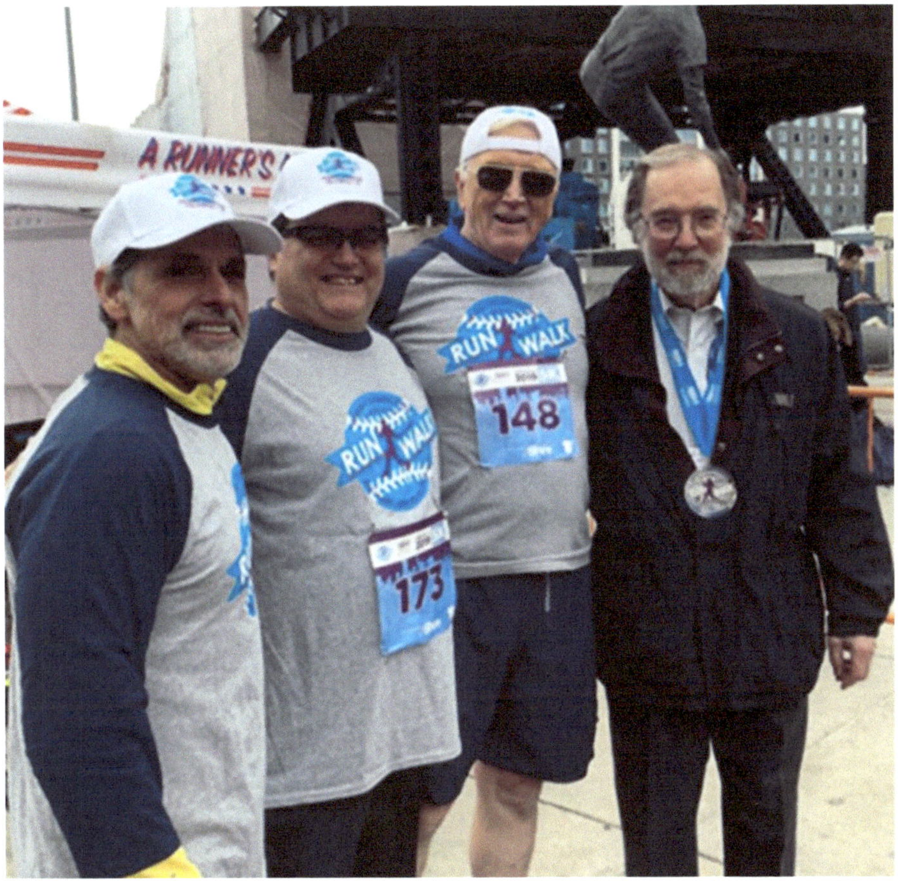

Left to right: Joseph D. Diaz, MD (1986-1988); Sean A. McKnight, MD (2002-2004); Dennis K. Ledford, M.D. (1983-1985); Bill Busse, MD. 2019 American Academy of Allergy Asthma & Immunology Foundation 7th Annual 5K Run/Walk, San Francisco, CA.

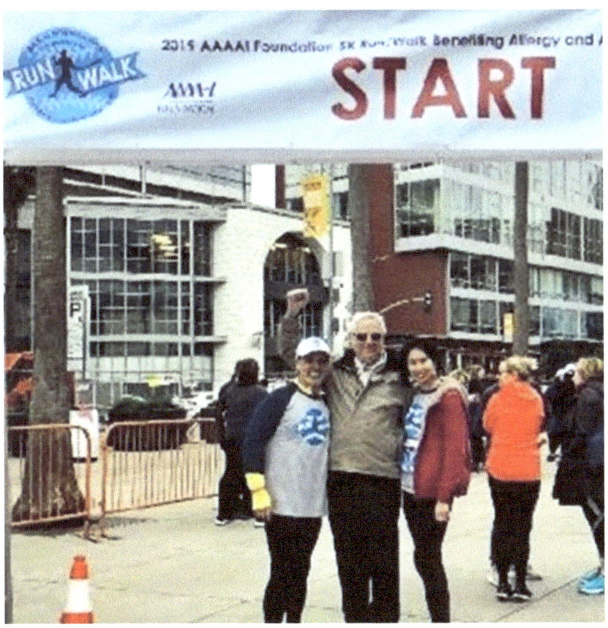

Left to right: Joseph D. Diaz, MD (1986-1988); Richard F. Lockey, MD, MS; Panida Sriaroon, MD (ACH, 2006-2009). 2019 American Academy of Allergy Asthma & Immunology Foundation 7th Annual 5K Run/Walk, San Francisco, CA.

Chapter 16: Christmas and New Year's Celebrations

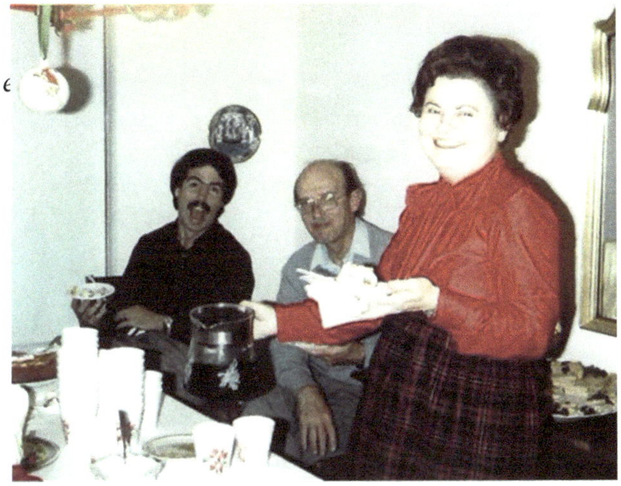

Left to right: John J. Stablein, MD (1979-1981); Jesse Stone Binford, PhD; Lolita Binford; circa 1981.

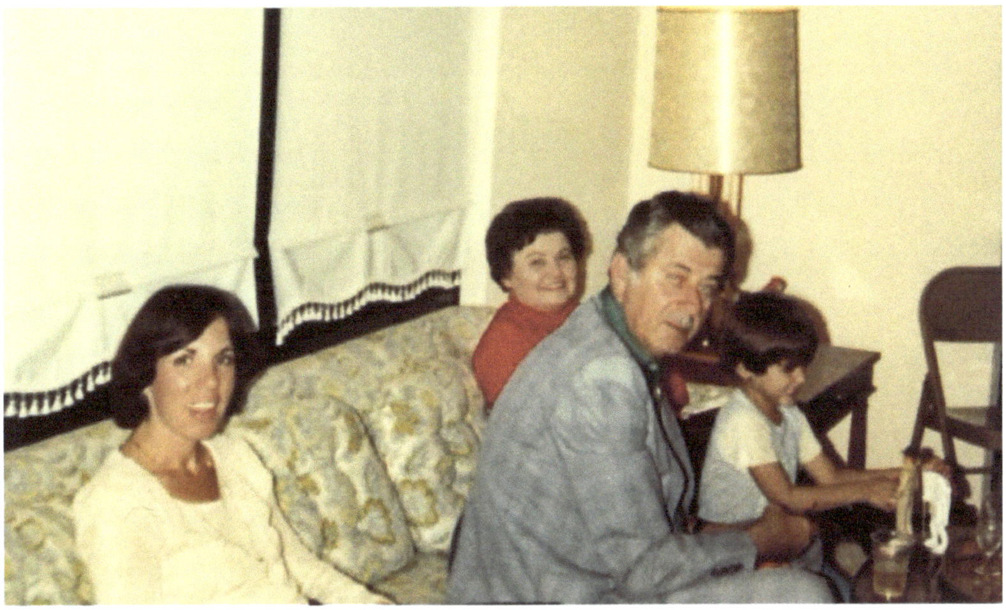

Left to right: Barbara Louie; Samuel C. Bukantz, MD; Lolita Binford; circa 1981.

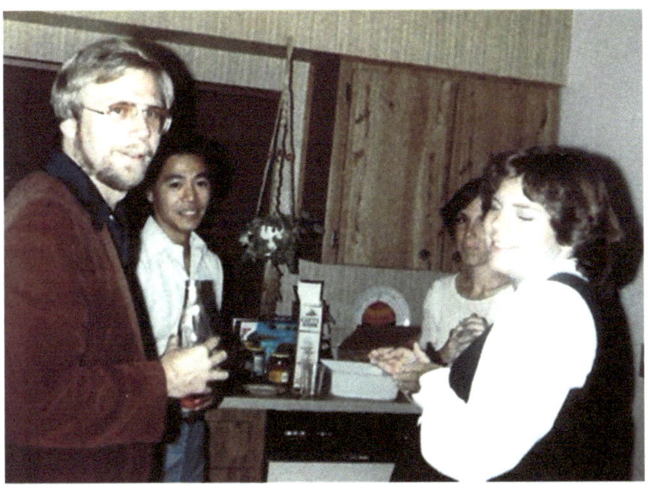

Front: Roger W. Fox, MD (1978-1980) and Cynthia Fox. Back: Steven J. Louie, MD (1981-1983) and Barbara Louie. Circa 1981.

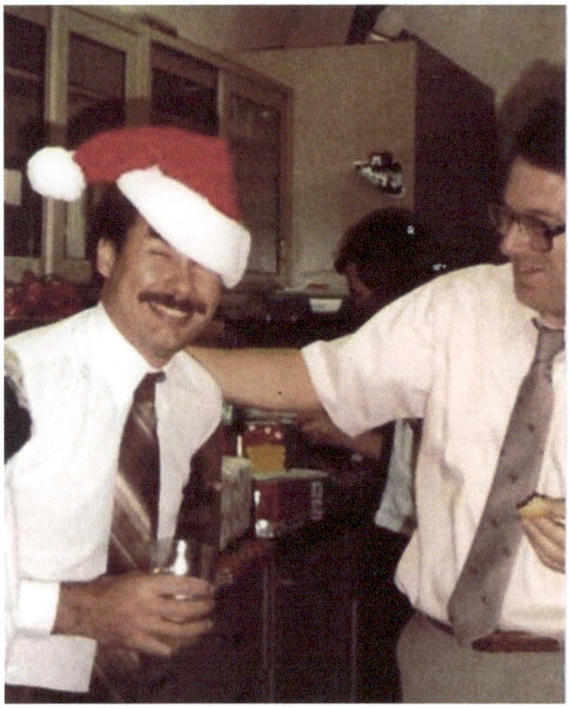

Left to right: Gerald A. Bucholtz, MD (1980-1982) and Richard F. Lockey, MD, MS; 1983.

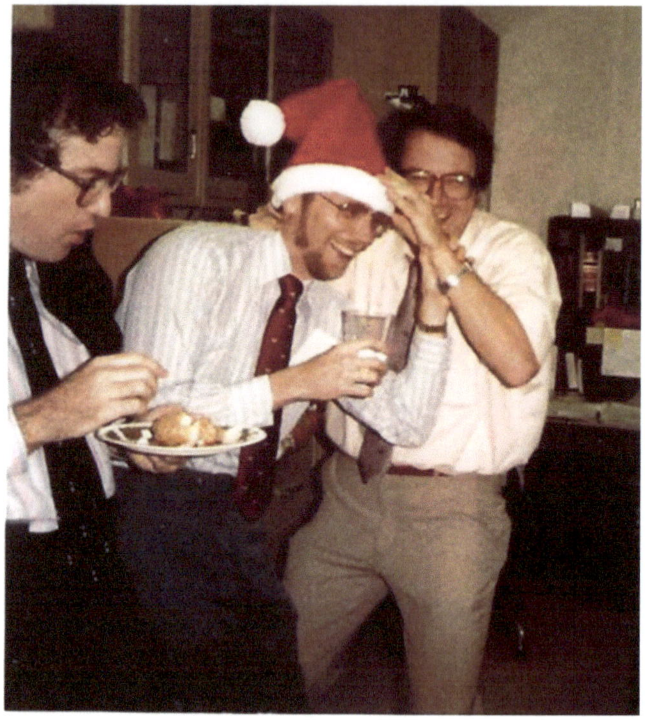

Left to right: R. Lawrence Siegel, MD, PhD; Roger W. Fox, MD (1978-1980); Richard F. Lockey, MD, MS; circa 1983.

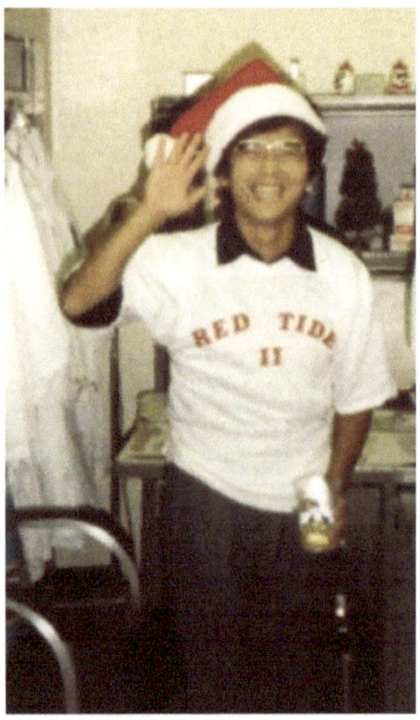

Yuji Sakamoto, MD; 1983.

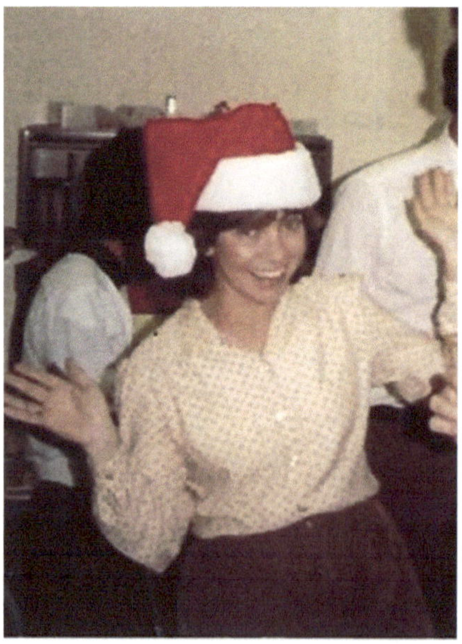

Ginger Montuoro; 1983.

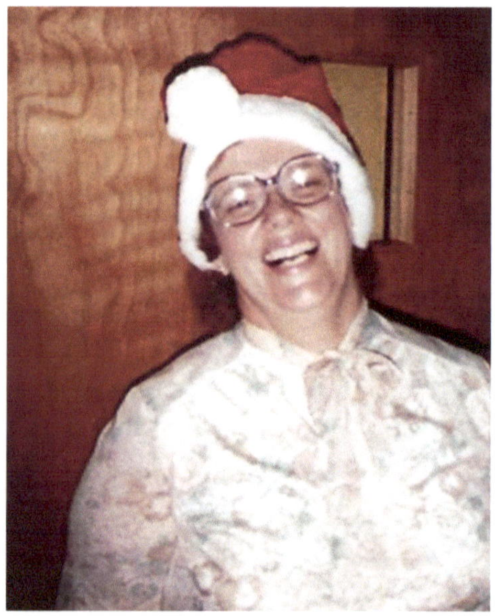

Irene Baird-Warren; 1983.

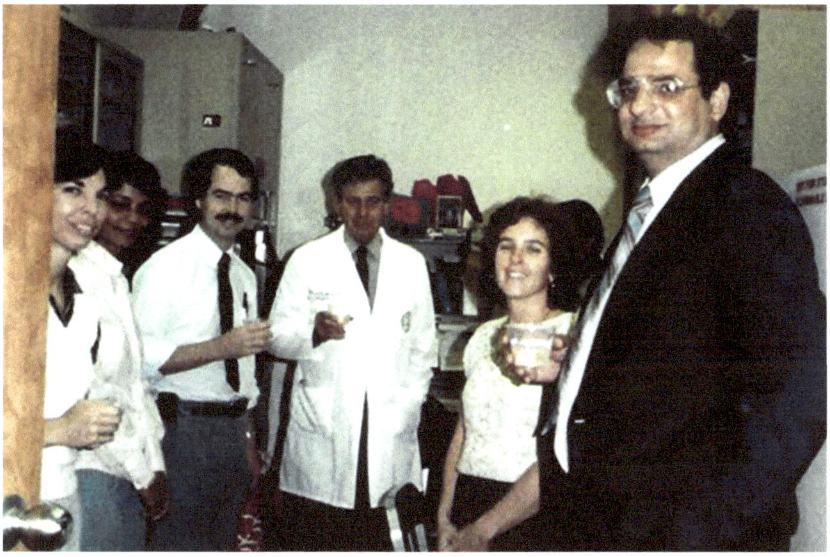

Left to right: Debbie Serbousek; Rama Ganguly, PhD; John J. Stablein, MD (1979-1981); Samuel C. Bukantz, MD; Pat Walsh; Saber Samaan, PhD; 1984.

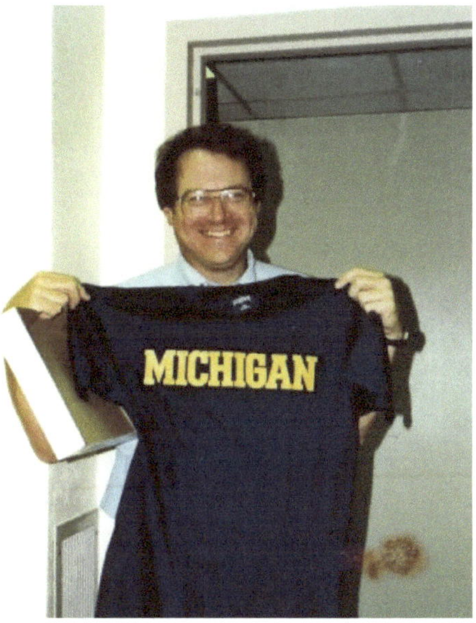

Richard F. Lockey, MD, MS; 1985.

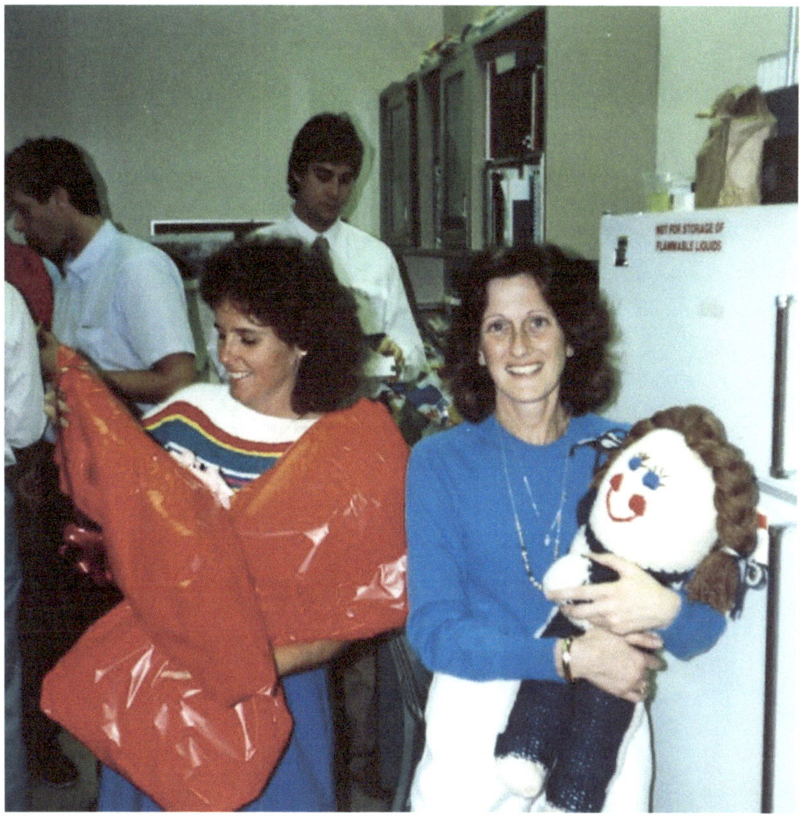

Left to right: Pat Walsh and Peggy Hales; 1986.

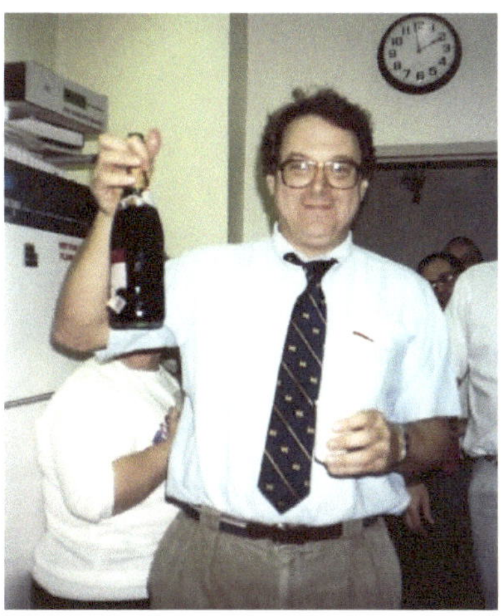

Richard F. Lockey, MD, MS; 1989.

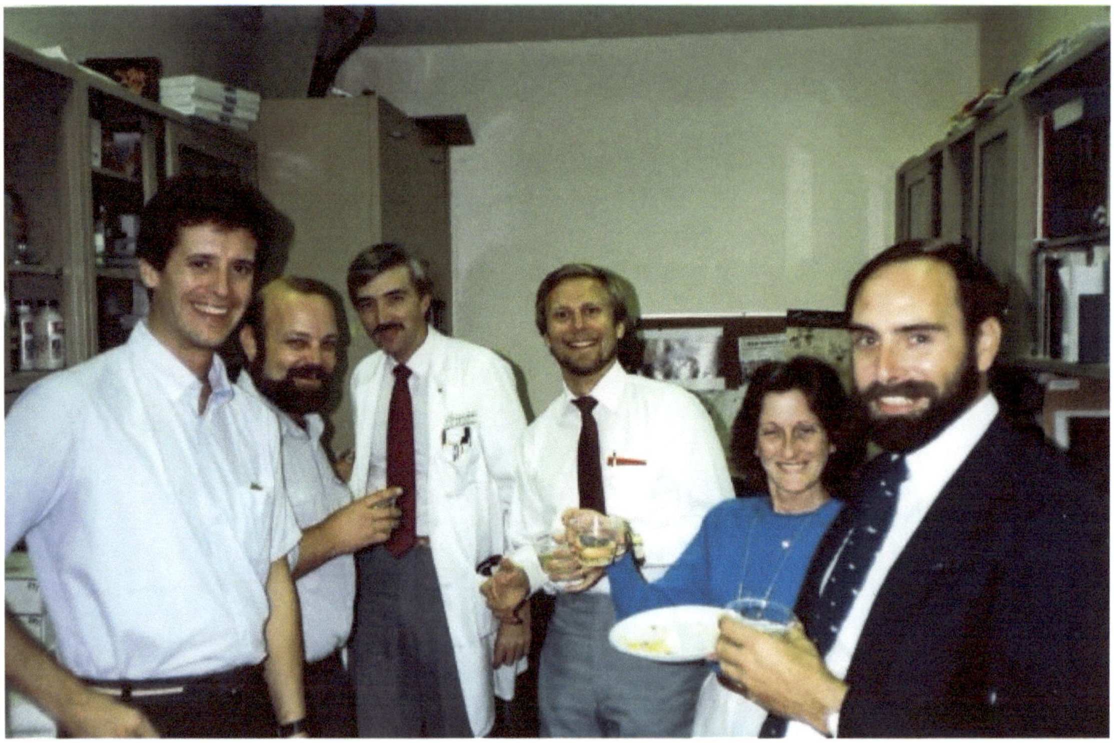

Left to right: Enrique Fernandez-Caldas, PhD; Walter Trudeau III, MS; Dennis K. Ledford, MD (1983-1985); Roger W. Fox, MD (1979-1980); Peggy Hales; Jim Keller (Schering Pharmaceuticals); 1987.

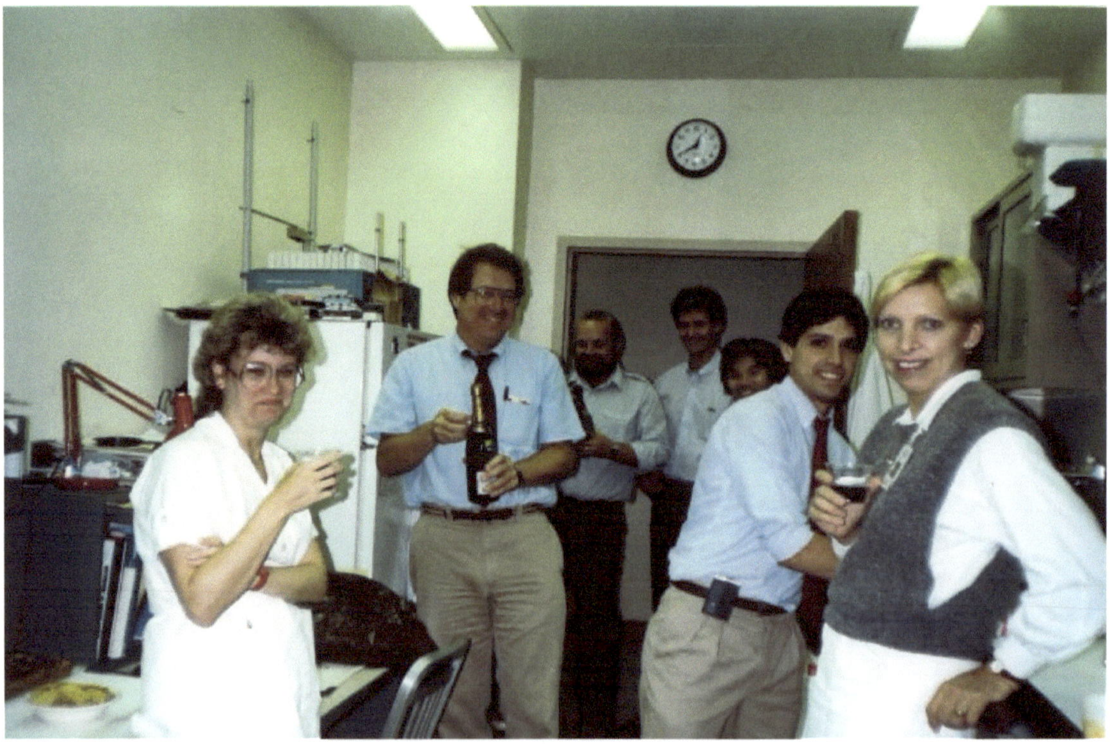

Left to right: Nancy (surname unknown) (VA nurse); Richard F. Lockey, MD, MS; Walter Trudeau III, MS; Enrique Fernandez-Caldas, PhD; name unknown; Joseph Diaz, MD (1986-1988); Ann Rogers (VA nurse);1987.

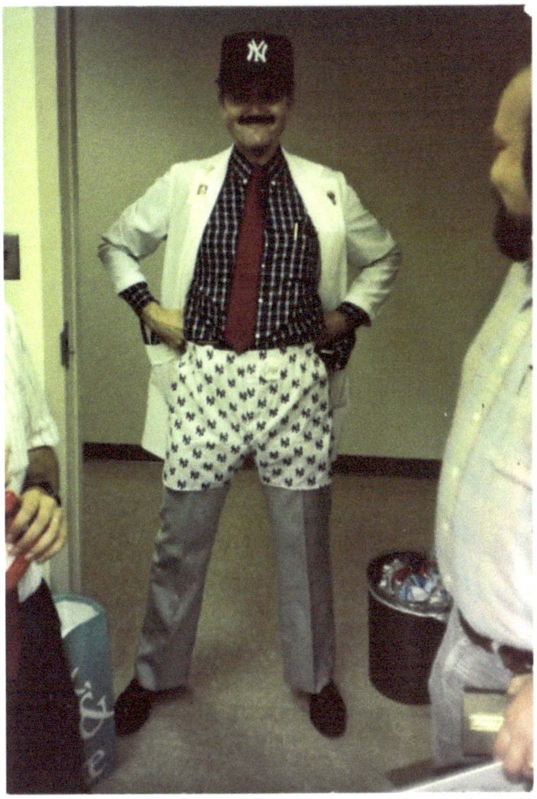

Dennis K. Ledford, MD (1983-1985); circa 1996.

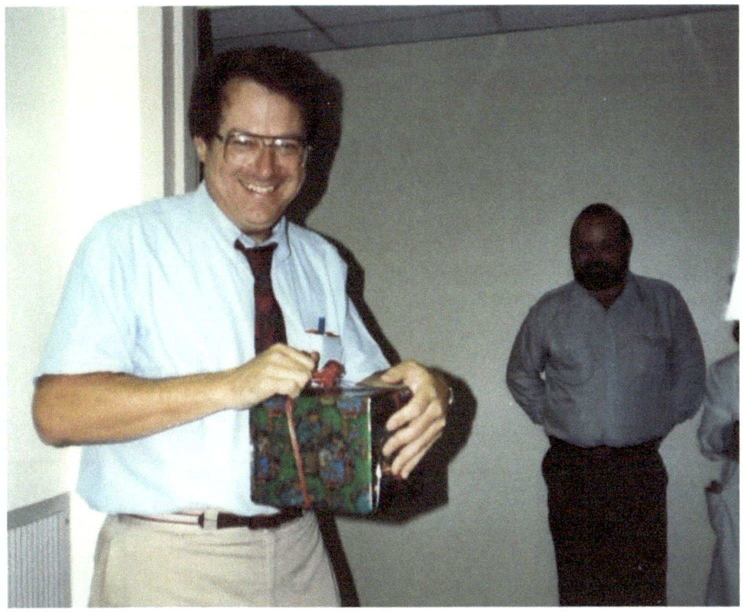

Richard F. Lockey, MD, MS and Walter Trudeau III, MS; 1995.

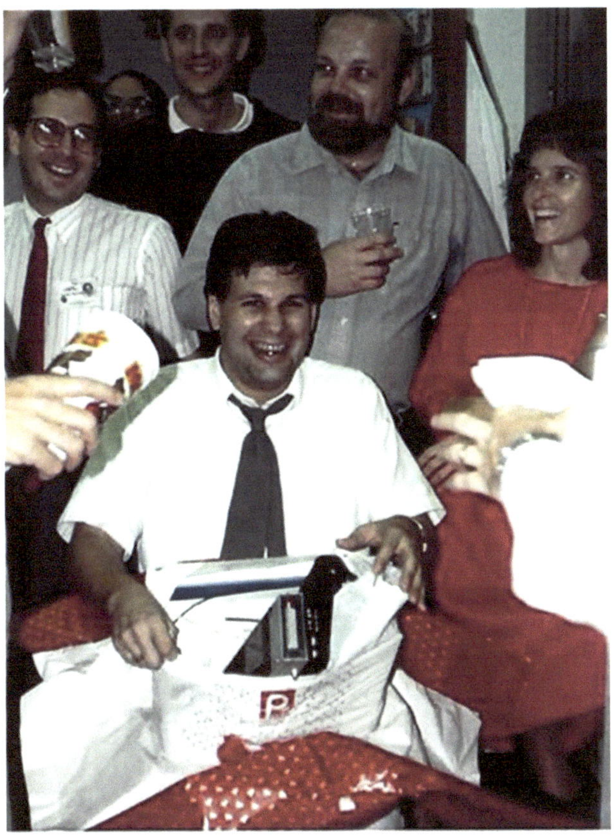

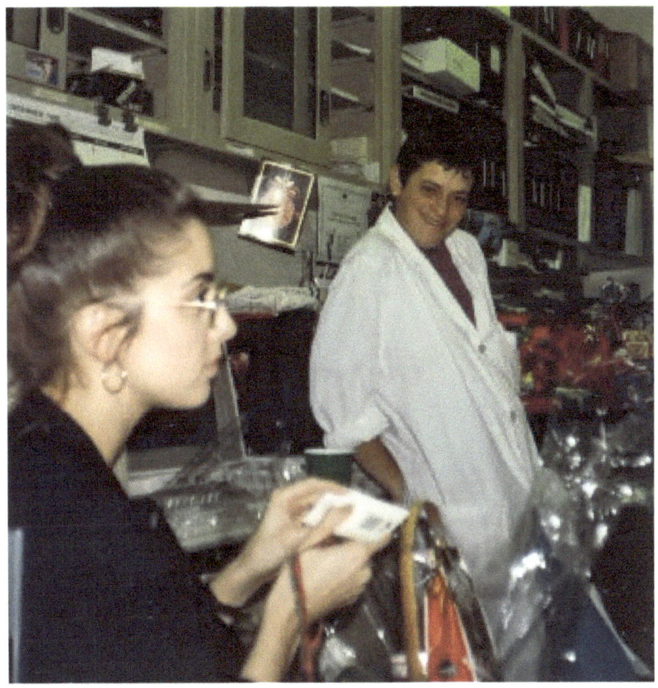

Above, left to right: Lizette S. Hernandez, MD (1994-1997) and Rosa Codina, PhD;1996.

Left, front: David N. Wright, MD (1988-1991). Back (left to right): Richard P. Silton, MD (1988-1990); Walter Trudeau III, MS; Pat Walsh. 1989.

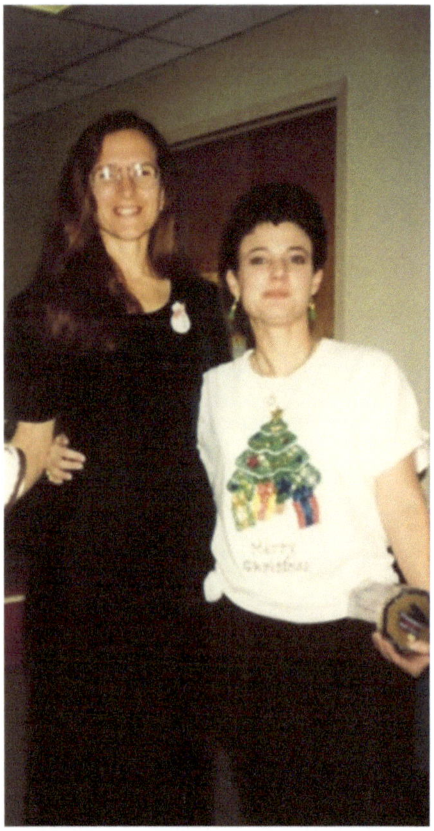

Michelle Twitmyer and Yvette Meunier; 1996.

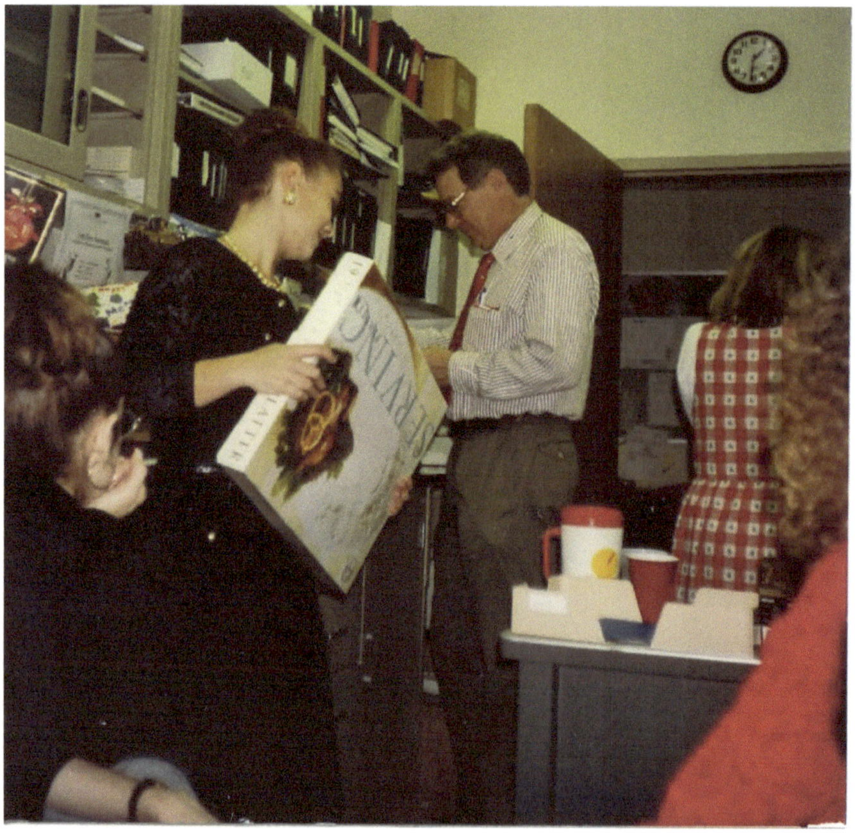

Left to right: Giana L. Nicoara-Kasti, MD (1996-1998) and Richard F. Lockey, MD, MS; 1996.

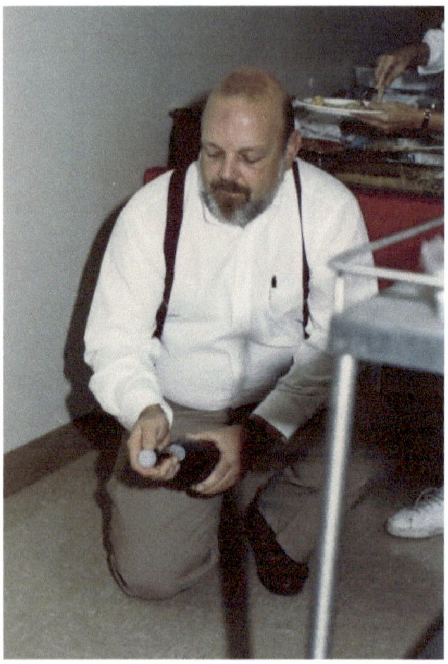

Walter Trudeau III, MS; 1996.

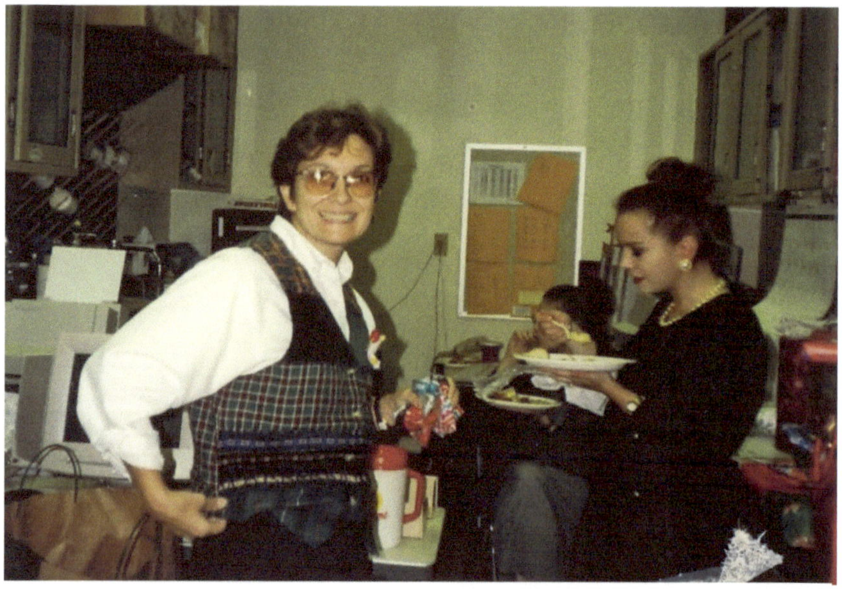

Left to right: Cindy Reichart and Giana L. Nicoara-Kasti, MD (1996-1998); 1996.

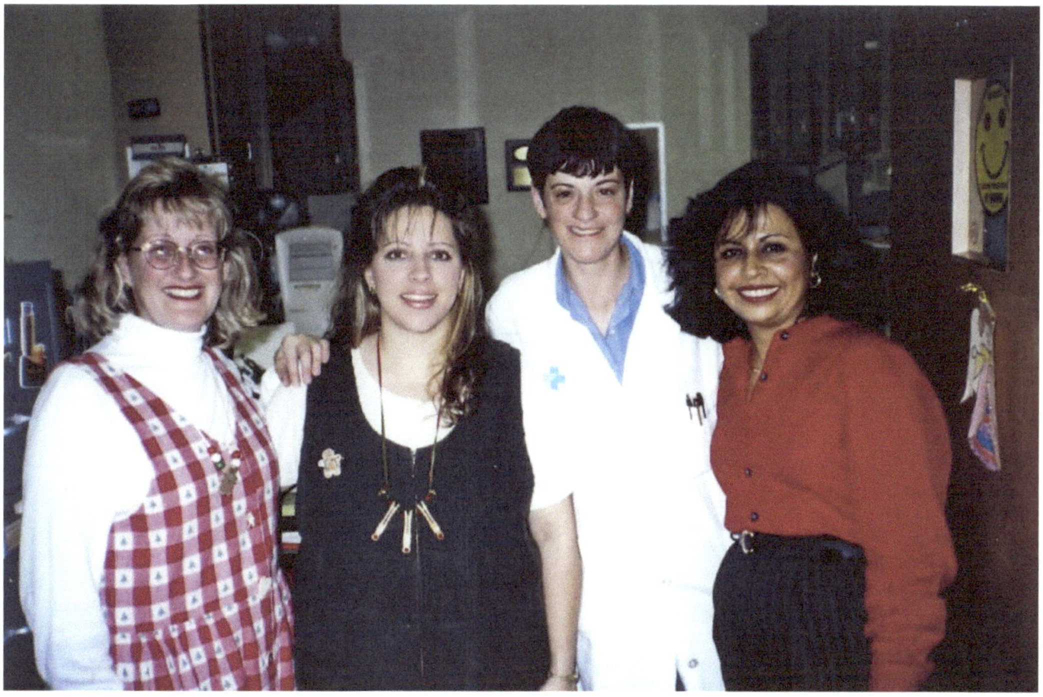

Left to right: Peggy Hales; Karen Collins; Rosa Codina, PhD; Geeta Gehi; circa 1996.

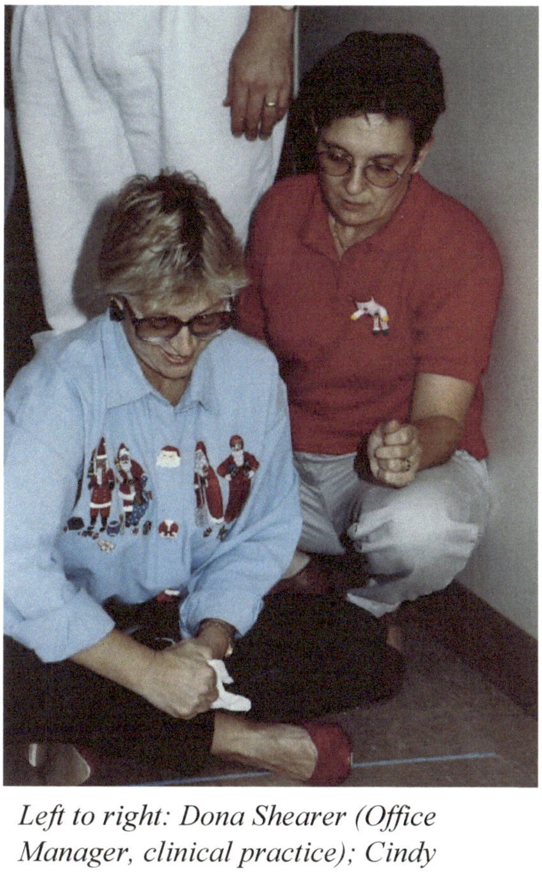

Left to right: Dona Shearer (Office Manager, clinical practice); Cindy Reichart; 1998.

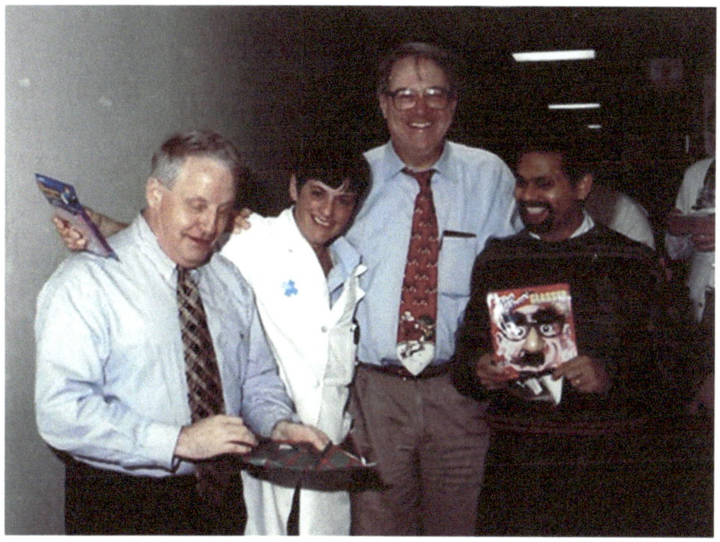

Left to right: David L. Vesely, MD, PhD (Endocrinology); Rosa Codina, PhD; Richard F. Lockey, MD, MS; Shyam S. Mohapatra, PhD; 1999.

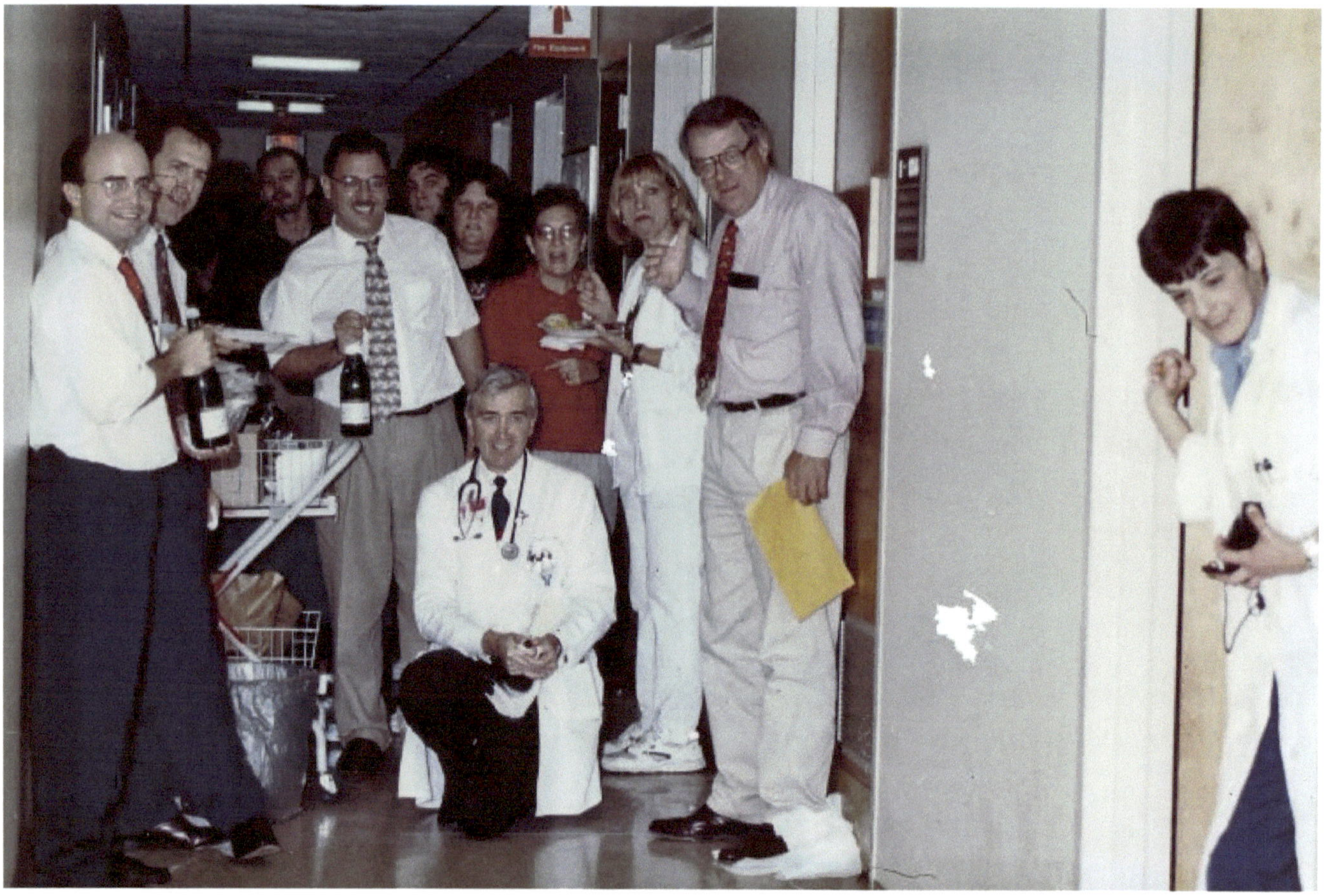

Standing (left to right): Kevin P. Rosenbach, MD (1995-1998); Hugh H. Windom, MD; Demetrios Theodoropoulos, MD (1997-2000); Cindy Reichart; Ann Rogers (VA nurse); Richard F. Lockey, MD, MS. Kneeling: Dennis K. Ledford, MD (1983-1985); Far right, standing in doorway: Rosa Codina, PhD. 1997

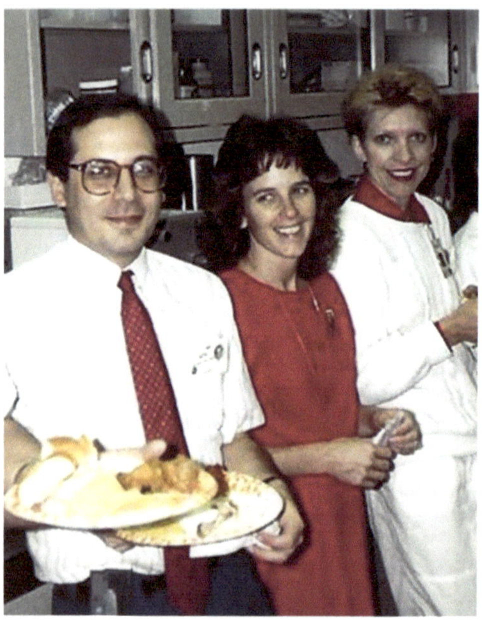

Left to right: Richard P. Silton, MD (1988-1990); Pat Walsh; Ann Rogers (VA nurse); 1989.

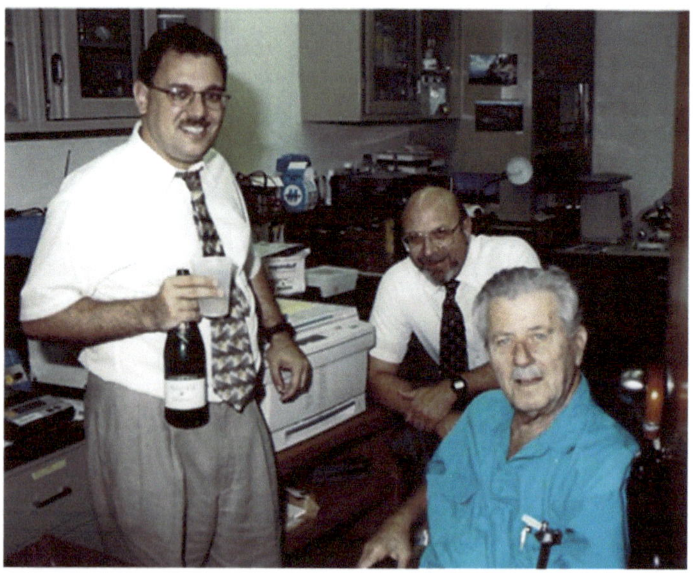

Standing: Demetrios Theodoropoulos, MD (1997-2000). Sitting, front: Samuel C. Bukantz, MD. Sitting, back: Joseph J. Krzanowski, PhD (Pharmacology and Therapeutics); 1999.

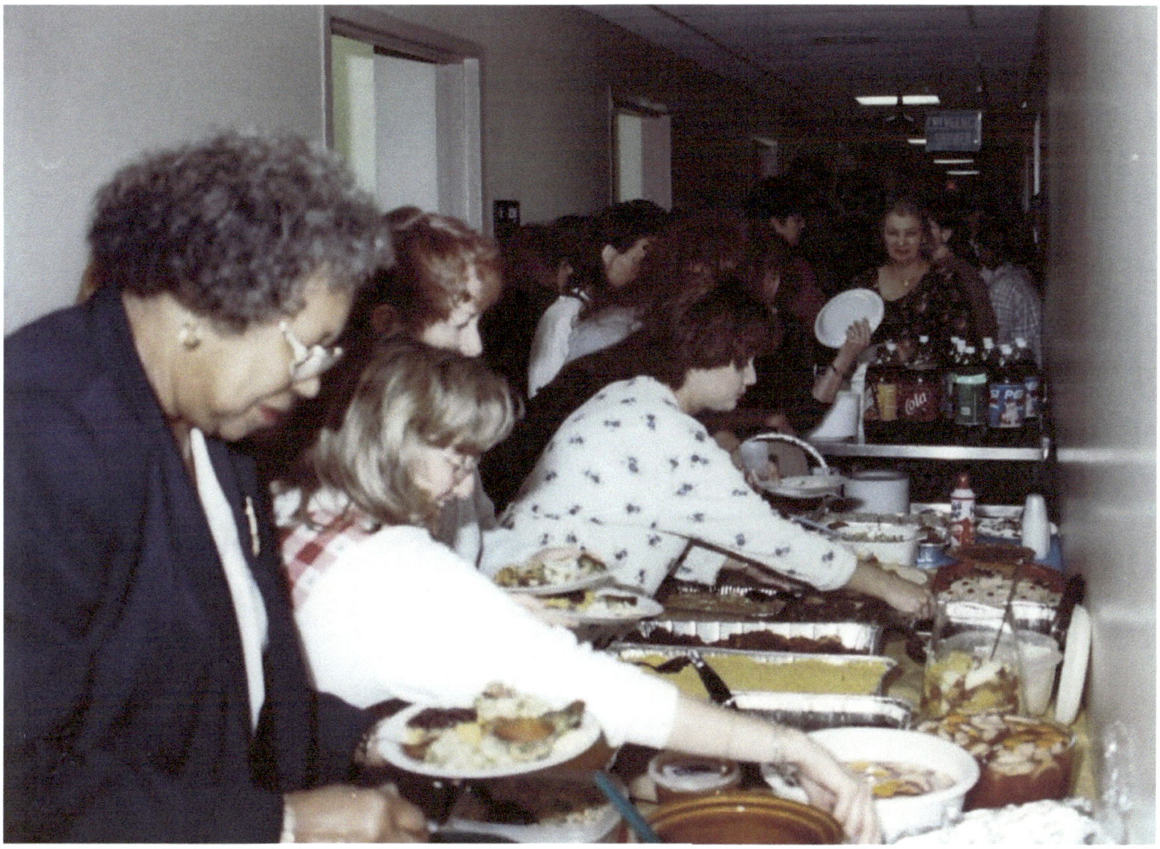

Buffet line in the hallway, Christmas 1999.

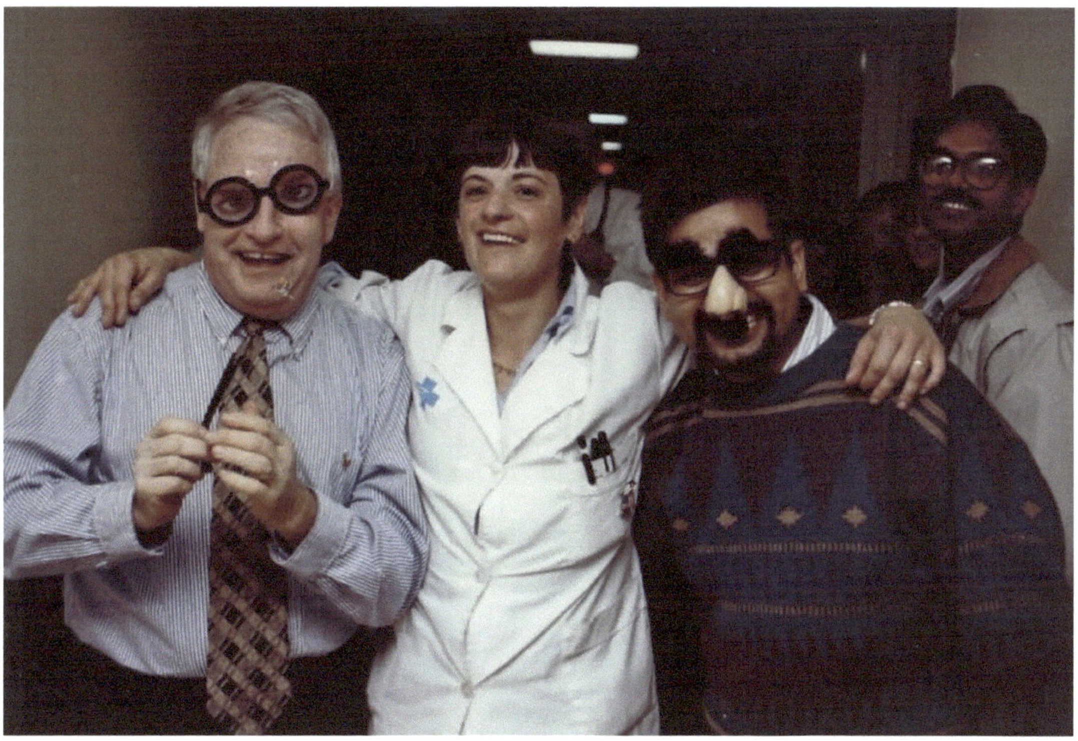

Left to right: David L. Vesely, MD, PhD (Endocrinology); Rosa Codina, PhD; Shyam S. Mohapatra, PhD; Mukesh Kumar, PhD (background); 1999.

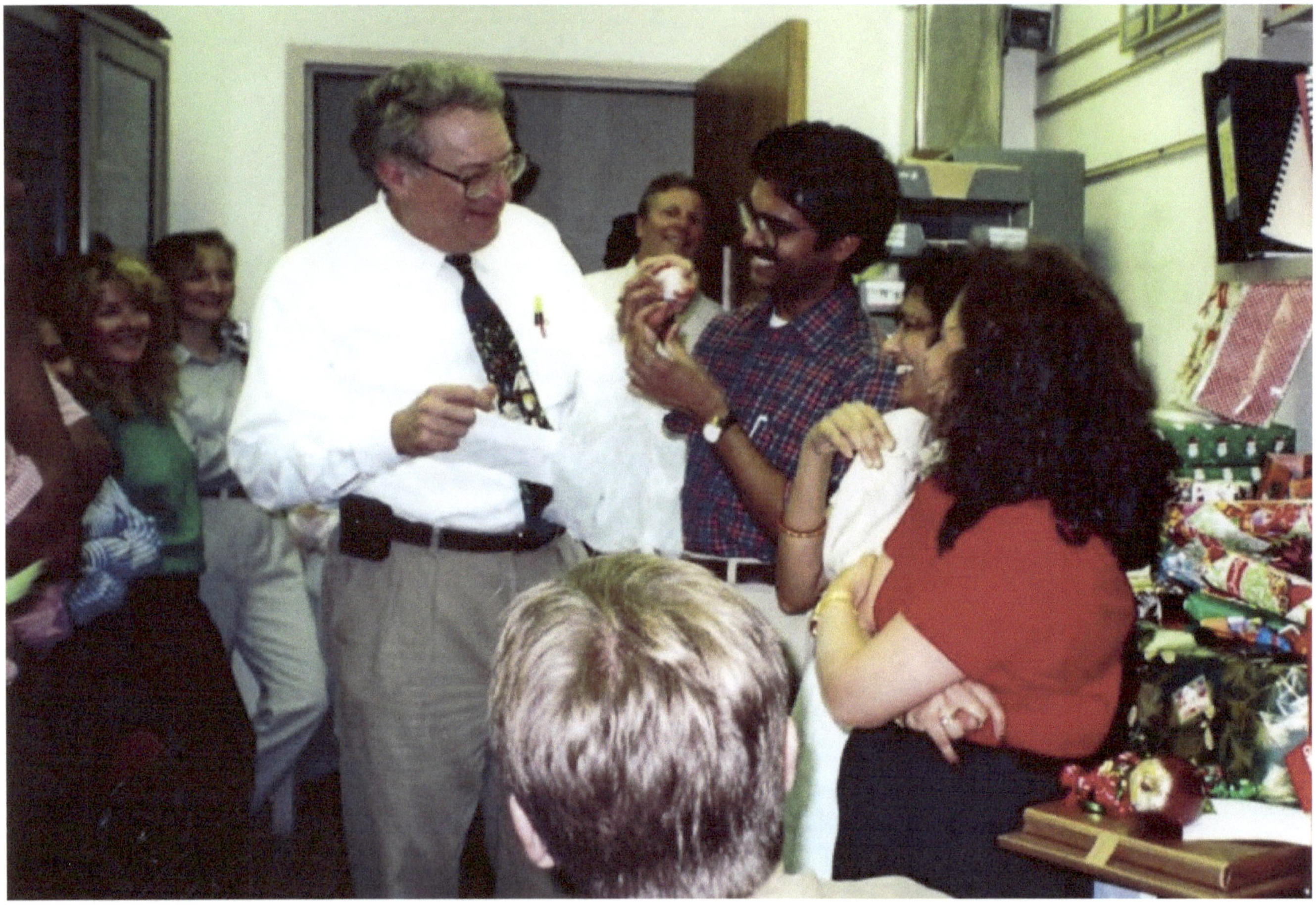

Left to right: Richard F. Lockey, MD, MS; Mukesh Kumar, PhD; Aruna Behera, PhD; Geeta Gehi; Christmas 2000.

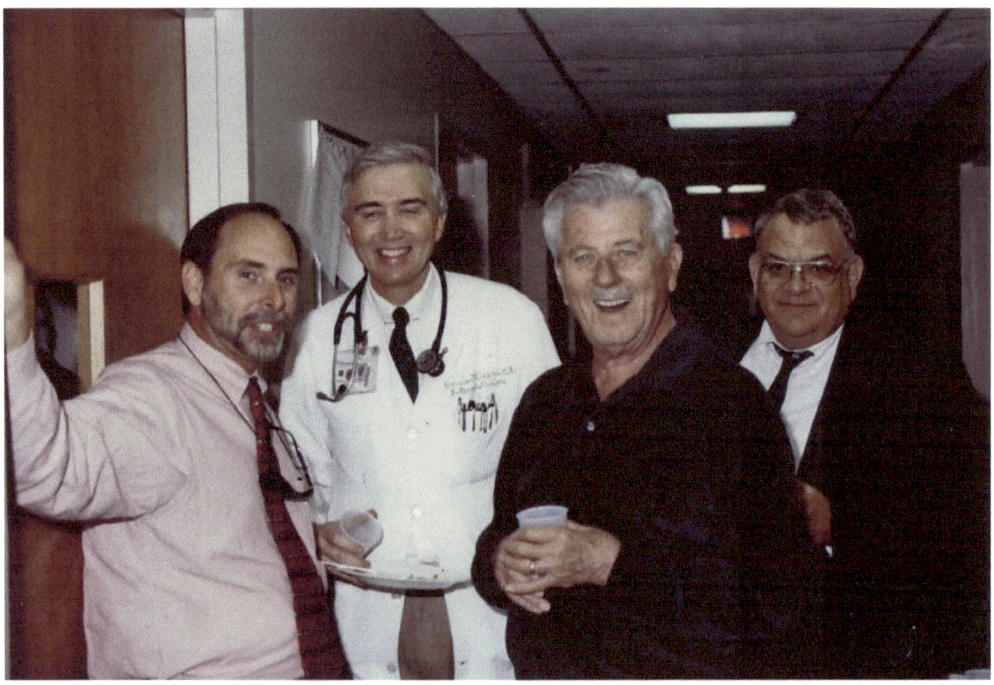

Left to right: Jim Keller (Schering Pharmaceuticals); Dennis K. Ledford, MD (1983-1985); Samuel C. Bukantz, MD; John W. Hadden, MD (Immunopharmacology).

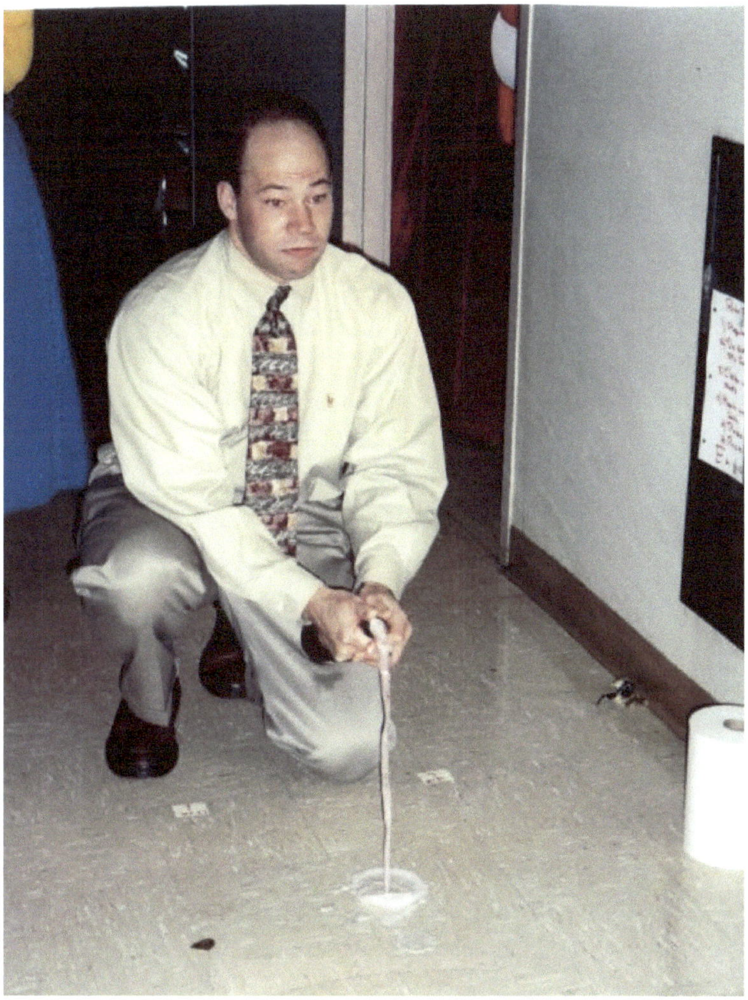

Daniel A. Reichmuth, MD (1999-2002); 2001.

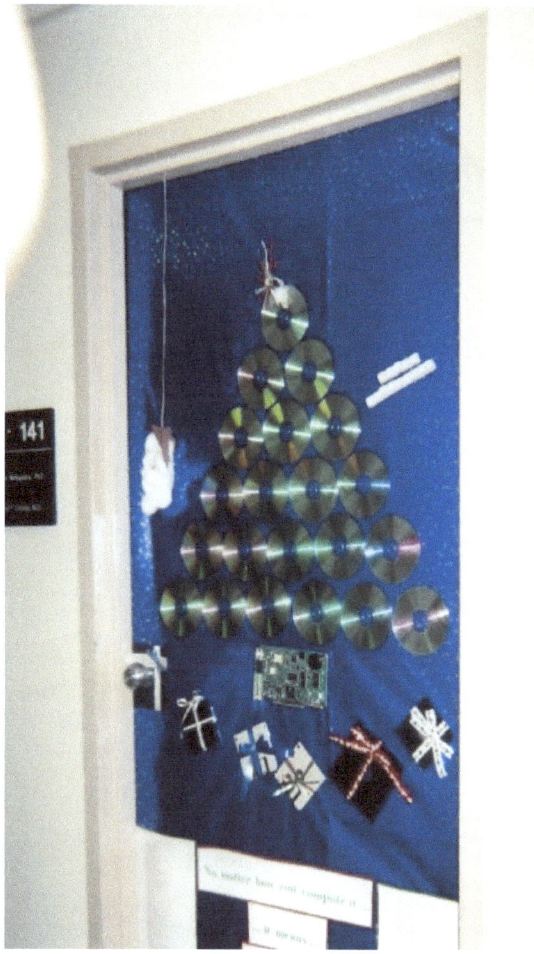

Research Building Door Decorating Contest; 2002.

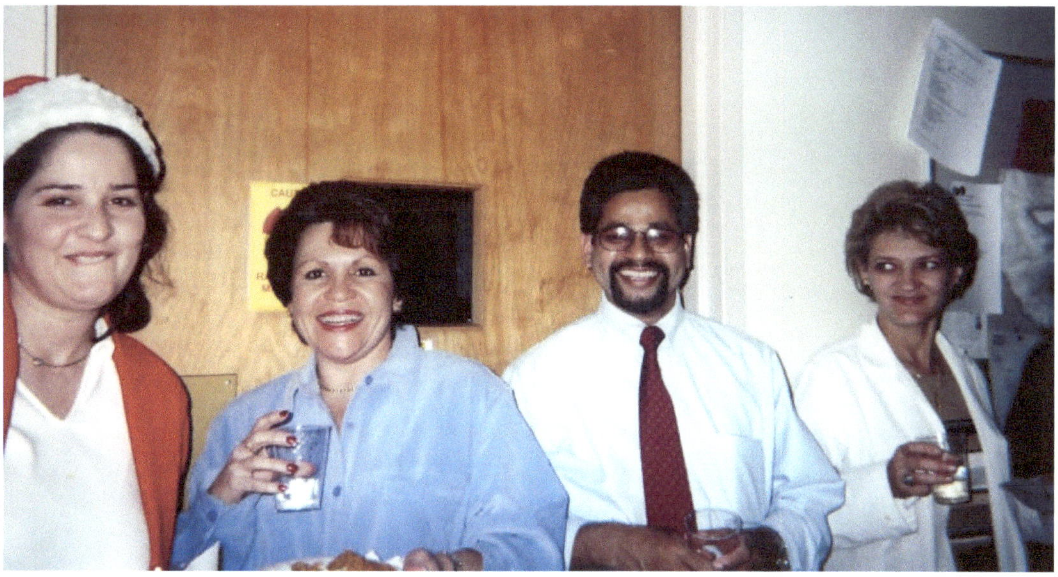

Menayra Caro; Nina C. Ramirez, MD (2000-2002); Shyam S. Mohapatra, PhD; Denise Cooper, PhD (Endocrinology); 2001.

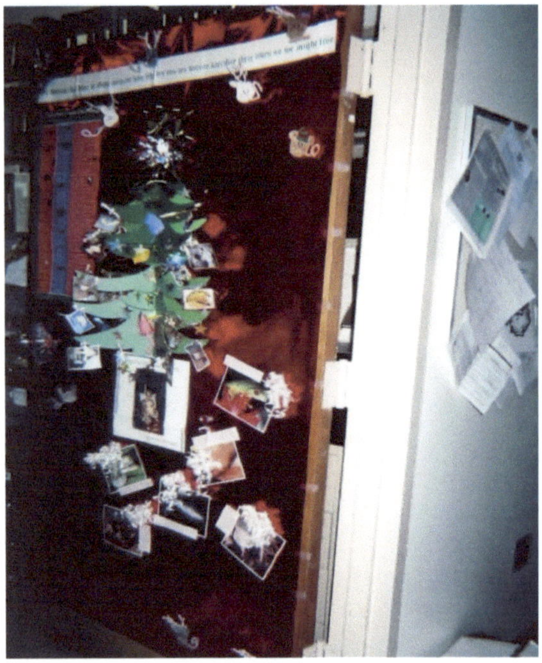

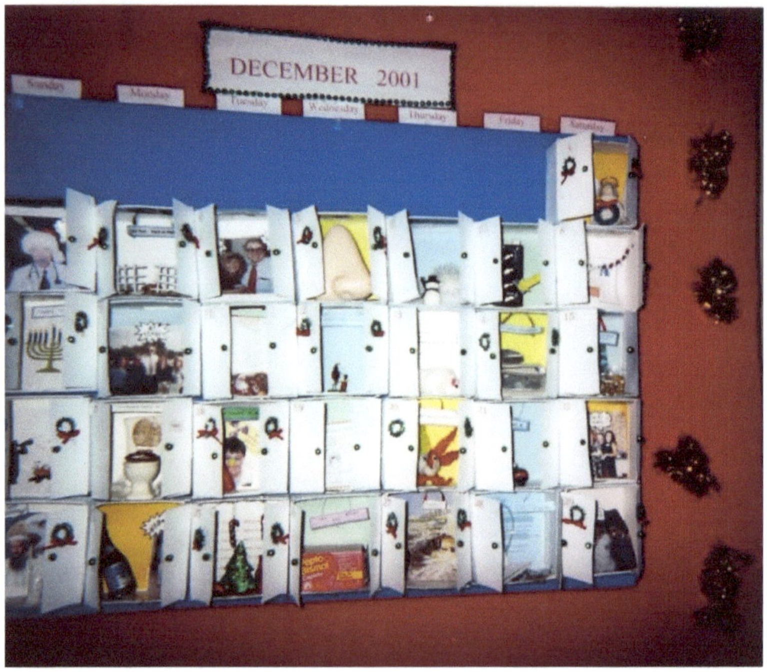

Research Building Door Decorating Contest, 2001.

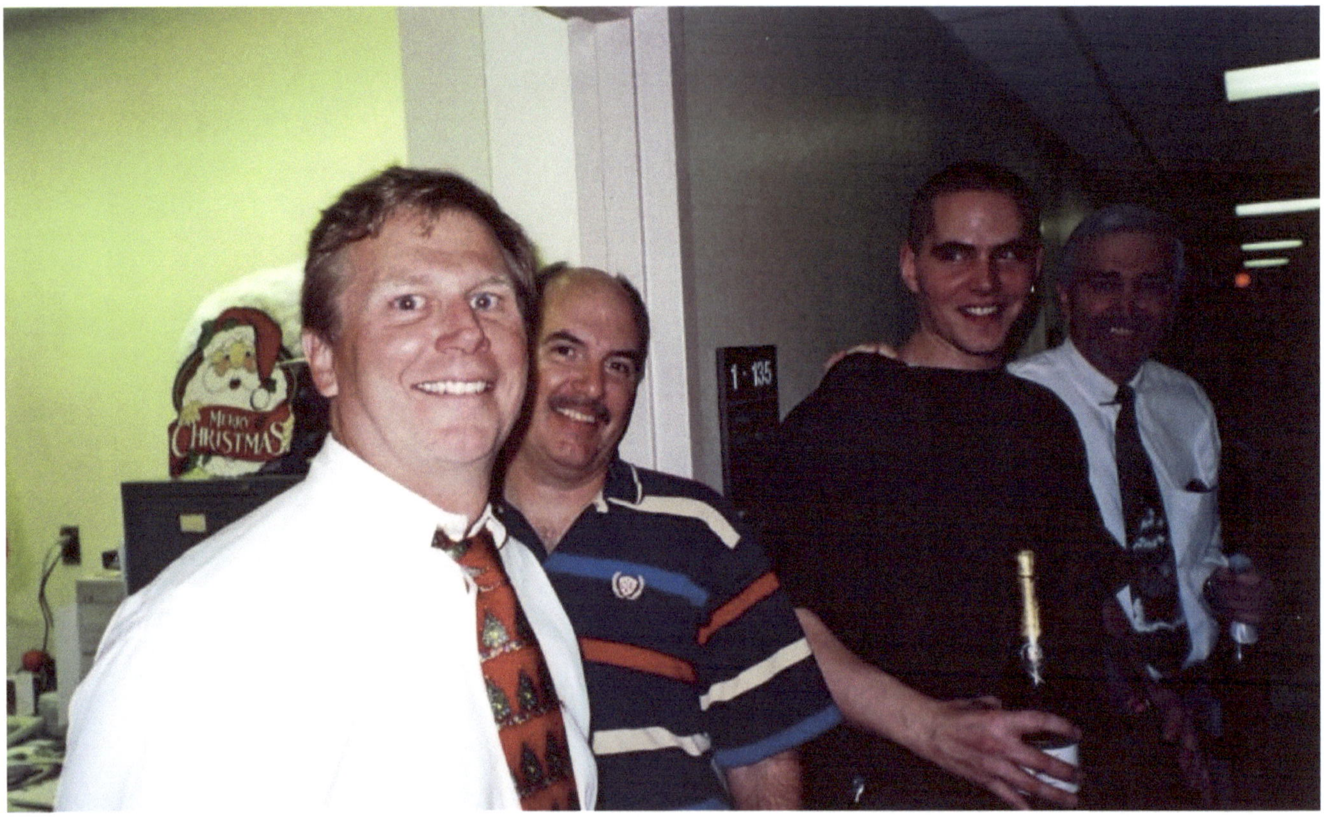

Left to right: Roger W. Fox, MD (1978-1980); William Gower, PhD (Surgery; Molecular Pharmacology & Physiology; Pathology & Cell Biology); Todd (surname unknown) (Neurology); Dennis K. Ledford, MD (1983-1985); 2002.

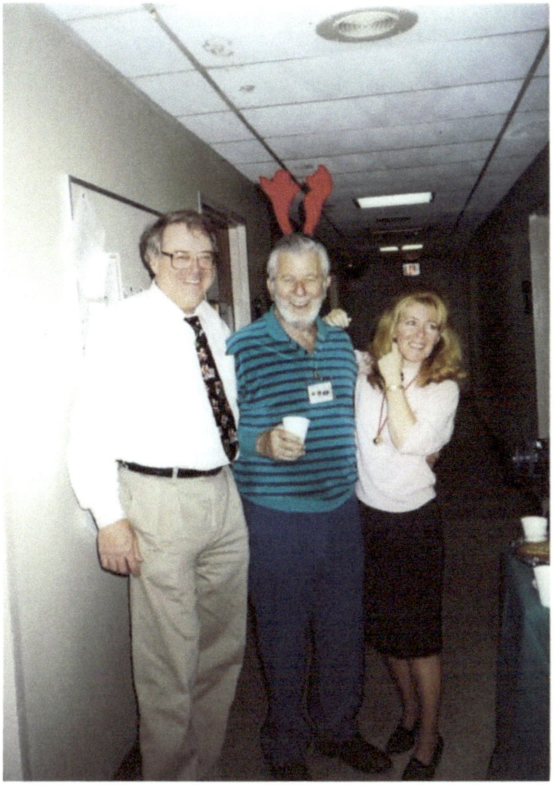

Left to right: Richard F. Lockey, MD, MS; Samuel C. Bukantz, MD; Sandra Rocha; circa 2002.

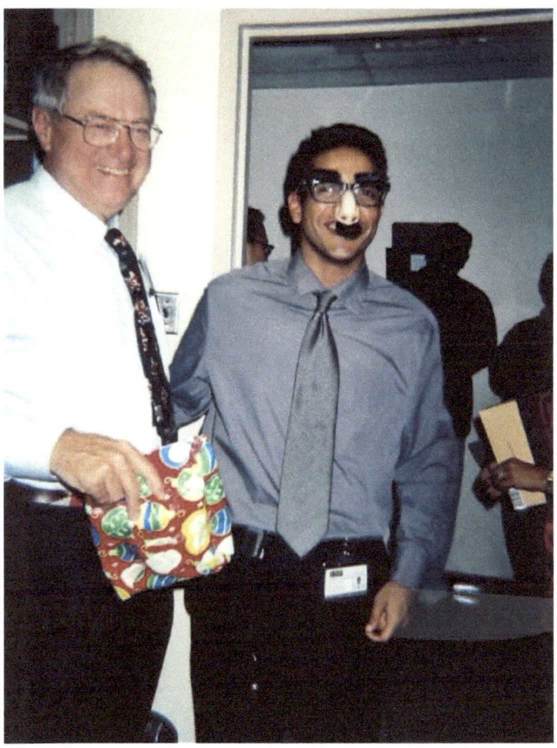

Left to right: Richard F. Lockey, MD, MS and Thomas Chacko, MD (2005-2007); 2005.

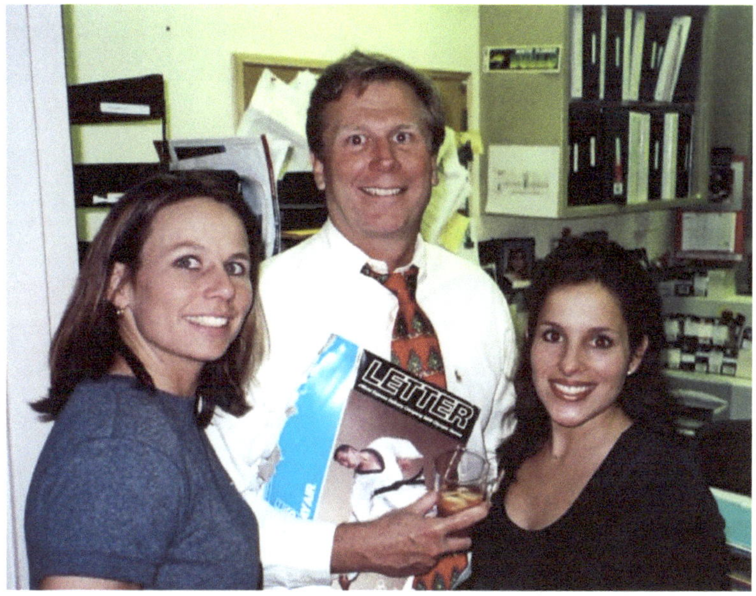

Left to right: Diana Miller; Roger W. Fox, MD; Alisa Diecidue; 2002.

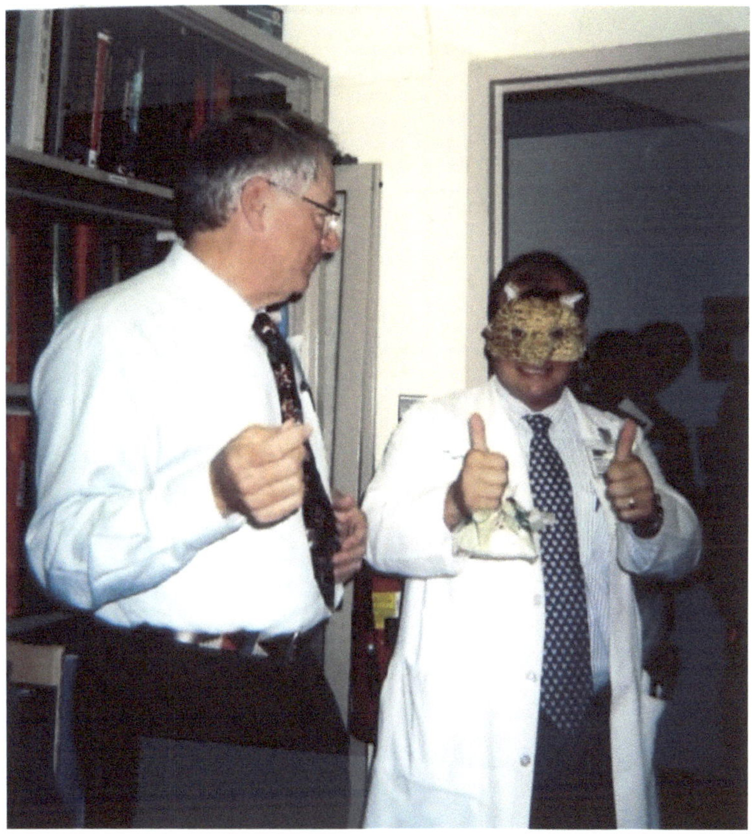

Left to right: Richard F. Lockey, MD, MS and Mark C. Glaum, MD, PhD; 2005.

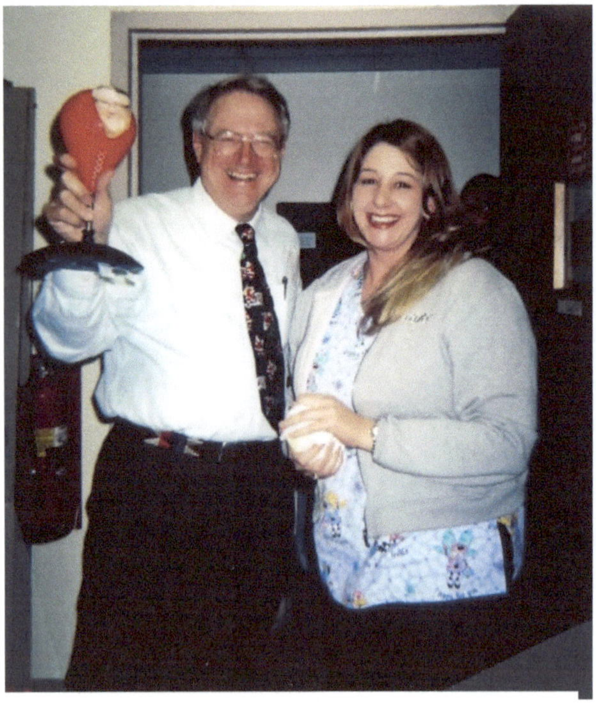

Richard F. Lockey, MD, MS and Michelle Grandstaff-Singleton; circa 2005.

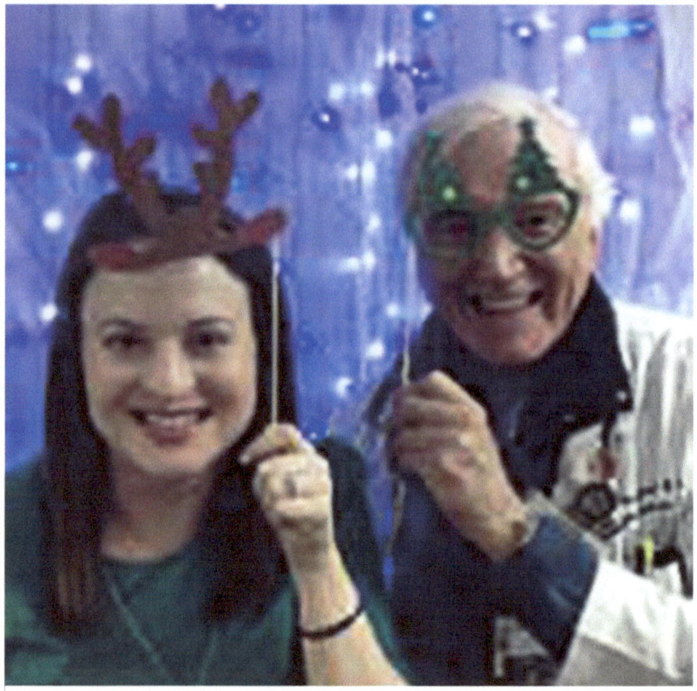

Amber N. Pepper, MD (2016-2018) and Dennis K. Ledford, MD (1983-1985);2017.

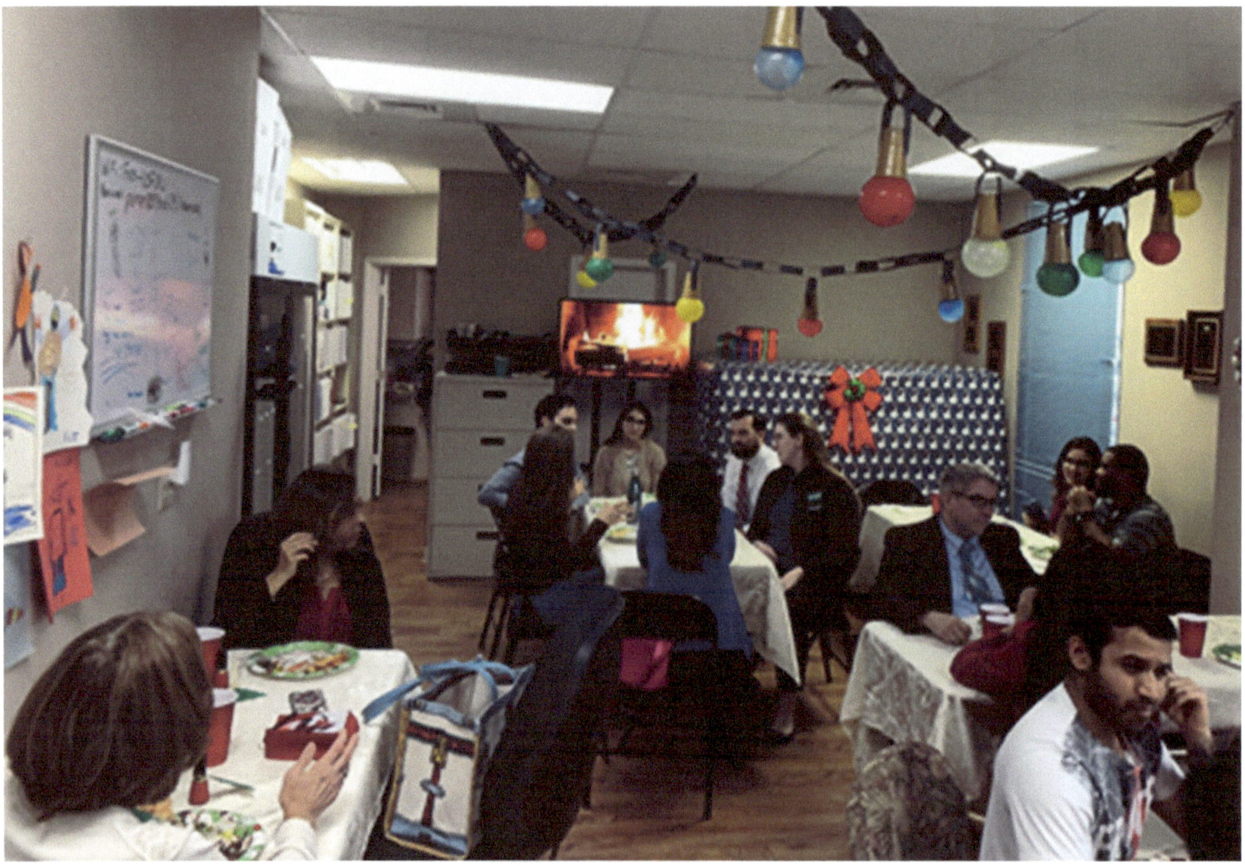

Division annual Christmas party at the Clinical Research Unit; 2019.

Chapter 17: Division Celebrations

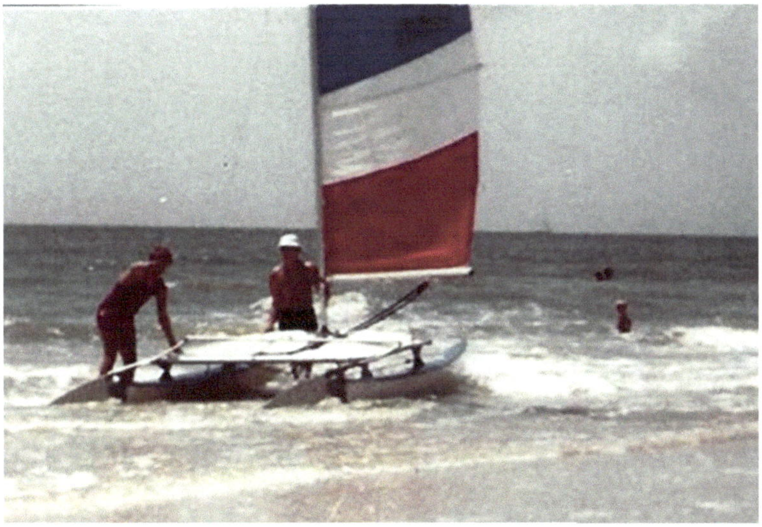

Dr. Fox's graduation party; summer 1980.

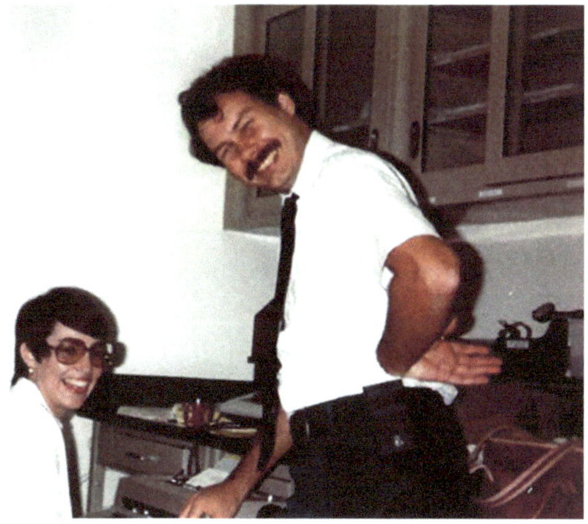

Left to right: Judy Bien; Gerald A. Bucholtz, MD (1980-1982); 1980.

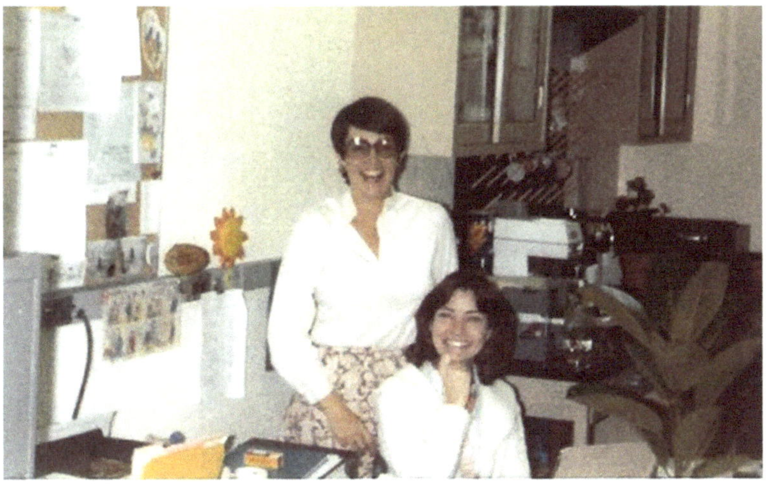

Ginger Montuoro (sitting); Judy Bien (standing); 1980.

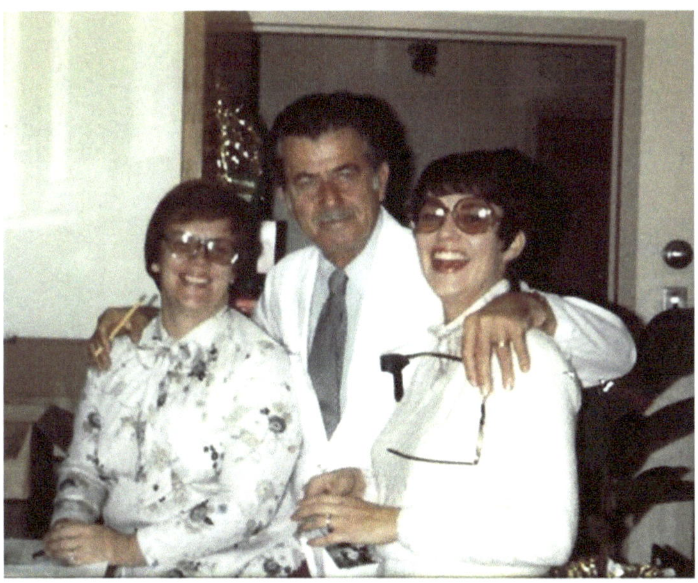

Left to right: Irene Baird-Warren; Samuel C. Bukantz, MD; Judy Bien; 1981.

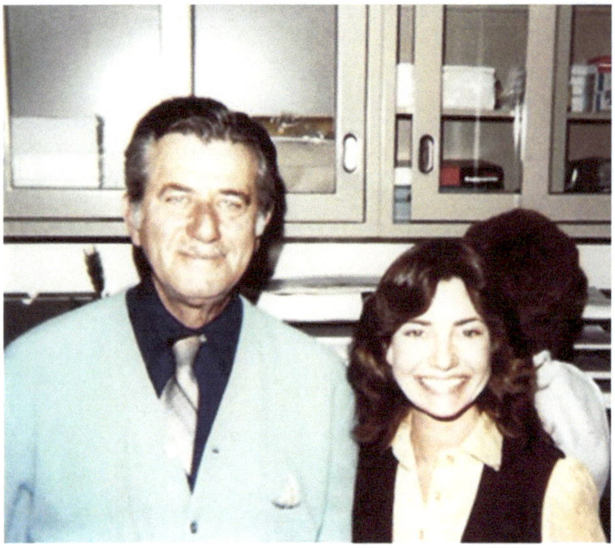

Left to right: Samuel C. Bukantz, MD and Ginger Montuoro; 1981.

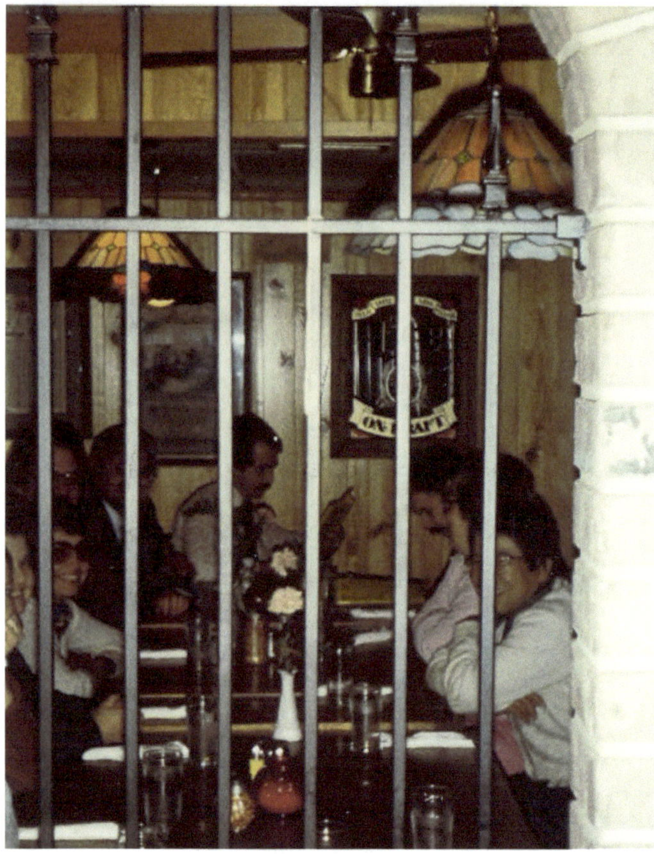

Birthday celebration; CDB Pizza; 1981.

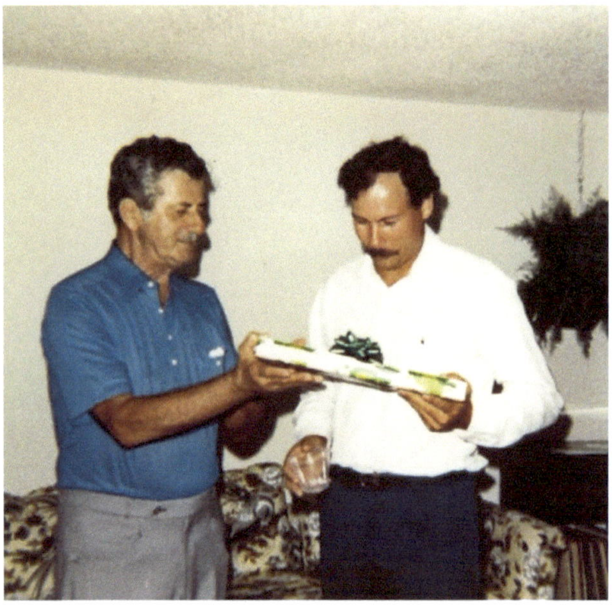

Left to right: Samuel C. Bukantz, MD and Gerald A. Bucholtz, MD (1980-1982); graduation party for Dr. Bucholtz; 1982.

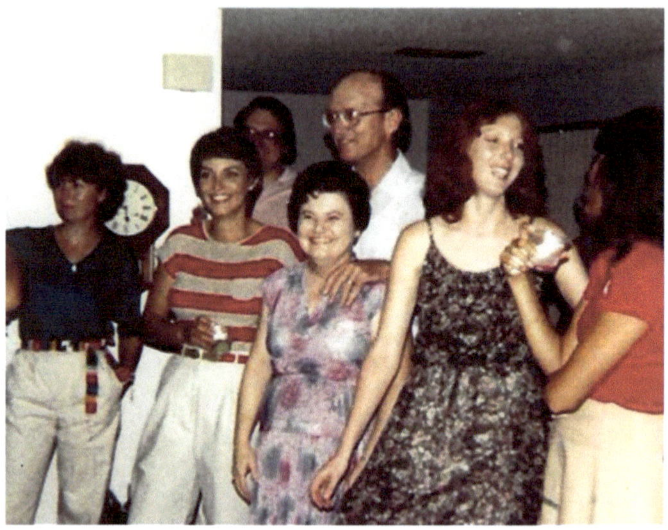

Front row (left to right): Carol Lee Lockey; Judy Bien; Lolita Binford; Cindy (surname unknown); Diane Stablein. Back row (left to right): Richard F. Lockey, MD, MS; Jesse Stone Binford, PhD. 1981.

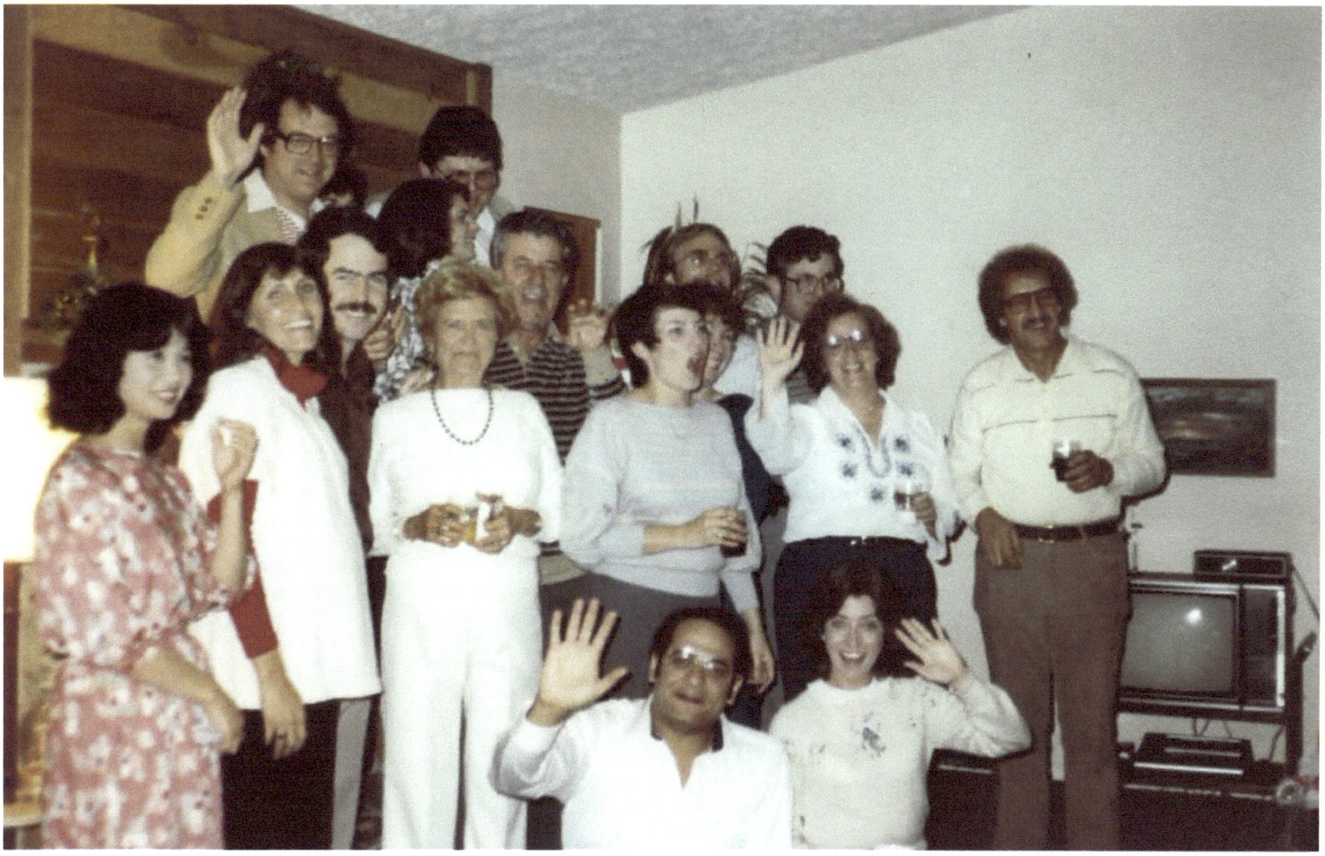

Front row (left to right): Saber Samaan, PhD; Ginger Montuoro. Second row (left to right): Jewell Bukantz; Judy Bien; Irene Baird-Warren; Bob Warren. Third row (left to right): guest; Diane Stablein; John J. Stablein, MD (1979-1981); guest; Samuel C. Bukantz, MD; Roger W. Fox, MD (1978-1980); R. Lawrence Siegel, MD, PhD. Fourth row (left to right): Richard F. Lockey, MD, MS; Albert E. Hensel, MD (1982-1984) in 1982.

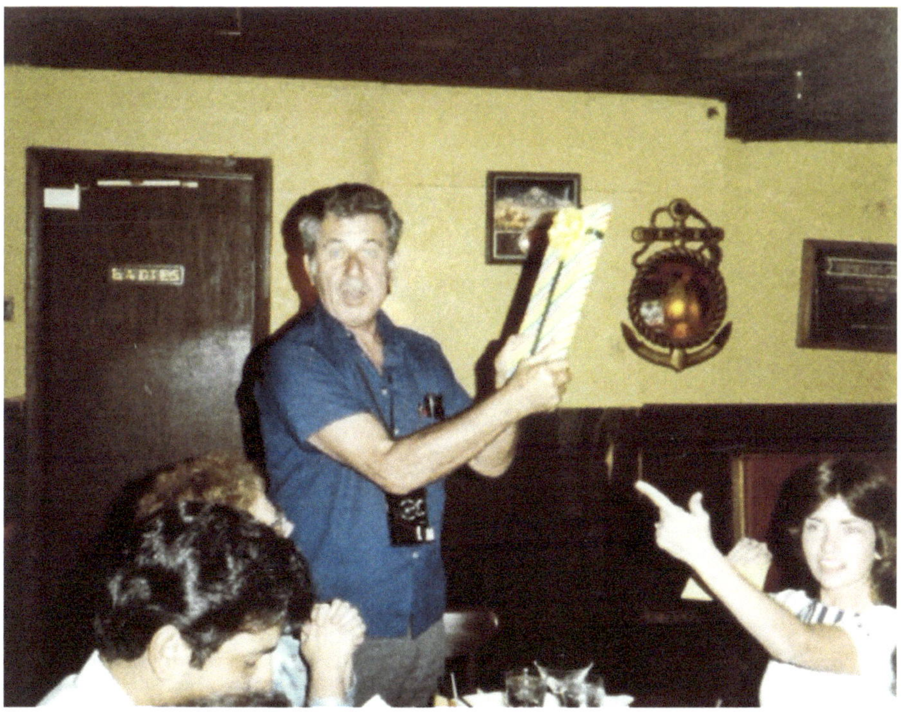

Samuel C. Bukantz, MD in 1983.

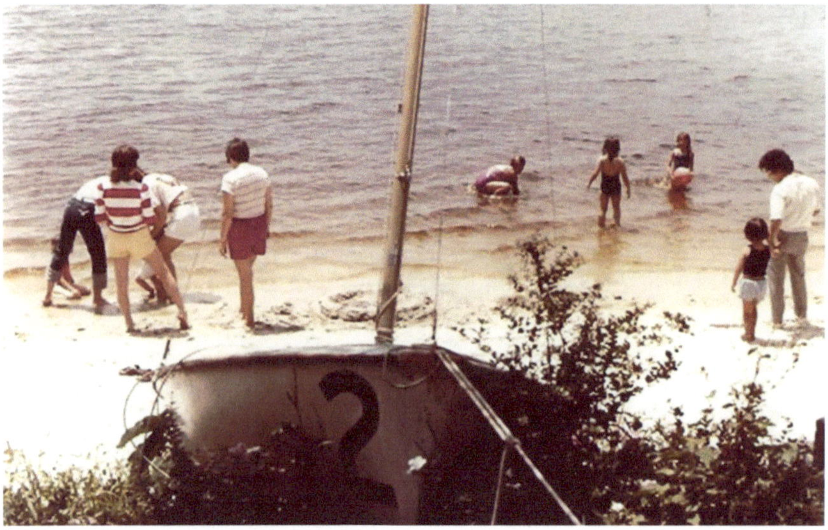

May Day Picnic; 1983.

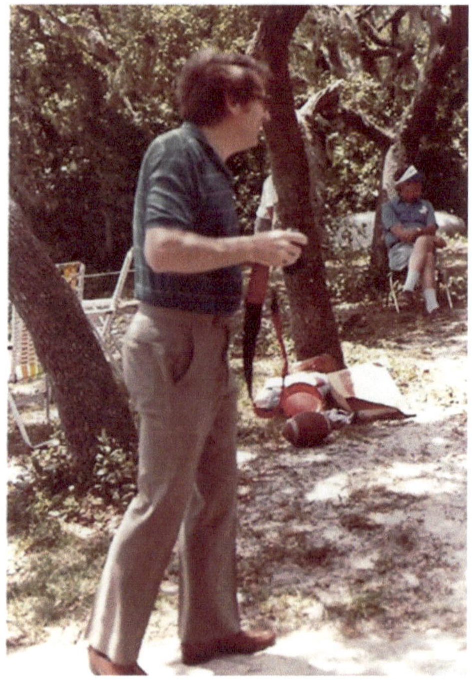

Richard F. Lockey, MD, MS; 1983.

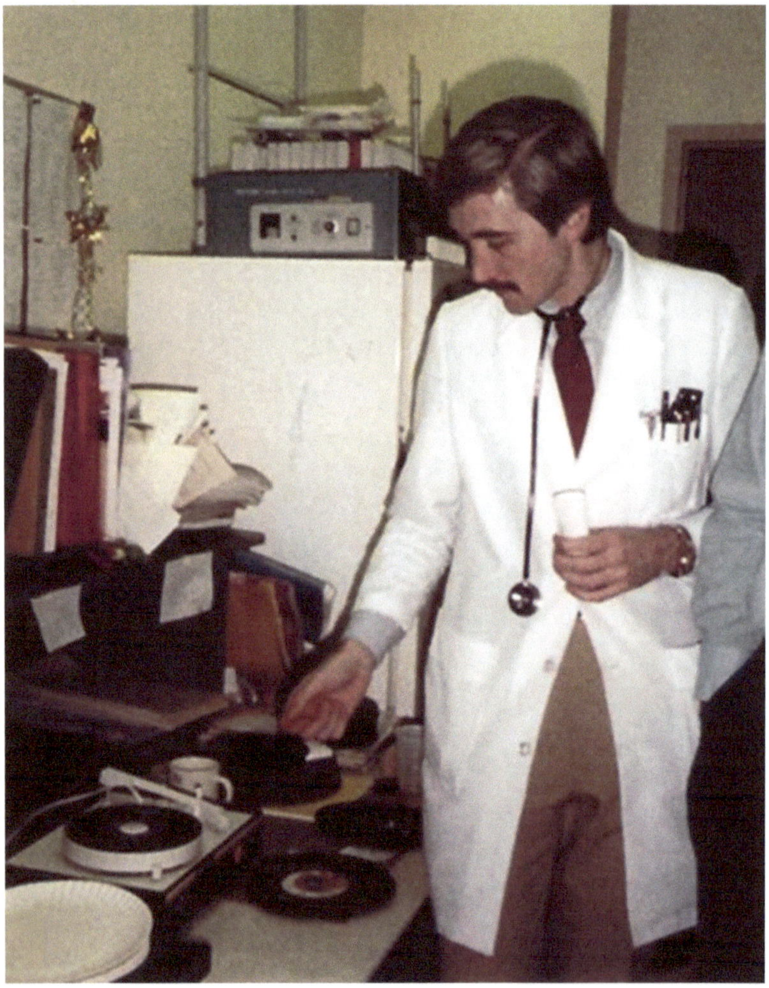

Dennis K. Ledford, MD (1983-1985); 1984.

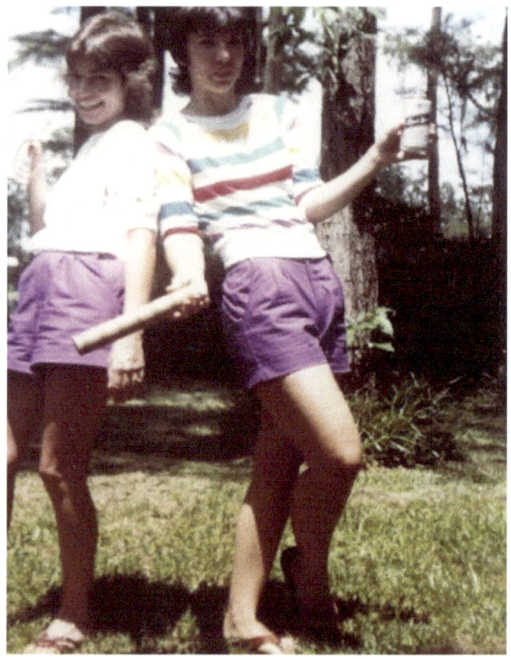

Left to right: Ginger Montuoro and Debbie Serbousek;1983.

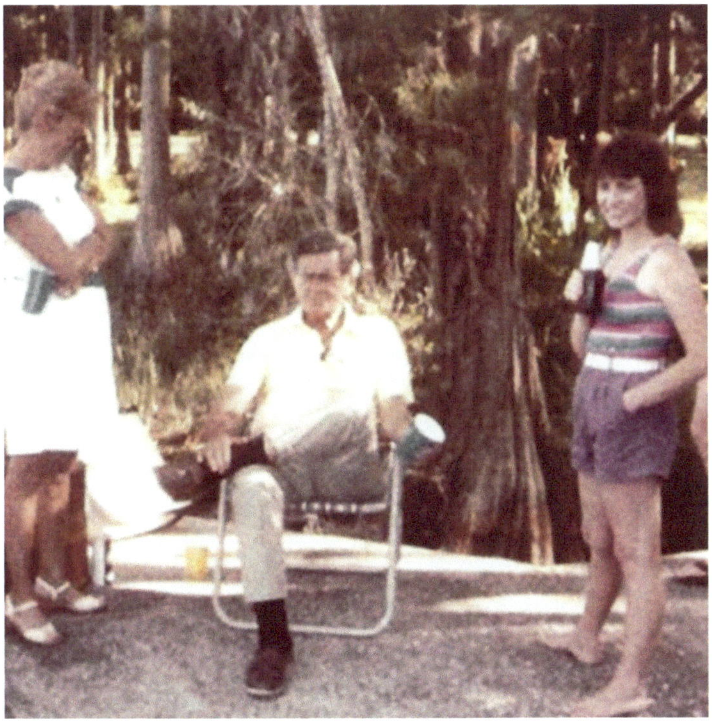

Left to right: Jewell Bukantz; Samuel C. Bukantz, MD; Ginger Montuoro; circa 1984.

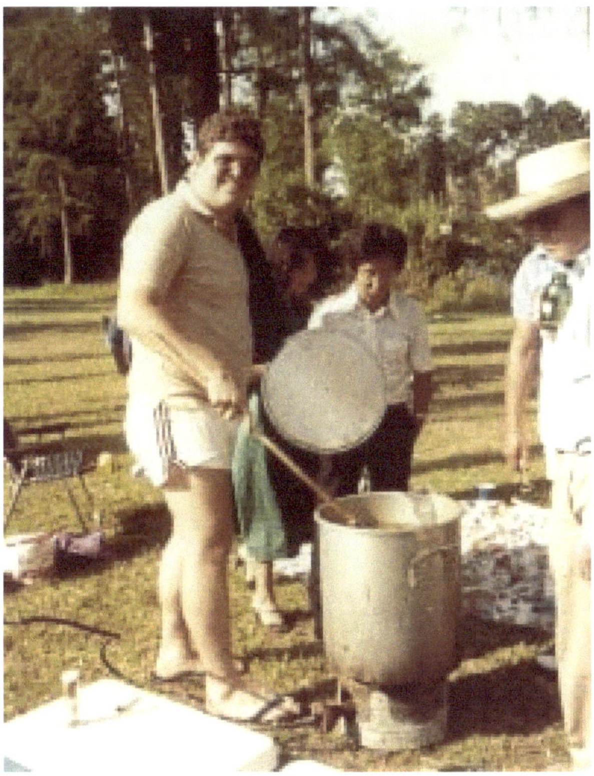

Albert E. Hensel, MD (1982-1984); May Day 1984.

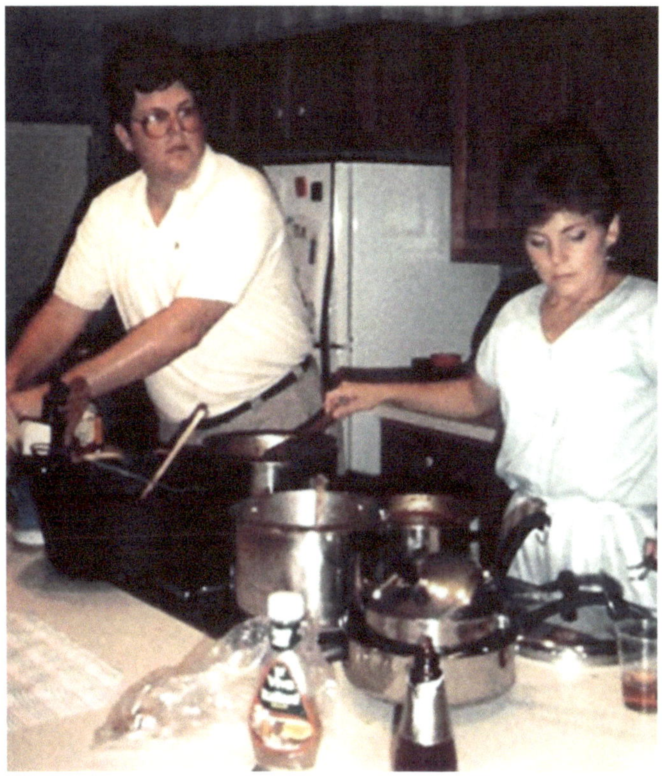

Left to right: Albert E. Hensel, MD (1982-1984) and Cynthia Fox; 1984.

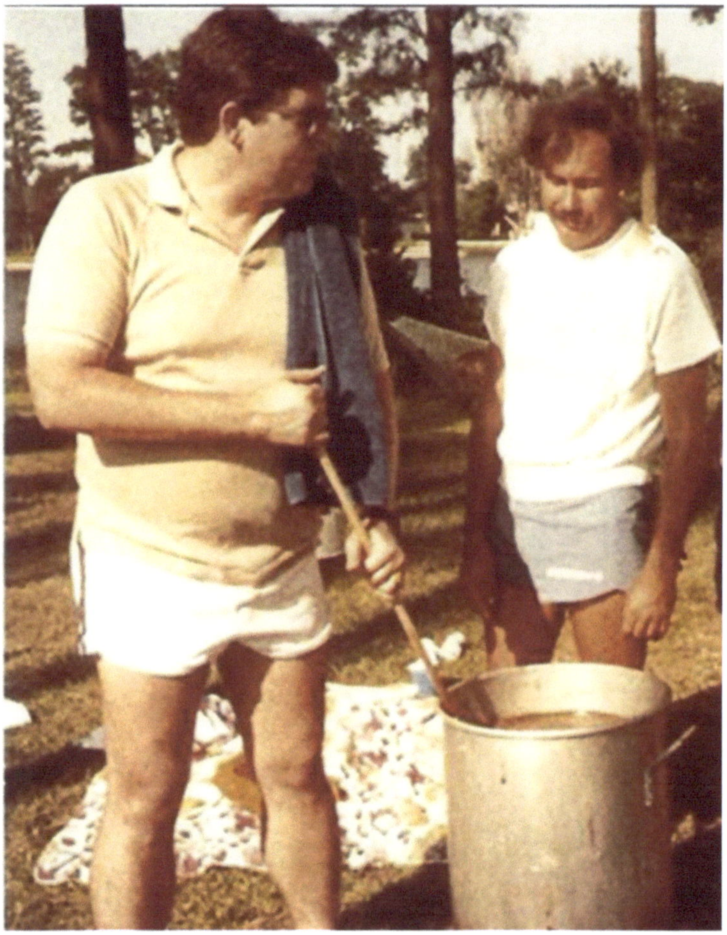

Left to right: Albert E. Hensel, MD (1982-1984) and Gerald A. Bucholtz, MD (1980-1982); May Day 1984.

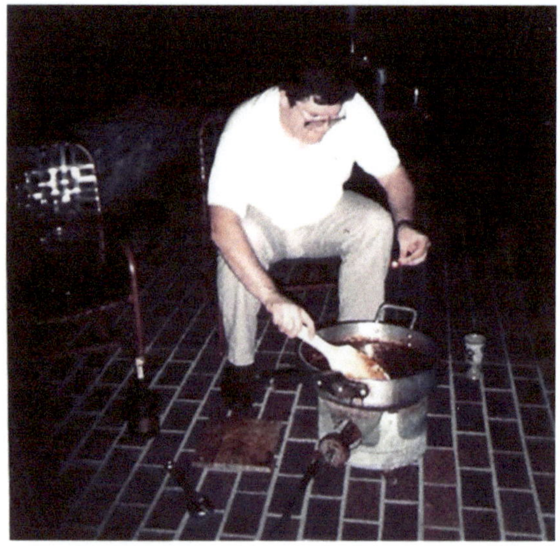

Albert E. Hensel, MD (1982-1984); preparing bananas Foster; 1984.

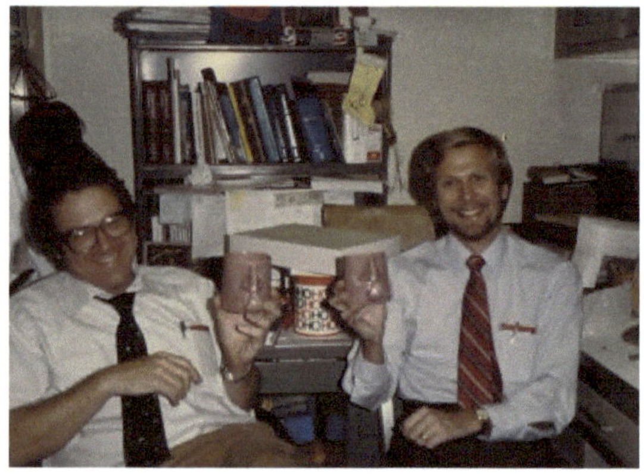

Left to right: Richard F. Lockey, MD, MS and Roger W. Fox, MD (1978-1980). Nose mug Christmas gift from Dr. Stablein; circa 1984.

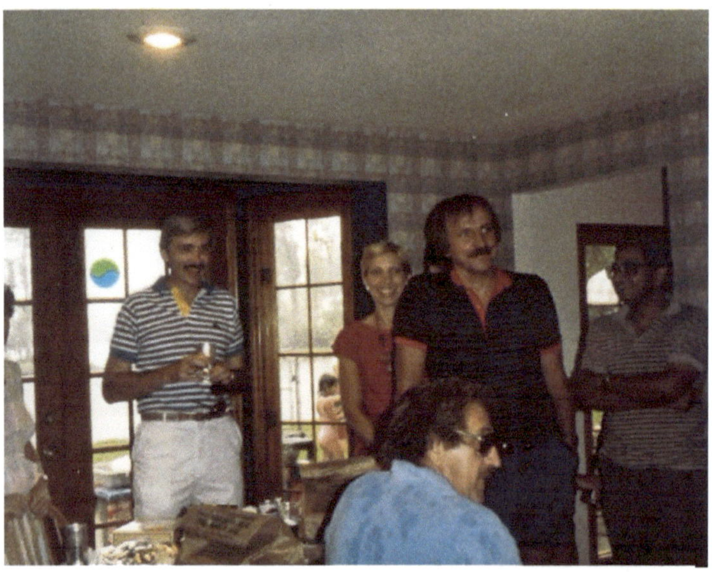

Front, sitting: Bob Warren. Standing (left to right): Dennis K. Ledford, MD (1983-1985); Ann Rogers (VA nurse); Ken Rogers; Donnie Banerji, MD., 1985.

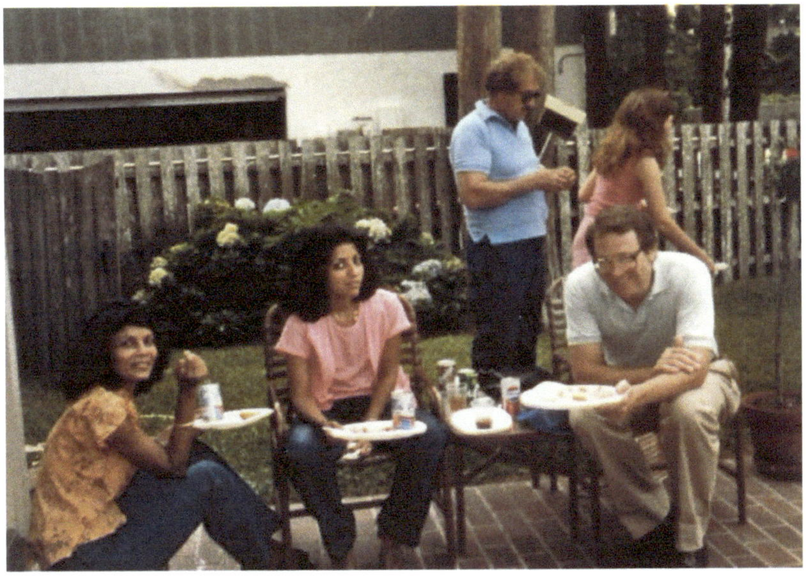

Sitting (left to right): Rama Ganguly, PhD; Sue Banerji; Richard F. Lockey, MD, MS; 1985.

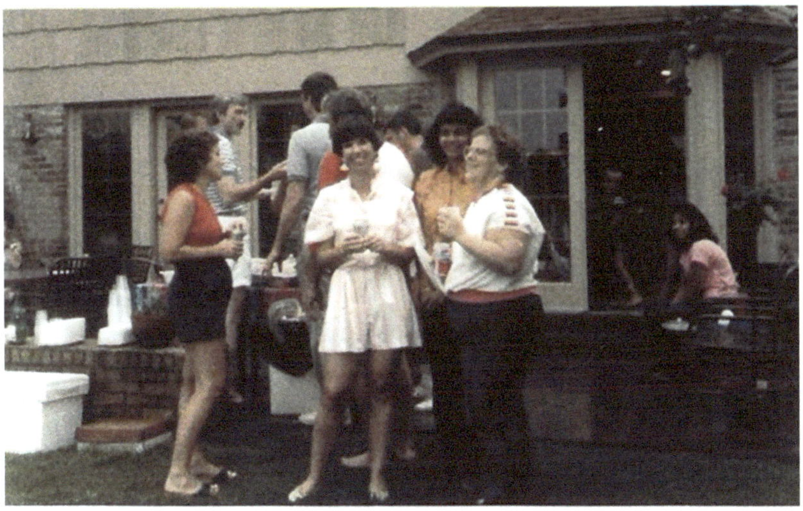

Left to right: Pat Walsh; Debbie Serbousek; Rama Ganguly, PhD; Irene Baird-Warren; 1985.

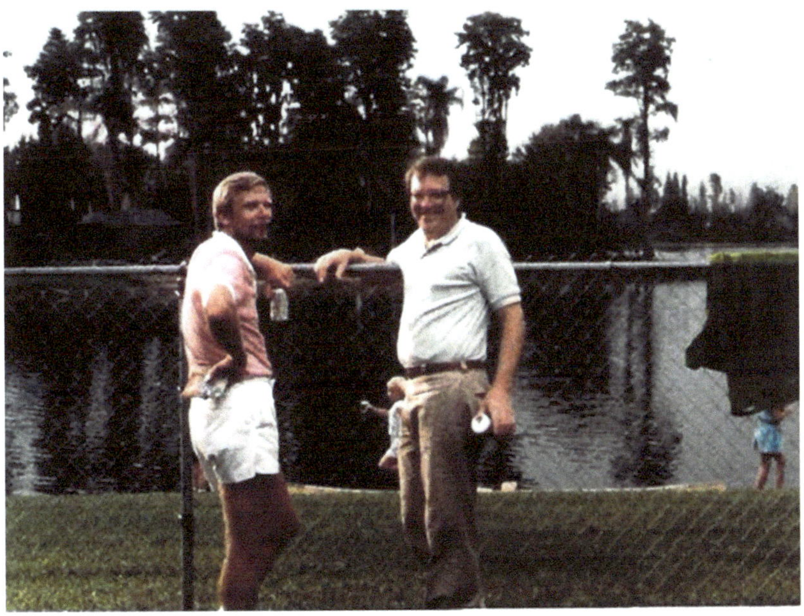

Left to right: Roger W. Fox, MD (1978-1980) and Richard F. Lockey, MD, MS; 1985.

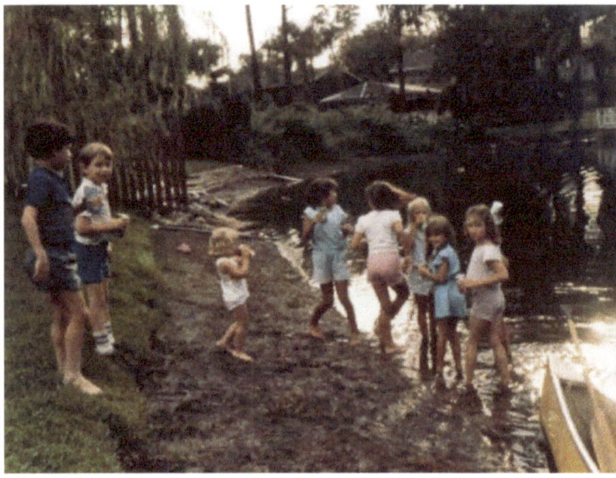

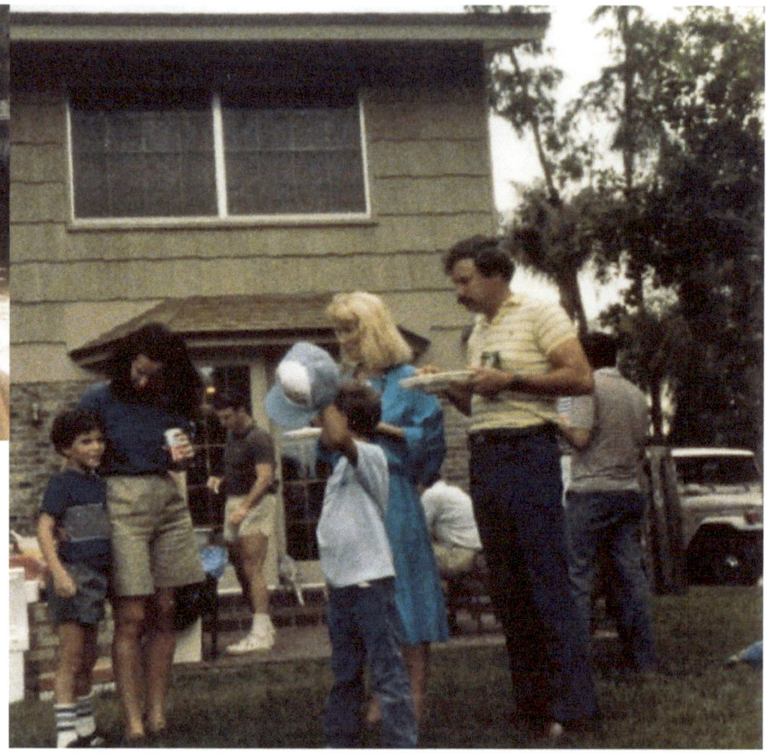

Left to right: Keith Ledford; Jennifer Ledford; Dr. Bucholtz's son; Randi Bucholtz; Gerald A. Bucholtz, MD (1980-1982); 1985.

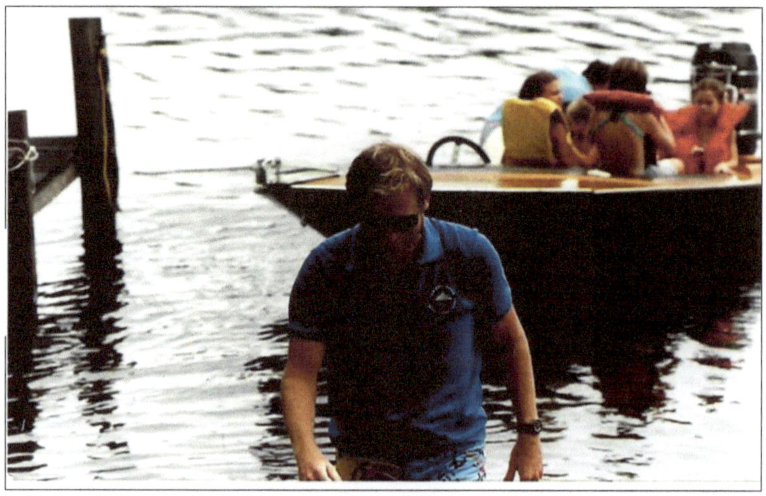

Roger W. Fox, MD (1978-1980); circa 1986.

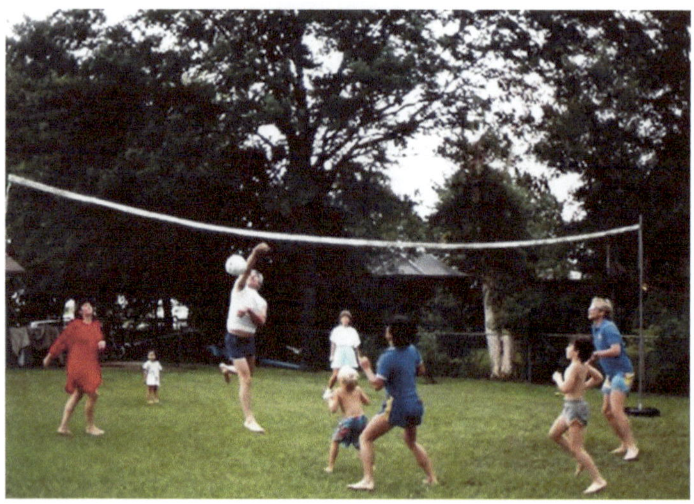

Picnic and volleyball; circa 1986.

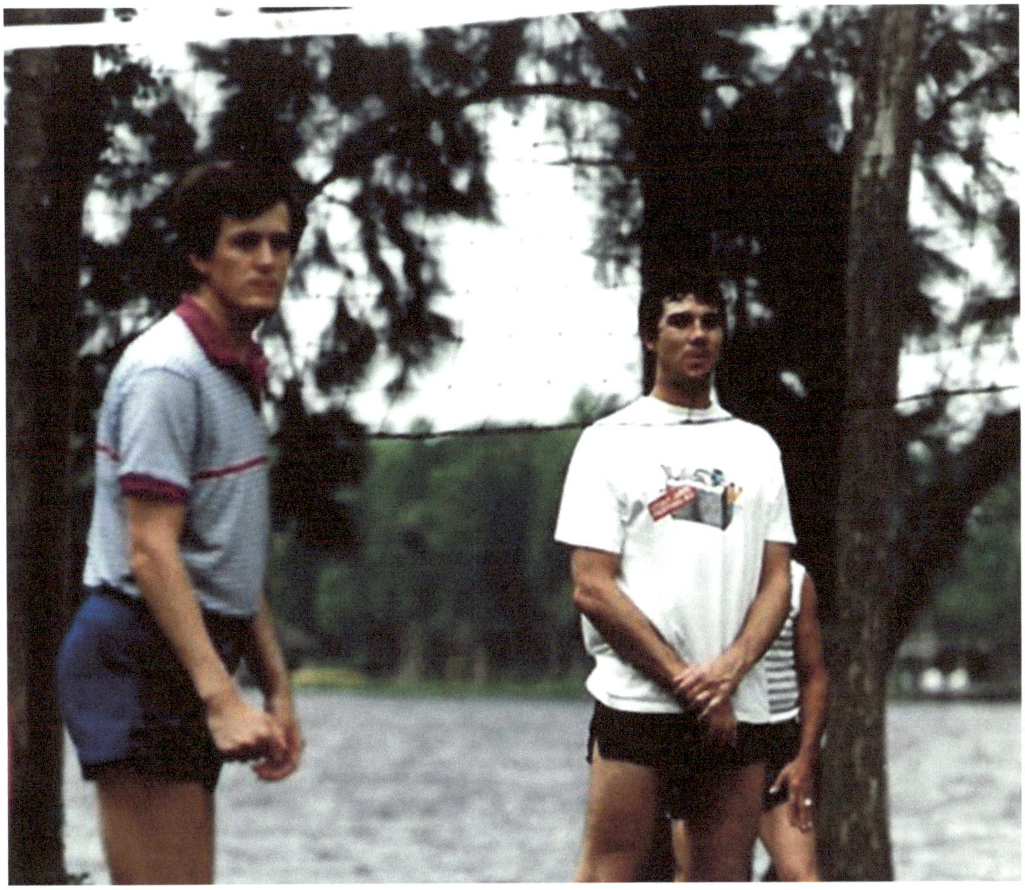

Left to right: Mark Minor, MD (1985-1987) and Robert P. Nelson, MD (1985-1987); circa 1986.

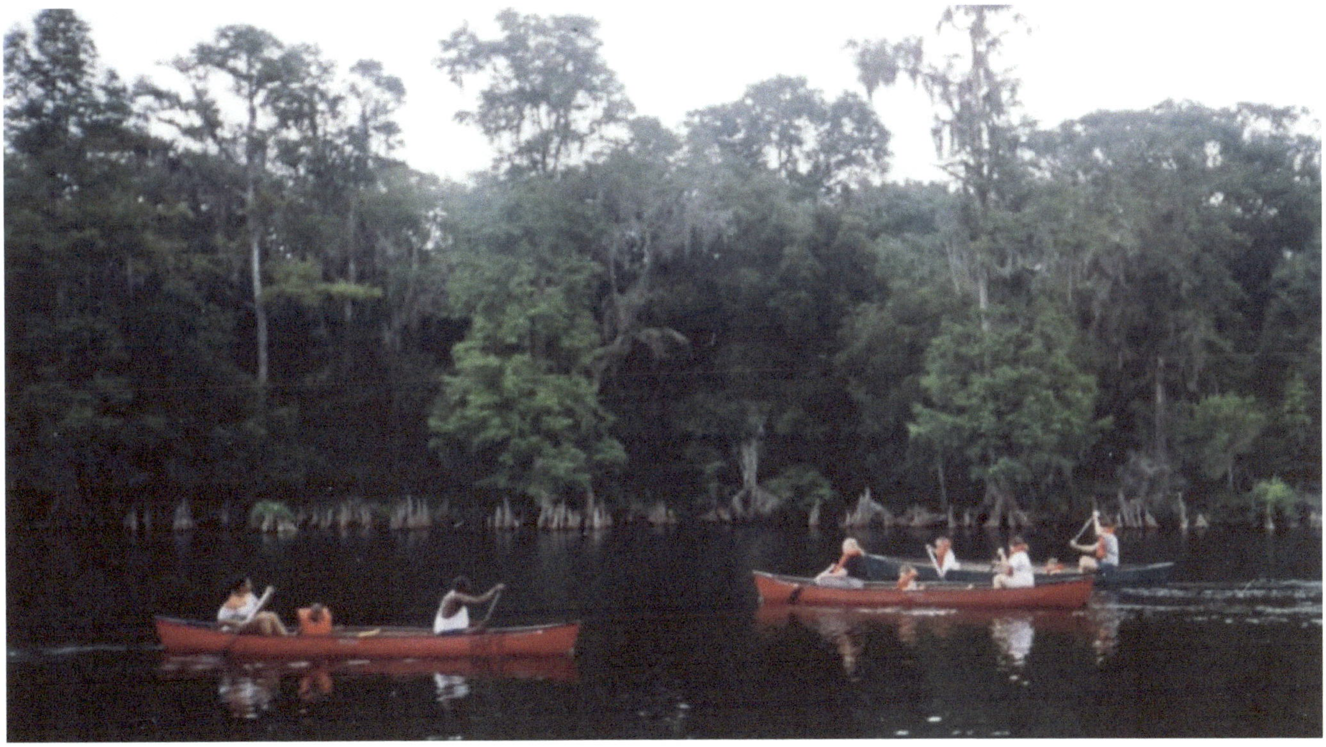

Division Picnic, USF Riverfront Park, May 1997.

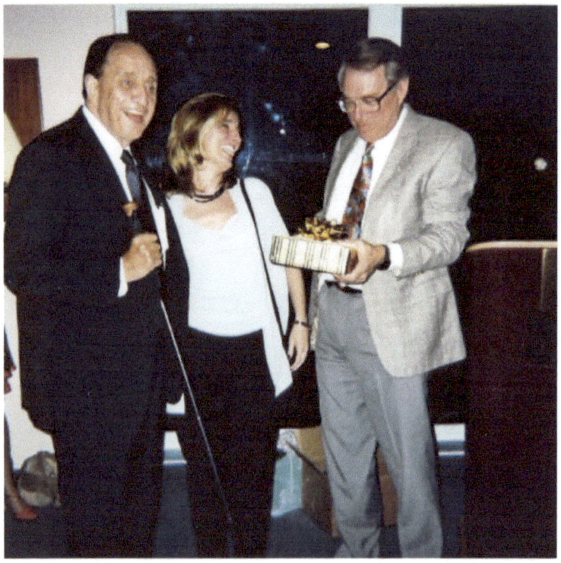

Left to right: Robert A. Good, MD, PhD, DSc; Maria (Maite) de la Morena, MD; Richard F. Lockey, MD, MS; circa 1999.

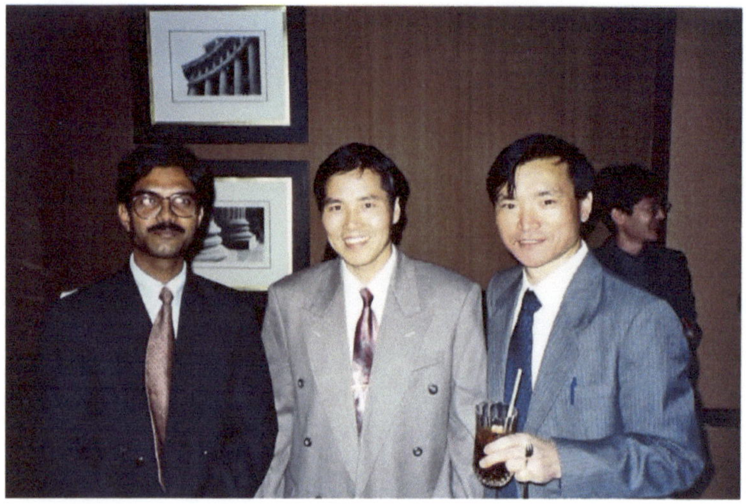

Left to right: Mukesh Kumar, PhD; Jianan Hu, MD; Jian Zhang, MD; circa 1999.

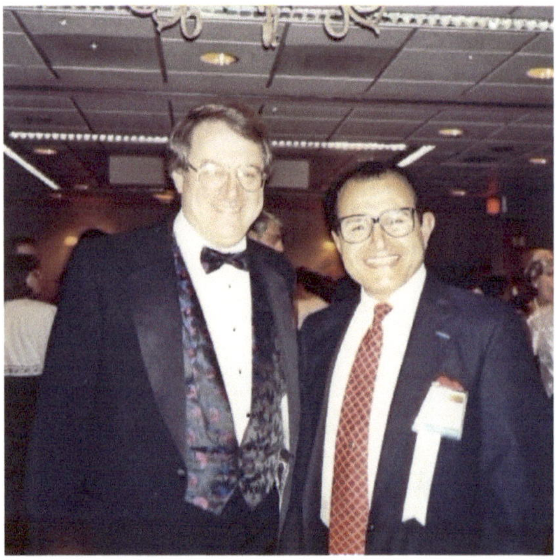

Left to right: Richard F. Lockey, MD, MS and Sami Bahna, MD, DrPH; 1994.

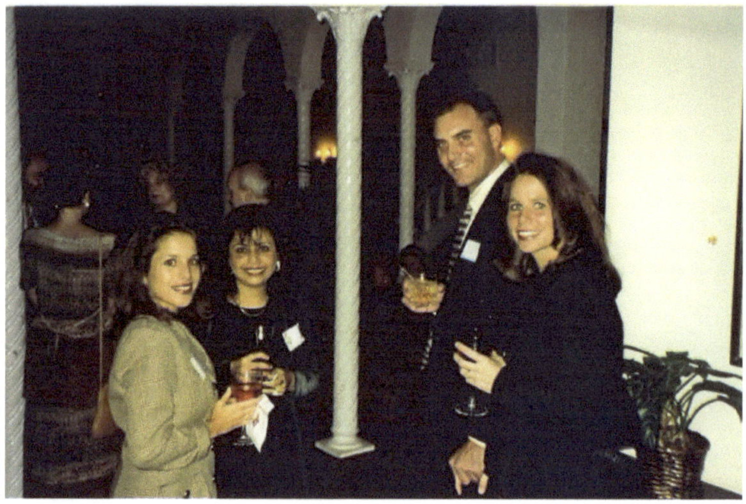

Left to right: Alisa Diecidue; Geeta Gehi; Mark and Diana Miller; 1999.

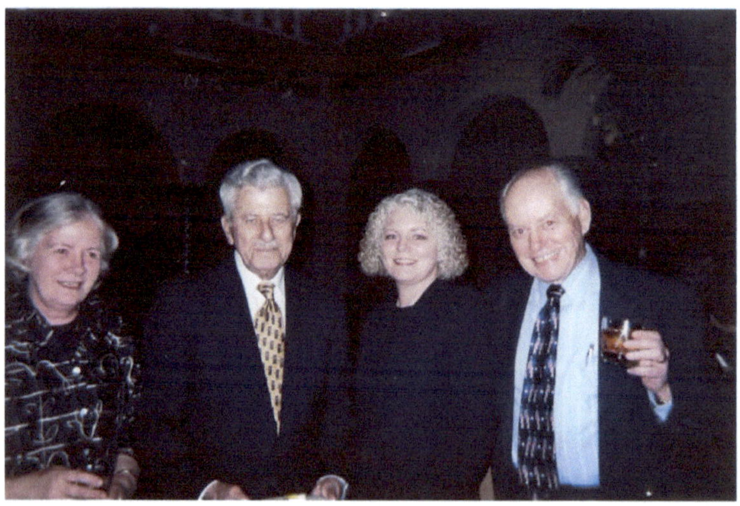

Left to right: Barbara King; Samuel C. Bukantz, MD; Cynthia Fox; Monroe J. King, DO; circa 1999.

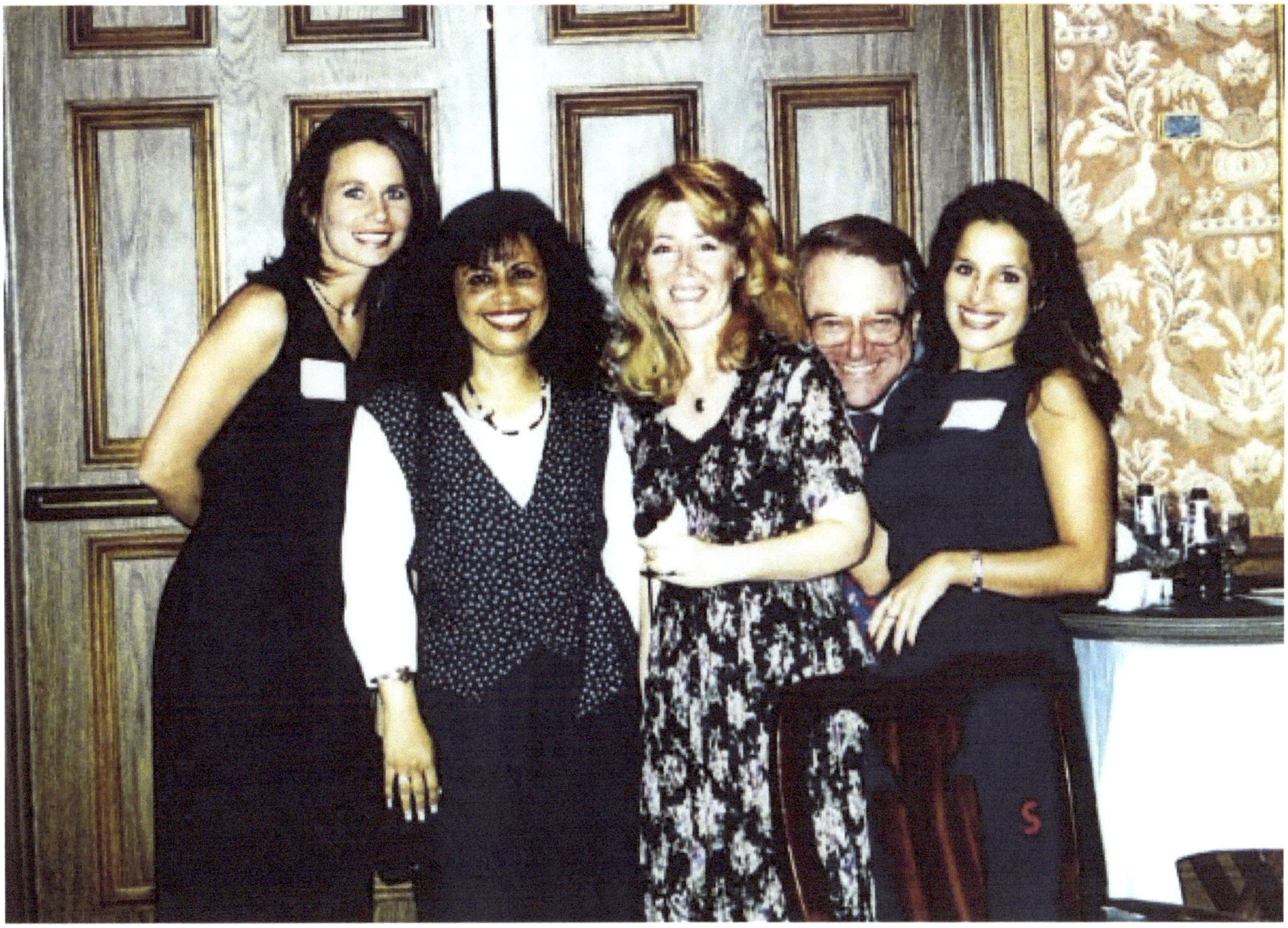

Left to right: Diana Miller; Geeta Gehi; Sandra Rocha; Richard F. Lockey, MD, MS; Alisa Diecidue; circa 1999.

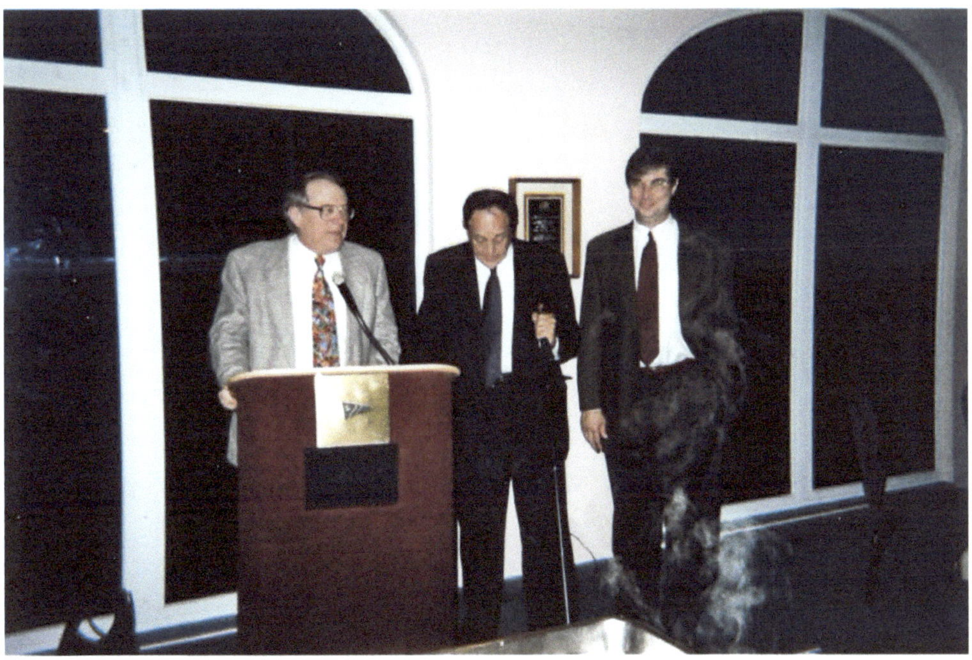

Left to right: Richard F. Lockey, MD, MS; Robert A. Good, MD, PhD, DSc; Robert P. Nelson, MD (1985-1987); circa 1999.

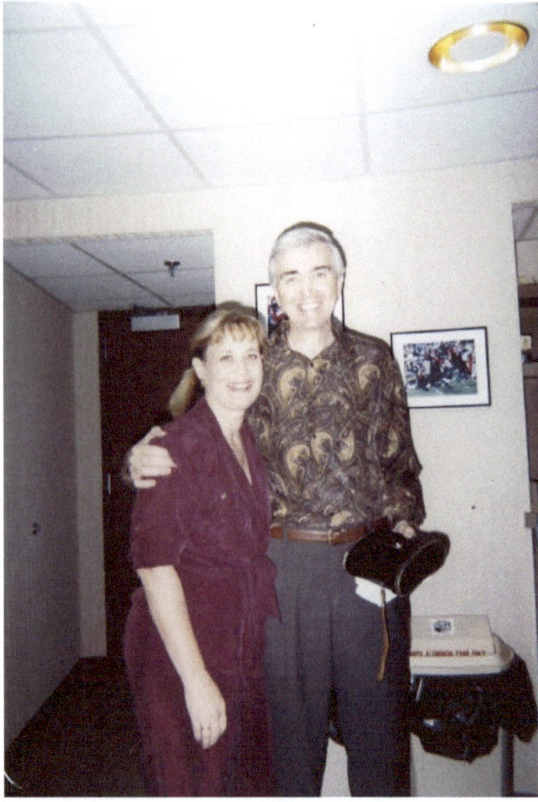

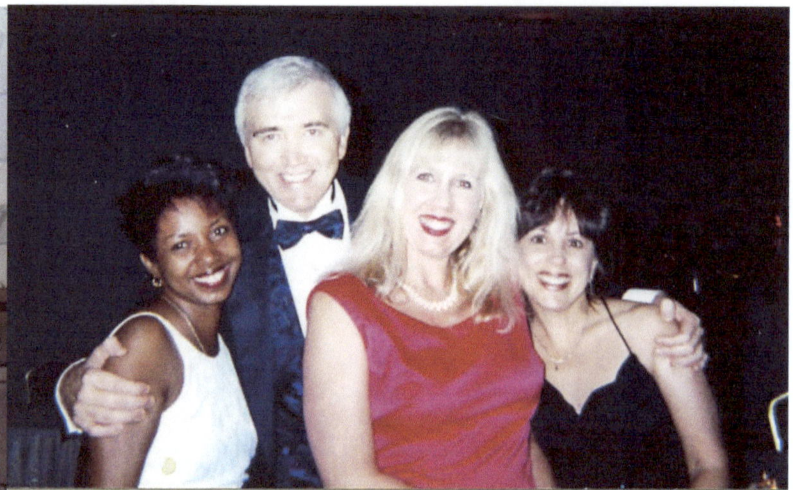

Above: left to right: Linda Livingston (nurse, clinical office); Dennis K. Ledford, MD; Janet O'Neill (nurse, clinical office); Mary Sosa (nurse, clinical office). 2000 Asthma & Allergy Foundation of America, Florida Chapter fundraising event.

Left: Jennifer and Dennis Ledford, MD.

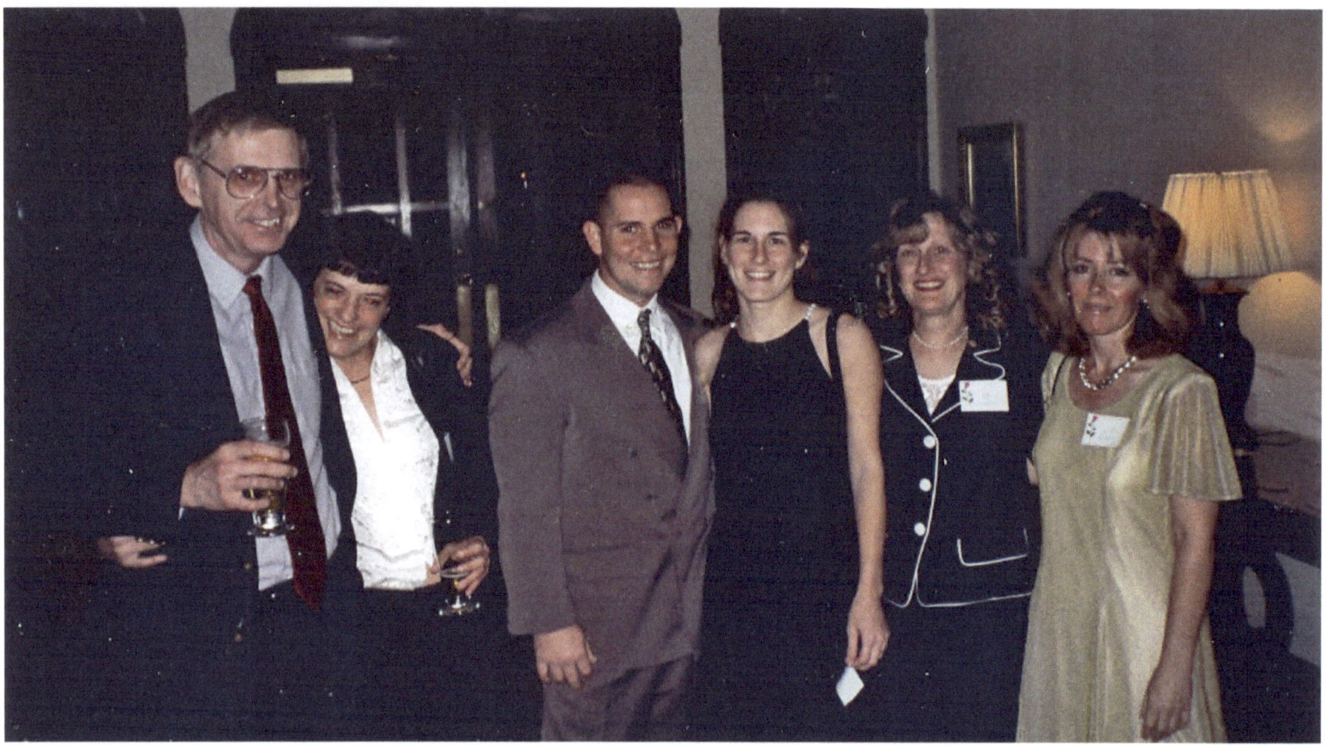

Left to right: Lee Overcash; Rosa Codina-Overcash; Darren Rose; Kimberly Rose; Peggy Hales, Sandra Rocha.

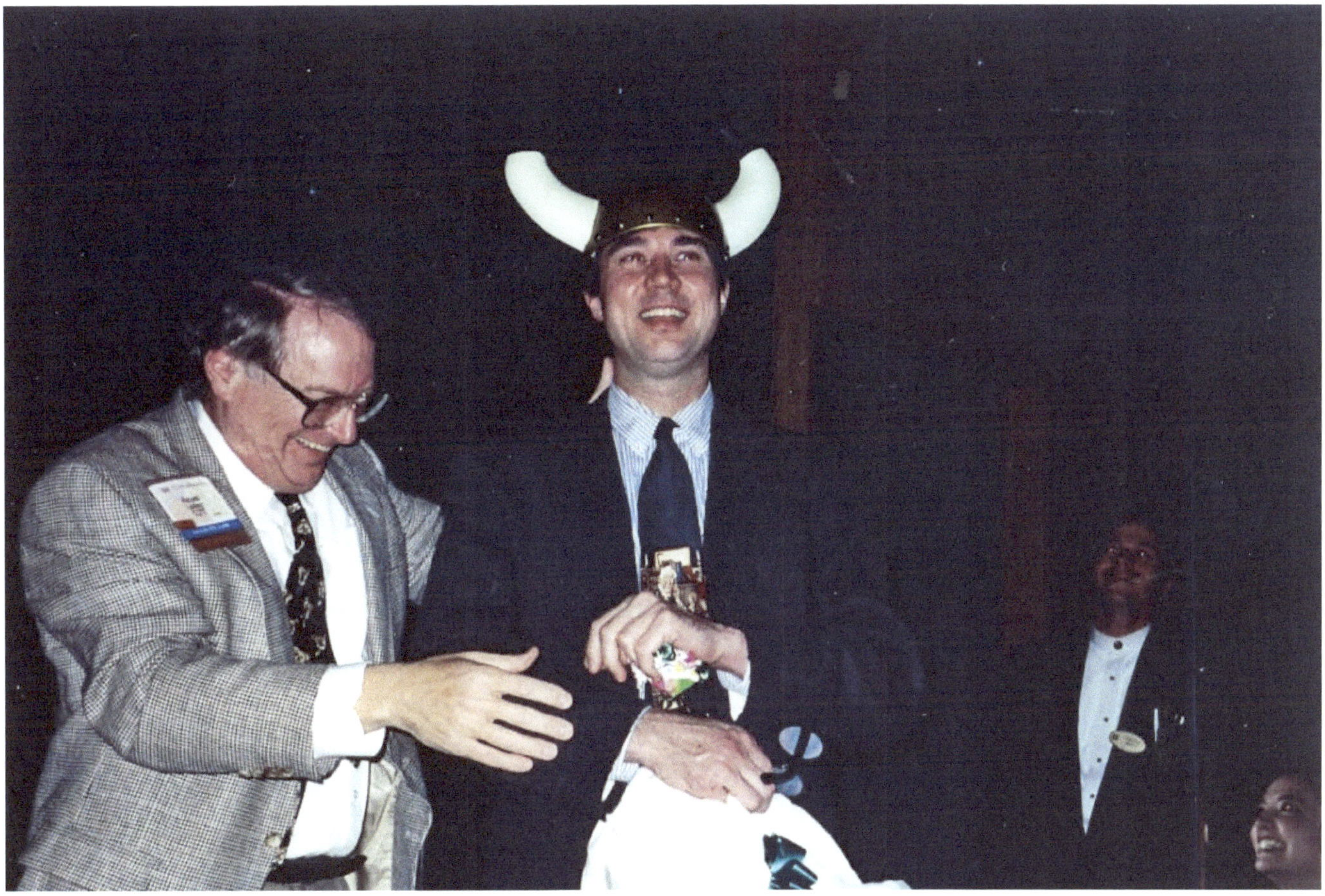

Left to right: Richard F. Lockey, MD, MS and Robert P. Nelson, MD (1985-1987).

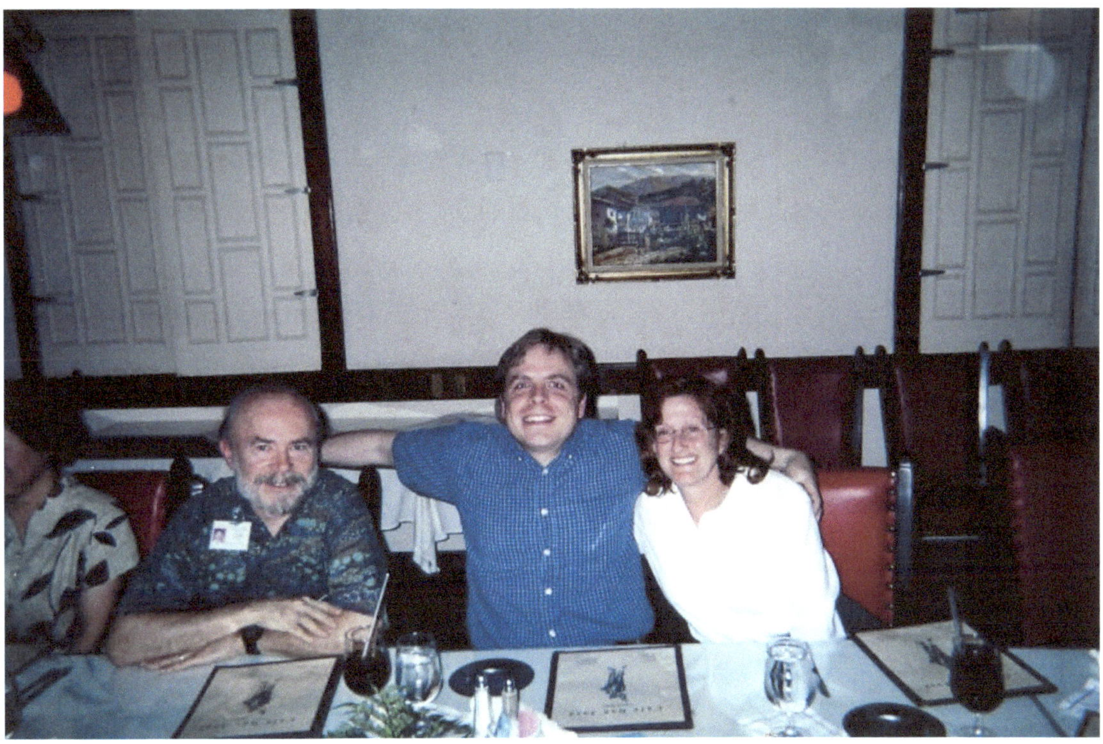

Left to right: Gary Hellermann, PhD; Richard E. Crockett, MD (2000-2003); Peggy Hales; circa 2001.

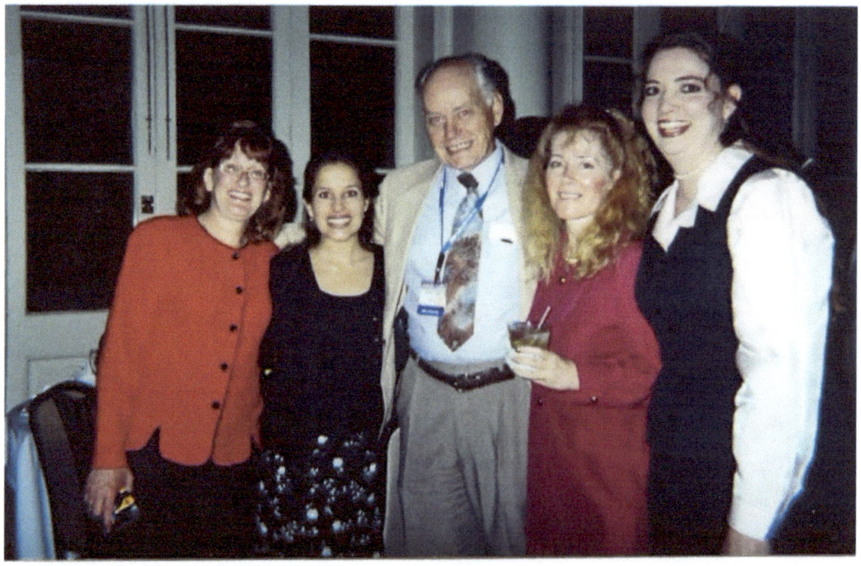

Left to right: Peggy Hales; Alisa Diecidue; Monroe J. King, DO; Sandra Rocha; Angie Renner; circa 2001.

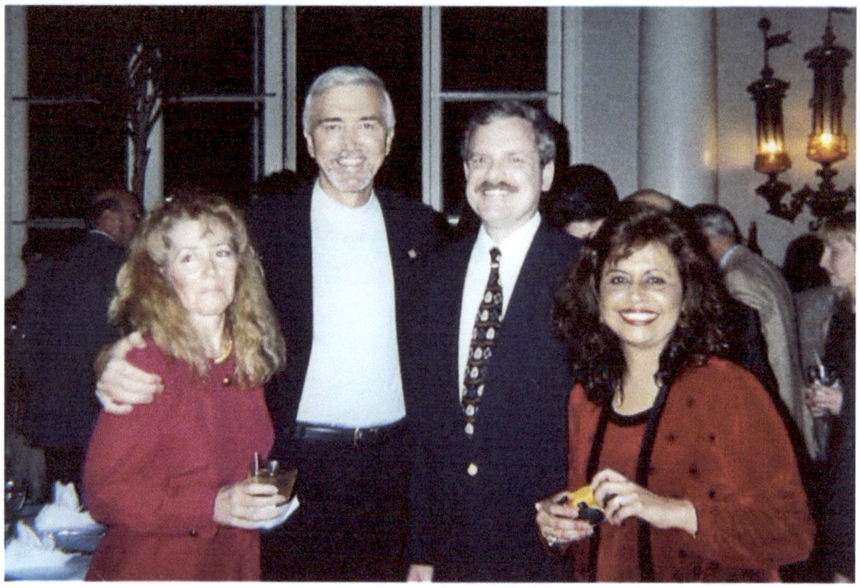

Left to right: Sandra Rocha; Dennis K. Ledford, MD (1983-1985); Stephen F. Kemp, MD (1993-1996); Geeta Gehi; 2001.

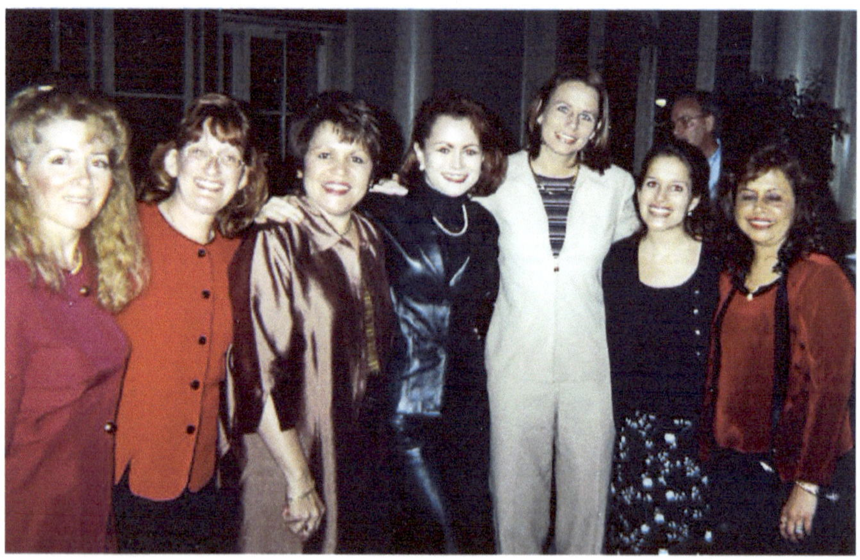

Left to right: Sandra Rocha; Peggy Hales; Nina Ramirez, MD (2000-2002); Giana L. Nicoara-Kasti, MD (1996-1998); Diana Miller; Alisa Diecidue; Geeta Gehi; 2001.

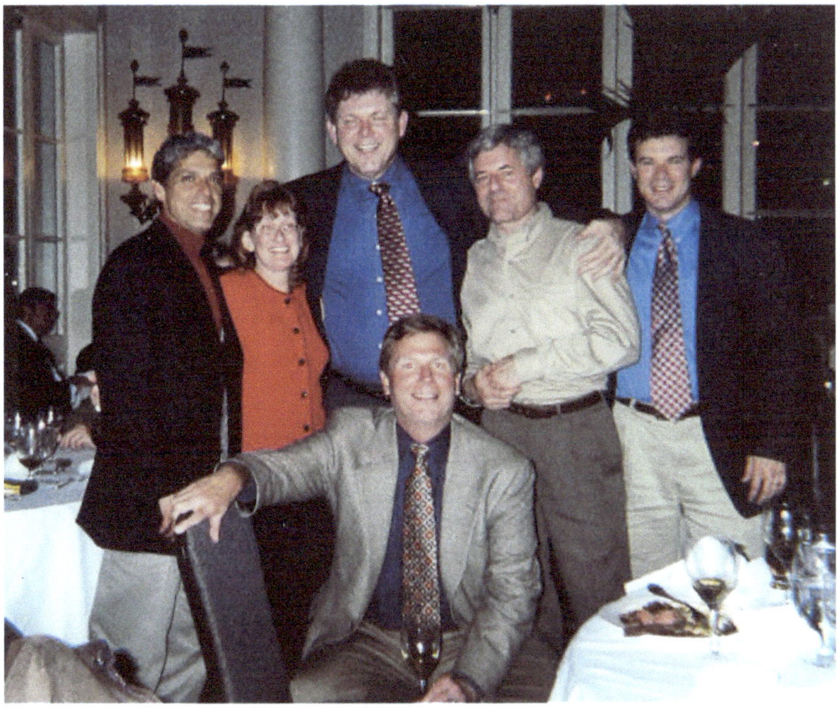

Front, sitting: Roger W. Fox, MD (1978-1980). Standing (left to right): Joseph D. Diaz, MD (1986-1988); Peggy Hales; Albert E. Hensel, MD (1982-1984); Donald W. Russell, MD (1987-1990); Brett E. Stanaland, MD (1992-1995). Circa 2001.

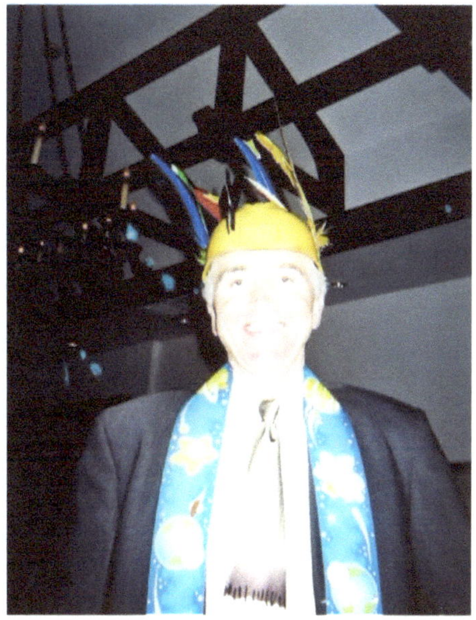

Dennis K. Ledford, MD (1983-1985). The helmet was a gift to Dr. Ledford following a pollen counting study where Dr. Ledford wore a helmet with a collecting rod and culture plates while mowing the grass; circa 2000.

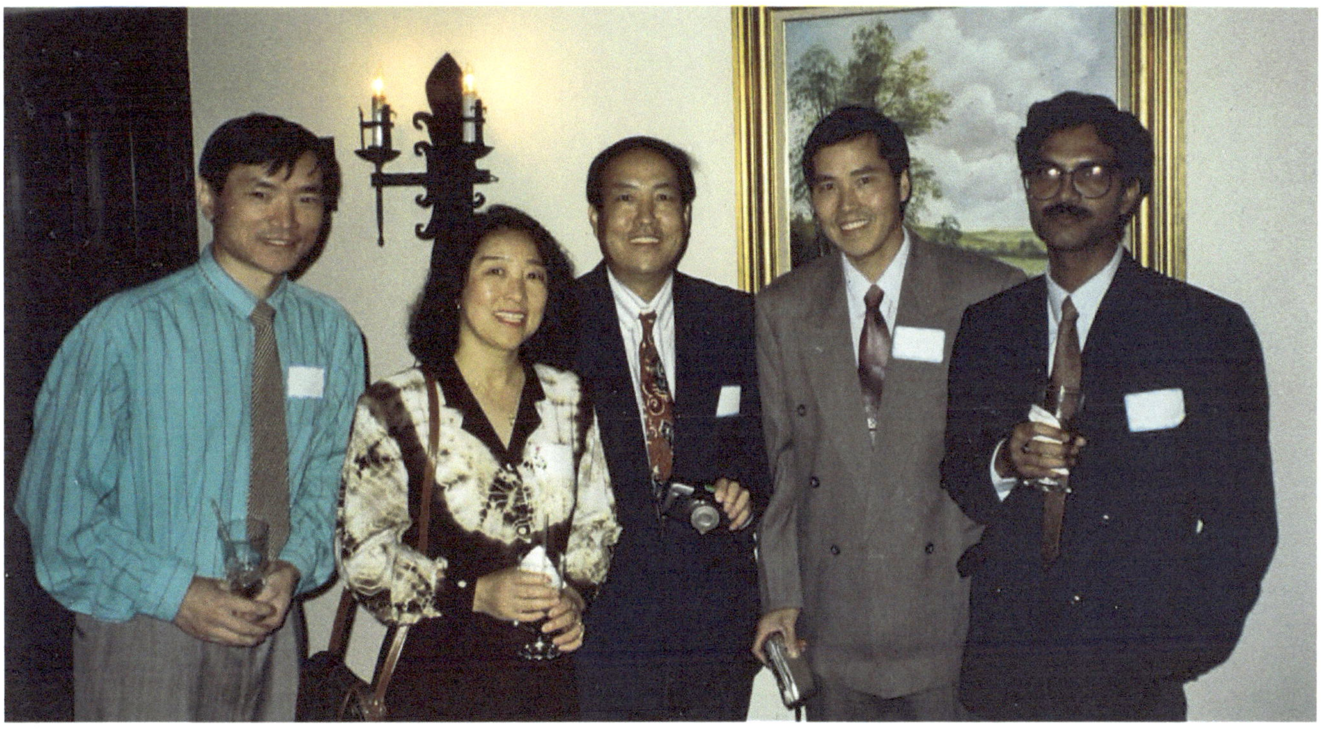

Left to right: Jian Zhang, MD; Xiaoyuan (Sonya) Kong, MD; Shijie Song, MD (Neurology); Jianan Hu, MD; Mukesh Kumar, PhD; circa 2001.

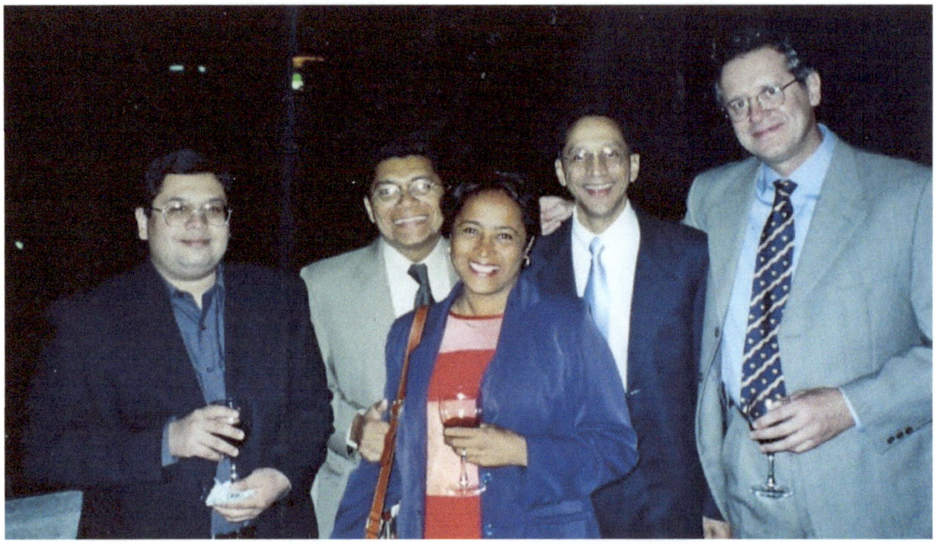

Left to right: Homero San Juan, MD, PhD; Leonardo Puerta, PhD; Mrs. Leonardo Puerta; Luis Caraballo, MD, PhD; Enrique Fernandez-Caldas, PhD.

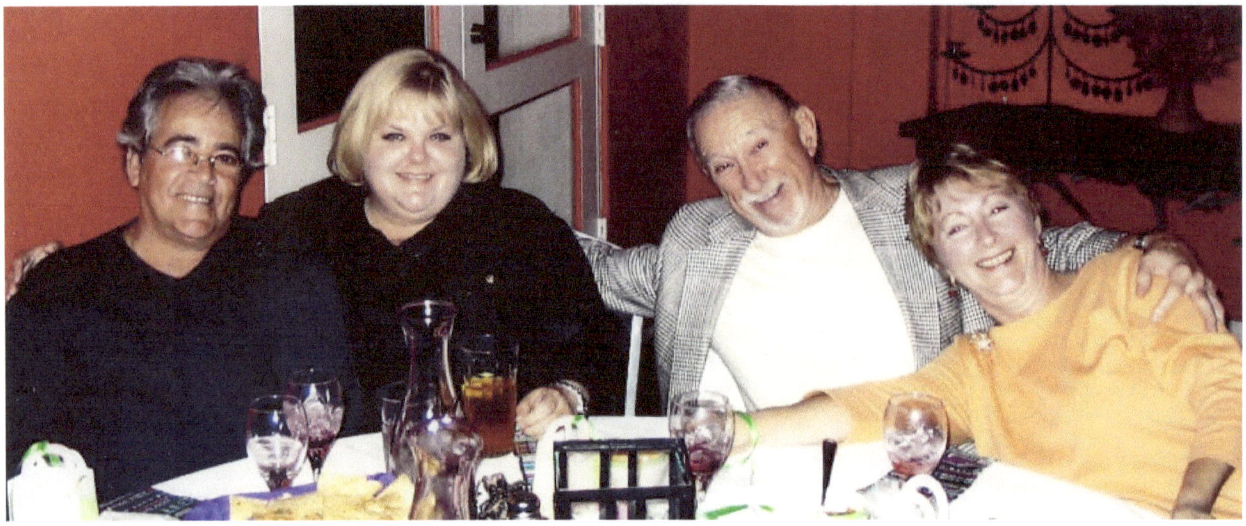

Left to right: husband of Anna Palles (USF nurse); Anna Palles; Paul Shearer; Dona Shearer; 2005.

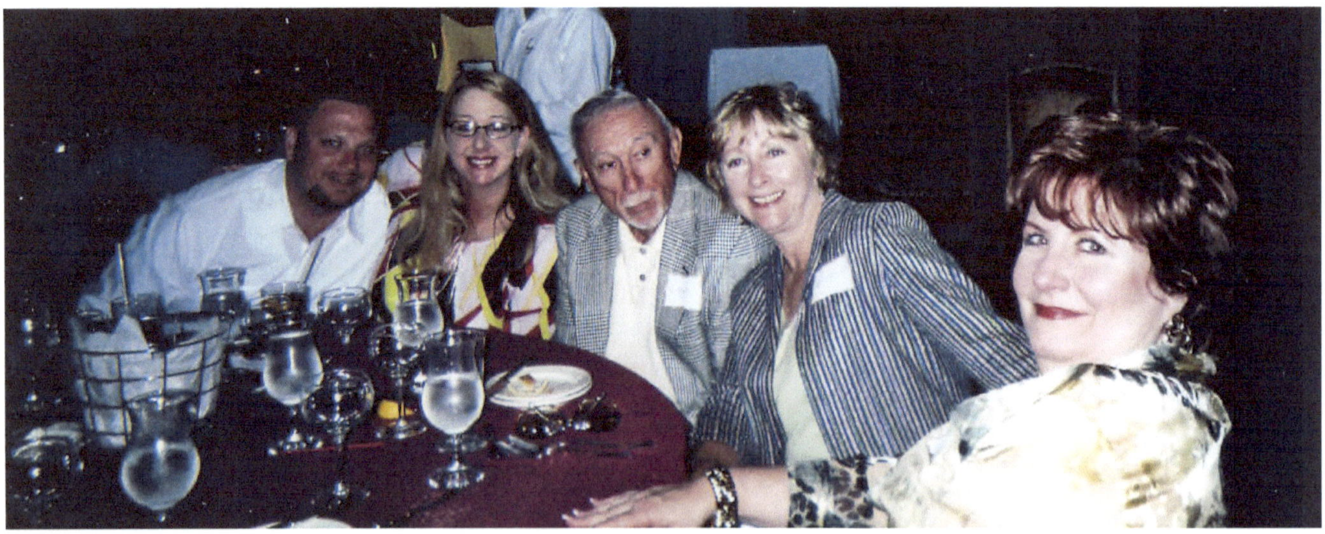

Left to right: Michael Singleton; Michelle Grandstaff-Singleton; Paul Shearer; Dona Shearer; Maryse Parrino; 2006.

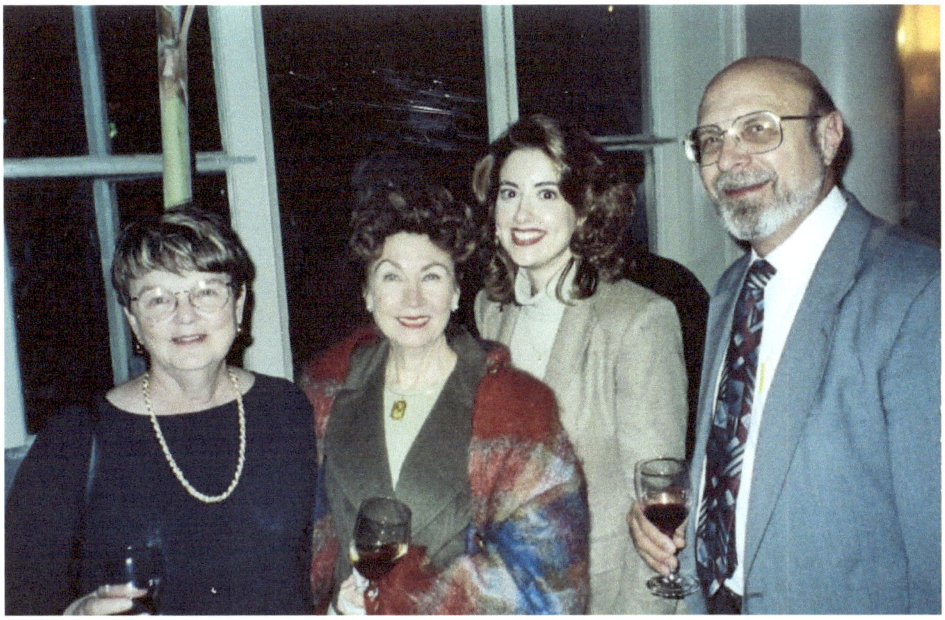

Left to right: Patricia Krzanowski; Carol Lee Lockey; Lizette Hernandez, MD (1994-1997); Joseph J. Krzanowski, PhD (Pharmacology and Therapeutics).

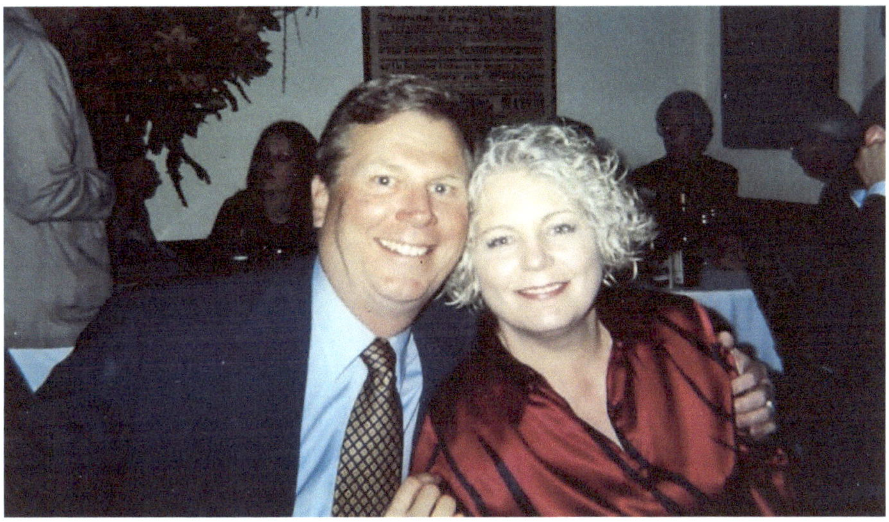

Left to right: Roger W. Fox, MD (1978-1980) and Cynthia Fox.

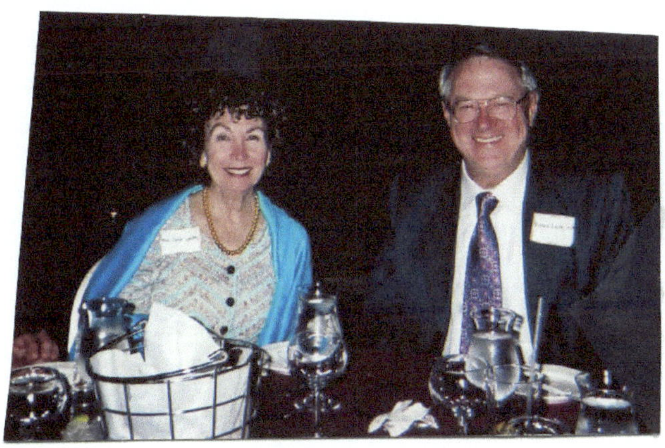

Left to right: Carol Lee Lockey and Richard F. Lockey, MD, MS; 2006.

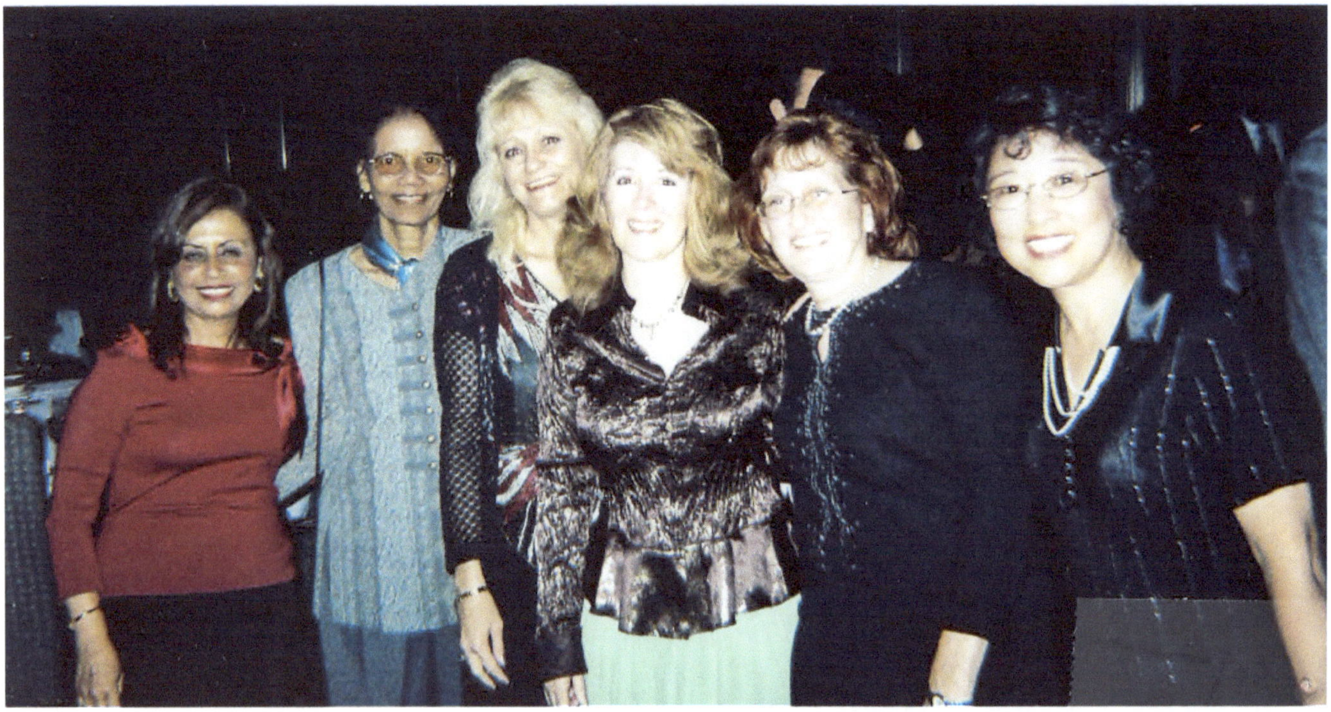

Left to right: Geeta Gehi; Rama Ganguly, PhD; Rebecca Carter-Muncey; Sandra Rocha; Peggy Hales; Xiaoyuan (Sonya) Kong, MD; 2006.

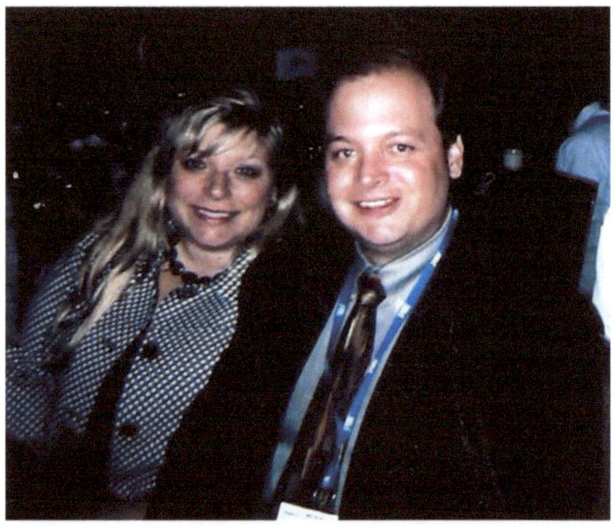

Left to right: Vicki Glaum and Mark C. Glaum, MD, PhD; 2009.

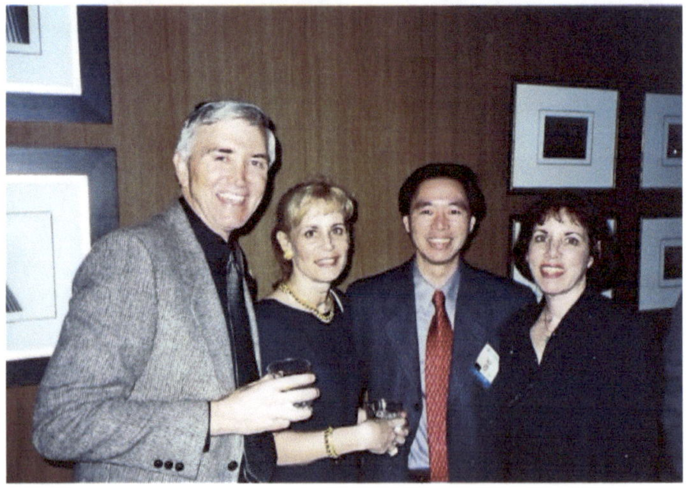

Left to right: Dennis K. Ledford, MD (1983-1985); Jennifer Ledford; Steven J. Louie (1981-1983); Barbara Louie.

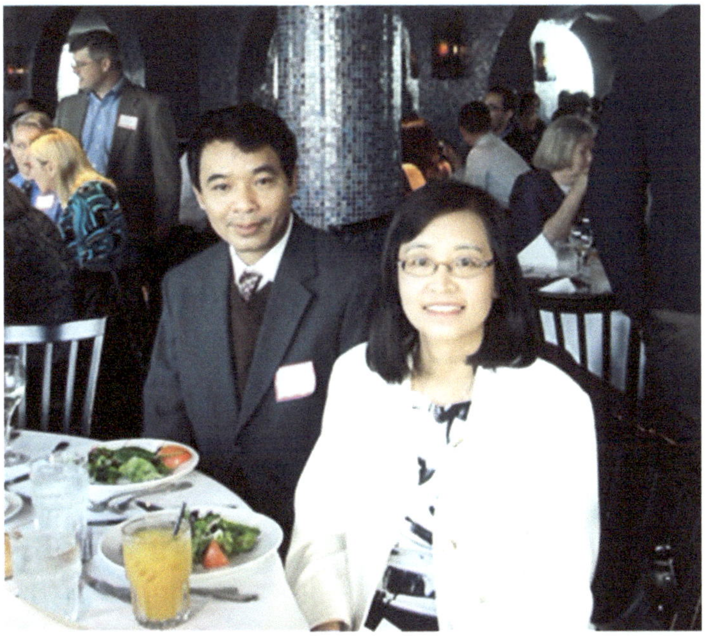

Left to right: Jia-Wang Wang, PhD and Kunyu Li; 2011.

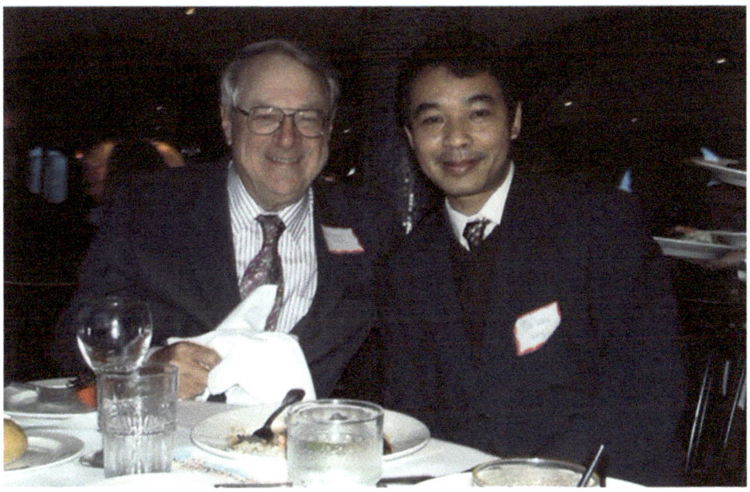

Left to right: Richard F. Lockey, MD, MS and Jia-Wang Wang, PhD; 2011.

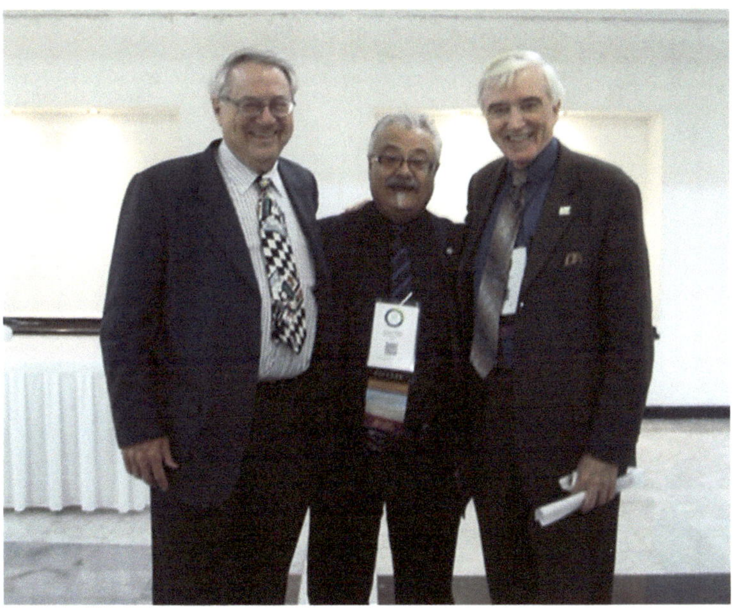

Left to right: Richard F. Lockey, MD, MS (President, World Allergy Organization); G. Walter Canonica, MD (Director, Allergy and Respiratory Diseases Clinic, Genoa University, Italy); Dennis K. Ledford, MD (1983-1985). XXII World Allergy Congress, Cancún Center & Fiesta Americana, December 4-8, 2011.

Left to right: Glenn Whelan, PharmD; Michael Teng, PhD; Narasaiah Kolliputi, PhD. XXII World Allergy Congress, Cancún Center & Fiesta Americana, December 4-8, 2011.

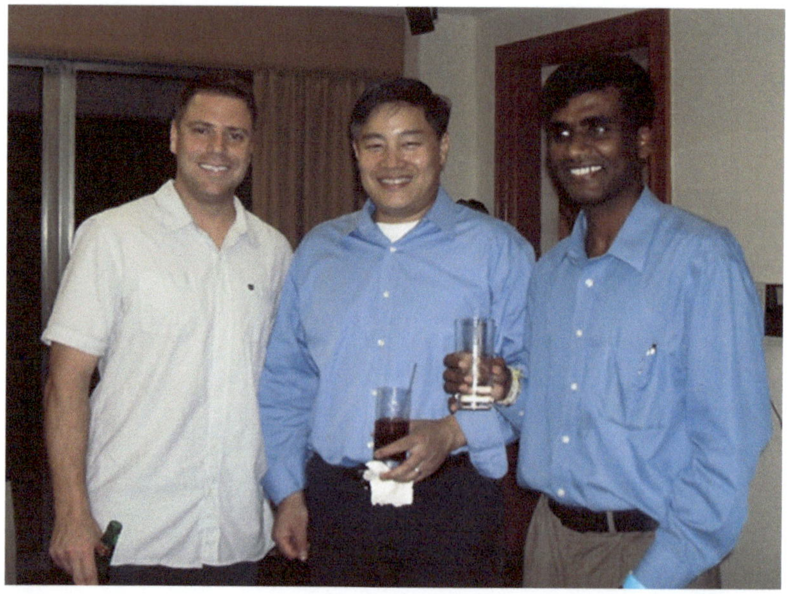

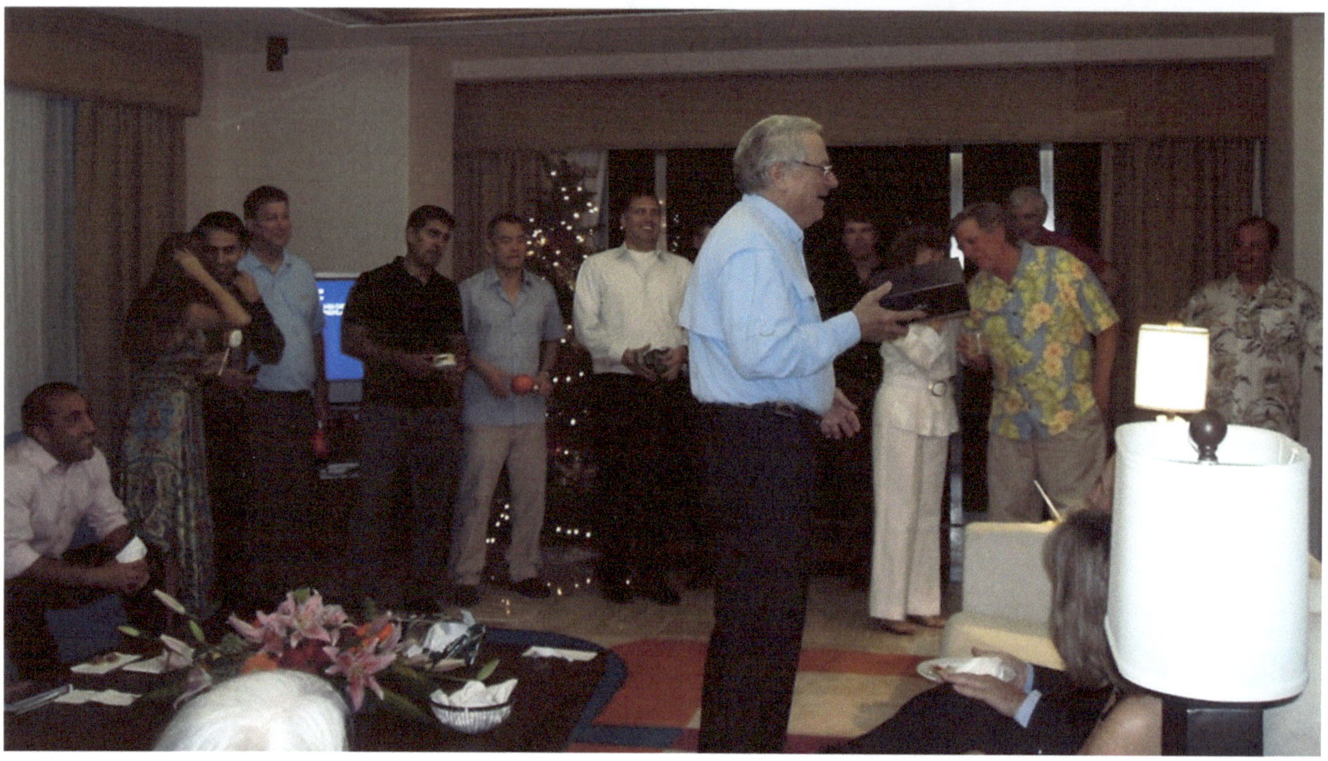

Front: Richard F. Lockey, MD, MS.

Standing to Dr. Lockey's right): Carol Lee Lockey; Roger W. Fox, MD (1978-1980); Mark C. Glaum, MD, PhD.

Back row; left to right: Michel Alkhalil, MD (2009-2011); Susan Culverhouse, MD (2011-2013); Salman Aljubran, MD (2010-2013); James Parkerson, DO (2010-2012); Ahmed Butt, MD (2010-2012); Doanh Nguyen, MD (ACH, 2010-2012); Patrick DeMarco, MD (2003-2005); David Fitzhugh, MD. (2010-2012) (hidden behind Dr. Lockey); Brett E. Stanaland, MD (1992-1995); Dennis K. Ledford, MD (1983-1985).

XXII World Allergy Congress, Cancún Center & Fiesta Americana, December 4-8, 2011.

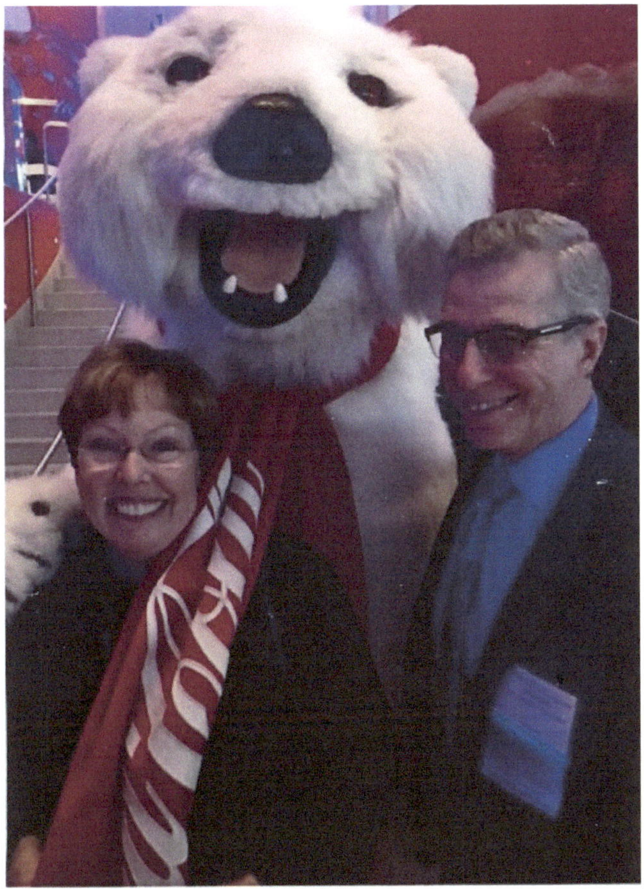

Left to right: Jean Casale and Thomas Casale, MD; circa 2015.

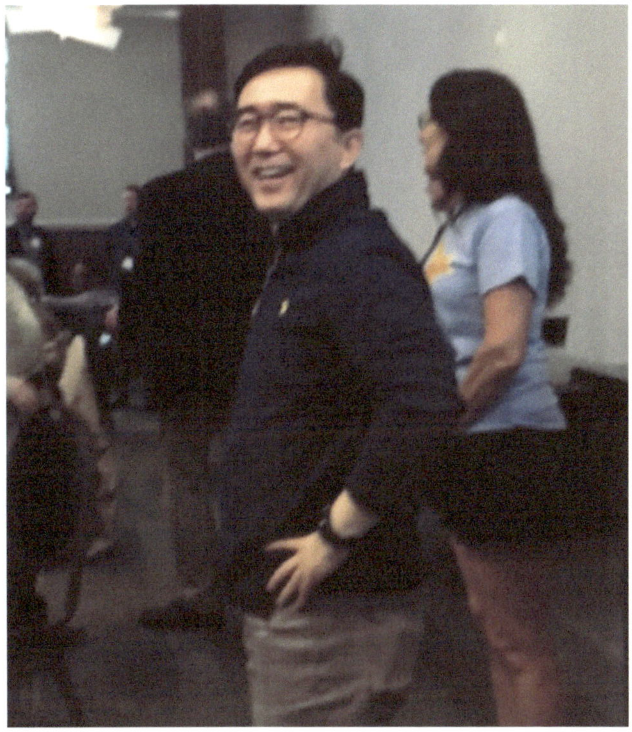

Seong Cho, MD; USF Alumni Dinner; Orlando, Florida; 2018.

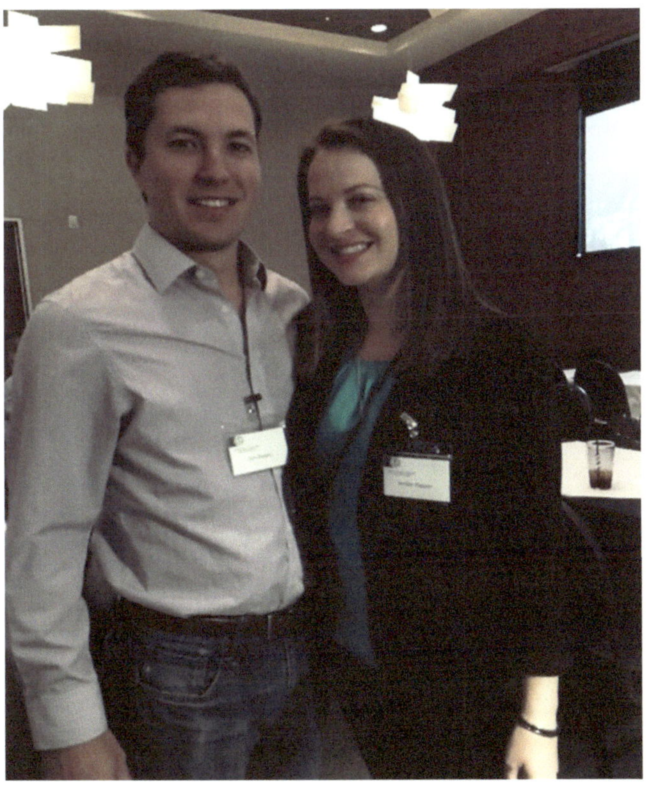

Left to right: Dan Pepper and Amber Pepper, MD (2016-2018); USF Alumni Dinner; Orlando, Florida; 2018.

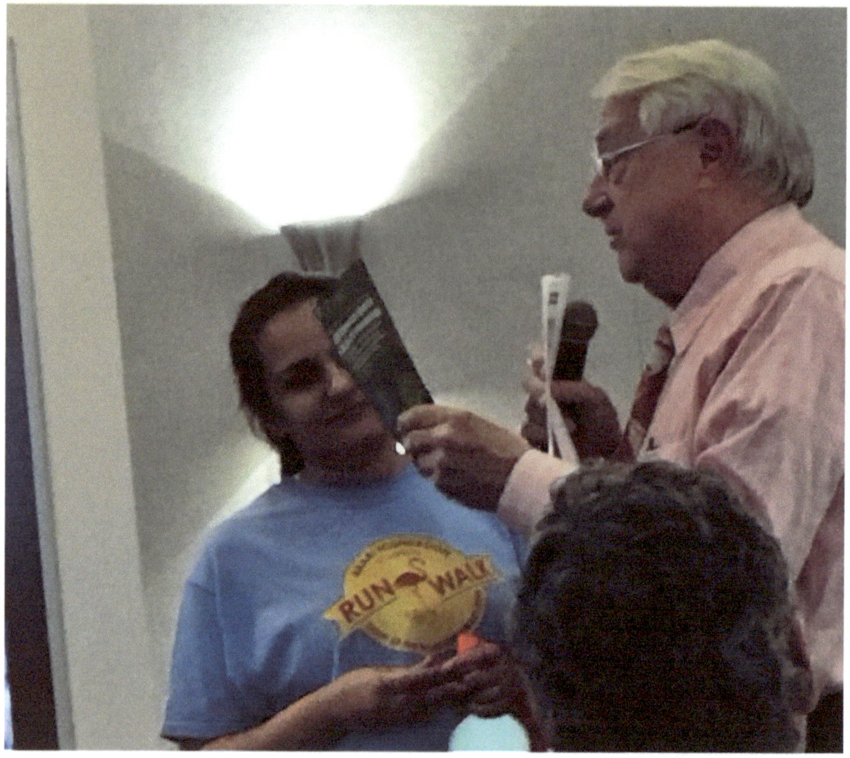

Left to right: Farnaz Tabatabaian, MD (ACH, 2013-2015) and Richard F. Lockey, MD, MS; USF Alumni Dinner; Orlando, Florida; 2018.

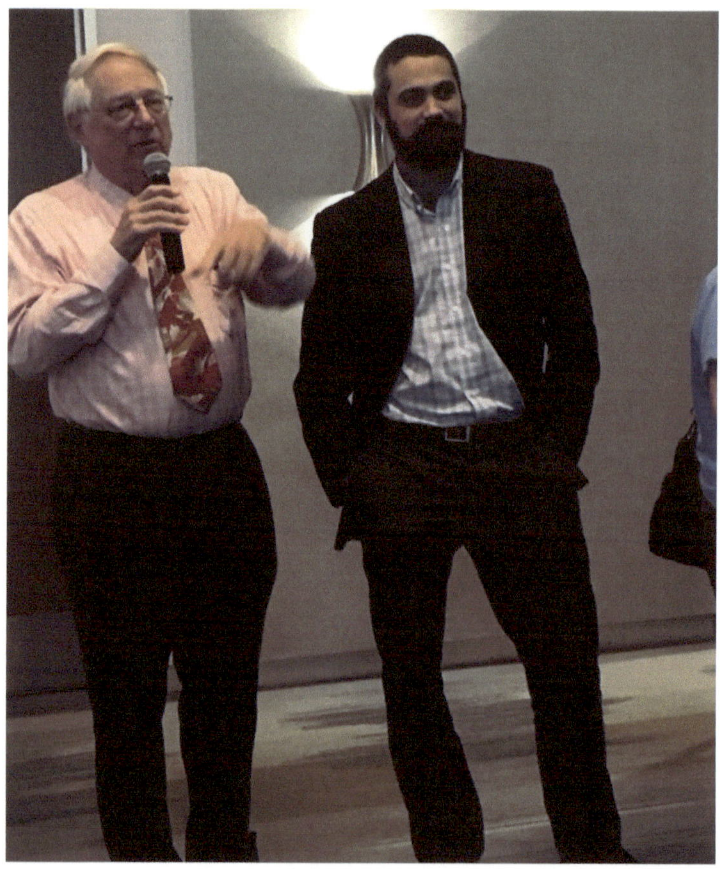

Left to right: Richard F. Lockey, MD, MS and Juan Carlos Cardet, MD, MPH; USF Alumni Dinner; Orlando, Florida; 2018.

Ingram Content Group UK Ltd.
Milton Keynes UK
UKHW052216100323
418412UK00003B/38